# MEIOSIS - MOLECULAR MECHANISMS AND CYTOGENETIC DIVERSITY

Edited by **Andrew Swan**

**Meiosis - Molecular Mechanisms and Cytogenetic Diversity**
**Edited by Andrew Swan**

**Published by InTech**

Janeza Trdine 9, 51000 Rijeka, Croatia



**Publishing Process Manager** Bojan Rafaj

**Technical Editor** Teodora Smiljanic

**Cover Designer** InTech Design Team

Additional hard copies can be obtained from orders@intechopen.com

Meiosis - Molecular Mechanisms and Cytogenetic Diversity, Edited by Andrew Swan
p. cm.
ISBN 978-953-51-0118-5

For EU product safety concerns:
IN TECH d.o.o., Prolaz Marije Krucifikse Kozulić 3, 51000 Rijeka, Croatia,
info@intechopen.com or visit our website at intechopen.com.

# Meet the editor

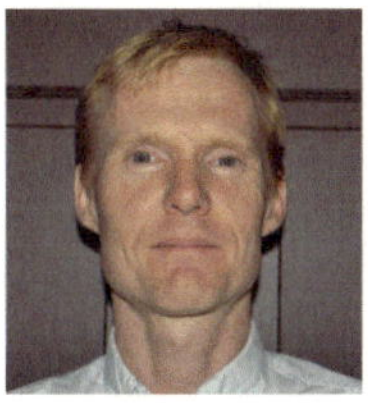

Dr. Andrew Swan is an Assistant Professor at the University of Windsor where he has been since 2007. He obtained his PhD from McGill University in 1999 and did his Postdoctoral studies at Princeton University. In his current research, Dr. Swan is studying the cell cycle and cell proliferation. A major focus of his lab is on the spatial and temporal control of meiosis. His research combines genetics, molecular biology and molecular imaging using the Drosophila (fruit fly) as a model system.

# Contents

**Preface XI**

**Part 1 Molecular and Comparative Study of Meiosis in Model Systems 1**

Chapter 1 **Epigenetics of the Synaptonemal Complex 3**
Abrahan Hernández-Hernández,
Rosario Ortiz Hernádez and Gerardo H. Vázquez-Nin

Chapter 2 **Facing the Correct Pole: The Challenge of Orienting Chromosomes for Meiotic Divisions 17**
Karishma Collette and Györgyi Csankovszki

Chapter 3 **Cohesins and Cohesin-Regulators in Meiosis 35**
Adela Calvente and José L. Barbero

Chapter 4 **Dynamics of Cellular Components in Meiotic and Premeiotic Divisions in *Drosophila* Males 67**
Yoshihiro H. Inoue, Chie Miyauchi,
Tubasa Ogata and Daishi Kitazawa

Chapter 5 **Sex Chromosomes and Meiosis in Spiders: A Review 87**
Douglas Araujo, Marielle Cristina Schneider,
Emygdio Paula-Neto and Doralice Maria Cella

Chapter 6 **How Does the Alteration of Meiosis Evolve to Parthenogenesis? - Case Study in a Water Flea, *Daphnia pulex* - 109**
Chizue Hiruta and Shin Tochinai

Chapter 7 **Avian Meiotic Chromosomes as Model Objects in Cytogenetics 123**
Katarzyna Andraszek and Elżbieta Smalec

**Part 2** **Molecular Biology of Mammalian Meiosis 149**

Chapter 8 **The Control of Meiotic Arrest and Resumption in Mammalian Oocytes 151**
Sylvie Bilodeau-Goeseels and Nora Magyara

Chapter 9 **Energy Metabolism Regulating Mammalian Oocyte Maturation 173**
N. Songsasen

Chapter 10 **PKC Regulation of Gametogenesis and Early Development 187**
James J. Faust, Madhavi Kalive, Anup Abraham and David G. Capco

Chapter 11 **Role of Bcl2l10 in Regulation of Meiotic Cell Cycle in the Mouse Oocyte 207**
Kyung-Ah Lee, Se-Jin Yoon, Eun-Young Kim, Jeehyeon Bae, Hyun-Seo Lee, Su-Yeon Lee and Eun-Ah Kim

Chapter 12 **Nuage Components and Their Contents in Mammalian Spermatogenic Cells, as Revealed by Immunoelectron Microscopy 216**
Yuko Onohara and Sadaki Yokota

Chapter 13 **Meiotic Behaviour of Chromosomes Involved in Structural Chromosomal Abnormalities Determined by Preimplantation Genetic Diagnosis 241**
L. Xanthopoulou and H. Ghevaria

Chapter 14 **OMICS for the Identification of Biomarkers for Oocyte Competence, with Special Reference to the Mare as a Prospective Model for Human Reproductive Medicine 257**
Maria Elena Dell'Aquila, Yoon Sung Cho, Nicola Antonio Martino, Manuel Filioli Uranio, Lucia Rutigliano and Katrin Hinrichs

Chapter 15 **Insight Into the Molecular Program of Meiosis 283**
Hiba Waldman Ben-Asher and Jeremy Don

**Part 3** **Molecular and Cytogenetic Studies of Plant Meiosis 301**

Chapter 16 **Quantifying Meiosis: Use of the Fractal Dimension, $D_f$, to Describe and Predict Prophase I Substages and Metaphase I 303**
Cynthia Ross Friedman and Hua-Feng Wang

Chapter 17 **Haploid Independent Unreductional Meiosis in Hexaploid Wheat 321**
Filipe Ressurreição, Augusta Barão, Wanda Viegas and Margarida Delgado

Chapter 18 **Meiotic Behavior in Intra- and Interspecific Sexual and Somatic Polyploid Hybrids of Some Tropical Species 331**
Maria Suely Pagliarini, Maria Lúcia Carneiro Vieira and Cacilda Borges do Valle

Chapter 19 **Meiotic Irregularities in Interspecific Crosses Within Edible Alliums 349**
Agnieszka Kiełkowska

Chapter 20 **Evaluation of Interspecific-Interploid Hybrids ($F_1$) and Back Crosses ($BC_1$) in *Hylocereus* Species (Cactaceae) 367**
Aroldo Cisneros and Noemi Tel-Zur

Chapter 21 **Embryology of Flowering Plants Applied to Cytogenetic Studies on Meiosis 389**
Jorge E. A. Mariath, André L. L. Vanzela, Eliane Kaltchuk-Santos, Karen L. G. De Toni, Célia G. T. J. Andrade, Adriano Silvério, Erica Duarte-Silva, Carlos R. M. da Silva, Juca A. B. San Martin, Fernanda Nogueira and Simone P. Mendes

Chapter 22 **Investigating Host Induced Meiosis in a Fungal Plant Pathogen 411**
B. J. Saville, M. E. Donaldson and C. E. Doyle

# Preface

Meiosis, the specialized cell cycle that results in the production of gametes for sexual reproduction, has a long history as a subject of scientific study. It is an important process on many levels with direct relevance to understanding of and treatment of human disease and anneuploidies, and the development of assisted reproductive technologies. A fundamental understanding of meiosis is also essential for the development of new strategies for improving economically important animal and plant species. From a more general perspective, the study of meiosis has also been driven by challenge of understanding such a complex process, and by the recognition of its importance in creating so much of the genetic diversity on our planet.

This book brings together a broad sampling of the current research on meiosis. Each chapter brings a unique perspective and introduces some of the many novel and interesting approaches that are being used in the study of meiosis. The book is divided into three sections. In the first section are chapters dealing with meiosis at the molecular level, using model system approaches. Many of these chapters deal with fundamental processes that are unique to meiosis. For example the first two chapters deal with the synaptonemal complex and lampbrush chromosomes respectively – two structures that have central roles in meiosis. The 3rd chapter deals with another process that is completely unique to meiosis, the bi-orientation of homologous chromosomes onto a spindle in meiosis I. Many processes that occur in meiosis represent complex variations on events in mitosis. An example of this is provided in chapter 4, which deals with the cohesins and their important role in ensuring proper homologue and sister chromatid segregation in meiosis. Chapter 5 discusses spermatogenesis in the genetically tractable Drosophila model system and highlights advances made in this meiotic system that have helped develop our understanding of basic cell biological processes such as cytokinesis. The first section closes with two examples of the amazing diversity of meiosis. Chapter 5 offers a thorough review of the many sex chromosome systems employed by spiders. Chapter 6 provides a fascinating examination of the molecular basis for the non-reductional meiosis that occurs in parthenogenic development of the water flea.

The 2nd section of this book deals with meiosis specifically in mammals. The first two chapters in this section deal with the hormonal and signal signaling pathways that regulate the meiotic cell divisions in mammalian cells. Chapter 3 deals with the unique energy requirements of growing oocytes. Chapters 4 and 5 provide examples of some of the unique cell biology of meiosis – the use of apoptotic machinery in meiosis and the use of cytoplasmic structure, the nuage and associated chromatoid bodies. Chapters 6, 7 and 8 all deal with some of the genomics and proteomics approaches and technologies that are being used both to study meiosis and to improve both animal breeding and medical diagnostics.

The 3rd section of this book deals with meiosis in the plants. The first two chapters deal with cytological approaches to the study of meiosis in plants. Chapter 1 looks specifically at meiosis in the flowering plants, while Chapter 2 gives an example of how the classic cytological approaches are being updated and given new power by advances in imaging and analysis methods. Several chapters here deal with issues of great importance in plant breeding. Chapters 3 and 4 deal with challenges in manipulating polyploid species, including some of the most agriculturally important food crops. Chapters 5 and 6 focus on challenges that are faced in generating interspecific hybrids – in edible alliums in Chapter 5 and in the cacti in Chapter 6. Chapter 7 deals with meiosis in a plant pathogen, the rust fungi. This final chapter deals with the rusts as both a model system for understanding host/pathogen interactions, and as an important agricultural pest for which an understanding of meiosis will provide new means of biological control.

The incredible breadth of research included in this volume reflects the great complexity and diversity of meiotic processes. It is also a reflection of the great diversity of motivations that have brought researchers to the study meiosis – from a desire to see improvements in medical treatments and diagnostics, to a desire to improve agricultural production, to a fascination with the complexity and diversity of a fundamental biological process.

**Dr. Andrew Swan**
Assistant Professor
University of Windsor
Canada

# Part 1

# Molecular and Comparative Study of Meiosis in Model Systems

# 1

# Epigenetics of the Synaptonemal Complex

Abrahan Hernández-Hernández[1],
Rosario Ortiz Hernádez[2] and Gerardo H. Vázquez-Nin[2]
[1]*Department of Cell and Molecular Biology, Karolinska Institute, Stockholm,*
[2]*Laboratory of Electron Microscopy, Faculty of Sciences,*
*National Autonomous University of Mexico,*
[1]*Sweden*
[2]*Mexico*

## 1. Introduction

Meiosis is a process composed of two divisions of the germ line cells without an intervenient S phase, thus there is no duplication of DNA between the first and the second meiotic divisions. The first meiotic division begins with the pre-leptotene that is the stage where the DNA replicates and chromosomes prepare to enter the meiotic prophase I in most of the organisms with sexual reproduction (Marston & Amon, 2004). The first meiotic division separates one homologue chromosome from the other member of the pair and in this way the two produced cells contain half number of chromosomes with two chromatids. During the metaphase of the first meiotic division the maternal and the paternal chromosomes of the bivalents are oriented at random, so the two new haploid cells receive a random number of chromosomes of each progenitor.

After a brief interphase the second division separates the sister chromatids of each chromosome and then the products of this division have the haploid number of chromosomes provided with one DNA double helix, frequently composed by segments of maternal and paternal DNA. In male mammals the final products of meiosis are four spermatids with half of the number of chromosomes of the species, with only one DNA double helix. However, in female organisms the final product of meiosis is one haploid oocyte and two small cells with a nucleus and a very small cytoplasm called polar bodies, which are not viable. During fecundation the union of two haploid gametes, the oocyte and the spermatozoa, recreates a diploid cell.

One of the biological significances of the meiosis is the production of genetic variability by the exchange of DNA between homologous chromosomes. Such exchange takes place during an extended meiotic prophase I and in most of the organisms proper meiotic genetic exchange depends on the accurate formation of a proteic structure between the homologous chromosomes, the synaptonemal complex (SC, for detailed revision see: Zickler & Kleckner 1998, 1999; Page & Hawley, 2004). There are several models used to study the SC and its importance for meiotic recombination, including yeast, Drosophila, C. elegans, plants and mice. Each model has its advantages and disadvantages. The mouse system has some advantages despite the low speed of genetics. Mouse genome and hence its chromosomes are larger than those of yeast and flies. This makes immunocytochemical analysis more powerful than in many other model organisms. Mouse genetics has been effectively used in combination with cytology to examine meiotic phenotypes produced as a result of targeted mutagenesis in embryonic stem cells.

## 2. Meiotic prophase I

Meiotic prophase I has been divided in five stages according to the chromosome morphology, meiotic recombination progression and the SC assembling. The interplay among these processes has been widely reviewed in different organisms (see Zickler & Kleckner 1998, 1999; Page & Hawley, 2004; Handel & Schimenti, 2010). Recently, with the identification of the histone code and its importance in gene regulation, chromatin structure and nuclear architecture (Turner, 2000; Jenuwein & Allis, 2001), old questions regarding chromosome structure and SC formation could be addressed. In this chapter we will focus our interest on the chromatin structure driven by epigenetic modifications and its relevance for SC formation and establishment, especially in mammals.

### 2.1 From chromosome homology recognition to synapsis

During the period G2 following meiotic phase S (some times called pre-leptotene) begins the recognition of similar sequences in the extended chromatin of homologous chromosomes. This process of recognition continues in leptotene and zygotene stages in microlampbrush chromosomes (Fig. 1).

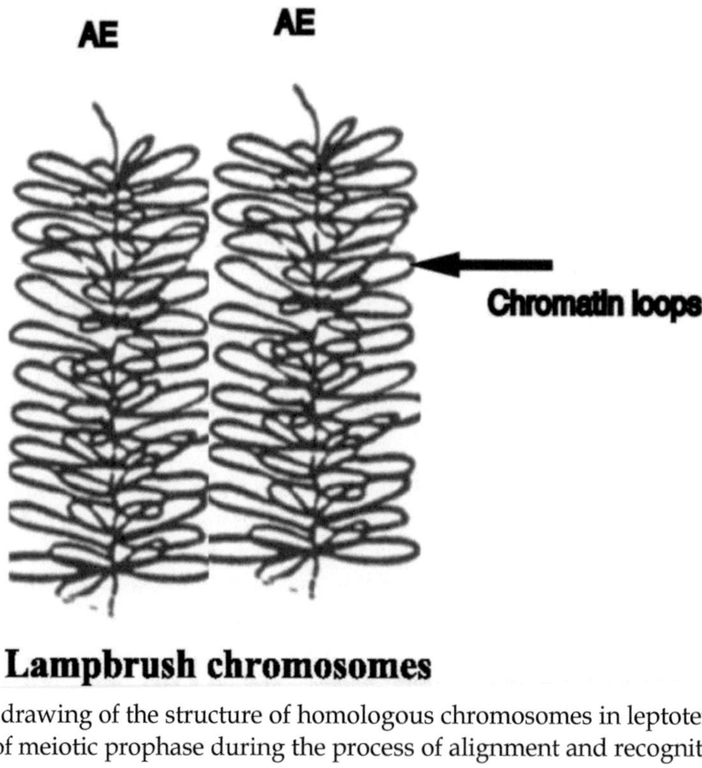


Fig. 1. Schematic drawing of the structure of homologous chromosomes in leptotene and zygotene stages of meiotic prophase during the process of alignment and recognition.

During pre-leptotene and leptotene the homologous chromosomes are not necessarily close to each other until the formation of the bouquet. The bouquet is a process that takes place during zygotene stage of the first meiotic prophase, the telomeres of the chromosomes slide associated to the nuclear membrane until they group in an area near the place of where the centrioles are located in the cytoplasm. In this way, the proximity of the chromosomes facilitates the recognition of homologies (Fig. 2)

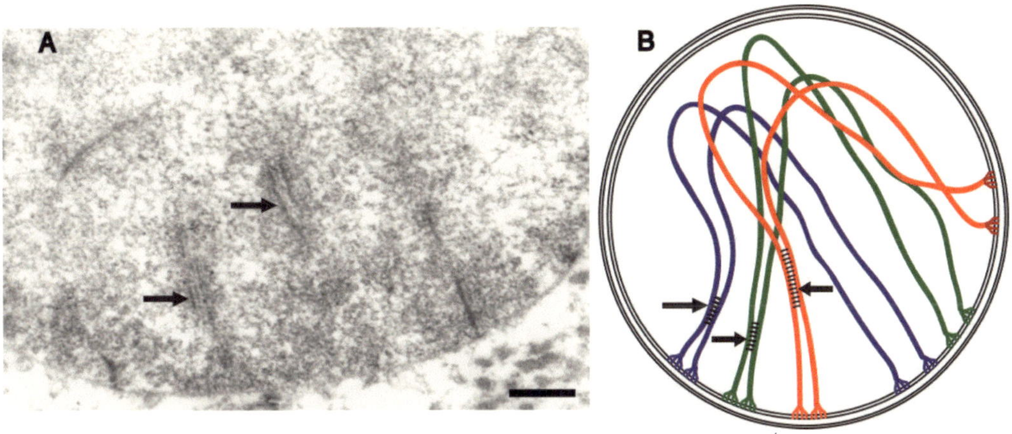


Fig. 2. A. - Electron microscopy image showing the pairing between homologous chromosomes (arrows) during the bouquet array and beginning of the formation of the synaptonemal complexes in zygotene stage. B. - Schematic representation of bouquet formation in zygotene stage. Homologous chromosomes migrate anchored to nuclear envelope until become close to each other, forming an array know as a bouquet. Synapsis takes place between homologous that are close enough to pair (arrows in A and B). Bar 500 nm.

The nature of the molecular mechanisms for this recognition of homologue sequences is not known, however, there are at least two processes proposed, one dependent on the distribution of transcription sites or factories (Cook, 1997) and the other dependent of non-spliced nascent RNA (Vázquez-Nin et al., 2003). According to the first view each chromosome has a unique array of transcription units along its length. Therefore, the chromatin fibrils with polymerases and transcription factors are folded into an array of loops, only the homologous chromosomes share similar distribution of loops with transcription factories and become zipped together (Cook, 1997). The second proposition also involves transcription as a possible mechanism of homology recognition. The study of the meiotic S phase (pre-leptotene), as well as leptotene and zygotene stages of meiotic prophase -that is the period of homology recognition and pairing- demonstrated an intense transcription but a very reduced pre-mRNA splicing. In this condition the newly synthesized mRNA could not be exported to the cytoplasm, as was demonstrated by quantitative autoradiography. So the function of newly synthesized mRNA must be inside the nucleus and in this period the main functions that were taking place inside the nuclei were homology recognition and pairing. Furthermore, electron microscope studies demonstrated a micro lampbrush structure of the chromosomes, which are in intense transcriptional activity. In pre-leptotene some loops of the micro lampbrush chromosomes contact loops of other chromosomes and the first parallel alignments of chromosomes take place (Fig. 1). Therefore, it was proposed that homologous chromosomes are in physical contact already at pre-leptotene stage (Vázquez-Nin et al., 2003). However it has not been shown a direct relationship of this chromosomal array with homology recognition.

During zygotene, as homologous chromosomes become aligned in pairs, the proteins of the lateral elements of the synaptonemal complex are incorporated to the chromosomal axis and the loops located between the axes leave the inter-axial space creating a region without DNA, which is the precursor of the central space of the synaptonemal complex.

## 3. The synaptonemal complex

The SC is a tripartite structure, which was described by Moses (1956) in spermatocytes of the crayfish. Since then it was found in all eukaryotic kingdoms (see reviews by Moses, 1956, 1968, 1969; Sotelo, 1969; Westergaard & von Wettstein 1972; Gillies, 1975; Loidl, 1990, 1991). SC morphology has been studied by means of electron microscopy. It is composed by two lateral elements (LEs) and a central region (CR). Each replicated homologous chromosome is anchored to one LE (Fig. 3), while completion of meiotic recombination (referred as crossover) takes place at late recombination nodules (RN) that are located in the CR (Fig. 3).

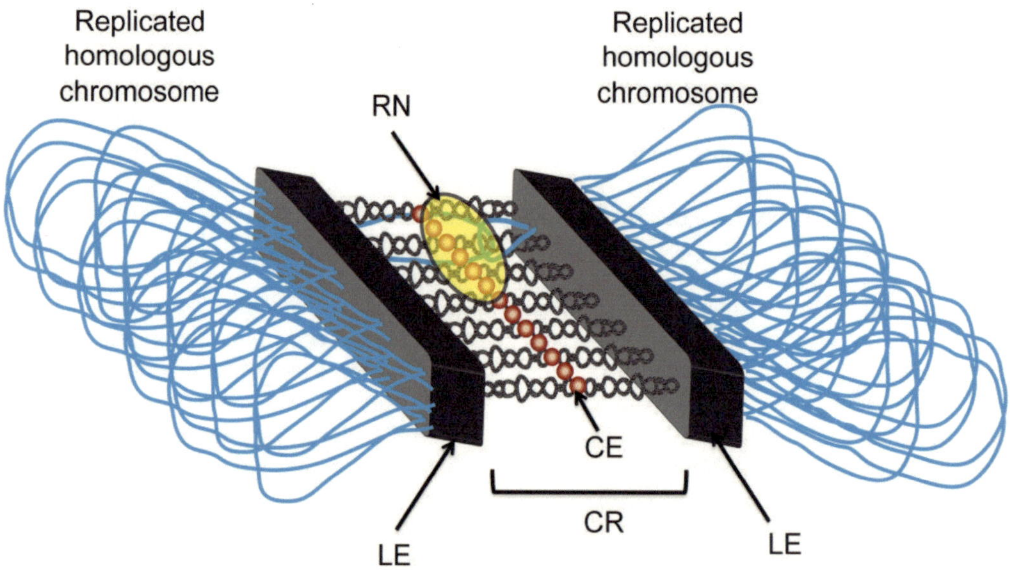


Fig. 3. Schematic representation of synaptonemal complex. The replicated homologous chromosomes are anchored to the lateral elements (LEs) of the synaptonemal complex (SC) while the genetic exchange between these homologous (referred as crossing over) takes place at the late recombination nodule (RN), that is tethered to the central region (CR).

The major protein components of the LEs are the meiosis specific proteins SYCP2 and SYCP3 (Dobson et al., 1994; Lammers et al., 1994; Offenberg et al., 1998; Winkel et al., 2009) as well as cohesion complexes (described below), whereas the CR is composed by SYCP1, SYCE1, SYCE2, SYCE3 and Tex12 (Figure 3) (Meuwissen et al., 1992; Costa et al., 2005; Hamer et al., 2008; Schramm et al., 2011). SYCP3 is a major structural component of vertebrate synaptonemal complexes. The evolutionary conserved domains of SYCP3, the alpha helix together with two flanking motif CM1 and CM2, are necessary and sufficient for SYCP3 polymerization and assembly of high order structures (Baier et al., 2007). Nevertheless, some differences in the SYCP3 expression have been found among mammals. In contrast to other vertebrates, rat and mouse SYCP3 exists in two isoforms. The short isoform is conserved among vertebrates. However, the longer isoform, which represents an N-terminal extension of the shorter one, most likely appeared about 15 millions years ago in a common ancestor of rat and mouse and after the separation of the hamster branch (Alsheimer et al., 2010). SYCP2 and SYCP3 incorporate to the axial elements of chromosomes during lepto-zygotene, forming fibrous cores in the homologous chromosomes (Hamer et al., 2008 and references therein).

The C-terminus of SYCP1 directly interacts with SYCP2 (Winkel et al., 2009). These authors proposed that SYCP2 acts as a linker between SYCP1 and SYCP3 and therefore it could be the connecting link between lateral elements and transverse filaments of the CR (Winkel et al., 2009). On the other hand, the N-terminus of SYCP1 is associated in the middle of the CR with another N-terminus of SYCP1 forming the central element (CE) of the CR. At the CE are also found the proteins SYCE1, SYCE2, SYCE3 and Tex12, which are important for the proper CR assembling and for the crossover resolution (Bolcun-Filas et al., 2007, 2009; Hamer et al., 2008, Schramm et al., 2011). Defects in the organization of the synaptonemal complex result in alterations of the meiotic recombination and infertility.

Cohesins are chromosomal proteins that form complexes involved in the maintenance of sister chromatid cohesion during division of somatic and germ cells. Three meiotic cohesins subunits have been reported in mammals, REC8, STAG3 and SMC1 beta, their expression has been found in mouse spermatocytes (Prieto et al., 2004) and human oocytes (García-Cruz et al., 2010). SMC1 beta, SMC3 and STAG3 are localized along axial fibers of leptotene-zygotene chromosomes and then to the LE of the SC. Cohesins are essential for completion of recombination, pairing, meiotic chromosome axis formation, and assembly of the SC. Rec8 is involved in several functions as cohesion, pairing, recombination, chromosome axis and SC assembly (Brar et al., 2009). At difference from meiosis in male mice, the cohesin axis is progressively lost in oocytes, with parallel destruction of the axial elements at dictyated arrest (Prieto et al., 2004).

The SC is important for the normal formation of crossovers. In many, but not all, organisms, the homology search, that occurs mediated by DNA-DNA interactions, is also intimately associated with the movement of homologous chromosomes to bring them into close juxtaposition (Székvölgyi & Nicolas, 2010).

Chiasmata formed by crossovers are central for the process of chromosome segregation as they hold together the homologous chromosomes at metaphase of the first meiotic division; at least one crossover per pair of homologs allows that each member of the pair migrates to an opposite pole of the spindle (Székvölgyi & Nicolas, 2010).

Most eukaryotes possess two recombinases, Rad51 and Dmc1. Homologues of these proteins are widely conserved in nature, from virus to humans. In eukaryotes Rad51 is required for most homologous recombination pathways in both mitotic and meiotic cells (Kagawa & Kurumizaka, 2009 and references therein).

## 4. Chromosome organization on the synaptonemal complex

As mentioned above, the SC is essential for meiotic recombination completion; this is because crossover formation depends in the accurate formation of the CR of the SC. The crossovers are observed as dense structures associated to the CR, as showed by electron microscopy. Crossovers are referred as late recombination nodules (RN, Fig. 3) and they are observed tether to the CR of the SC (Carpenter, 1975, 1979, 1981). Therefore, the SC is considered as the scaffold to which the chromosomes are anchored while they exchange genetic material.

After DNA replication at pre-leptotene stage, replicated sister chromatids are held together at specific points by the cohesion component SMC3 and the meiosis-specific cohesin Rec8 is incorporated to this scaffold. As the cells progress to leptotene stage, the chromosomes undergo condensation and SMC1 beta/STAG3, other meiosis-specific cohesins, are incorporated to the cohesion scaffold. At this stage fine filaments formed by the cohesin scaffold can be identified by immunocytochemical approaches. These filaments, called axial elements (AEs) are the precursors of the LEs and are surrounded by chromatin loops protruding out of them (Fig. 1). In this stage, SYCP2 and SYCP3 are incorporated to the AEs and in zygotene stage SYCP1 and accessory proteins begin to synapse the aligned AEs. During pachytene the SC is fully formed throughout the whole length of LEs. The homologous chromosomes are anchored to the AEs in early stages and to the LEs in pachytene stage. However the mechanism of association of the chromosomes to the AEs/LEs has been controversial and poorly understood.

The presence of DNA in the LEs was documented by enzymatic digestion followed by staining methods almost at the same time as the SC was observed (Coleman & Moses, 1964) and corroborated by immunocytochemical approaches in later studies (Vázquez-Nin et al., 1993). There have been few studies trying to identify DNA sequences associated to the LEs of the SC. In C. elegans, the chromosomes pair at specific areas known as pairing centers, recently it has been shown that repeat sequences motifs are at these pairing centers (Phillips et al., 2009). It has been suggested that in mammals repeat sequences interspersed through the genome, are responsible to anchor the chromosomes to the LEs (Pearlman et al., 1992; Hernández-Hernández et al., 2008). However not all the bulk of repeat sequences are incorporated into the LEs, suggesting a mechanism of selection of specific sequences to be anchored to the LE. Further experiments have shown that the chromatin structure at these lateral element-associated repeated sequences (LEARS) is in part responsible for their association to the SC (Hernández-Hernández et al., 2010).

### 4.1 Chromosomes anchor to the lateral elements by means of specific DNA sequences

The presence of DNA in the inner part of the LEs suggested that chromosomes are anchored by means of specific sequences. Two different studies have shown that LEs contain specific DNA sequences. One of the studies suggested that LEs associate DNA consist in repeat sequences like long and short interspersed elements (LINE/SINE) (Pearlman et al., 1992). In the second study the authors used chromatin immunoprecipitation (ChIP) using anti-sycp3 antibody to pull down DNA sequences associated to the LE (Hernández-Hernández et al., 2008). All the immunoprecipitated sequences consisted of repeat DNA, like LINE, SINE, long terminal repeats (LTR), satellite, and simple repeats. The presence of these sequences in the LEs has been corroborated by means of DNA in situ hybridization at the optical and electron microscope level (Hernández-Hernández et al., 2008; Spangenberg et al., 2010). Therefore, these specific sequences have been called lateral element-associated repeat sequences or LEARS. However the presence of some other sequences can not be ruled out with these studies, more analysis are needed to determinate whether these are the only sequences helping the chromosomes to anchor to the LEs.

## 5. Chromatin structure in the LEs of the SC

Chromatin immunoprecipitation experiment using the LEs specific protein SYCP3, demonstrated enrichment of repeat DNA sequences, which localize to the LEs, as well as in the bulk of the chromatin, as shown by in situ hybridization (Hernández-Hernández et al., 2008). However, features in the primary structure of LEARS did not reveal any obvious consensus sequence, suggesting that secondary structure might be responsible for recruitment of LEARS to the LEs. In somatic cells, most of these transcriptionally inactive repeat sequences are subject to epigenetic modifications favoring their organization in heterochromatin (Martens et al., 2005). Furthermore, chromatin structure dictated by epigenetic modifications during meiosis is critical for accurate SC assembly and meiosis progression (Hernández-Hernández et al., 2009). Therefore, it is possible that specific epigenetic modifications of LEARS influence their interaction with LEs. To address this hypothesis our group has performed immunofluorescent detection (IF) of histone post translation modifications (PTM) that are associated to repeat sequences in somatic cells (Martens et al., 2005). We found specific association of PTM with the SC during pachytene stage. Tri-methylation of histone H3 on lysine 9 and tri-methylation of histone H4 on lysine 20 (H3K9me3 and H4K20me3 respectively) co-localize with one extreme of the SCs (Fig. 4), whereas tri-methylation of histone H3 on lysine 27 (H3K27me3) co-localizes to the SC in almost all its length (Fig. 4). We then followed the dynamics of co localization of these specific marks throughout the meiotic prophase I.

Leptotene stage: at this stage, sycp3 antibody stains fine filaments that correspond to the axial elements. H3K9me3 and H4K20me3 are already co-localizing with one of the extremities of the AE. Centromeres are located close to the end of acrocentric chromosomes and in rat they are mainly composed of minor and mayor satellite DNA repeats. These sequences are enriched with the PTMs H3K9me3 and H4K20me3 (Martens et al., 2005). In cells undergoing meiosis and SC assembling, the centromeres are located near one of the extremes of the AE nearby the nuclear envelope. The staining pattern of H3K9me3 and H4K20me3 in the AE therefore may correspond to the satellite repeats present in the centromeric and pericentromeric region. H3K27me3 was absent from the whole nucleus at this stage.

Zigotene: the AEs of homologous chromosomes start to synapse. H3K9me3 and H4K20me3 are located in the extreme of the SC in formation.

Pachytene: The SC between homologous chromosomes is completely formed. H3K9me3 and H4K20me3 continue associated to one of the extremes of the SC (Fig. 4). In this stage

H3K27me3 staining pattern is visible and this PTM is co-localizing with SYCP3 throughout patches of the SC (Fig. 4). The results of these IFs suggest that these three histone marks may be involved in the chromatin structure at the LEARS in the LEs.

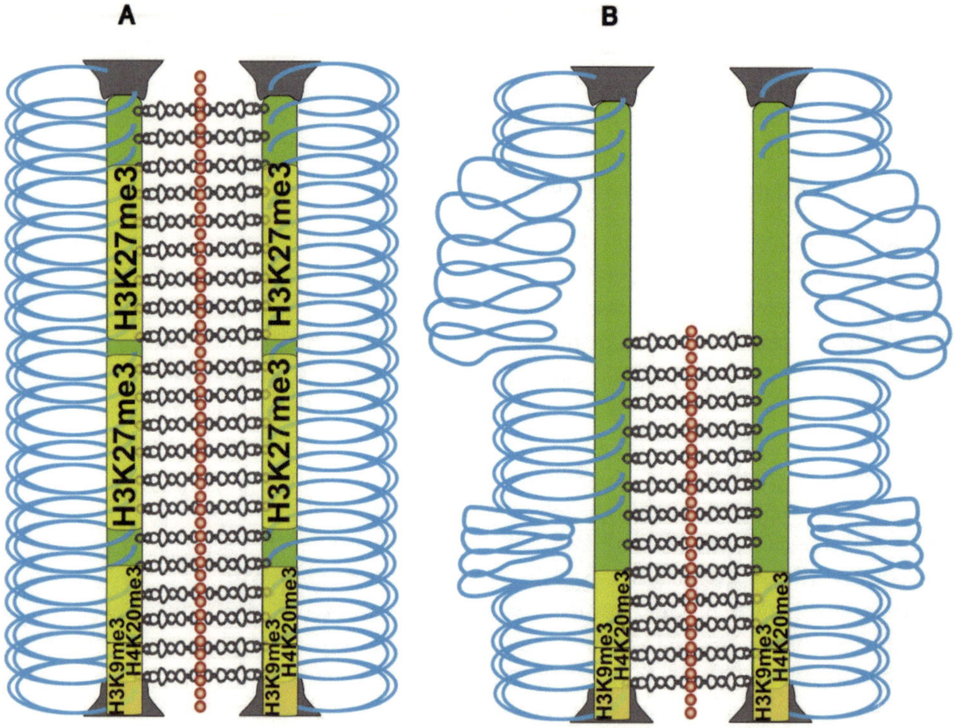


Fig. 4. Model of chromatin structure in the LEs of the SC. A. - Homologous chromosomes are attached to the LEs of the SC by means of specific DNA sequences (LEARS). These anchorage DNA sequences are enriched with histone PTMs that determinate their chromatin structure. B. - Blocking of chromatin structure leads to a defective chromosome anchorage to the LEs. H3K27me3 is not longer associated with SINE and LTR sequences producing their detachment from the LEs.

### 5.1 Epigenetic profile of LEARS

In order to understand whether the specific PTM are associated with the LEARS, we performed two rounds of ChIP assays (re-ChIP). The first round of ChIP analyses was done using the SYCP3 antibody to pull down the LEARS and the chromatin proteins associated to them. As a template for the second round of ChIP, we used the pulled down complexes from the first round of ChIP (SYCP3 and chromatin of LEARS) and pulled down DNA sequences associated with the distinct PTM of interest (H3K9me3, H3K27me3 and H4K20me3). Enrichment of the different LEARS with PTM marks was assessed by semi quantitative polymerase chain reaction (sqPCR) (Hernandez-Hernandez et al., 2010). Table 1 summarizes the enrichment of PTM in the different LEARS. Satellite repeats are enriched with H3K9me3 and H4K20me3, whereas LINE sequences are enriched with H4K20me3. SINE and LTR sequences are enriched with H3K27me3.

| LEARS | Histone mark (PTM) | | |
|---|---|---|---|
| | H3K9me3 | H4K20me3 | H3K27me3 |
| LINE | - | Enriched | |
| SINE | - | | Enriched |
| LTR | - | | Enriched |
| Satellite | Enriched | Enriched | |

Table 1. LEARS and their enrichment with histone marks

By analyzing the patterns of IF for PTMs/SC proteins during the meiotic prophase and the enrichment of PTM in the LEARS, we can predict whether or not histone PTMs have a role in the recruitment of LEARS to the LE of the SC.

H3K9me3 and H4K20me3 are already enriched in the satellite repeats of the centromeric region when the AE is formed during leptotene stage. Probably these marks are constitutive for satellite repeats, since in somatic cells this enrichment has been reported before (Marten et al., 2005). Therefore the likelihood that these PTMs are important for LEARS recruitment is scarce. LINE sequences are enriched with H4K20me3, the same PTM present in satellite sequences. However the staining pattern only resembles that for satellite sequences. LINE sequences are not confined to centromeric regions, rather they are present all along the chromosomes, therefore it would be expected that the staining pattern would be co localizing with SYCP3 not only at one of the extremes, but to the entire length of the SC. A possible explanation for the absence of IF signal for H3K20me3 in the whole length of the SC is that LINE sequences are not highly clustered as the satellite sequences in specific regions of the chromosome. The clustered satellite regions in one of the extremities of the SC produce a strong IF signal, making difficult to detect the signal of LINE sequences in regions were there is not clustering, for example along the LEs. Thus, LINE sequences are enriched with H4K20me3, but they are masked by the signal from satellite DNA regions.

### 5.2 A specific histone mark appears at the time the SC is mature

H3K27me3 colocalizes with SYCP3 along patches through the whole length of the SC. Strikingly; this pattern is only seen in pachytene stage when the SC is mature (Hernández-Hernández et al., 2010). Furthermore, this histone mark was enriched in SINE- and LTR-LEARS. These evidences suggest that SINE and LTR sequences are enriched with H3K27me3, conferring a specific chromatin structure that in turn is contributing to the LE structure, probably anchoring and/or maintaining the attachments of these sequences to the LEs.

To address this hypothesis, we decided to treat rat testicles with tricostatin-A (TSA), a histone desacetylase (HDACs) inhibitor, during nine days. After this period of treatment, pachytene cells have received the treatment since leptotene stage, according to the duration of meiotic prophase I (Adler, 1996). TSA has been shown to effectively inhibit HDACs, blocking downstream reactions and finally methylation of histone lysine residues (Ekwall et al., 1997). Then we perform IF, ChIP and re-ChIP experiments to assess the effect of HDACs inhibition on the SC structure (Hernández-Hernández et al., 2010).

H3K9me3 and H4K20me3 IF signal was reduced at pachytene stage, but the pattern is the same as that of non-treated animals. Suggesting that most of these marks were deposited on centromers before leptotene stage. In agreement with this, leptotene and zygotene cells, which have been treated since they were at pre-leptotene stages, showed reduced signal and more scattered IF pattern that in non-treated animals. TSA treatment therefore, partially affected deposition of these PTMs and chromatin structure as well. Enrichment of H3K9me3 and H4K20me3 in satellite sequences and H4K20me3 in LINE sequences was significantly reduced. However these two classes of LEARS are still attached to the LEs of the SC as shown by ChIP assays in treated and control animals (Hernández-Hernández et al., 2010). In summary, TSA affected enrichment of H3K9me3 and H4K20me3 in satellite and LINE sequences, but this loss of enrichment does not produce loss of these two LEARS from the LE of the SC. Implying that satellite and LINE sequences may have another unidentified PTM that is involved in their association to the LE or that these sequences do not associate to the LE via histone modifications. Moreover, staining pattern in treated animal at one of the extremes of the EA/LE, suggest that most of this mark was not altered during such a short period of treatment (Hernández-Hernández et al., 2010).

The most striking result was the observed for H3K27me3. The staining pattern for H3K27me3 is specific for pachytene cells, co localizing with SYCP3 along stretches of the SC. This PTM is also enriched in the SINE and LTR sequences attached to the LEs. After TSA treatment, the IF signal for H3K27me3 almost disappears from the nucleus of pachytene cells. Furthermore, the enrichment of this PTM in SINE and LTR was significantly reduced and these sequences were not longer associated to the LEs of the SC. These results suggest that H3K27me3 appears in pachytene stage and is important for attachment and/or maintenance of SINE and LTR sequences in the LEs o the SC (Hernández-Hernández et al., 2010).

### 5.3 Failures in pairing between homologous chromosomes and loss of DNA-associated to the LE

To evaluate the direct effect of loss of LEARS from the LEs of the SC, we analyzed the ultrastructure of the SC by means of optical and electron microscopy. IF staining of LEs and CR of the SC in sections allowed us to identify that homologous chromosomes are paired but synapsis is not complete. By means of electron microscopy we found a high incidence of LEs that were not synapsed. These defects in SC formation in turn activate the programmed cell death of spermatocytes in late pachytene stage observed in sections of seminiferous tubules. Furthermore, when homologous were partially synapsed, we identified failures in the CR structure. The CR was formed between the homologous but not throughout the entire length of the SC. By means of a specific ultrastructural DNA staining, we observed that the DNA pattern was less dense in the LEs of treated animals than in the LEs from non-treated rats (Hernández-Hernández et al., 2010). This suggested that DNA association to the LEs was altered and that the CR in not completely formed between the homologous chromosomes.

## 6. A model of the chromatin structure in the LEs of the SC

Taking in account all the evidences, we proposed that chromatin structure of a sub set of LEARS (SINE and LTR) is important for LEARS recruitment and/or maintenance in the LEs of the SC. Blocking of this specific chromatin structure leads to failures in SC structure, detachment of DNA sequences form the LEs (SINE, LTR DNA sequences) and finally to cell death. Therefore we suggest that H3K27me3 is an indispensable histone PTM important for chromosome attachment to the LEs and hence SC structure.

## 7. References


Adler, ID. (1996). Comparison of the duration of spermatogenesis between male rodents and humans. *Mutat Res,* 10,352(1-2):169-72.

Alsheimer, M., Baier, A., Schramm S., Shütz, W., & Benavente, R. (2010). Synaptonemal complex protein SYCP3 exists in two isoforms showing different conservation in mammalian evolution. *Cytogenetics and Genome Research,* 128(1-3):162-8.

Baier, A., Alsheimer, M., Voiff, JN., & Benavente, R. (2007). Synaptonemal complex protein SYCP3 of the rat: evolutionarily conserved domains and the assembly of higher order structures. *Sex Dev,* 1(3):161-168.

Bolcun-Filas, E., Costa, Y., Speed, R., Taggart, M., Benavente, R., De Rooij, DG., & Cooke, HJ. (2007). SYCE2 is required for synaptonemal complex assembly, double strand break repair, and homologous recombination. *J Cell Biol,* 176(6):741-7.

Bolcun-Filas, E., Hall, E., Speed, R., Taggart, M., Grey, C., de Massy, B., Benavente, R., & Cooke, HJ. (2009). Mutation of the mouse Syce1 gene disrupts synapsis and suggests a link between synaptonemal complex structural components and DNA repair. *PLoS Genet,* 5(2):e1000393.

Brar, GA., Hochwagen, A., Ee, LS., & Amon, A. (2009). The multiple roles of cohesin in meiotic chromosome morphogenesis and pairing. *Mol Biol Cell,* 20(3):1030-47.

Carpenter, ATC. (1975). Electron microscopy of meiosis in Drosophila melanogaster females: II: The recombination nodule-a recombination-associated structure at pachytene? *Proc Nat Acad Sci USA,* 72(8):3186-3189.

Carpenter, ATC. (1979). Synaptonemal complex and recombination nodules in wild-type Drosophila melanogaster females. *Genetics,* 92(2):511-541.

Carpenter, ATC. (1981). EM autoradiographic evidence that DNA synthesis occurs at recombination nodules during meiosis in Drosophila melanogaster females. *Chromosoma,* 83:59-80.

Coleman, JR., & Moses, MJ. (1964). DNA and the fine structure of synaptic chromosomes in the domestic rooster (gallus domesticus). *J Cell Biol,* 23:63-78.

Costa, Y., Speed, R., Ollinger, R., Alsheimer, M., Semple, CA., Gautier, P., Maratou, K., Novak, I., Höög, C., Benavente, R., & Cooke, HJ. (2005). Two novel proteins recruited by synaptonemal complex protein 1 (SYCP1) are at the center of meiosis. *J Cell Sci,* 118:2755-2762.

Cook, PR. (1997). The transcriptional basis of chromosome pairing. *J Cell Sci,* 110(9):1033-1040.

Dobson, MJ., Pearlman, RE., Karaiskakis, A., Spyropoulos, B., & Moens, PB. (2007). Synaptonemal complex proteins: occurrence, epitope mapping and chromosome disjunction. *J Cell Sci*, 107:2749-2760.

Ekwall, K., Olsson, T., Turner, BM., Cranston, G., & Allshire, RC. (1997). Transient inhibition of histone deacetylation alters the structural and functional imprint at fission yeast centromeres. *Cell*, 91:1021–1032

García-Cruz, R., Brieño, MA., Roig, I., Velilla, E., Pujol, A., Cabero, L., Pessarronda, A., Barbero, JL., & García Caldés, M. (2010). Dynamics of cohesin proteins REC8, STAG3, SMC1 beta and SMC3 are consistent with a role in sister chromatid cohesion during meiosis in human oocytes. *Hum Reprod*, 25:2316-2327.

Gillies, CB. (1975). Synaptonemal complex and chromosome structure. *Annu Rev Genet* 9:91-109.

Hamer, G., Wang, H., Bolcun-Filas, E., Cooke, HJ., Benavente, R., & Höög, C. (2008). Progression of meiotic recombination requires structural maturation of the central element of the synaptonemal complex. *J Cell Sci*, 121:2445-2451.

Handel MA., & Schimenti, JC. (2010) Genetics of mammalian meiosis: regulation, dynamics and impact on fertility. *Nat Rev Genet*, 11(2):124-36.

Hernández-Hernández, A., Rincón-Arano, H., Recillas-Targa, F., Ortiz, R., Valdes-Quezada, C., Echeverría, OM., Benavente, R., & Vázquez-Nin, GH. (2008). Differential distribution and association of repeat DNA sequences in the lateral element of the synaptonemal complex in rat spermatocytes. *Chromosoma*, 117(1):77-87.

Hernández-Hernández, A., Vázquez-Nin, GH., Echeverría, OM., & Recillas-Targa, F. (2009). Chromatin structure contribution to the synaptonemal complex formation. *Cell Mol Life Sci*, 66:1198-1208.

Hernández-Hernández, A., Ortiz, R., Ubaldo, E., Martínez, OM., Vázquez-Nin, GH., & Recillas-Targa, F. (2010). Synaptonemal complex stability depends on repressive histone marks of the lateral element-associated repeat sequences. *Chromosoma*, 119(1):41-58.

Jenuwein, T., & Allis, CD. (2001). Translating the histone code. *Science*, 293(5532):1074-80.

Kagawa, W., & Kurumizaka, H. (2009). From meiosis to postmeiotic events: Uncovering the molecular roles of the meiosis-specific recombinase Dmc1. *FEBS J*, 277(3):590-598.

Lammers, JH., Offenberg, HH., van Aalderen, M., Vink, AC., Dietrich, AJ., & Heyting, C. (1994). The gene encoding a major component of the lateral elements of synaptonemal complexes of the rat is related to X-linked lymphocyte-regulated genes. *Mol Cell Biol*, 14(2): 1137-1146.

Loidl, L. (1990). The initiation of meiotic pairing: the cytological view. *Genome*, 33: 759-778.

Loidl, L. (1991). Coming to grips with a complex matter. A multidisciplinary approach to the synaptonemal complex. *Chromosoma*, 100:289-292.

Marston, AL., & Amon, A. (2004). Meiosis: cell-cycle controls shuffle and deal. *Nat Rev Mol Cell Biol*, 5(12):983-997.

Martens, JH., O'Sullivan, RJ., Braunschweig, U., Opravil, S., Radolf, M., Steinlein, P., & Jenuwein, T. (2005). The profile of repeat-associated histone lysine methylation states in the mouse epigenome. *EMBO J*, 24(4):800-812.

Meuwissen, RL., Offenberg, HH., Dietrich, AJ., Riesewijk, A., van Iersel, M., & Heyting, C. (1992). A coiled-coil related protein specific for synapsed regions of meiotic prophase chromosomes. *EMBO J*, 11(13): 5091-5100.

Moses, MJ. (1956). Chromosomal structures in crayfish spermatocytes. *J Biophys Biochem Cytol*, 2:215-218.

Moses, MJ. (1968). Synaptonemal complex. *Annu Rev Genet*, 2:363-412.

Moses, MJ. (1969). Structure and function of the synaptonemal complex. *Genetics*, 67:41-51.

Offenberg, HH., Schalk, JA., Meuwissen, RL., van Aalderen, M., Kester, HA., Dietrich, AJ., & Heyting, C. (1998). SCP2: a major protein component of the axial elements of synaptonemal complexes of the rat. *Nuclei Acid Res*, 26:2572-2579.

Page, SL., & Hawley, RS. (2004). The genetics and molecular biology of the synaptonemal complex. *Annu Rev Cell Dev Biol*, 20:525-58.

Pearlman, RE., Tsao, N., & Moens, PB. (1992). Synaptonemal complexes from DNase-treated rat pachytene chromosomes contain (GT)n and LINE/SINE sequences. *Genetics*, 130(4):865-872.

Phillips, CM., Meng, X., Zhang, L., Chretien, JH., Urnov, FD., & Dernburg, AF. (2009). Identification of chromosome sequence motifs that mediate meiotic pairing and synapsis in C. elegans. *Nat Cell Biol*, 11(8):934-942.

Prieto, I., Tease, C., Pezzi, N., Buesa, JM., Ortega, S., Kremer, L., Martínez, A., Martínez-A, C., Hultén, MA., & Barbero, JL. (2004). Cohesin component dynamic during meiotic prophase I in mammalian oocytes. *Chromosome Res*, 12(3):197-213.

Schramm, S., Fraune, J., Naumann, R., Hernandez-Hernandez, A., Höög, C., Cooke, HJ., Alsheimer, M., & Benavente, R. (2011). A novel mouse synaptonemal complex protein is essential for loading of central element proteins, recombination, and fertility. *PLoS Genet*, 7(5):e1002088.

Sotelo, JR. (1969). Ultrastructure of the chromosomes in meiosis. In: *Handbook of Molecular Cytology*, Ed. Lima de Faria A, pp 412-434; 1969, North Holland Pub. Co. Amsterdam.

Székvölgyi, L. & Nicolas, A. (2010). From meiosis to postmeiotic events: Homologous recombination is obligatory but flexible. *FEBS J*, 277:571-589.

Spangenberg, VE., Dadashev, SIa., Matveevskii, SN., Kolomiets, OL., & Bogdanov, IuF. (2010). How do chromosomes attach to synaptonemal complexes? *Genetika*, 46(10):1363-6.

Turner, BM. (2000). Histone acetylation and an epigenetic code. *Bioessays*, 22(9):836-845.

Vázquez-Nin, GH., Flores, E., Echeverría, OM., Merkert, H., Wettstein, R., & Benavente, R. (1993). Immunocytochemical localization of DNA in synaptonemal complexes of rat and mouse spermatocytes, and chick oocytes. Chromosoma, 102(7):457-463.

Vázquez-Nin, GH., Echeverría OM., Ortiz, R., Scassellati, C., Martín, TE., Ubaldo, E., & Fakan, S. (2003). Fine structural cytochemical analysis of homologous chromosome recognition, alignment, and pairing in guinea pig spermatogonia and spermatocytes. *Biol Reprod*, 69(4):1362-1379.

Westergaard, M., & von Wettstein, D. (1972). The synaptonemal complex. Annu Rev Genet, 6:71-110.

Winkel, K., Alsheimer, M., & Benavente, R. (2009). Protein SYCP2 provides a link between transverse filaments and lateral elements of mammalian complexes. Chromosoma, 118(2): 259-267.

Zickler, D., & Kleckner, N. (1998). The leptotene-zygotene transition of meiosis. *Annu Rev Genet*, 32:619-97.

Zickler, D., & Kleckner, N. (1999). Meiotic chromosomes: integrating structure and function. *Annu Rev Genet*, 33:603-754.

# 2

# Facing the Correct Pole: The Challenge of Orienting Chromosomes for Meiotic Divisions

Karishma Collette and Györgyi Csankovszki
*Department of Molecular, Cellular and Developmental Biology, University of Michigan, USA*

## 1. Introduction

Meiosis is a specialized cell division that directs a diploid germ cell to produce haploid gametes (reviewed in Schvarzstein et al, 2010; Sakuno and Watanabe, 2009). Meiosis differs from mitosis, in that one round of DNA replication is followed by two rounds of chromosome segregation. In the first round, meiosis I, homologous chromosomes separate (reductional division), and in the second round, meiosis II, sister chromatids separate (equational division). Meiosis II is similar to mitosis in that in both processes, replicated sister chromatids orient away from each other (are said to be bioriented), and will be separated at the metaphase to anaphase transition. By contrast, meiosis I, represents special challenges to the cell. In the first meiotic division, sister chromatids must face the same pole (are monooriented), and instead homologs, connected by the chiasma, are oriented away from each other toward opposite poles (Fig. 1). This chapter discusses our current understanding of how sister chromatid monoorientation and homolog biorientation are achieved during meiosis I.

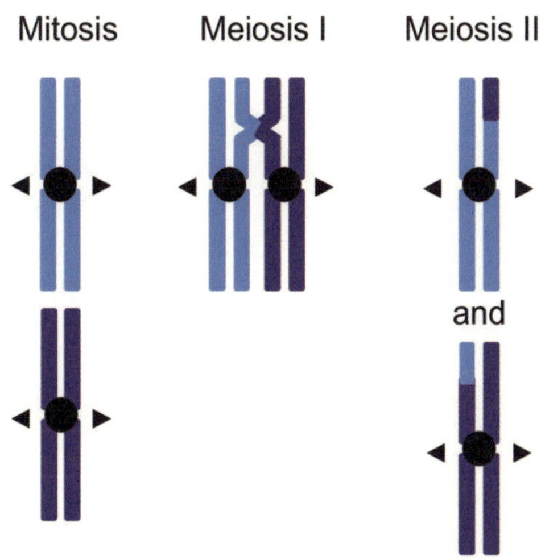


Fig. 1. Orientation of sister chromatids and homologous chromosomes in mitosis and meiosis. Arrowheads indicate the direction chromatids or chromosomes face.

Organisms with different chromosomal organization deal with this challenge differently. The majority of eukaryotic model organisms studied (such as yeast, flies and mammals) have monocentric chromosomes. Monocentric chromosomes have a single centromere, the region on the chromosomes where the kinetochore assembles. During mitosis and meiosis the kinetochores serve as site of attachment for spindle microtubules (Sakuno and Watanabe, 2009). In monocentric organisms, the centromere is where many meiotic events are coordinated, including orientation of chromosomes. Holocentric chromosomes (in organisms such as the nematode *C. elegans*) lack a localized centromere. On these chromosomes the kinetochore assembles along the entire length of the chromosomes during mitosis and forms cup-like structures encompassing each homolog during meiosis (Schvarzstein et al., 2010) (Fig. 2). Comparisons of the strategies used on chromosomes with such diverse organizational features highlight the common themes and the conserved molecular factors implementing these strategies.

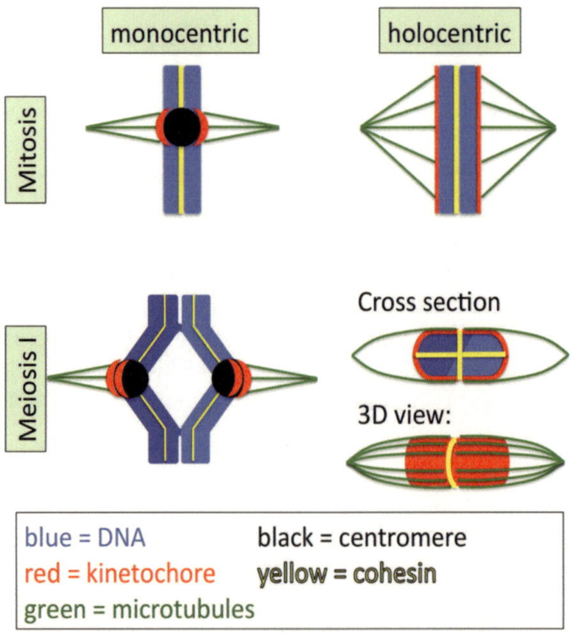


Fig. 2. The organization of kinetochores on monocentric and holocentric chromosomes during mitosis and meiosis I. During mitosis on monocentric chromosomes the kinetochore assembles at the region defined by the centromere. On holocentric chromosomes the kinetochores assemble along the entire length of the chromosomes. During meiosis I on monocentric chromosomes, kinetochores of sister chromatids function as one unit and orient toward the same pole. On holocentric chromosomes the kinetochore cups the volume of the sister chromatid pair.

One crucial player in the process of chromosome orientation is the chromosomal passenger complex (CPC), which monitors and regulates kinetochore-microtubules attachments. The CPC is composed of Aurora B kinase, inner centromere protein INCENP, Survivin and Borealin/Dasra B. Homologs of CPC subunits have been identified in organisms from yeast to humans. CPC proteins first associate with condensing chromatin at prophase, accumulate at the centromere during prometaphase and metaphase, relocate to the spindle midzone at the metaphase-anaphase transition, and finally associate with the midbody during telophase and cytokinesis (Vagnarelli and Earnshaw, 2004). This characteristically dynamic localization of the CPC likely reflects movement of Aurora B to act on different substrates. While on chromosomes, the CPC has important functions in condensin recruitment, facilitation of accurate microtubule-kinetochore attachments, spindle checkpoint function, and cohesin regulation. After the CPC transfers onto the central spindle and midbody, it is needed for the successful execution of cytokinesis (Vagnarelli and Earnshaw 2004).

The Structural Maintenance of Chromosomes (SMC) protein containing complexes condensin and cohesin, influence many aspects of chromosome organization and segregation and play roles in regulating chromosome orientation as well. Condensin is composed of a heterodimer of an SMC2 class and an SMC4 class ATPase protein, and three regulatory subunits referred to as chromosome associated polypeptide (CAP) proteins (Hirano, 2004; Hudson et al., 2009, Losada and Hirano, 2005). Budding and fission yeasts have a single condensin complex, but higher eukaryotes have two: condensin I and II. Condensins I and II differ in the identity of their CAP subunits. Condensin I contains CAP-G, -D2, and –H, while condensin II contains CAP-G2, -D3, and –H2. The single yeast condensin is most similar to the condensin I complex of higher eukaryotes. Although their exact molecular contribution to chromosome packaging remains a mystery, condensin complexes are essential for the precise organization and structural integrity of chromosomes (Bhat et al., 1996; Chan et al., 2004; Cobbe et al., 2006; Coelho et al., 2003; Dej et al., 2004; Gerlich et al., 2006; Hagstrom et al., 2002; Hartl et al., 2008; Hirota et al., 2004; Hudson et al., 2003; Lieb et al., 1998; Oliveira et al., 2003, 2005; Ono et al., 2003, 2004; Ribeiro et al., 2009; Samoshkin et al., 2009; Savvidou et al., 2005; Siddiqui et al., 2003; Stear and Roth, 2002; Steffensen et al., 2001; Vagnarelli et al., 2006; Watrin and Legagneux, 2005; Wignall et al., 2003; Yu and Koshland, 2003, 2005). SMC2 and 4 were originally identified as structural components of mitotic chromosomes in *Xenopus* and chicken cells (Hirano and Mitchison, 1994; Saitoh et al., 1994) and as important regulators of chromosome condensation and segregation in budding and fission yeast (Saka et al., 1994; Strunnikov et al., 1995).

Cohesin contains two SMC ATPase proteins of the SMC1 and SMC3 subclasses, and two regulatory subunits, Scc1 and Scc3 (Hirano, 2002, Jessberger, 2002). In meiosis, Scc1 is replaced by its paralog, Rec8 (Watanabe and Nurse, 1999). Cohesin mediates sister chromatid cohesion from the time they are replicated in S phase until sister chromatids separate at anaphase of mitosis and meiosis (Hirano, 2000; Nasmyth et al., 2001). Condensin and cohesin functions have been recently reviewed elsewhere. In this chapter we will concentrate on their role in regulating chromosome orientation.

## 2. Biorientation of sister chromatids in mitosis

Regulation of kinetochore orientation has been most extensively studied in mitosis. As the principle forces orientating chromosomes in mitosis and meiosis are likely mediated by the same factors, we will begin with a brief review of mitotic chromosome orientation. Mitotic chromosome segregation is preceded by a round of DNA replication, resulting in identical sister chromatids held together by cohesin. At entry into mitosis, or early during mitosis, condensin complexes associate with chromosomes to facilitate their compaction and segregation. In higher eukaryotes, the bulk of cohesin is removed from chromosomes arms in prophase, while centromeric cohesin is released at the metaphase to anaphase transition. In yeast, cohesin is removed from chromosomes in a single step, at the metaphase to anaphase transition (Nasmyth, 2002).

Prior to their separation, chromosomes align on the metaphase plate. Chromosome alignment and orientation is complete when all kinetochores are under tension, as a result of two opposing forces. Tension is generated because kinetochore microtubules are pulling sister chromatids toward opposite poles, and this poleward force is opposed by cohesion between sister chromatids in the centromeric region (Hauf and Watanabe, 2004; Sakuno and Watanabe, 2009). Sister kinetochores are arranged back-to-back, an arrangement that naturally facilitates biorientation. Kinetochore-microtubule attachments occur via trial and error, and are stabilized only when tension is established. An ideal attachment in mitosis, with two sister kinetochores attached to microtubules from opposite poles, is called an amphitelic attachment. Erroneous chromosome-spindle attachments, such as attachment of both sister kinetochores to the same pole (syntelic attachment), or attachment of only one sister kinetochore to a pole (monotelic attachment), result in insufficient tension. Merotelic attachment (one sister attached to both poles) could, in principle, establish tension, but must also be corrected (Fig. 3) (Cimini, 2007).

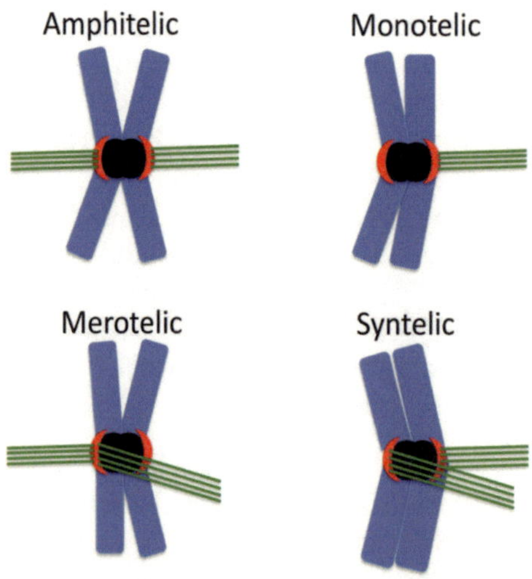


Fig. 3. Various forms of kinetochore-microtubule attachments at mitosis. Chromosomes are shown in blue, centromeres in black, kinetochores in red, and microtubules in green.

During mitosis, the CPC is enriched at the inner centromere where it is perfectly situated to monitor and correct aberrant kinetochore-microtubule attachments. (Tanaka, 2002; Vagnarelli and Earnshaw, 2004; Ruchaud et al. 2007; Watanabe, 2010) CPC depletion drastically disrupts metaphase chromosome alignment and orientation and subsequent anaphase segregation (Biggins et al., 1999; Biggins and Murray, 2001; Carvalho et al., 2003; Cimini et al., 2006; Ditchfield et al., 2003; Hauf et al., 2003, 2007; Honda et al., 2003; Kallio et al., 2002; Knowlton et al., 2006; Lens et al., 2003; Liu et al., 2009; Tanaka et al., 2002; Zhu et al., 2005). Aurora B and the CPC detect inappropriate or reduced tension at sites of incorrect attachment, and facilitate the release of these ill-fated connections. Aurora B appears to assume a more emphatic role in regulating syntely (Hauf, 2003, 2007; Lampson, 2004), but merotely is also fixed by the kinase (Cimini et al., 2006; Hauf et al., 2007; Knowlton et al., 2006). Hesperadin (a specific Aurora B inhibitor) treated HeLa cells showed a high incidence of syntelic attachments, and monotelic attachments were reduced six fold compared to control. These results led to a model whereby kinase function is required for the conversion of syntelic into temporary monotelic connections, such that the newly released kinetochore can search for microtubules from the correct pole (Hauf et al., 2003). A study in budding yeast suggests that centromeric INCENP-survivin (another CPC subunit) is a tension sensor that communicates with Aurora B to specifically destroy attachments under aberrant tension (Sandall et al., 2006).

Recent research has suggested that the spatial distribution of Aurora B is key to coupling tension sensing with the stability of kinetochore-microtubule attachments. Aurora B kinase influences microtubule interactions via phosphorylation of various centromeric/kinetochore targets. The phosphorylation status of Aurora B substrates depends on the extent of spatial separation from Aurora B at the inner centromere. Targets experiencing low tension (for example, in a syntelic connection) are physically closer to the kinase at the inner centromere, and undergo phosphorylation, whereas targets subjected to high tension (as seen in a bioriented attachment) are pulled away from Aurora B and escape phosphorylation (Tanaka et al., 2002; Liu et al., 2009).

Aurora B targets include the centromere associated kinesin MCAK (Andrews et al., 2004; Lan et al., 2004) and kinetochore proteins Dam1p, Ndc80p (Cheeseman et al., 2002) and Ndc10p (Biggins et al., 1999). Aurora B activation abolishes incorrect kinetochore-microtubule attachments by promoting microtubule fiber turnover and disassembly (Lampson et al., 2004; Cimini et al., 2006). Paradoxically, the microtubule-depolymerizing activity of MCAK, a major regulator of microtubule dynamics, is suppressed by Aurora B phosphorylation (Andrews et al., 2004; Lan et al., 2004). Perhaps phosphorylation of MCAK temporarily turns off its depolymerizing activity and supports new attempts at establishing kinetochore-microtubule connections, once incorrect attachments have been resolved (Knowlton et al., 2006; Lan et al., 2004).

Phosphorylation by Aurora B reduces the microtubule binding affinity of its kinetochore substrates (Cheeseman et al., 2006; DeLuca et al., 2006; Ciferri et al., 2008). Phosphorylation by Aurora B also disrupts subunit interactions within the multiprotein kinetochore and may thus contribute to the elimination of inappropriate kinetochore-microtubule connections (Shang et al., 2003). Thus, phosphorylation of the kinetochore targets of aurora B reduces their affinity for microtubules, causing them to relinquish wrong connections, and seek out fibers coming from the appropriate pole.

The CPC functions not only to detect and dissolve improper attachments, but it also activates the spindle attachment checkpoint (SAC) (Biggins and Murray, 2001; Carvalho et la., 2003; Ditchfield et al., 2003; Lens et al., 2003). SAC is activated in response to insufficient tension or unattached kinetochores. Checkpoint activation delays anaphase onset, so that bipolar attachments can be achieved for all chromosomes.

Tension is only established if the pulling forces of the spindle are counteracted by cohesion between sister centromeres. Centromeric cohesin function is needed for bipolar attachment of sister kinetochores (Sonoda et al., 2001; Tanaka et al., 2000). In fission yeast, cohesin localizes specifically to pericentric regions, and less to the core centromere (Bernard et al.,

2001; Nonaka et al., 2002; Tomonaga et al., 2000). These results support a model in which reduced levels of cohesin at the core centromere allow core regions to open up and assume back-to-back orientation, while pericentric cohesion ensures proper establishment of tension (Sakuno et al., 2009; Sakuno and Watanabe, 2009).

In addition to cohesin, condensin also seems to play a role in ensuring proper biorientation of sisters. In *C. elegans,* condensin depletion results in disorganized centromeres, and merotelic attachment (Hagstrom et al., 2002; Stear and Roth, 2002). In condensin depleted vertebrate cells, sister kinetochores move closer to each other and they do not face opposite poles anymore (Ono et al., 2004). It is likely that if the underlying chromosome structure is disrupted, especially at the centromeric regions, kinetochore function is perturbed as well.

## 3. Chromosomes are restructured extensively in preparation for meiosis

During meiosis I, sister chromatids orient toward the same pole and paired homologs (called bivalents) held together by the chiasma, become bioriented at metaphase instead (See Fig. 1). Differences in chromosome orientation during mitosis and meiosis could, in principle, be due to differences in the structure of the chromosomes themselves, or differences in the spindle. Micromanipulation experiments support the former possibility (Paliulis and Nicklas, 2000). Meiotic chromosomes placed on a mitotic spindle orient like meiotic chromosomes, and vice versa.

In both monocentric and holocentric organisms, chromosomes are extensively restructured during prophase of meiosis I to facilitate their proper segregation (reviewed in (Page and Hawley, 2003; Schvarzstein et al., 2010). Homologous chromosomes first pair, synapse (form a structure called the synaptonemal complex (SC) along the entire length of the homolog interface), and undergo crossing over, leading to the formation of bivalents. Metaphase chromosome alignment faces two challenges. First, sister kinetochores must be held together and orient toward the same pole. Second, homologs must be oriented away from each. As in mitosis, tension must be established. This tension is mediated by the pulling forces of the spindle microtubules exerted on kinetochores of homologs. Unlike in mitosis, the pulling forces of spindle microtubules are not counterbalanced by cohesion between sister kinetochores, but by the physical linkage of homologs mediated by the chiasma (see Fig. 2). Although research thus far has primarily focused on the importance of the CPC for sister chromatid biorientation in mitosis, recent evidence suggests that its role in destabilizing improper kinetochore-microtubule attachments may be conserved in meiosis as well (see below).

To deal with the special challenges of meiosis, the distribution and/or composition of chromosomal proteins can be different on meiotic chromosomes, as compared to mitosis. In mouse oocytes at metaphase I, condensin II concentrates within the core of individual sister chromatids, while condensin I is enriched at the centromere (Lee et al., 2011). This is in contrast to the mitotic distribution of these complexes. During mitosis in HeLa cells, the two condensin complexes alternate along chromosome axes, with condensin II being enriched at the centromere (Ono et al., 2004) (See Fig. 4). An additional difference between mitosis and meiosis is the subunit composition of cohesin. In meiosis, Rec8 (and other Rec8 paralogs) replace the mitotic paralog Scc1 (Watanabe and Nurse, 1999).

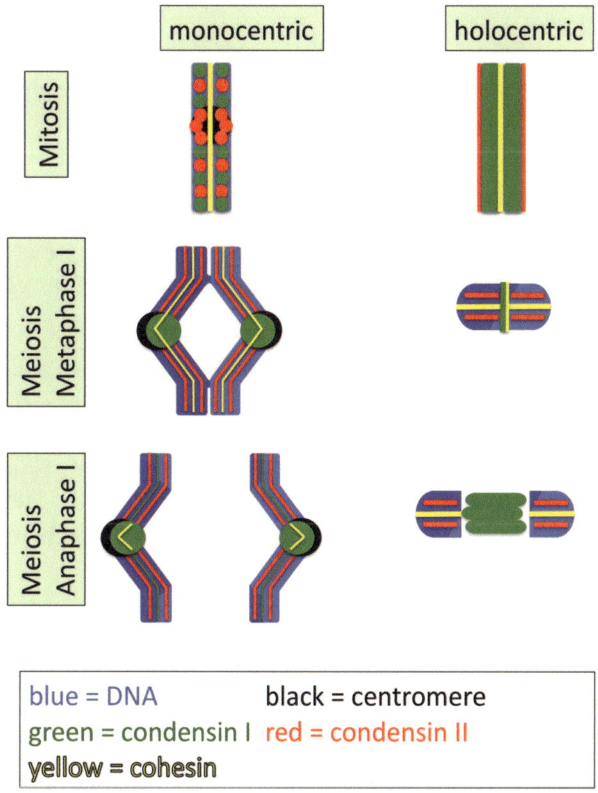


Fig. 4. The distribution of condensin I, condensin II, and cohesin on monocentric and holocentric chromosomes during mitosis and meiosis I.

In monocentric organisms, during prophase I of meiosis, cohesin molecules surrounding the site of crossover hold homologous chromosomes together until initiation of anaphase I. Homolog separation in meiosis I requires the resolution of sister chromatid cohesion distal to the chiasma. At the same time, sister chromatids must be held together until anaphase II by sister chromatid cohesion at the centromere. To achieve sequential loss of cohesin, in meiosis I arm cohesion is released, but centric cohesion is protected from degradation by Shugoshin/MEI-S322 (Kitajima et al., 2004; Resnick et al, 2006; Sakuno and Watanabe, 2009). This ensures that homologous chromosomes are no longer tethered, and can migrate to opposite poles, but sister chromatids travel together (Fig. 4) At anaphase II, centromeric cohesion is lost, and sister chromatids separate (Petronczki et al., 2003).

Holocentric organisms do not have a localized centromere, and phrases such as arm cohesion and centromeric cohesion do not apply. During *C. elegans* meiosis, the kinetochores form cup-like structures surrounding the entire volume of each homolog (Dumont et al., 2010) (See Fig. 2). Differentiation of domains within bivalents must therefore be coordinated in a different manner. Research in the last decade revealed that the formation of the crossover provides the primary clue for bivalent differentiation (Chan et al., 2004; Nabeshima et al., 2005). In *C. elegans*, each pair of homologs typically undergoes one crossover event in the terminal one-third of the chromosome. Toward the end of prophase I, bivalents are restructured into cross-shaped structures, in which the short arm is formed from the domain between the crossover and the closer chromosome end, and the long arm is formed from the domain between the crossover and the more distant chromosome end. Cohesin along the short arm is released in meiosis I to separate homologs, while cohesin along the long arm must be protected until anaphase II (reviewed in (Schvarzstein et al., 2010). Cohesion protection in C. elegans appears to be independent of Shugoshin, and instead is regulated by the HORMA domain containing protein HTP-1 and worm specific PP1 phosphatase interacting protein LAB-1 (de Carvalho et al., 2008; Martinez-Perez et al,. 2008). Note that while cohesion protection in meiosis I in monocentric organisms is performed at the centromere, in *C. elegans* cohesion is protected along the long arms of bivalents (Fig. 4).

As in monocentric organisms, distribution of chromosomal proteins differs between mitosis and meiosis in holocentric organisms as well. Our laboratory recently described the distinct distribution of condensin complexes in *C. elegans,* and compared their distributions in mitosis and meiosis (Collette et al., 2011). As in mouse oocytes, *C. elegans* condensin II occupies the core domain within each sister chromatid (Chan et al., 2004). Condensin I, on the other hand, is found at the midbivalent at the interface between homologs (Csankovszki et al., 2009; Collette et al., 2011) (Fig. 4).

## 4. Holding sister together: Monopolin and Rec8

Sisters are usually monooriented in meiosis I, even if homologs are not connected due to lack of chiasma formation. In most genetic backgrounds with defective crossover formation, homologs are not held together, but sister chromatids still segregate together toward the same pole (or are lost) during the first meiotic division. This finding implies that holding sisters together is not simply a consequence of keeping homologs apart. In budding yeast, a pair of sister kinetochores appears to be captured by a single microtubule (Winey et al., 2005). In higher eukaryotes, multiple microtubule attachments are made and both sister kinetochores are captured but they are connected to the same pole (Goldstein, 1981; Lee et al., 2000; Moore and Orr-Weaver, 1998; Parra et al., 2004.) Two possible mechanisms have been suggested to explain these findings: either sister kinetochores are fused into a single entity or one of the sisters is inactivated (Monje-Casas et al., 2007). Indeed, electron microscopy studies indicate that in meiosis I sister kinetochores are arranged side-by-side, as opposed to the back-to-back orientation seen in mitosis or meiosis II (Goldstein, 1981; Lee et al., 2000; Parra et al., 2004).

Studies of sister chromatid monoorientation in different model organisms have uncovered some interesting similarities and differences. Budding yeast makes use of a complex called monopolin to monoorient sisters. Monopolin is made up of Mam1, Csm1, Lrs4 and Hrr25 (Petronczki et al., 2003, 2006; Rabitsch et al., 2003; Toth et al., 2000). While in other model organisms the meiosis specific cohesin subunit Rec8 plays an important role in the process (see below), in budding yeast the function of Rec8 is not required for monoorientation (Toth et al., 2000, Yokobayashi et al., 2003), and monopolin appears to glue sisters together independent of cohesin function (Monje-Casas et al., 2007) On the other hand, condensin function is important for proper chromosome orientation, perhaps via correct localization of monopolin. In condensin depleted cells, monopolin association with kinetochores is reduced and a portion of sister kinetochores biorient (Brito et al., 2010).

Monocentric organisms other than budding yeast do not use Monopolin for sister chromatid monoorienation, and instead make use of cohesin and other meiosis specific factors. Rec8 seems to play an especially important role. Rec8 deficiency in fission yeast and plants leads to biorientation of sister chromatids, resulting in equational rather than reductional division in meiosis I (Chelysheva et al., 2005; d'Erfurth et al., 2009; Watanabe and Nurse, 1999, Yu and Dawe, 2000). Replacement of Rec8 with its mitotic paralog also results in biorientation, indicating that Rec8 function is specifically required (Yokobayashi et al., 2003). While Rec8 is necessary for sister monoorientation, it is not sufficient (Watanabe and Nurse, 1999; Yokobayashi et al., 2003). In fission yeast at least one other meiosis specific factor, Moa1, assists Rec8 in the process (Yokobayashi and Watanabe, 2005). In fission yeast, Rec8 has a distinct localization pattern, and is also found at the central core region of the centromere, in addition to chromosome arms and pericentric regions (Yokobayashi et al., 2003). This is different from the localization pattern of mitotic cohesin, which is specifically reduced at the centromere core (see above). According to current models, cohesion at the core centromere induces sister kinetochore monorientation, and cohesion at pericentric regions (as in mitosis and meiosis II) allows kinetochores to move away from each other promoting biorientation (Sakuno et al., 2009; Sakuno and Watanabe, 2009).

Since holocentric organisms do not have a localized centromere, they must use a different method to hold sister chromatids together during meiosis I. Recent studies suggest that despite the difference in chromosomal organization, REC-8 plays an important role in sister monoorientation in *C. elegans* as well (Severson et al., 2009). In *rec-8* mutant oocytes, homologs are not held together by a chiasma at metaphase due to an earlier defect in meiosis. However, *rec-8* mutant univalents (a pair of sister chromatids) become bioriented and separate from each other in meiosis I. Therefore *C. elegans* uses the same factor as monocentric organisms (REC-8), but this protein is functioning to promote sister monoorientation at different chromosomal domains: at the centromere in monocentric organisms and at the long arm of bivalents in *C. elegans.*

## 5. Regulating kinetochore-microtubule attachments: Aurora B function promotes homolog biorientation

As discussed above, in meiosis I homologous chromosomes become bioriented at the metaphase plate, as opposed to the biorientation of sister chromatids seen in mitosis and meiosis II. In principle, the problem to be solved is similar: tension must be established between two kinetochore entities that are connected. The difference is that this connection is centric cohesin in mitosis and chiasma between homologs during meiosis. During mitosis, Aurora B plays a crucial role in biorienting sister chromatids. During meiosis in fission yeast, budding yeast and mouse, Aurora B also localizes to the centromeric regions (Monje Casas et al., 2007; Parra et al., 2003, Petersen et al., 2001), therefore the protein is present at the right place and at the right time to regulate kinetochore-microtubule attachments in meiosis as well.

The first indication that Aurora B homologs are functioning in meiotic chromosome orientation came from studies in yeast. In budding yeast, Ipl1/Aurora B is needed for biorientation of homologs (Monje-Casas et al., 2007, Yu and Koshland, 2007). The results obtained in this system are consistent with the primary role of Aurora B to regulate turnover of kinetochore-microtubule attachments, similar to its role in mitosis. The fission yeast Aurora B homolog, Ark1, is also crucial for homolog biorientation during the first meiotic division (Hauf et al., 2007). Ark1 can promote biorientation of homologs, but it is also needed for biorientation of Rec8-deficient univalents (Hauf et al., 2007). In fact, Aurora B can promote biorientation even on kinetochores that are only loosely connected by a DNA thread (Dewar et al., 2004). These findings led to the suggestion that Aurora B can promote biorientation of any two kinetochores that are connected, further supporting the hypothesis that the molecular function of Aurora B is the same in mitosis and meiosis: correcting faulty kinetochore-microtubule attachments (Hauf et al., 2007).

Fission yeast Ark1 kinase appears to promote not only homolog biorientation, but also sister monoorientation. Ark1 can correct attachment of a unified pair of sister chromatids to both poles (merotelic attachment). While corrections of these merotelic attachments ultimately promote sister monoorientation, this mechanism is fundamentally different from the mechanism used by Rec8 and Moa1 to alter kinetochore geometry discussed above (Hauf et al., 2007).

On the holocentric chromosomes of *C. elegans*, Aurora B/AIR-2 is also located in an ideal position for regulating chromosome orientation, although this role has not been formally demonstrated yet. When bivalents orient at the metaphase plate, their long arms are parallel to spindle microtubules, and the midbivalent domains line up at the metaphase plate. Surprisingly, microtubule density on the poleward end of bivalents is low. Instead chromosomes are ensheathed by lateral microtubule bundles (Wignall and Willeneuve, 2009) (See Fig. 4). This ensheathment by lateral microtubules naturally promotes the orientation of homologs away from each other (Schwarzstein et al., 2010). Importantly, Aurora B/AIR-2 is found at the midbivalent domain, at the homolog interface (Kaitna et al., 2002; Rogers et al., 2002). Aurora B is perfectly situated here to promote homolog biorientation by performing its usual function: destabilizing incorrectly attached microtubules. Ensuring that microtubules do not attach at the zone of high Aurora B activity, coupled with ensheathment of bivalents by lateral microtubules provides an attractive model for biorientation of holocentric homologs.

## 6. Regulating chromosome orientation: a role for condensin?

Condensin I during mouse (Lee et al., 2011) and *C. elegans* meiosis (Collette et al., 2011) colocalizes with Aurora B. In the mouse, both condensin I and Aurora B are enriched at the centromere during metaphase I—at the domain important for regulating chromosome orientation. We recently demonstrated that in *C. elegans* AIR-2/Aurora B and condensin I colocalize at metaphase and anaphase of both meiotic divisions. Interestingly, condensin I occupies the same domain as AIR-2 not just on chromosomes at metaphase I and II, but also on the spindle between separating chromosomes at anaphase (Fig. 5). In addition, we also showed that correct targeting of condensin I to the midbivalent in meiosis I is dependent on AIR-2 (Collette et al., 2011). These results raise the interesting possibility that condensin I may aid Aurora B in performing its functions in regulating chromosome orientation in meiosis.

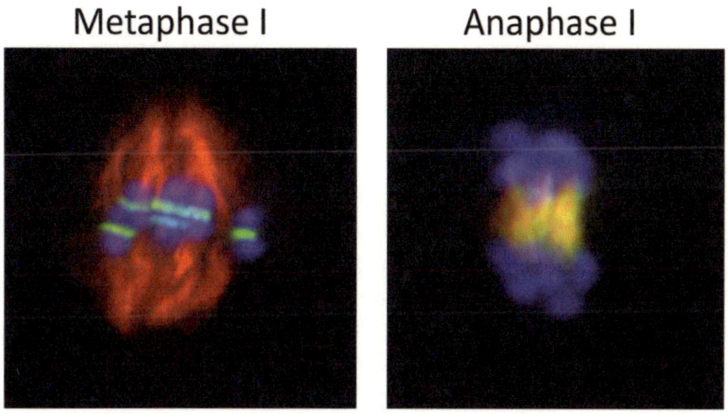


Fig. 5. Fluorescence microscopy images of condensin I distribution during *C. elegans* meiosis. During metaphase I, condensin I associates with the midbivalent domain, and during anaphase it is found on spindle microtubules between separating chromosomes. Microtubules are shown in red, condensin I in green, and chromosomes in blue.

Condensin depletion experiments support a role for condensin in regulating chromosome orientation. In budding yeast, condensin depletion leads to reduced localization of Monopolin subunit Mam1 to kinetochores and increased incidence of sister chromatid biorientation (Brito et al., 2010). In mouse oocytes, injections of SMC2 antibodies (which interfere with the function of both condensin complexes) led to a portion of sister chromatids assuming back-to-back, rather than side-by-side orientation. Anti-CAP-H injection (which interferes with condensin I only) caused disorganized centromeres and chromosome alignment problems (Lee et al., 2011). Condensin function may influence kinetochore structure, or may affect the underlying structure of centromeric chromatin (Bernad et al., 2011; Lee et al., 2011; Ono et al., 2004). Whether similar defects will be seen upon condensin I depletion in holocentric organisms as well remains to be demonstrated. However, given the colocalization of Aurora B and condensin I in mouse and *C. elegans* meiosis, the role for Aurora B in chromosome orientation in yeast and mouse meiosis, and the apparently conserved function of Aurora B in different organisms, we would like to propose that condensin I may aid chromosome orientation in *C. elegans* meiosis as well.

## 7. Conclusion

During meiosis in monocentric organisms, the centromere is used as a site where kinetochore-microtubule attachments, and therefore chromosome orientation, are regulated. In organisms other than budding yeast, enrichment of meiotic Rec8-containing cohesin at core centromeric regions promote monoorientation of sister chromatids. Aurora B at centromeric region appears to function to correct aberrant kinetochore-microtubule attachments to promote biorientation of homologs and prevent merotelic attachment of unified sister kinetochores. During meiosis in *C. elegans*, the site of the crossover, and not a localized centromere, ultimately determines the plane of chromosome orientation. During metaphase, the short arms of bivalents are lined up along the metaphase plate and the long arms point toward opposite poles. The kinetochore "cups" the entire volume of sister chromatids along the long arms. The activities that monoorient sisters and biorient homologs are concentrated at opposite domains of the bivalents. REC-8 promotes sister chromatid monoorientation along the long arms. By contrast, Aurora B is restricted to the short arm, where by preventing microtubules from "crossing the plane" of the bivalent short arm, it can ensure that sisters stay together, and homologs stay apart.

One way to conceptualize the differences between holocentric and monocentric chromosome orientation in meiosis is to think of holocentric bivalents as one large centromere without extended chromosome arms. The entire holocentric chromosome is cupped by the kinetochore. One domain within the kinetochore-bound domain (the long arm) contains REC-8, and according to this analogy, is comparable to core centromeric regions of monocentric chromosomes. Another domain (the short arm) is comparable to regions of Aurora B enrichment at centromeres. The organization of holocentric chromosomes magnifies the distinction between the various specialized chromosomal domains and makes it an ideal setting in which to examine these differences.

## 8. References

Andrews, P. D., Y. Ovechkina, et al. (2004). Aurora B regulates MCAK at the mitotic centromere. *Dev Cell* 6(2): 253-268.

Bernad, R., P. Sanchez, et al. (2011). Xenopus HJURP and condensin II are required for CENP-A assembly. *J Cell Biol* 192(4): 569-582.

Bernard, P., J. F. Maure, et al. (2001). Requirement of heterochromatin for cohesion at centromeres. *Science* 294(5551): 2539-2542.

Bhat, M. A., A. V. Philp, et al. (1996). Chromatid segregation at anaphase requires the barren product, a novel chromosome-associated protein that interacts with Topoisomerase II. *Cell* 87(6): 1103-1114.

Biggins, S. and A. W. Murray (2001). The budding yeast protein kinase Ipl1/Aurora allows the absence of tension to activate the spindle checkpoint. *Genes Dev* 15(23): 3118-3129.

Biggins, S., F. F. Severin, et al. (1999). The conserved protein kinase Ipl1 regulates microtubule binding to kinetochores in budding yeast. *Genes Dev* 13(5): 532-544.

Brito, I. L., H. G. Yu, et al. (2010). Condensins promote coorientation of sister chromatids during meiosis I in budding yeast. *Genetics* 185(1): 55-64.

Carvalho, A., M. Carmena, et al. (2003). Survivin is required for stable checkpoint activation in taxol-treated HeLa cells. *J Cell Sci* 116(Pt 14): 2987-2998.

Chan, R. C., A. F. Severson, et al. (2004). Condensin restructures chromosomes in preparation for meiotic divisions. *J Cell Biol* 167(4): 613-625.

Cheeseman, I. M., S. Anderson, et al. (2002). Phospho-regulation of kinetochore-microtubule attachments by the Aurora kinase Ipl1p. *Cell* 111(2): 163-172.

Cheeseman, I. M., J. S. Chappie, et al. (2006). The conserved KMN network constitutes the core microtubule-binding site of the kinetochore. *Cell* 127(5): 983-997.

Chelysheva, L., S. Diallo, et al. (2005). AtREC8 and AtSCC3 are essential to the monopolar orientation of the kinetochores during meiosis. *J Cell Sci* 118(Pt 20): 4621-4632.

Ciferri, C., S. Pasqualato, et al. (2008). Implications for kinetochore-microtubule attachment from the structure of an engineered Ndc80 complex. *Cell* 133(3): 427-439.

Cimini, D. (2007). Detection and correction of merotelic kinetochore orientation by Aurora B and its partners. *Cell Cycle* 6(13): 1558-1564.

Cimini, D., X. Wan, et al. (2006). Aurora kinase promotes turnover of kinetochore microtubules to reduce chromosome segregation errors. *Curr Biol* 16(17): 1711-1718.

Cobbe, N., E. Savvidou, et al. (2006). Diverse mitotic and interphase functions of condensins in Drosophila. *Genetics* 172(2): 991-1008.

Coelho, P. A., J. Queiroz-Machado, et al. (2003). Condensin-dependent localisation of topoisomerase II to an axial chromosomal structure is required for sister chromatid resolution during mitosis. *J Cell Sci* 116(Pt 23): 4763-4776.

Collette, K. S., Petty, E. L., et al., Different roles for Aurora B in condensin targeting during mitosis and meiosis. (2011). *J Cell Sci*: in press

Csankovszki, G., K. Collette, et al. (2009). Three distinct condensin complexes control C. elegans chromosome dynamics. *Curr Biol* 19(1): 9-19.

d'Erfurth, I., S. Jolivet, et al. (2009). Turning meiosis into mitosis. *PLoS Biol* 7(6): e1000124.

de Carvalho, C. E., S. Zaaijer, et al. (2008). LAB-1 antagonizes the Aurora B kinase in C. elegans. *Genes Dev* 22(20): 2869-2885.

Dej, K. J., C. Ahn, et al. (2004). Mutations in the Drosophila condensin subunit dCAP-G: defining the role of condensin for chromosome condensation in mitosis and gene expression in interphase. *Genetics* 168(2): 895-906.

DeLuca, J. G., W. E. Gall, et al. (2006). Kinetochore microtubule dynamics and attachment stability are regulated by Hec1. *Cell* 127(5): 969-982.

Dewar, H., K. Tanaka, et al. (2004). Tension between two kinetochores suffices for their bi-orientation on the mitotic spindle. *Nature* 428(6978): 93-97.

Ditchfield, C., V. L. Johnson, et al. (2003). Aurora B couples chromosome alignment with anaphase by targeting BubR1, Mad2, and Cenp-E to kinetochores. *J Cell Biol* 161(2): 267-280.

Dumont, J., K. Oegema, et al. (2010). A kinetochore-independent mechanism drives anaphase chromosome separation during acentrosomal meiosis. *Nat Cell Biol* 12(9): 894-901.

Gerlich, D., T. Hirota, et al. (2006). Condensin I stabilizes chromosomes mechanically through a dynamic interaction in live cells. *Curr Biol* 16(4): 333-344.

Goldstein, L. S. (1981). Kinetochore structure and its role in chromosome orientation during the first meiotic division in male D. melanogaster. *Cell* 25(3): 591-602.

Hagstrom, K. A., V. F. Holmes, et al. (2002). C. elegans condensin promotes mitotic chromosome architecture, centromere organization, and sister chromatid segregation during mitosis and meiosis. *Genes Dev* 16(6): 729-742.

Hartl, T. A., S. J. Sweeney, et al. (2008). Condensin II resolves chromosomal associations to enable anaphase I segregation in Drosophila male meiosis. *PLoS Genet* 4(10): e1000228.

Hauf, S., A. Biswas, et al. (2007). Aurora controls sister kinetochore mono-orientation and homolog bi-orientation in meiosis-I. *EMBO J* 26(21): 4475-4486.

Hauf, S., R. W. Cole, et al. (2003). The small molecule Hesperadin reveals a role for Aurora B in correcting kinetochore-microtubule attachment and in maintaining the spindle assembly checkpoint. *J Cell Biol* 161(2): 281-294.

Hauf, S. & Watanabe, Y. (2004). Kinetochore Orientation in Mitosis and Meiosis. Cell 119:317-327.

Hirano, T. (2000). Chromosome cohesion, condensation, and separation. *Annu Rev Biochem* 69: 115-144.

Hirano, T. (2002). The ABCs of SMC proteins: two-armed ATPases for chromosome condensation, cohesion, and repair. *Genes Dev* 16(4): 399-414.

Hirano, T. (2004). Chromosome shaping by two condensins. *Cell Cycle* 3(1): 26-28.

Hirano, T. and T. J. Mitchison (1994). A heterodimeric coiled-coil protein required for mitotic chromosome condensation in vitro. *Cell* 79(3): 449-458.

Hirota, T., D. Gerlich, et al. (2004). Distinct functions of condensin I and II in mitotic chromosome assembly. *J Cell Sci* 117(26): 6435-6445.

Honda, R., R. Korner, et al. (2003). Exploring the functional interactions between Aurora B, INCENP, and survivin in mitosis. *Mol Biol Cell* 14(8): 3325-3341.

Hudson, D. F., K. M. Marshall, et al. (2009). Condensin: Architect of mitotic chromosomes. *Chromosome Res* 17(2): 131-144.

Hudson, D. F., P. Vagnarelli, et al. (2003). Condensin is required for nonhistone protein assembly and structural integrity of vertebrate mitotic chromosomes. *Dev Cell* 5(2): 323-336.

Jessberger, R. (2002). The many functions of SMC proteins in chromosome dynamics. *Nat Rev Mol Cell Biol* 3(10): 767-778.

Kaitna, S., P. Pasierbek, et al. (2002). The aurora B kinase AIR-2 regulates kinetochores during mitosis and is required for separation of homologous Chromosomes during meiosis. *Curr Biol* 12(10): 798-812.

Kallio, M. J., M. L. McCleland, et al. (2002). Inhibition of aurora B kinase blocks chromosome segregation, overrides the spindle checkpoint, and perturbs microtubule dynamics in mitosis. *Curr Biol* 12(11): 900-905.

Kitajima, T. S., Kawashima, S. A. et al. (2004). The conserved kinetochore protein shugoshin protects centromeric cohesion during meiosis. *Nature* 427: 510-517.

Knowlton, A. L., W. Lan, et al. (2006). Aurora B is enriched at merotelic attachment sites, where it regulates MCAK. *Curr Biol* 16(17): 1705-1710.

Lampson, M. A., K. Renduchitala, et al. (2004). Correcting improper chromosome-spindle attachments during cell division. *Nat Cell Biol* 6(3): 232-237.

Lan, W., X. Zhang, et al. (2004). Aurora B phosphorylates centromeric MCAK and regulates its localization and microtubule depolymerization activity. *Curr Biol* 14(4): 273-286.

Lee, J., T. Miyano, et al. (2000). Specific regulation of CENP-E and kinetochores during meiosis I/meiosis II transition in pig oocytes. *Mol Reprod Dev* 56(1): 51-62.

Lee, J., S. Ogushi, et al. (2011). Condensin I and II are essential for construction of bivalent chromosomes in mouse oocytes. *Mol Biol Cell.*

Lens, S. M., R. M. Wolthuis, et al. (2003). Survivin is required for a sustained spindle checkpoint arrest in response to lack of tension. *EMBO J* 22(12): 2934-2947.

Lieb, J. D., M. R. Albrecht, et al. (1998). MIX-1: an essential component of the C. elegans mitotic machinery executes X chromosome dosage compensation. *Cell* 92(2): 265-277.

Liu, D., G. Vader, et al. (2009). Sensing chromosome bi-orientation by spatial separation of aurora B kinase from kinetochore substrates. *Science* 323(5919): 1350-1353.

Losada, A. and T. Hirano (2005). Dynamic molecular linkers of the genome: the first decade of SMC proteins. *Genes Dev* 19(11): 1269-1287.

Marston, A. L. and A. Amon (2004). Meiosis: cell-cycle controls shuffle and deal. *Nat Rev Mol Cell Biol* 5(12): 983-997.

Martinez-Perez, E., M. Schvarzstein, et al. (2008). Crossovers trigger a remodeling of meiotic chromosome axis composition that is linked to two-step loss of sister chromatid cohesion. *Genes Dev* 22(20): 2886-2901.

Monje-Casas, F., V. R. Prabhu, et al. (2007). Kinetochore orientation during meiosis is controlled by Aurora B and the monopolin complex. *Cell* 128(3): 477-490.

Moore, D. P. and T. L. Orr-Weaver (1998). Chromosome segregation during meiosis: building an unambivalent bivalent. *Curr Top Dev Biol* 37: 263-299.

Nabeshima, K., A. M. Villeneuve, et al. (2005). Crossing over is coupled to late meiotic prophase bivalent differentiation through asymmetric disassembly of the SC. *J Cell Biol* 168(5): 683-689.

Nasmyth, K. (2002). Segregating sister genomes: the molecular biology of chromosome separation. *Science* 297(5581): 559-565.

Nasmyth, K., J. M. Peters, et al. (2001). Splitting the chromosome: cutting the ties that bind sister chromatids. *Novartis Found Symp* 237: 113-133; discussion 133-118, 158-163.

Nonaka, N., T. Kitajima, et al. (2002). Recruitment of cohesin to heterochromatic regions by Swi6/HP1 in fission yeast. *Nat Cell Biol* 4(1): 89-93.

Oliveira, R. A., P. A. Coelho, et al. (2005). The condensin I subunit Barren/CAP-H is essential for the structural integrity of centromeric heterochromatin during mitosis. *Mol Cell Biol* 25(20): 8971-8984.

Ono, T., Y. Fang, et al. (2004). Spatial and temporal regulation of Condensins I and II in mitotic chromosome assembly in human cells. *Mol Biol Cell* 15(7): 3296-3308.

Ono, T., A. Losada, et al. (2003). Differential contributions of condensin I and condensin II to mitotic chromosome architecture in vertebrate cells. *Cell* 115(1): 109-121.

Page, S. L. & Hawley, R. S. (2003). Chromosome choreography: The meiotic ballet. *Science* 310: 785-789.

Paliulis, L. V. and R. B. Nicklas (2000). The reduction of chromosome number in meiosis is determined by properties built into the chromosomes. *J Cell Biol* 150(6): 1223-1232.

Parra, M. T., A. Viera, et al. (2004). Involvement of the cohesin Rad21 and SCP3 in monopolar attachment of sister kinetochores during mouse meiosis I. *J Cell Sci* 117(Pt 7): 1221-1234.

Parra, M. T., A. Viera, et al. (2003). Dynamic relocalization of the chromosomal passenger complex proteins inner centromere protein (INCENP) and aurora-B kinase during male mouse meiosis. *J Cell Sci* 116(Pt 6): 961-974.

Petersen, J., J. Paris, et al. (2001). The S. pombe aurora-related kinase Ark1 associates with mitotic structures in a stage dependent manner and is required for chromosome segregation. *J Cell Sci* 114(Pt 24): 4371-4384.

Petronczki, M., J. Matos, et al. (2006). Monopolar attachment of sister kinetochores at meiosis I requires casein kinase 1. *Cell* 126(6): 1049-1064.

Petronczki, M., M. F. Siomos, et al. (2003). Un menage a quatre: the molecular biology of chromosome segregation in meiosis. *Cell* 112(4): 423-440.

Rabitsch, K. P., M. Petronczki, et al. (2003). Kinetochore recruitment of two nucleolar proteins is required for homolog segregation in meiosis I. *Dev Cell* 4(4): 535-548.

Resnick, T. D., Satinover, D. L. et al., (2006) INCENP and Aurora B promote meiotic sister chromatid cohesion through localization of the Shugoshin MEI-S322 in Drosophila. *Dev Cell* 11: 57-68.

Ribeiro, S. A., J. C. Gatlin, et al. (2009). Condensin regulates the stiffness of vertebrate centromeres. *Mol Biol Cell* 20(9): 2371-2380.

Rogers, E., J. D. Bishop, et al. (2002). The aurora kinase AIR-2 functions in the release of chromosome cohesion in Caenorhabditis elegans meiosis. *J Cell Biol* 157(2): 219-229.

Ruchaud, S., M. Carmena, et al. (2007). Chromosomal passengers: conducting cell division. *Nat Rev Mol Cell Biol* 8(10): 798-812.

Saitoh, N., I. G. Goldberg, et al. (1994). ScII: an abundant chromosome scaffold protein is a member of a family of putative ATPases with an unusual predicted tertiary structure. *J Cell Biol* 127(2): 303-318.

Saka, Y., T. Sutani, et al. (1994). Fission yeast cut3 and cut14, members of a ubiquitous protein family, are required for chromosome condensation and segregation in mitosis. *EMBO J* 13(20): 4938-4952.

Sakuno, T., K. Tada, et al. (2009). Kinetochore geometry defined by cohesion within the centromere. *Nature* 458(7240): 852-858.

Sakuno, T. K. & Watanabe Y. (2009) Studies of meiosis disclose distinct roles of cohesion in the core centromere and pericentric regions. *Chromosome Res* 17:239-249.

Samoshkin, A., A. Arnaoutov, et al. (2009). Human condensin function is essential for centromeric chromatin assembly and proper sister kinetochore orientation. *PLoS ONE* 4(8): e6831.

Sandall, S., F. Severin, et al. (2006). A Bir1-Sli15 complex connects centromeres to microtubules and is required to sense kinetochore tension. *Cell* 127(6): 1179-1191.

Savvidou, E., N. Cobbe, et al. (2005). Drosophila CAP-D2 is required for condensin complex stability and resolution of sister chromatids. *J Cell Sci* 118(Pt 11): 2529-2543.

Schumacher, J. M., A. Golden, et al. (1998). AIR-2: An Aurora/Ipl1-related protein kinase associated with chromosomes and midbody microtubules is required for polar body extrusion and cytokinesis in Caenorhabditis elegans embryos. *J Cell Biol* 143(6): 1635-1646.

Schvarzstein, M., S. M. Wignall, et al. (2010). Coordinating cohesion, co-orientation, and congression during meiosis: lessons from holocentric chromosomes. *Genes Dev* 24(3): 219-228.

Severson, A. F., L. Ling, et al. (2009). The axial element protein HTP-3 promotes cohesin loading and meiotic axis assembly in C. elegans to implement the meiotic program of chromosome segregation. *Genes Dev* 23(15): 1763-1778.

Shang, C., T. R. Hazbun, et al. (2003). Kinetochore protein interactions and their regulation by the Aurora kinase Ipl1p. *Mol Biol Cell* 14(8): 3342-3355.

Siddiqui, N. U., P. E. Stronghill, et al. (2003). Mutations in Arabidopsis condensin genes disrupt embryogenesis, meristem organization and segregation of homologous chromosomes during meiosis. *Development* 130(14): 3283-3295.

Sonoda, E., T. Matsusaka, et al. (2001). Scc1/Rad21/Mcd1 is required for sister chromatid cohesion and kinetochore function in vertebrate cells. *Dev Cell* 1(6): 759-770.

Stear, J. H. and M. B. Roth (2002). Characterization of HCP-6, a C. elegans protein required to prevent chromosome twisting and merotelic attachment. *Genes Dev* 16(12): 1498-1508.

Steffensen, S., P. A. Coelho, et al. (2001). A role for Drosophila SMC4 in the resolution of sister chromatids in mitosis. *Curr Biol* 11(5): 295-307.

Strunnikov, A. V., E. Hogan, et al. (1995). SMC2, a Saccharomyces cerevisiae gene essential for chromosome segregation and condensation, defines a subgroup within the SMC family. *Genes Dev* 9(5): 587-599.

Tanaka, T., J. Fuchs, et al. (2000). Cohesin ensures bipolar attachment of microtubules to sister centromeres and resists their precocious separation. *Nat Cell Biol* 2(8): 492-499.

Tanaka, T. U. (2002). Bi-orienting chromosomes on the mitotic spindle. Curr Opin *Cell Biol* 14(3): 365-371.

Tanaka, T. U., N. Rachidi, et al. (2002). Evidence that the Ipl1-Sli15 (Aurora kinase-INCENP) complex promotes chromosome bi-orientation by altering kinetochore-spindle pole connections. *Cell* 108(3): 317-329.

Tomonaga, T., K. Nagao, et al. (2000). Characterization of fission yeast cohesin: essential anaphase proteolysis of Rad21 phosphorylated in the S phase. *Genes Dev* 14(21): 2757-2770.

Toth, A., K. P. Rabitsch, et al. (2000). Functional genomics identifies monopolin: a kinetochore protein required for segregation of homologs during meiosis i. *Cell* 103(7): 1155-1168.

Vagnarelli, P. and W. C. Earnshaw (2004). Chromosomal passengers: the four-dimensional regulation of mitotic events. *Chromosoma* 113(5): 211-222.

Vagnarelli, P., D. F. Hudson, et al. (2006). Condensin and Repo-Man-PP1 co-operate in the regulation of chromosome architecture during mitosis. *Nat Cell Biol* 8(10): 1133-1142.

Watanabe, Y. (2010). Temporal and spatial regulation of targeting aurora B to the inner centromere. *Cold Spring Harb Symp Quant Biol* 75: 419-423.

Watanabe, Y. and P. Nurse (1999). Cohesin Rec8 is required for reductional chromosome segregation at meiosis. *Nature* 400(6743): 461-464.

Watrin, E. and V. Legagneux (2005). Contribution of hCAP-D2, a non-SMC subunit of condensin I, to chromosome and chromosomal protein dynamics during mitosis. *Mol Cell Biol* 25(2): 740-750.

Wignall, S. M., R. Deehan, et al. (2003). The condensin complex is required for proper spindle assembly and chromosome segregation in Xenopus egg extracts. *J Cell Biol* 161(6): 1041-1051.

Wignall, S. M. and A. M. Villeneuve (2009). Lateral microtubule bundles promote chromosome alignment during acentrosomal oocyte meiosis. *Nat Cell Biol* 11(7): 839-844.

Winey, M., G. P. Morgan, et al. (2005). Three-dimensional ultrastructure of Saccharomyces cerevisiae meiotic spindles. *Mol Biol Cell* 16(3): 1178-1188.

Yokobayashi, S. and Y. Watanabe (2005). The kinetochore protein Moa1 enables cohesion-mediated monopolar attachment at meiosis I. *Cell* 123(5): 803-817.

Yokobayashi, S., M. Yamamoto, et al. (2003). Cohesins determine the attachment manner of kinetochores to spindle microtubules at meiosis I in fission yeast. *Mol Cell Biol* 23(11): 3965-3973.

Yu, H. G. and R. K. Dawe (2000). Functional redundancy in the maize meiotic kinetochore. *J Cell Biol* 151(1): 131-142.

Yu, H. G. and D. Koshland (2005). Chromosome morphogenesis: condensin-dependent cohesin removal during meiosis. *Cell* 123(3): 397-407.

Yu, H. G. and D. Koshland (2007). The Aurora kinase Ipl1 maintains the centromeric localization of PP2A to protect cohesin during meiosis. *J Cell Biol* 176(7): 911-918.

Yu, H. G. and D. E. Koshland (2003). Meiotic condensin is required for proper chromosome compaction, SC assembly, and resolution of recombination-dependent chromosome linkages. *J Cell Biol* 163(5): 937-947.

Zhu, C., E. Bossy-Wetzel, et al. (2005). Recruitment of MKLP1 to the spindle midzone/midbody by INCENP is essential for midbody formation and completion of cytokinesis in human cells. *Biochem J* 389(Pt 2): 373-381.

3

# Cohesins and Cohesin-Regulators in Meiosis

Adela Calvente and José L. Barbero
*Cell Proliferation and Development Department, Centro de Investigaciones Biológicas, Spain*

## 1. Introduction

Cells have rigorous mechanisms controlling sister chromatid cohesion during cell division to ensure proper distribution of genetic material to daughter cells. Errors in these mechanisms often lead to aneuploidy, frequently implicated in cell death, tumour development and infertility. The main actor in this process is a four-protein complex called the cohesin complex. The role of cohesin complex in chromosome segregation is mediated by the formation of a ring-like structure, which entrapped replicated DNA. The dynamic of the cohesin ring is regulated by a still undetermined number of cohesin-interacting proteins. These cohesin-regulators were essentially identified and studied in relation with the cohesion function of cohesin complexes. In the last years, we have improved our understanding of the key players in the regulation of sister chromatid cohesion during cell division in mitosis and meiosis. During meiosis the formation and disassemble of synaptonemal complex (SC), the recombination between homologue chromosomes and the maintenance of sister chromatid cohesion until metaphase II - anaphase II transition require unique features and players participating in the control of chromosome segregation. While in mammalian mitosis there are essentially two cohesin complexes, which only differ in the STAG subunit (STAG1 or STAG2), in meiosis several cohesin complexes composed by specific and unspecific meiotic cohesins coexist and probably they develop different functions depending of their spatio-temporal chromosome localization. On the other hand, a correct control of chromosome cohesion in meiosis involves specific regulators that monitor the sequential cohesin release during both meiotic divisions. Recently excellent papers have appeared in the literature looking in depth on the molecular control of sister chromatid cohesion and cohesins in cell division. In this chapter, we review the implication of cohesins and cohesin-interacting proteins in meiosis-specific processes and chromosome dynamic. Furthermore due to the increasing relevance of cohesins in human syndromes, we briefly point how problems in their tasks during mammalian mitotic and meiotic cycle drive to pathological situations.

## 2. Cohesin basic concepts

The pair of sister chromatids produced after DNA replication must be maintained together throughout the G2 phase and until its segregation to ensure a correct cell division. Thus, the sister chromatid cohesion is established during S phase (Miyazaki & Orr-Weaver, 1994) and although in mitosis the cohesion is released during prophase and prometaphase in arms (Hauf et al., 2005), the sister chromatid are joined at centromeres until the onset of anaphase. In meiosis, there are two consecutive chromosome divisions, segregating homologous chromosomes in anaphase I and sister chromatids in anaphase II. Thus the cohesion regulation presents specific characteristics of this kind of cell division, and whereas the arm cohesion is lost at anaphase I, the centromere cohesion is released at anaphase II (Watanabe, 2004). Since both cohesion releases follow the same pathway in meiosis, the meiotic centromere cohesin complexes must be protected until the second meiotic division (Kitajima et al., 2004). At any case, mitosis and meiosis, the multi-protein complex responsible of sister chromatid cohesion is called cohesin complex and it was first characterized in *Saccharomyces cerevisiae* and *Xenopus laevis* (Losada et al., 1998, Michaelis et al., 1997). The cohesin complex is composed by four subunits: two structural maintenance of chromosomes family proteins (SMC1 and SMC3), one α-kleisin subunit (SCC1/RAD21), and a HEAT-repeat domain protein (SCC3/SA/STAG) (Nasmyth & Haering, 2005). The most of components of the cohesin complex are conserved from yeast to humans (Uhlmann, 2001) but there are specific subunits depending on the species or the cell division type. The most conserved cohesins are the SMC proteins, which form a V-shaped heterodimer, representing the core of the cohesin complex (Haering et al., 2002). Higher eukaryotes have two mitotic SA/STAG family members, SA1/STAG1 and SA2/STAG2 (Carramolino et al., 1997), which do not coexist and are present in different cohesin complexes (Losada et al., 2000). In germ cells have been characterized distinct meiosis-specific subunits of cohesin complex in different organisms. In mammals, a meiotic paralogue of SMC1 has been described, the SMC1β, thus the subunit presents in mitosis and meiosis is called SMC1α (Revenkova et al., 2001). In yeast and mammals REC8 is the meiotic paralogue of SCC1/RAD21 subunit (Eijpe et al., 2003, Molnar et al., 1995, Watanabe & Nurse, 1999) and in mice a new α-kleisin has been identified recently, the RAD21L, a paralogue of RAD21 (Gutierrez-Caballero et al., 2011, Ishiguro et al., 2011, Lee & Hirano, 2011). RAD21L interacts with STAG3 (meiosis-specific SCC3 subunit) and with the three described SMC cohesin subunits, SMC1α, SMC1β and SMC3. STAG3 is the meiosis-specific paralogue for STAG1/2 in mammals (Pezzi et al., 2000, Prieto et al., 2001). Whereas these cohesin subunits, RAD21L, REC8, STAG3 and SMC1β, are meiosis-specific and they are present specifically in spermatocytes and oocytes (Garcia-Cruz et al., 2010, Herran et al., 2011, Prieto, et al., 2001), different cytological and molecular analysis show the participation of the SMC1α, RAD21 and STAG2 in mammalian mitosis and meiosis (Prieto et al., 2002, Revenkova et al., 2004, Revenkova & Jessberger, 2006). Characterization of distinct meiotic cohesin complexes containing REC8, RAD21 or RAD21L as α-kleisin subunits, which have distinct localization patterns and dynamics, as well as the simultaneous presence of SMC1α and β-containing complexes and the presence of STAG2 and STAG3 in mammalian meiosis suggest a large variety of putative cohesin complexes formed by combinations of cohesin subunits (Suja & Barbero, 2009). The most accepted model of the cohesin complex organization describes a heterodimer of SMC proteins jointed by their hinge domains. The ATPase heads of SMC1 and SMC3 are connected by the α-kleisin, forming a tripartite ring and finally the SCC3 subunit interacts with SCC1 via SCC1's C-terminus (Fig. 1A) (Haering, et al., 2002). Two major models, which are not mutually exclusive, have been proposed for the cohesin complex function in sister chromatid cohesion and its interaction with the DNA molecules. The first one is based on the electronic microscopy results and structural characteristics of SMCs and described a cohesin complex forming a ring-like structure (Fig. 1B), which mediates cohesion by embracing chromatin fibers of both sister chromatids (Gruber et al., 2003). The second model was named handcuff model, it involves the participation of two cohesin rings formed by SMC1/SMC3/SCC1 subunits which interacts in an SCC3-dependent manner (Fig. 1C). In this model each sister chromatid is encircled by a tripartite cohesin ring (Zhang et al., 2008a).

The activity of the cohesin complex is closely related to the action of three cohesin cofactors: PDS5, WAPL (Fig. 1A) and Sororin. PDS5 is associated with cohesins but in a less tightly bound manner than the cohesin complex proteins. In vertebrates there are two PDS5 homologues, PDS5A and PDS5B. The role of PDS5 is related to the maintenance of cohesion and the modulation of the interaction of cohesin complex with the chromatin (Losada et al., 2005). WAPL is involved in heterochromatin organization in *Drosophila melanogaster* (Verni et al., 2000) and in human cells regulates the resolution of sister chromatid cohesion during prophase (Gandhi et al., 2006).

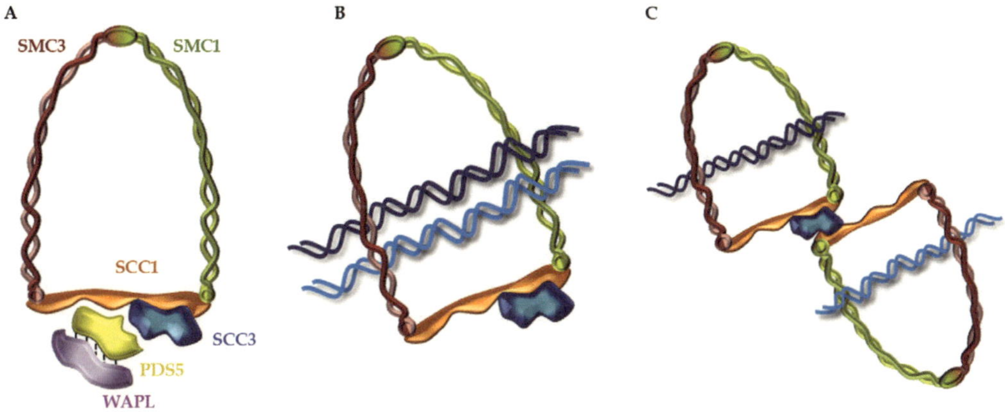


Fig. 1. Cohesin complex organization and cohesion models.
**A.** The cohesin complex is formed by four proteins: SMC1, SMC3, SCC1 and SCC3 (green, red, orange and blue piece respectively). The SMC1, SMC3 and SCC1 subunits form a ring-like structure. The SCC3 protein interacts with SCC1 to complete the cohesin complex. The cofactors PDS5 (yellow piece) and WAPL (purple piece) interact to form a protein complex, which is associated to the cohesin complex by SCC3 interaction. **B.** Ring-embraced model of cohesion. A single cohesin complex hugs the two sister chromatids. **C.** Handcuff model of cohesion. Two cohesin rings interacts by a single SCC3 molecule. Each cohesin ring encircles a single chromatid.

Regarding to the Sororin, it has been described in culture cells that this protein have a role in centromere cohesion, probably it is implicated in the protection of centromeric cohesin complexes (Diaz-Martinez et al., 2007). Moreover Sororin seems to have a role in the cohesion establishment during replication (Lafont et al., 2010). The implication of all these cofactors in meiosis is a wide field of study nowadays. The importance of cohesins, cohesin complex and cohesion cofactors not only consists in keeping jointed both sister chromatid and then ensure the bipolar attachment and the chromosomal segregation (Tanaka et al., 2000) in mitosis and meiosis, but the cohesins acquire a pivotal role in many different aspects of meiosis and chromosome dynamics such as the modulation of gene expression, the double strand breaks (DSBs) repair, axial elements (AEs) formation or pairing and synapsis of homologous chromosomes. In this chapter some of those different roles of cohesins and cohesion cofactors are reviewed, giving special attention to the specificity of some cohesin subunits to specific functions.

## 3. Loading, establishment, maintenance and release of cohesin complexes

Chromosome segregation control is managed by an intricate network of events, which assures that each daughter cell receives the right chromosome number, equal amount of chromosomes in mitosis and a haploid recombined chromosomal pack in meiosis. On one hand, fails in mitotic chromosome segregation compromises the viability of the organism, on the other hand fails in meiotic chromosome segregation jeopardizes the fertility of individuals. The importance of cohesion must be taken into account from the loading of cohesins to the establishment of cohesion, maintenance of cohesive function and finally the removal of cohesin complexes. In this context, the association/dissociation of sister chromatids is a well-controlled process that involves the role of different cohesin-interacting proteins. The loading of cohesin complexes to chromosomes occur near the G1 to S phase previous to cell division, thus it would be easy to think that the regulators of cohesin loading would be similar in mitosis and meiosis. In fact, most of them have been first described in yeast mitosis and afterwards a similar meiotic function was identified in some cases. Although we do not should forget that the transition from mitosis to meiosis could be trigger from the premeiotic S phase, and taking into account the presence of meiotic cohesin complexes and the special regulation of meiotic cohesion release, crucial differences might exist between mitosis and meiosis. It was described in *S. cerevisiae* that the loading of cohesin complexes depends on the SCC2/SCC4 adherin complex (Ciosk et al., 2000). This loading is not sufficient for the cohesion function in chromosome segregation and the Eco1/Ctf7p acetyltransferase is required for the establishment of cohesion in mitotic yeast chromosomes (Skibbens et al., 1999, Toth et al., 1999). In humans, two Eco1 orthologues have been identified: ESCO1 and ESCO2. Both proteins exhibit not redundant acetyltransferase activity and the depletion of any of them by siRNA cause defects in sister chromatid cohesion and chromosome segregation. However, in S-phase the role of both proteins seems to be directly related to the cohesion establishment and do not with the cohesin loading (Hou & Zou, 2005). The substrate of Eco1/ESCO1 is SMC3 in both human and yeast cells, being required the acetylation of SMC3 for sister chromatid cohesion. The acetylation of SMC3 could regulate its interaction with SCC1, promoting the turn from a chromosome-bound cohesin complex into a cohesive complex (Zhang et al., 2008b), suggesting that the cohesin complexes with acetylated SMC3 may be stably bound to chromosomes (Unal et al., 2008). The activity of Eco1 could be facilitated due to its interaction with PCNA (proliferating cell nuclear antigen) (Moldovan et al., 2006). The acetylation of SMC3 is maintained until metaphase - anaphase transition and its deacetylation in yeast mitosis depends on Hos1, but this deacetylase cannot act until the SCC1 cohesin subunit is cleaved by a protease called Separase, recycling then the tripartite open ring of cohesin (Beckouet et al., 2010, Borges et al., 2010). In mammalian mitosis the deacetylase responsible for SMC3 deacetylation has not been identified, moreover the cycle of SMC3 acetylation/deacetylation in meiosis is still poorly known.

The release of cohesion in mitotic prophase and anaphase follows different pathways of resolution (Waizenegger et al., 2000). In mitosis, the arm cohesion is released during prophase in a Separase-independent manner, it depends on the phosphorylation of SCC3/SA2/STAG2 subunit by Aurora B and Polo-like kinases (Hauf, et al., 2005), but the correct chromosome segregation depends on the centromeric cohesion, which is maintained until anaphase onset and then released by the Separase activity. The release of cohesin complexes from centromeric chromatin at mitotic metaphase - anaphase transition is mediated by the Separase, a specific protease that cleaves the SCC1 subunit of the cohesin complex (Uhlmann et al., 1999), destabilizing the association of cohesins to chromatin. Before anaphase, Separase remains inactivated by binding to its specific inhibitor Securin (Ciosk et al., 1998). Activation of the anaphase promoting complex/cyclosome (APC/C) leads to ubiquitination of Securin, allowing cleavage of SCC1/RAD21 by Separase and triggering the onset of anaphase (Uhlmann et al., 2000). In meiosis there are two consecutive chromosome segregations which are triggered by a Separase-dependent mechanism of lost of cohesion. During first meiotic division, the cohesin complexes at chromosome arms are removed during the metaphase I - anaphase I transition, allowing segregation of recombined homologues to opposite poles. In the second meiotic division, the cohesion is released from centromeres and sister chromatids are segregated to opposites poles to generate haploid gametes. Then, this type of cell division presents unique characteristics in sister chromatid cohesion removal and centromere cohesion protection. This is necessary to prevent premature separation of sister chromatids in order to avoid aneuploidy in the resulting gametes. Related to the centromere protection a protein family was indentified in fission yeast, the Shugoshins: Sgo1 and Sgo2 (Kitajima, et al., 2004). In these organisms Sgo1 seems to be essential in meiosis and Sgo2 is mostly implicated in mitotic division. The activity of Sgo1 and Sgo2 is related to the recruitment of a serine/threonine protein phosphatase 2A (PP2A) (Kitajima et al., 2006). In humans these proteins are called SGOL1 and SGOL2 and in mitosis they also collaborate with PP2A. In mice it has been described the localization of SGOL2 in male meiosis and it corresponds with a protection function of centromeric cohesion during first meiotic division (Gomez et al., 2007). An interesting model is the SGOL2-deficient mouse, where a precocious dissociation of the meiosis-specific REC8 cohesin complexes from anaphase I centromeres was observed (Llano et al., 2008), demonstrating the specific implication of SGOL2 in centromere protection during meiosis.

The cohesin-regulators PDS5 and WAPL are also involved in the opening/closing of cohesin ring by interactions with different cohesin subunits. These cofactors are not required for cohesin association to chromosomes but they are necessary for cohesin complex dynamics. The action of PDS5 is related to its interaction with the SA1 and SA-containing complexes in somatic cells (Sumara et al., 2000). In vertebrates two PDS5 proteins have been characterized: PDS5A and PDS5B. Both are large HEAT-repeat proteins that bind to chromatin in a cohesin-dependent manner in human cells and *Xenopus* egg extracts. RNAi depletion of PDS5A and PDS5B show that both are needed for maintaining cohesion, altering preferentially centromeric cohesion in *Xenopus* egg extracts. (Losada, et al., 2005). Mice lacking PDS5B function die shortly after birth and exhibit multiple developmental anomalies that resemble those found in humans with Cornelia de Lange syndrome (CdLS), indicating a relevant function for PDS5B beyond chromosome segregation, but there are no discernible defects in sister chromatid cohesion (Zhang et al., 2007). Despite of these contradictory results, the function of PDS5 has been related with the maintenance of sister chromatid cohesion during G2 (Panizza et al., 2000). Although, whether PDS5 also has a function in sister chromatid resolution remains to be determined. Another interesting cohesin cofactor is the product of the previously identified *Drosophila* wings apart-like (*Wapl*) gene, involved in heterochromatin organization (Verni, et al., 2000). Human WAPL regulates the resolution of sister chromatid cohesion and promotes cohesin complex removal by direct interaction with the RAD21 and SA/STAG cohesin subunits (Gandhi, et al., 2006). Thus, WAPL seems to destabilize cohesins. It has been proposed that PDS5 and WAPL form a protein complex, which in association with SCC3 cohesin subunit antagonizes the establishment of cohesion, calling the WAPL-PDS5 anti-establishment complex.

Skibbens proposed a model of cohesion establishment where the recruitment of PDS5-WAPL complex onto SCC3 subunit prevents the binding of cohesin complexes by destabilizing cohesin-cohesin association. During S phase, Eco1/ESCO1 acetylates SMC3, which inhibits the WAPL-PDS5 activity temporally (Skibbens, 2009). After S phase, PDS5 would stabilize the cohesin complexes activity.

Sororin has been implicated in centromere cohesion. This protein was firstly identified in a screen for substrates of the APC in vertebrates and no homologues have been described in other organisms. Different results in somatic cells suggested that Sororin interacts with the cohesin complex and it is essential for the maintenance of sister chromatid cohesion. Sororin is ubiquitinized and degraded after sister chromatid cohesion is dissolved (Rankin, 2005). Studies on Sororin-depleted and Shugoshin-depleted cells indicate that both proteins might act in concert in the protection of centromeric cohesion (Diaz-Martinez, et al., 2007). Sororin is also needed for maintaining stable chromatin-bound cohesin and DSBs repair in G2 (Schmitz et al., 2007). The Sororin recruitment depends on Eco2/ESCO2, both are subtrates of APC and its activity is related to the DNA replication (Lafont, et al., 2010). In agreement with these findings, Nishiyama reported that DNA replication and cohesin acetylation promote binding of Sororin to cohesin complex and that Sororin displaces WAPL from its binding partner PDS5, thus it would contribute to maintenance of a stable binding of cohesin to chromatin (Nishiyama et al., 2010).

Despite of the relevant roles in chromosome cohesion control suggested by all these results, there are few data regarding to the putative functions of cohesion cofactors such as SCC2/SCC4, Eco1/ESCO1, Eco2/ESCO2, WAPL, PDS5 or Sororin in chromosome segregation in meiosis.

## 4. Roles of the cohesin-regulators in meiosis

Updates there are no many evidences regarding to the specific implication of all the cohesion cofactors in meiosis. It is predictable that all of them might act in meiosis in a similar way to that described in mitotic cells or perhaps they acquire specific roles due to the particular regulation of meiotic division. Update the unique indication that ESCO2 have a role in meiosis was the identification of *Esco2* gene as a candidate to be a potential regulator of the transition from mitosis to meiosis in mammals, identifying by means microarray database in both testis and ovary of mouse (Hogarth et al., 2011). The data are supported not only by a pattern of mRNA expression but also by protein immunolocalization, showing on one hand that *Esco2* is expressed in testis and ovary, specifically in the embryonic gonad, and on the other hand that ESCO2 localized to the nucleus of spermatocytes at early prophase I. This last probe was performed by immunofluorescence techniques over testis sections at different ages. At 10dpp (days post-partum) male mice, ESCO2 was presented at preleptotene and leptotene diffusely and from 15dpp this protein is located at pachytene in a discrete domain within the nuclei. Our laboratory is actually studying the ESCO2 implications in meiosis and using the same antibody (Bethyl Laboratories, A301-689A) we have identified that the discrete domain observed by Hogarth et al., is in fact the XY body (Figs. 2 and 3). We have analyzed the male mice meiosis over squashes of seminiferous tubules (Page et al., 1998, Parra et al., 2004) and spreads of meiocytes (Peters et al., 1997, Viera et al., 2009a) and performed the double-immunolocation of ESCO2 and SYCP3 (Santa Cruz Biotechnology, sc-74569). Our results indicate that the ESCO2 acetyltranferase is present over the chromatin of XY body from zygotene to late stages of prophase I, detecting a more intense signal at pachytene (Fig. 2 and 3 A). We distinguish the XY body in squashed spermatocytes because of it usually is located at nuclear periphery and its AEs are partially unsynapsed due to this pair of chromosomes share only a homologue region called pseudoatosomal region, which the SC is exclusively formed in. Also the DAPI chromatin staining led us to identify the XY body undoubtedly in squashes (Fig. 2D). At pachytene nucleus the synapsis between autosomes is completed, which can be detected by SYCP3 immunolabeling (Fig. 2 and 3 B).

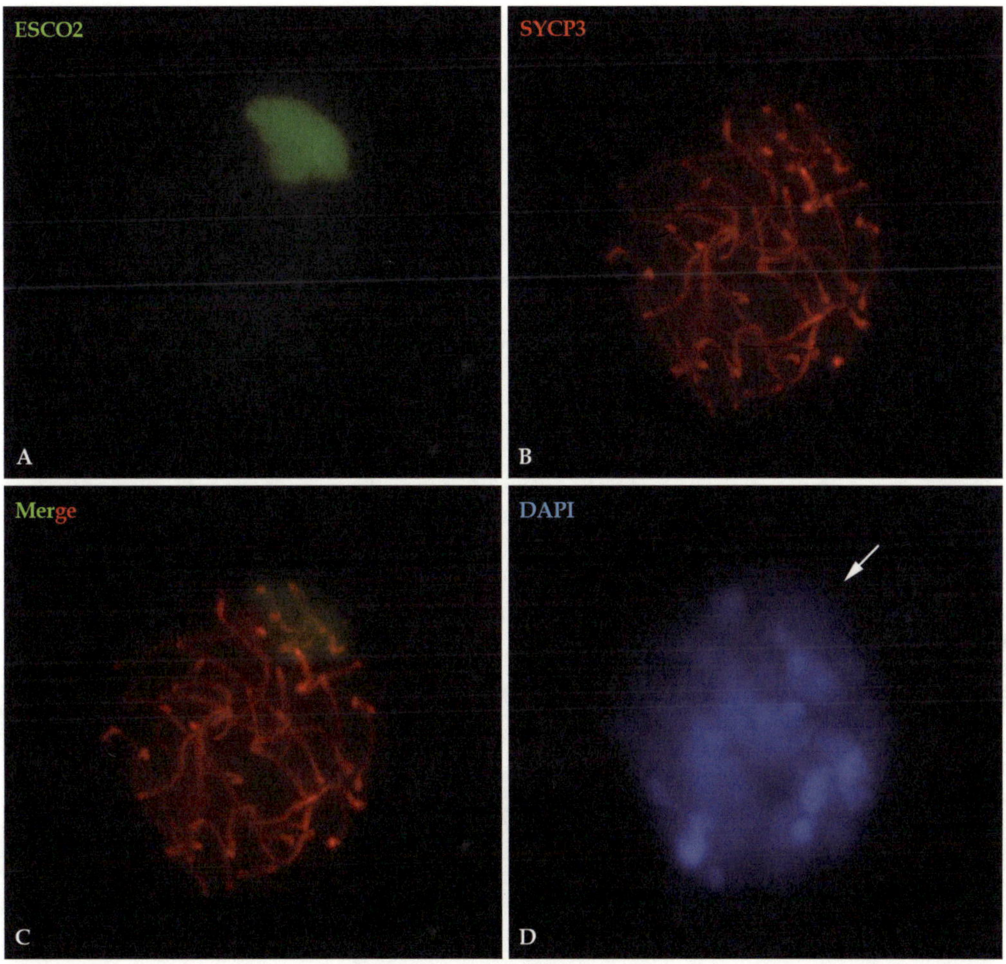


Fig. 2. Immunolabeling of ESCO2 (green) and SYCP3 (red) at pachytene after squasing of spermatocytes.

**A.** ESCO2 immunolabeling (rabbit anti-ESCO2 Bethyl Laboratories, A301-689A; 1:50 dilution) mark the XY body at pachytene. FITC-conjugated anti-rabbit IgG secondary antibody (Jackson Laboratories) was used at 1:150 dilution. **B.** SYCP3 (mouse monoclonal antibody anti-SYCP3. Santa Cruz Biotechnology, SCP-3 (D-1): sc-74569; 1:100 dilution) mark the LEs of synapsed autosomes and the AE/LEs of the XY body. DyLight594-conjugated anti-mouse IgG secondary antibody (Jackson Laboratories) was used at 1:150 dilution. **C.** The merge image of ESCO2 and SYCP3 signals is shown. **D**. The chromatin was counterstaining with DAPI in blue (4′,6-diamidino-2-phenylindole, SIGMA). The XY body is indicated (white arrow). After mounting the preparations with Vectashield (Vector Laboratories), the meiocytes were visualized using a Leica AFX6000LX multidimensional microscopy. The images were captured with LAS_AF software and analyzed and processed with public domain ImageJ and Adobe Photoshop CS3 softwares. All images are the result of superimposition of all the focal planes occupying the total volume of a pachytene mouse spermatocyte after squashing of seminiferous tubules.

We have not detected any ESCO2 labelling over the autosomas at any stage of meiosis. Since the X and Y chromosomes in all eutherian mammals preserve only a small region of homology, the genetic and morphological differentiation of sex chromosomes mark the XY behaviour during meiosis, which cannot be comparable with autosomes. Thus, structural modifications in the unsynapsed AEs of XY pair have been identified. Moreover, modifications in the distribution of different cohesin subunits have been also observed, as the preferential location of REC8 in the synapsed region of the XY body at pachytene (Page et al., 2006). However, our results show that the ESCO2 labelling embrace all the chromatin of sex chromosomes, similar signals have been detected after immunostaining of γ-H2AX and surprisingly the cohesin subunit RAD21L has been also observed in the XY chromatin at pachytene and diplotene (Herran, et al., 2011, Ishiguro, et al., 2011).

The presence of RAD21L over the XY chromatin has been explained as part of the sexual dimorphism observed regarding to the detection of RAD21L in mice and the authors pointed to a specific role of this meiotic cohesin subunit in the pairing and development of the sex body (Herran, et al., 2011), although deep studies should be performed to understand the role of a cohesin subunit in all sex chromatin. γ-H2AX is the histone variant derived from the phosphorylation of H2AX at serine 139 as consequence of DSBs (Mahadevaiah et al., 2001), however the presence of this chromatin modification in XY pair has been related to the transcriptional repression associated with the sex body (Fernandez-Capetillo et al., 2003).

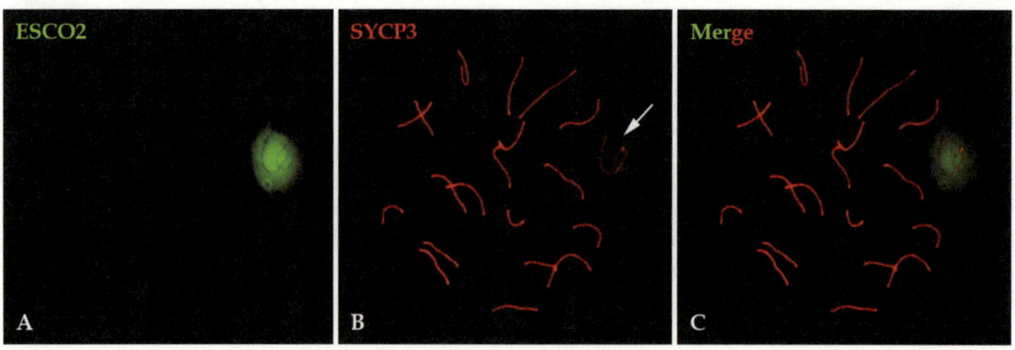


Fig. 3. Immunolabeling of ESCO2 (green) and SYCP3 (red) at pachytene after spreading of spermatocytes.

**A.** The immunolabeling of ESCO2 (rabbit anti-ESCO2 Bethyl Laboratories, A301-689A; 1:50 dilution ) mark the XY body at pachytene. FITC-conjugated anti-rabbit IgG secondary antibody (Jackson Laboratories) was used at 1:150 dilution. **B.** The LEs of synpased autosomes and the AE/LEs of the sex chromosomes (white arrow) are detected with an anti-SCYP3 antibody (mouse monoclonal antibody anti-SYCP3. Santa Cruz Biotechnology, SCP-3

(D-1): sc-74569; 1:100 dilution). DyLight594-conjugated anti-mouse IgG secondary antibody (Jackson Laboratories) was used at 1:150 dilution. **C.** Merge image of ESCO2 and SYCP3 signals. After mounting the preparations with Vectashield (Vector Laboratories), the meiocytes were visualized using a Leica AFX6000LX multidimensional microscopy. The images were captured with LAS_AF software and analyzed and processed with public domain ImageJ and Adobe Photoshop CS3 softwares.

During male meiosis, X and Y chromosomes are silenced in a process called Meiotic Sex Chromosome Inactivation (MSCI), it has been described that this chromosome inactivation is essential for male meiosis progression, thus the disruption of MSCI arrest the male meiosis at pachytene, being essential for male fertility (Fernandez-Capetillo, et al., 2003, Royo et al., 2010). According to the formation of XY body and its transcriptionally silenced status during spermatogenesis different histone modifications have been described at pachytene such as H3 and H4 deacetylation or H3-K9 dymethylation (Khalil et al., 2004). The specific function of ESCO2 in the sex chromatin of male mice is not known. However it has been described that this acetyltransferase could play a role in regulating transcription, specifically it has been suggested a transcriptional repression activity through the interaction of ESCO2 with chromatin modifying enzymes and with the CoREST complex, achieving the repression by means of histone modification (Kim et al., 2008). Moreover, the authors talk about an ESCO2-containing complex, which has histone methyltransferase activity in culture cells. These evidences could link the presence of ESCO2 in sex chromatin and the MSCI process. Another cytological example of the specific presence of a cohesion cofactor in meiosis is related to WAPL localization. WAPL was found on axial and lateral elements of chromosomes (AE/LEs) in some prophase I stages in mouse spermatocytes (Kuroda et al., 2005) and oocytes (Zhang et al., 2008c) colocalizing with SYCP3, a constitutive protein of the SC; however, no more extensive study has been carried out on the role of WAPL in meiosis. It has been established that WAPL and PDS5 act as a protein complex during cohesion establishment and maintenance (see Skibbens, 2009 for further details); but there is no data about the possible presence of PDS5 in mammalian prophase I. However in budding yeast meiosis has been described that Pds5 is required for pairing of homologous chromosomes and this cofactor could have a role inhibiting the synapsis between sister chromatids. Depletion of Pds5 gives raise to fails in synapsis, hypercondense chromosomes and blocking meiocytes at pachytene-like stage (Jin et al., 2009). This result was preceded by the *Pds5* fission yeast mutant that showed absence of SC formation (Ding et al., 2006). The action of Pds5 in pairing and synapsis could be related with the interaction between both proteins and the Pds5 capacity of modulating Rec8 activity in both fission and budding yeast (Ding, et al., 2006, Jin, et al., 2009). Although these studies point out to the importance of the structural organization of meiotic chromosomes and the implication of cohesin complexes and cohesion cofactor in such important process as synapsis of homologous chromosomes, further cytological and biochemical studies are needed to characterize the role of PDS5 and WAPL during meiosis. Are those cohesion cofactors acting in unknown manner or their activity is related to the cohesion modulation? This is an unresolved question yet. Finally a recent molecular-genetic approach have shown that the cohesin-loading factor Scc2 and the subunits Scc3 and Smc1 of the cohesin complex are required for activating the production of the meiosis-specific subunit Rec8 in the *S. cerevisiae* (Lin et al., 2011). This result suggests that Scc2 could play a dual role in gene regulation and sister-chromatid cohesion during meiotic differentiation. Although the mechanism is poorly understood yet, the role of cohesins and cohesion cofactors in gene regulation has been largely studied in the somatic line (Chien et al., 2011, Dorsett, 2011,

Newman & Young, 2010, Ong & Corces, 2011). However, meiosis-specific gene regulation is a future field of study where probably different groups are work in.

## 5. To form bivalents: Cohesion, synapsis and recombination

Two of the most important phenomena that characterize the meiosis are the SC formation and the reciprocal homologous recombination. Both are meiosis-specific and are implicated in the physical connexion of homologous chromosomes to form and maintain the bivalents. In this context, the cohesion is the third pivotal factor. Since the cohesion stabilizes the joint between sister chromatids from S phase until their segregation, it is easy to think that the cohesin complexes are needed to ensure that both sister chromatids of each homologous chromosome act in a single manner during prophase I, in a cellular context where the AEs formation, the synapsis and the meiotic recombination between homologous chromosomes is taking place. This would be the role of cohesin complexes in sister chromatid cohesion, its canonical function. Thus, during first meiotic division these three events: cohesion, synapsis and recombination, must be perfectly coordinated. However, the existence of meiotic-specific cohesins and its specific localization during first meiotic division become evident that the meiotic cohesin complexes could be implicated in SC formation and recombination directly further than the canonical function of chromatid cohesion.

### 5.1 The importance of individual cohesin subunits to synapsis

The SC is a meiosis-specific proteinaceous structure formed by two lateral elements (LEs), derivate from AEs of chromosomes, and a central element (CE) connected by transverse filaments (TFs). It is known that this meiotic structure play important roles in the condensation and pairing of chromosomes and also has a close relationship to the programmed DSBs formation and resolution (Page & Hawley, 2004). The formation of SC between homologous chromosomes is highly conserved in evolution, it derivates in the synapsis of homologous chromosome during the meiotic prophase I. One of the first references of the close relationship between the SC and cohesion was observed in budding yeast (Klein et al., 1999). In these organisms the cohesin subunit Smc3p presents a continuous localization along chromosome cores similar to that described for SC proteins in rat (Schalk et al., 1998). Klein et al., included a functional analysis, they studied the *Smc3* and *Rec8* mutants and observed that both were defective in cohesion, formation of AEs and SC assembly, demonstrating in yeast that the cohesins were essential not only for the meiotic sister chromatid cohesion but also for the synapsis. Moreover they postulated that the meiotic cohesin complexes were in fact part of AEs of chromosomes. However, two years later Pelttari et al., went farther and proposed that the cohesin axis was preformed along each chromosome and might act as the organizing framework for AE/LEs formation. This proposal was based on the evidences that *Sycp3*$^{-/-}$ mice were able to form a cohesin axis even in the absence of AEs (Pelttari et al., 2001). Contrary, the *Rec8*$^{-/-}$ and *Smc1β*$^{-/-}$ mice showed AEs partially assembled (Revenkova, et al., 2004, Xu et al., 2005). In rat spermatocytes the interaction between SMC cohesin subunits and SYCP2 and SYCP3, the main components of AEs and LEs, was also studied, concluding that the cohesin axes were essential in the SC formation and synapsis progression during early stages of prophase I (Eijpe et al., 2000, Eijpe, et al., 2003). These first observations pointed to the contribution of cohesins not only to form the AEs but also as part of AEs/LEs and then to its function in synapsis. Since then we have known different examples which closely relate the SC proteins and the synapsis progression to cohesin localization and function in meiosis. In the table 1 we summarize some of examples of the contribution of cohesin to SC formation and synapsis that we detail forward.

| Organism | Cohesin | Role in AE/LEs formation or synapsis | Reference |
|---|---|---|---|
| *C. elegans* | REC-8 | Chromosome pairing<br>AE component<br>SC assembly | Chan 2003<br>Colaiacovo 2006<br>Pasierbek 2001 |
| *S. cerevisiae* | SMC3p<br>REC 8 | AE/LEs localization<br>SC assembly | Klein 1999 |
| Rat | SMC1α/β<br>SMC3 | AE/LEs formation<br>Interaction with SYCP2 and SYCP3 | Eijpe 2000<br>Revenkova 2001 |
| | REC8 | AEs assembly | Eijpe 2003 |
| | SMC1α<br>SMC3 | Part of AEs | |
| Tomato | SMC3<br>SMC1<br>SCC3<br>REC8 | AE/LEs localization<br>Sequential assembly | Qiao 2011<br>Stack 2009 |
| Grasshoppers | SMC3 | AE/LEs localization | Valdeolmillos 2007 |
| | SA1<br>RAD21 | Present in synapsed regions exclusively | |
| Mice | STAG3 | Association to SC | Prieto 2001 |
| | REC8 | Homologous SC assembly | Xu 2005 |
| | RAD21L | AEs formation and synapsis | Herrán 2011 |
| | SMC1α | Synapsis | James 2002 |
| | SMC1β | AEs formation and SC assembly | Revenkova 2004 |

Table 1. Role of different cohesin subunits in AE/LEs formation and synapsis

The evidences of the implications of cohesin complexes in SC assembly, pairing and/or AEs formation came from many different organisms and scientific approaches. In plants, a specific and intermittently localization of SMC3 in the AE/LEs has been observed in tomato by means immunogold labeling and electron microscopy in zygotene microsporocytes (Qiao et al., 2011, Stack & Anderson, 2009), similar to that observed by light microscopy after the immunolabeling of SMC1, SMC3, SCC3 and REC8, although no all subunits presented the same pattern of accumulation and appearance during prophase I (Qiao, et al., 2011). In this vegetal species REC8, SMC1 and SMC3 are localized as foci from preleptotene which are arranged to AEs at leptotene but do not colocalize. However they exhibit colocalization in synapsed regions at zygotene and pachytene. SCC3 appears later than the other three cohesin subunits, observing a substantial amount of SCC3 foci along AE/LEs from zygotene through pachytene, according with the SC assembly. There is no a functional analysis about the implication of this vegetal cohesin in SC formation and synapsis, but this sequential loading shows a possible change of cohesin complexes composition or organization at a meiotic stage which is key in the correct progression of synapsis . This non-homogenous timing and spatial localization of different cohesin proteins has been reported in other organisms such as *C. elegans* (Chan et al., 2003) or male grasshoppers (Valdeolmillos et al., 2007). Males of grasshoppers *Locusta migratoria* and *Eyprepocnemis plorans* species represent another cytological example of the contribution of cohesins to synapsis. In grasshoppers the SMC3 subunit appeared as a dotted signal in preleptotene to form continuous lines in leptotene, meanwhile the non-SMC subunits RAD21 and SA1 were not localized until zygotene and only on synapsed regions. This means that in grasshoppers the incorporation of non-SMC cohesins would be spatially and temporally concomitant with the progression of synapsis. In zygotene and pachytene SMC3 and RAD21 present a continuous and linear pattern, similar to what would be expected of AE/LEs proteins and both cohesin subunits present a complete colocalization until diplotene, coinciding with the stages of disassemble of SC. It is relevant that the single X chromosome of grasshopper males, which remains unsynapsed, presents neither RAD21 nor SA1 during prophase I. Further than the possible implication of RAD21 and SA1 in the complete assembly of SC or *vice-versa*, these observations open new questions: Would this synapsis-dependent sequential loading of cohesin during prophase I have an effect on the distribution of cohesins in metaphase I? Could we talk about a presence of cohesin depending on the synaptic history of chromosomes? At any case, these kind of studies pointed not only that cohesin subunits can be loaded onto meiotic chromosomes at different time or as part of different complexes, but also relate the loading of specific cohesin subunits with the timing of AEs formation and SC assembly. The idea of specific synapsis cohesin complexes is also supported by the evidence that SMC1α is mainly located along synapsed regions in mice spermatocytes, whereas SMC3 subunit localizes along the synapsed and unsynased AEs (James et al., 2002), in front of SMC1β which is mainly required for sister chromatid cohesion (Revenkova, et al., 2004). In addition, *Sycp3*$^{-/-}$ and *Smc1β*$^{-/-}$ single and double oocytes mice mutants show that both proteins contribute to meiotic chromosome axis organization (Novak et al., 2008). The authors propose a several layers axis association, which contributed to the formation of meiotic chromosome axes in an independent manner. The basic layer would be formed by the same proteins that form the mitotic chromosome axis, the scaffold proteins (Maeshima & Laemmli, 2003). SMC1β would be part of the second layer, it contributes to axes length but is not essential (Revenkova, et al., 2004). Finally SYCP3 would represent the third layer as basic component of AE/LEs. Thus a cohesin axis would be defined as a base axis before the AE/LEs in mammals, a similar organization has been proposed in grasshoppers (Valdeolmillos, et al., 2007). *Smc1β* $^{-/-}$ mice spermatocytes do not progress further than mid-pachytene and the cells present abnormalities in chromosome structure (Revenkova, et al., 2004). The analysis of SC proteins showed that the AEs were shortened, but the synapsis occurred between the 19 couples of homologous chromosomes. Thus, despite of the close relationship of the cohesins and SC proteins and the evident interdependence between both groups of proteins, there are examples in mice where the absence of a cohesin subunit does not inhibit the complete formation of SC, albeit its structure is compromised (Revenkova, et al., 2004, Xu, et al., 2005). This could be explaining due to the presence of different cohesin complexes in mammal meiotic cells (Revenkova & Jessberger, 2005, Revenkova & Jessberger, 2006, Suja & Barbero, 2009) which could act in a redundancy manner. All these evidences suggest that the cohesins and specifically the SMC cohesin provide a basis for AE assembly. Based on the description of the new cohesin subunits and regarding to its role in SC formation and synapsis, diverse authors have develop models of incorporation of new cohesin complexes or replacement of specific cohesin subunits during the early prophase I that we summarize in figure 4.

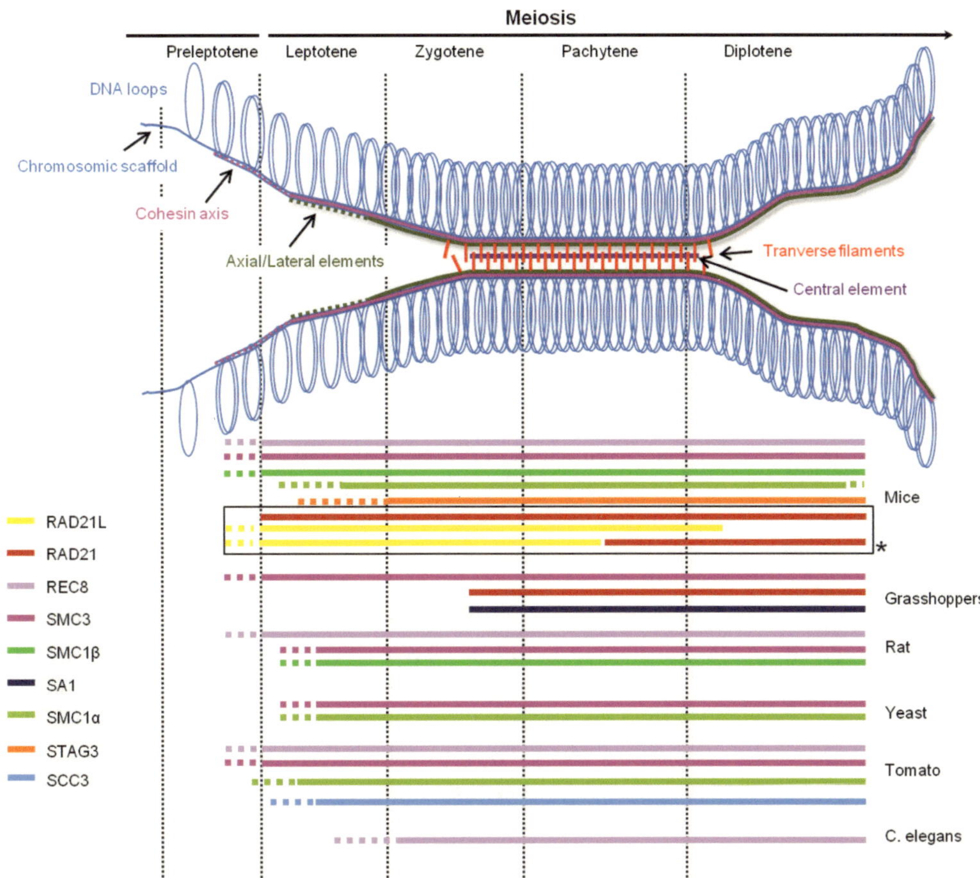


Fig. 4. Temporal meiotic appearance of cohesin subunits from preleptotene and its relationship with SC formation.

At the top of the figure a temporal line of early stages of meiosis progression is shown. The diagram positioned under this line is represented the cohesin axis formation and the SC assembly taking into account the data observed in mice. The blue lines represent the chromosomic scaffold and the blue circles are the chromatin loops. The pink color represents the cohesin organization, which is usually detected as a dotted pattern at preleptotene and from leptotene form axis that would the base for the AEs proteins. The AE/LEs are represented in green, the FTs in red and the CE of SC in purple. At the bottom of the figure, under the diagram of SC assembly, the temporal localization of different cohesin subunits in different species is shown. The colour code for each cohesin subunit is situated at the left.

* This box shows the disagreement regarding to the RAD21 and RAD21L dynamic. See text for further detail.

In the nematode *C. elegans*, REC-8 and HIM-3, a component of meiotic chromosomes axes required for synapsis (Zetka et al., 1999), overlap during leptotene, zygotene and pachytene, suggesting that REC-8 is a component of AE/LEs (Pasierbek et al., 2001). SMC-1 and SMC-3 loaded onto chromatin independently of REC-8 and SCC-3. On the other hand the depletion of *Rec-8* by RNAi did not cause change in SMC-1 or SMC-3 localization but a mislocalization of SCC-3 was detected (Chan, et al., 2003). The importance of REC-8 as an associated component of AEs in *C. elegans* derives from the evidence that this protein is presented along the axes of unsynapsed chromosomes and this meiosis-specific cohesin subunit seems to be necessary for the assembly of SC components such as HIM-3, SYP-1 and SYP-2 (Colaiacovo, 2006, MacQueen et al., 2002, Nabeshima et al., 2005, Pasierbek, et al., 2001). Moreover, the analysis of *Rec-8* (RNAi) mutants showed that this protein is implicated in the chromosome pairing and SC assembly during leptotene/zygotene stage and the meiotic chromosomes are reorganized before diplotene into pachytene-like arrangement but they fail to achieve a normal lengthwise alignment (Chan, et al., 2003). Probably REC8 is the subunit of cohesin more widely studied in meiosis, it is a meiotic-specific cohesin variant of the subunit SCC1/RAD21. REC8 has orthologs in different organisms, it is present in mammals (Xu, et al., 2005), yeast (Klein, et al., 1999, Molnar, et al., 1995), plants (Qiao, et al., 2011, Zhang et al., 2006) and *C. elegans* (Pasierbek, et al., 2001). Although it has not been defined an obvious REC8 homologue in *Drosophila melanogaster*, C(2)M is a protein distantly related to REC8 which has not play a cohesion role but localized to LEs and interacts with SMC3 (Anderson et al., 2005). In rat spermatocytes the meiosis-specific REC8 protein was observed as axial structures during premeiotic S phase, earlier than SMC1β and SMC3 which appeared during leptotene along with SYCP2 and SYCP3, suggesting an special role of REC8 in AEs formation (Eijpe, et al., 2003, Revenkova, et al., 2001). The meiocytes of males and females *Rec8* null mice do not complete the prophase I and presents SC assembly between sister chromatids (Xu, et al., 2005). Thus, in mammals REC8 seems to be necessary to the formation of SC between homologous chromosomes instead of the properly assembly of SC, albeit its structure is altered. Recently a new meiosis-specific SCC1 cohesin subunit has been identified in vertebrates, it is closely related to RAD21 and it has been named RAD21L (RAD21-like) (Gutierrez-Caballero, et al., 2011, Ishiguro, et al., 2011, Lee & Hirano, 2011). RAD21L interacts with other cohesin subunits such as SMC1α/β, SMC3 or STAG3 but does not interact with REC8, thus both kleisins subunits form distinct meiosis-specific cohesin complexes (Gutierrez-Caballero, et al., 2011, Ishiguro, et al., 2011). There is no agreement regarding to the localization of RAD21L from mid-pachytene/diplotene, thus meanwhile some authors ensure that RAD21L disappears from chromosomes axes at mid-pachytene when the SC is still formed (Lee & Hirano, 2011), others have found that RAD21L is dissociated from AEs on autosomes in a progressive manner, during SC disassembly at diplotene (Herran, et al., 2011, Ishiguro, et al., 2011) and it is accumulated at centromeres until anaphase II (Herran, et al., 2011). Similarly, there are different results in relation with the coexistence of RAD21 and RAD21L complexes during early prophase I stages. Lee and Hirano (2011) ensure that RAD21L seems to replace RAD21 from leptotene, finding that RAD21L localizes along AE/LEs until pachytene, accompanying the SC formation and homologous synapsis. However, RAD21 has been previously detected by immunolocalization during leptotene, zygotene and pachytene in mouse spermatocytes by other authors (Parra, et al., 2004, Xu et al., 2004) and at least in the first case, the antibody used in Parra's et al., study does not cross-react with RAD21L as it is shown in Herran's et al., paper., suggesting the presence of both RAD21 and RAD21L at the same time. At any case REC8, RAD21 and RAD21L are detected in a mutually exclusive manner, forming part of different cohesin complexes. The definitive evidence to ensure that RAD21L is directly implicated in AEs formation and synapsis is the *Rad21L*$^{-/-}$ male mouse which exhibits discontinuous AEs stretches and fails in homologous synapsis, moreover the mutants present defects in DSBs processing (Herran, et al., 2011). The RAD21L knockout males are sterile but females are fertile although develop age-dependent sterility is observed. On the other hand, there are evidences of the interaction of RAD21L and SYCP1, main component of TFs of SC (Meuwissen et al., 1992), and the centromere protein CENP-C (Ishiguro, et al., 2011, Lee & Hirano, 2011). In a general manner, there is a rising common idea about the specific implication of RAD21L in pairing and the initiation of synapsis between homologous chromosomes (Herran, et al., 2011, Ishiguro, et al., 2011, Lee & Hirano, 2011, Polakova et al., 2011). However, many questions are still open and new interesting doubts have been joined the fray regarding to the regulation of RAD21L cohesin complexes (Uhlmann, 2011).

In mouse testis the meiotic protein STAG3 was first identified as a stromalin member associated to SC (Pezzi, et al., 2000) and after that was described its participation in the cohesin complex and its specificity to cohesion of sister chromatid arms during first meiotic division (Prieto, et al., 2001), however the authors pointed that STAG3 could be a component of SC, being detectable on chromatin paralleling to AEs appearance. This is an interesting example because STAG3 is the fourth component of the cohesin complex, it is not a kleisin and does not interact with SMC proteins which might be the base of the cohesin axes formed during the early stage of prophase I. Thus in a general model it has been observed a correlation between the progression of AE/LEs formation and synapsis and the localization of several cohesin subunits. According to the studied organisms the localization of cohesin subunits during prophase I has been observed continuous or discontinuous; however this could be related with the preparation method or the meiotic stage. In any case, all cohesin subunit are associated with AE/LEs during prophase I. What we consider more relevant is the sequential loading of cohesins observed during the first stages of prophase I and how the appearance of some subunits seems to be closely related with the progression of AE/LEs and SC formation and synapsis progression. In this sense, it is important to consider if the association of the cohesin subunits with the AE/LEs could be in an independent manner one to another. These cases would be possible only if we consider that in these species different cohesin complexes exist, as different author postulated before (Chan, et al., 2003, Eijpe, et al., 2003, Qiao, et al., 2011, Suja & Barbero, 2009, Valdeolmillos, et al., 2007), being some of them more intimately related with the progression of synapsis or the SC formation. But then, we should think about if the cohesins loaded during early prophase I are really exerted a cohesin function or are related with AE/LEs formation and/or synapsis progression. Different analysis in mitotic cells showed that only the cohesins loaded during S phase are effective in the cohesion of sister chromatids (Austin et al., 2009, Guacci, 2007), despite of evidences about new cohesion at DBSs point (Strom & Sjogren, 2005). Generally, the SMC cohesins seems to be more closely related with the AE/LEs formation, derivates from the evidences that this cohesin subunits are the base of the cohesin complexes then they would be the base of a cohesin axis and appear during the stages where SYCP2 and SYCP3 are incorporated or a bit early (Eijpe, et al., 2000, Klein, et al., 1999, Novak, et al., 2008, Qiao, et al., 2011, Revenkova, et al., 2001, Valdeolmillos, et al., 2007). However, the non-SMC proteins seem to have more specific roles before AEs formation (Eijpe, et al., 2003, Gutierrez-Caballero, et al., 2011, Ishiguro, et al., 2011, Molnar, et al., 1995) or during SC assembly (Valdeolmillos, et al., 2007). Especially we are thinking in the SCC1 subunits and all its variants, and then a cohesin complex would acquire a specific role depending on the SCC1 which is formed with. It is difficult to split out the study of cohesin distribution during first meiotic division and the function of SC as the physical connector of homologous chromosomes at prophase I. More and more the scientists notice that the cohesins present function or contribute to function that historically had been attributed to the SC or to specific SC proteins and different cohesin complexes acquire specific functions in meiosis.

### 5.2 Cohesins and meiotic recombination

The first evidence that sister chromatid cohesion is required for DNA damage repair was the observation that the expression of mutated cohesins or the deletion of some subunits cause hypersensitivity and fails in DNA repair after induced or spontaneous DSBs in somatic line (Birkenbihl and Subramani, 1992; Sonoda et al., 2001). Cohesin complexes are preferred loaded at intergenic sites (Lengronne et al., 2004) onto the replicating chromosomes during S phase. However, now it is clear that in somatic cells the DNA damage induces the recruitment of cohesins after replication and lead to the formation of new cohesion (Strom and Sjogren, 2005), which is essential for DNA repair (Strom et al., 2004). Since the ability of SMC proteins to promote reannealing of complementary DNA strand was described, a role of cohesins in resolving DSBs was suggested (Jessberger et al., 1996). Different authors have studied and reviewed the role of cohesins in DSBs repair in S and G2 periods in mitotic cells (Cortes-Ledesma & Aguilera, 2006; Nagao et al., 2004; Strom & Sjogren, 2007; Watrin & Peters, 2006), however, during meiosis the DSBs are programmed, in front of the spontaneous breaks that can alter the genome during the rest of the cell cycle. Basically mitotic/somatic and meiotic recombination have different purposes, thus whereas the meiotic recombination is initiated to generate a crossover (CO) on each bivalent at least, the mitotic recombination is used to repair DNA damage to ensure the fidelity of DNA sequence and cell surveillance. This important difference affects the repair pathway (Andersen & Sekelsky, 2010). We do not pretend to review all the literature regarding to the function of cohesin in all kinds of DNA damage, we will focus our attention in those cohesin subunits that have a specific role in meiotic DSBs and recombination.

Most of current models of meiotic recombination are based in the model that Szostak and colleagues proposed in yeast in 1983. This model is based on the generation of DSBs at early prophase I, the strand invasion at zygotene, the formation of double Holliday junction (dHJ) intermediate and its resolution at pachytene/diplotene. Obviously the repair mechanisms of DNA molecules act in an organized chromosome, where protein axial structures such as AEs and cohesin axis exist. The DSBs may be resolved toward CO between homologous chromatids or NCO (non-crossover), this decision can be made at different steps or repair pathway (see Heyer et al., 2010 for further details). Meiotic COs are essential for ensuring chromosome segregation. Chiasmata, points of genetic interchange between non-sister chromatids, keep the homologous chromosomes as a single structure after the disassembly of SC. Chiasmata and sister chromatid cohesion ensure the correct orientation of bivalents at metaphase I. Thus, in a similar way that fails in cohesion lead premature separation of chromatids, fails in meiotic recombination promote the generation of univalents at metaphase I. In both cases a high probability of aneuploidy exists. Meiotic recombination is initiated after a replication period, thus the sister chromatids are linked by cohesins when the recombination process begins. It has been established that cohesins are needed for the formation and stabilization of DNA interconnections (Buonomo et al., 2000; Klein et al., 1999).

Meiotic recombination begins via DSBs formation by the Topoisomerase II-like enzyme SPO11 (Grelon et al., 2001; Keeney et al., 1997). As consequence of SPO11 activity a great amount of DSBs are generated during early meiotic prophase I and most of them are repaired as NCO. Thus the cohesins take part in bivalent stabilization and recombination to ensure that the excess of programmed DSBs do not alter the chromosome organization. On the other hand specific roles of different cohesin subunits in DSBs formation and regulation have been also described. As we stated above the basic difference between meiotic and mitotic recombination lies in the generation of DSBs, thus SPO11 has a pivotal role in the activation of meiotic recombination machinery and the regulation of this enzyme is one of the most interesting topics of meiotic recombination analysis. SPO11 has the key to begin all the process of genetic exchange between non-homologous chromosomes. Different studies have shown a non-random distribution of meiotic DSBs (Baudat & Nicolas, 1997; de Massy, 2003; de Massy et al., 1995; Gerton et al., 2000), giving raise to hot and cold-spots recombination sites. Different factors, as some histone variants (Buard et al., 2009) or the DNA sequence (Grey et al., 2009), determine and regulate the action of SPO11. In this context the cohesins have also been implicated. In budding yeast the initial centromeric entry of SPO11 depends on REC8 and this subunit of cohesin complex choreographs the distribution of SPO11 to DSBs sites (Kugou et al., 2009). On the other hand, in *S. pombe*, the *Rec8Δ* mutant shows a marked reduction of meiosis-specific DNA breakage by REC12 (the *S. pombe* SPO11 homologue) (Ellermeier & Smith, 2005) and in *C. elegans* has been proposed that REC-8 could be implicated in limiting the activity of SPO-11 (Hayashi et al., 2007). However, whereas in *S. cerevisiae Rec8* mutants the chromosome segregation is at random (Klein et al., 1999), similar mutants in *S. pombe* present a equational segregation of sister chromatids at anaphase I (Watanabe & Nurse, 1999). These discordant results suggest that the regulation of meiotic cohesin complexes containing REC8 and its role in recombination depends on the species. After the formation of DSBs by SPO11, modifications on chromatin as the phosphorylation of histone variants H2AX, H2Av and H2B occur (Fernández-Capetillo et al., 2004; Madigan et al., 2002; Redon et al., 2002) and a cascade of repair proteins are loaded onto damage sites in order to restore the DNA properly. The first recombinases that bind to chromatin after DSBs are RAD51 and DMC1. The last one is a meiosis-specific protein. Usually the recruitment of recombinases has been associated to the AEs (Plug et al., 1998; Tarsounas et al., 1999), but the cohesin axis is also functional in recruiting DNA recombination proteins. This issue was observed in *Sycp3*$^{-/-}$ mice spermatocytes, where the recombinase RAD51 is recruited in the absence of AEs (Yuan et al., 2000) suggesting a higher level of organization which is probably related to the cohesins. The resection of single-strand DNA allows the single-end invasion promoted by both recombinases RAD51 and DMC1 (Neale and Keeney, 2006; Shinohara and Shinohara, 2004). The extended invading strands are then processed to form CO or NCO. At this point the most of DBSs are resolved by Synthesis-Dependent Strand Annealing (SDSA) through NCO (Allers & Lichten, 2001). Some points of strand invasion are stabilized to form a D loop and double Holliday junctions (dHJ) intermediate, which can be resolved through CO or NCO depending on the cleavage of dHJ. The DSBs formation and the CO/NCO decision are two relevant items in meiotic recombination studies. In mice, before the AEs formation a cohesin core is observed as we reviewed above, but the action of SPO11 is not required for the formation of cohesin cores as it was observed in *Spo11*$^{-/-}$ spermatocytes, being SMC1α mostly associated to homologous or non-homologous synapsed regions meanwhile SMC3 localized both to AEs of unsynapsed and synapsed cores at arrested zygotene cells (James et al., 2002). In mammals, the absence of REC8 does not affect the timing of DSBs formation and the recruitment of the recombinases RAD51/DMC1, suggesting than DSBs and the early recombination events occur properly. But, the persistence of RAD51/DMC1 foci in *Rec8*$^{-/-}$ mice spermatocytes and the absence of MLH1 foci might reflect the inability to repair the DSBs (Xu et al., 2005). MLH1 and MLH3 protein are implicated in resolution of recombination to chiasma (Hunter & Borts, 1997; Wang et al., 1999). It is not clear if REC8 has a specific role in resolving the meiotic DNA damage or the persistence of unresolved DSBs is a consequence of that the *Rec8*$^{-/-}$ cells do not reach the meiotic stage where the recombination resolution takes place. In this rodent REC8 seems to have a pivotal role in sister chromatid cohesion and synapsis but its relationship with recombination is not clear, despite of a small proportion of REC8 coprecipitate with RAD51/DMC1. Moreover a small proportion of RAD50 coimmunoprecipitate with REC8 from spermatocyte lysates but REC8 does not coprecipitate with RAD50 (Eijpe et al., 2003). RAD50, MRE11 and NBS1 proteins form the MRN complex which is implicated in the early response to DNA damage. The action of MRN complex is related to nuclease activity at the 5′ ends, releasing SPO11 from DNA (Lichten, 2001). After the action of MRN, RAD51 and DMC1 can bind to single-strand DNA. These results which relate REC8 with recombination repair proteins would indicate that protein complexes that contain both REC8 and RAD51/DMC1 and some RAD50 exist in spermatocytes (Eijpe et al., 2003). The authors proposed that after S phase, cohesins would attract protein complexes that are involved in the early steps of homologous recombination. Recent results in yeast proposed that Rec8 could have a role in maintaining the homolog bias of recombination (Kim et al., 2010). In *Rad21L*$^{-/-}$ mice spermatocytes an accumulation of unrepaired DSBs has been described, but the cells are arrested at zygotene-like stage (Herran et al., 2011). Although, in sight of the cytological results of appearance and disappearance of RAD21L in wild type mice, a role in meiotic recombination has been suggested for this cohesin subunit (Herran et al., 2011; Ishiguro et al., 2011), deeply studies are needed to corroborate the implication of RAD21L in the processing of recombination intermediates. However, in this context we might probably talk about a role of SMC1β in recombination. Initially this protein was found at bridges between homologous AEs, and it was supposed that these represented the chiasmata sites (Revenkova et al., 2001). In *Smc1β*$^{-/-}$ spermatocytes early markers of recombination as RAD51 and γ-H2AX localize properly. The cells progress through mid-pachytene and MLH1 and MLH3 foci were not detected in males, additionally the *Smc1β*$^{-/-}$ oocytes develop further and also fail to form the normal number of MLH1 foci (Revenkova et al., 2004). Probably the effects observing in cohesin mutants regarding to recombination proteins could be explain due to improper sister chromatid cohesion, an incorrect formation of AEs or synaptic fails. Perhaps we have to analyze the relationship between cohesin and meiotic recombination in a cohesin-dependent chromatin organization. An example is found in *S. pombe*, in this organism Rec8 and Rec11, meiosis-specific cohesin subunits, are essential for DSBs only in some regions of the genome (Ellermeier & Smith, 2005). On the other hand the loading of Rec25 and Rec27, two recombination proteins in yeast, depends on the previous incorporation of Rec8 (Davis et al., 2008). This issue could be explained because of Rec8 is required for the normal chromosome compaction during meiotic prophase I (Ding et al., 2006), thus it has been proposed that the regional effect on DSBs production might be related to the meiotic chromosomal organization formed by the cohesins (Davis et al., 2008). Thus the role of cohesins in meiotic recombination should be at different levels, chromosomal organization, providing the proximity between sister chromatid to ensure a correct repair with an undamaged template and as individual proteins that form complexes with recombination proteins.

Finally we would like to comment two interesting cytological examples of the relationship between cohesin axis development, synapsis and recombination. The males of *Stethophyma grossum* exhibit a delay in cohesin axis formation in the eight longest bivalents of its complement and in the single X chromosome (Calvente et al., 2005). These regions remain unsynapsed, presenting three different synaptic situations: an unsynapsed sex chromosome, three bivalents with complete synapsis and eight bivalents with incomplete synapsis (Jones, 1973; Wallace & Jones, 1978). In this species the DSBs and the recruitment of first recombinases occur before the beginning of synapsis, detecting RAD51 foci over the cohesin axis at leptotene. But the most interesting event is that γ-H2AX and RAD51 foci are polarized to the nuclear region where the cohesin axis are formed in advanced and these regions correspond with the ulterior synapsed chromosomal regions. Thus, those chromosomal regions that at leptotene do not exhibit a formed cohesin axes do not present DSBs and then do not recruit RAD51 (Calvente et al., 2005). A similar case has been observed in *Paratettix meriodinalis*, another grasshopper species with an incomplete synapsis pattern. The spermatocytes of this species show a polarization of cohesin axes maturation and the initiation of meiotic recombination, suggesting that the early development of cohesin axis would drive the loading of recombination machinery (Viera et al., 2009b). Obviously the study of AEs proteins would clarify the real relationship among SC formation, cohesin axis development and recombination in this special organism but these examples show the relevance of a cohesin axis formed by at least SMC proteins not only in the beginning of meiotic recombination but also in synapsis progression.

## 6. Cohesins and cohesin-regulators in human cancer and cohesinophaties

As we commented before, dysfunction of chromosome cohesion during meiosis frequently gives fertility problems. However, now we know that cohesins participate in other important cell processes, such as mitotic DNA damage repair and control of gene expression. One of the most surprising findings was the discovery of a link between cohesin mutations and human diseases. Two groups, (Krantz et al., 2004, Tonkin et al., 2004), found that the *Nipbl* gene, the homologue to yeast *Scc2* adherin gene, is mutated in the human CdLS (OMIM: 122470, 300590, 610759). This pathology is a multiple neuro-developmental disorder characterized by facial dysmorphisms, mental retardation, growth delay, and upper limb abnormalities. Subsequent studies of several cases of this syndrome showed that mutations in SMC1α and SMC3 (Musio et al., 2006, and Deardorff et al., 2007) cause a mild variant of CdLS. Roberts syndrome/SC phocomelia (RBS; OMIM: 268300) is an autosomal recessive disorder phenotypically related to CdLS; RBS patients present craniofacial abnormalities, growth retardation, and limb reduction. Cells from RBS patients show a lack of cohesion at the heterochromatic regions around the centromeres and at the Y chromosome long arm (Van Den Verg and Francke, 1993). It has been described that RBS is caused by mutations in *ESCO2* gene (Vega et al., 2005) and analyses of different mutations in RBS patients pointed to the loss of ESCO2 acetyltransferase activity as the molecular mechanism involved in RBS pathology (Gordillo et al., 2008). On the other hand, in the last years have been published different studies and experimental data that links cancer development with disorders in the core cohesin subunit and cohesin- interacting proteins genes. Although, we do not mind to review this field here, the following paragraphs reveal the importance of cohesins, including meiotic-specific cohesin genes in tumorogenesis. The study of 11 somatic mutations in 132 human colorectal cancers identified 6 of them mapping to 3 cohesin, *SMC1a*, *SMC3* and *STAG3*, genes and 4 to a cohesin-regulator *SCC2* gene (Barber et al., 2008). Colorectal cancer cells are characterized by chromosomal instability, resulting in chromosome gain or loss. It is possible to argue that abnormal cohesin pathway activity leads to chromosome missegregation and chromosome instability. This hypothesis is supported by the observation that colorectal cancer cells exhibit up to 100-fold higher rates of missegregation than normal cells (Lengauer et al., 1997). In adittion, using a microcell mediated chromosome transfer and expression microarray analysis the cohesin *STAG3* gene was identified as one of the nine genes associated with functional suppression of tumorogenicity in ovarian cancer cell lines (*AIFM2, AKTIP, AXIN2, CASP5, FILIP1L, RBBP8, RGC32, RUVBL1* and *STAG3*) and as a candidate gene associated with risk and development of epithelial ovarian cancer (Notaridou et al., 2011). The future research on the molecular mechanisms surrounding the cell regulation of cohesin is crucial to understand the relationship between the cohesin-interacting proteins and cohesin post-translational modification with developmental alterations and cancer. These studies probably will help to understand the relationships between this interesting ring protein complex and the formation/development of tumors in humans.

## 7. Conclusions

In the late 90's, cohesins were discovered and characterized are the main actors in controlling the sister chromatid joint until the chromosomic segregation. This important issue ensures a correct distribution of chromosomes to daughter cells and then the viability and continuity of all organisms. Undoubtedly the cohesion regulation leads the chromosomic segregation in mitosis and meiosis. However, whereas a correct regulation of cohesion in mitosis is crucial for development, in meiosis this process is vital for the fertility of the individuals. The complexity of meiosis arises from the necessity of generate haploids cells and the magic of this type of cell division is that all the daughters cells are different among them and to the mother cell. In order to carry out this great objective, the homologous chromosomes form bivalents, recombine, organize a complex protein structure between them, the SC, and go through two consecutive segregations. In this context the cohesion and the cohesin complex in meiosis present different specializations such as meiosis-specific cohesin subunits or a strict regulation of the release of arm and centromeric cohesion during both chromosomic segregations. As an example of this complexity, nowadays four meiosis-specific cohesin subunits have been identified in mice: SMC1β, STAG3, REC8 and RAD21L. These subunits do not exclude the presence of other mitotic proteins, forming then a high number of different cohesin complexes. However, further than the role of cohesin complex in cohesion, all the specializations observed in meiosis seem to have an effect on functions of the cohesins. In this scenario we are now discovering the action of this fascinating group of proteins in the formation of AE/LEs, the progression of synapsis, the formation of programmed DSBs and the regulation of gene expression in meiosis. In a same way, we begin to understand the role of cohesins in developmental diseases and cancer. It have been identifying a growing number of proteins that interact with the cohesin complex and modulate the dynamics of cohesins and its binding to chromatin. Since the cohesins do not act in a single manner but they need different proteins to regulate their action, the cohesins-regulators have reached the attention of the scientific community. In addition, today we know that mutations in genes encoding cohesin regulators could give pathological conditions in humans. Update we do not know meiosis-specific regulators, but the action of the cohesin-interacting proteins must be regulated in a meiosis-specific manner and probably there are meiotic factors, which are waiting to be discovered. Many doubts are still unresolved and many doubts will appear later, but at any case we cannot study the cohesion and the cohesins as a single concept but a complex process and a versatile group of proteins which are implicated in the correct progress of the cell cycle in a global manner.

## 8. Acknowledgments

We thank Dr. Mónica Pradillo for her sincere and critical comments. We apologize to all colleagues whose important contributions have not been referenced due to space restrictions. This work was supported by the Spanish Ministerio de Ciencia e Innovación (grant BFU2009-08975/BMC) and CSIC (grant PIE-201120E020).

## 9. References

Allers, T. & Lichten, M. (2001). Differential timing and control of noncrossover and crossover recombination during meiosis. *Cell*. Vol.106, No.1, pp.47-57, ISSN:0092-8674

Andersen, S.L. & Sekelsky, J. (2010). Meiotic versus mitotic recombination: two different routes for double-strand break repair: the different functions of meiotic versus mitotic DSB repair are reflected in different pathway usage and different outcomes. *Bioessays*. Vol.32, No.12, pp.1058-1066, ISSN:1521-1878

Anderson, L.K., Royer, S.M., Page, S.L., McKim, K.S., Lai, A., Lilly, M.A. & Hawley, R.S. (2005). Juxtaposition of C(2)M and the transverse filament protein C(3)G within the central region of Drosophila synaptonemal complex. *Proc Natl Acad Sci U S A*. Vol.102, No.12, pp.4482-4487, ISSN:0027-8424

Austin, C., Novikova, N., Guacci, V. & Bellini, M. (2009). Lampbrush chromosomes enable study of cohesin dynamics. *Chromosome Res*. Vol.17, No.2, pp.165-184, ISSN:1573-6849

Barber, T.D., McManus, K., Yuen, K.W., Reis, M., Parmigiani, G., Shen, D., Barrett, I., Nouhi, Y., Spencer, F., Markowitz, S., Velculescu, V.E., Kinzler, K.W., Vogelstein, B., Lengauer, C. & Hieter, P. (2008). Chromatid cohesion defects may underlie chromosome instability in human colorectal cancers. *Proc Natl Acad Sci U S A.* Vol.105, No.9, pp.3443-3448, ISSN:1091-6490

Baudat, F. & Nicolas, A. (1997). Clustering of meiotic double-strand breaks on yeast chromosome III. *Proc Natl Acad Sci U S A.* Vol.94, No.10, pp.5213-5218, ISSN:0027-8424

Beckouet, F., Hu, B., Roig, M.B., Sutani, T., Komata, M., Uluocak, P., Katis, V.L., Shirahige, K. & Nasmyth, K. (2010). An Smc3 acetylation cycle is essential for establishment of sister chromatid cohesion. *Mol Cell.* Vol.39, No.5, pp.689-699, ISSN:1097-4164

Birkenbihl, R.P. & Subramani, S. (1992). Cloning and characterization of rad21 an essential gene of Schizosaccharomyces pombe involved in DNA double-strand-break repair. *Nucleic Acids Res.* Vol.20, No.24, pp.6605-6611, ISSN:0305-1048

Borges, V., Lehane, C., Lopez-Serra, L., Flynn, H., Skehel, M., Rolef Ben-Shahar, T. & Uhlmann, F. (2010). Hos1 deacetylates Smc3 to close the cohesin acetylation cycle. *Mol Cell.* Vol.39, No.5, pp.677-688, ISSN:1097-4164.

Buard, J., Barthes, P., Grey, C. & de Massy, B. (2009). Distinct histone modifications define initiation and repair of meiotic recombination in the mouse. *EMBO J.* Vol.28, No.17, pp.2616-2624, ISSN:1460-2075

Buonomo, S.B., Clyne, R.K., Fuchs, J., Loidl, J., Uhlmann, F. & Nasmyth, K. (2000). Disjunction of homologous chromosomes in meiosis I depends on proteolytic cleavage of the meiotic cohesin Rec8 by separin. *Cell.* Vol.103, No.3, pp.387-398.

Calvente, A., Viera, A., Page, J., Parra, M.T., Gomez, R., Suja, J.A., Rufas, J.S. & Santos, J.L. (2005). DNA double-strand breaks and homology search: inferences from a species with incomplete pairing and synapsis. *J Cell Sci.* Vol.118, No.Pt 13, pp.2957-2963

Carramolino, L., Lee, B.C., Zaballos, A., Peled, A., Barthelemy, I., Shav-Tal, Y., Prieto, I., Carmi, P., Gothelf, Y., Gonzalez de Buitrago, G., Aracil, M., Marquez, G., Barbero, J.L. & Zipori, D. (1997). SA-1, a nuclear protein encoded by one member of a novel gene family: molecular cloning and detection in hemopoietic organs. *Gene.* Vol.195, No.2, pp.151-159, ISSN:0378-1119

Ciosk, R., Zachariae, W., Michaelis, C., Shevchenko, A., Mann, M. & Nasmyth, K. (1998). An ESP1/PDS1 complex regulates loss of sister chromatid cohesion at the metaphase to anaphase transition in yeast. *Cell.* Vol.93, No.6, pp.1067-1076, ISSN:0092-8674

Ciosk, R., Shirayama, M., Shevchenko, A., Tanaka, T., Toth, A. & Nasmyth, K. (2000). Cohesin's binding to chromosomes depends on a separate complex consisting of Scc2 and Scc4 proteins. *Mol Cell.* Vol.5, No.2, pp.243-254, ISSN:1097-2765

Colaiacovo, M.P. (2006). The many facets of SC function during C. elegans meiosis. *Chromosoma.* Vol.115, No.3, pp.195-211, ISSN:0009-5915

Cortes-Ledesma, F. & Aguilera, A. (2006). Double-strand breaks arising by replication through a nick are repaired by cohesin-dependent sister-chromatid exchange. *EMBO Rep.* Vol.7, No.9, pp.919-926, ISSN:1469-221X

Chan, R.C., Chan, A., Jeon, M., Wu, T.F., Pasqualone, D., Rougvie, A.E. & Meyer, B.J. (2003). Chromosome cohesion is regulated by a clock gene paralogue TIM-1. *Nature.* Vol.423, No.6943, pp.1002-1009,

Chien, R., Zeng, W., Kawauchi, S., Bender, M.A., Santos, R., Gregson, H.C., Schmiesing, J.A., Newkirk, D.A., Kong, X., Ball, A.R., Jr., Calof, A.L., Lander, A.D., Groudine, M.T. & Yokomori, K. (2011). Cohesin mediates chromatin interactions that regulate mammalian beta-globin expression. *J Biol Chem*. Vol.286, No.20, pp.17870-17878, ISSN:1083-351X

Davis, L., Rozalen, A.E., Moreno, S., Smith, G.R. & Martin-Castellanos, C. (2008). Rec25 and Rec27, novel linear-element components, link cohesin to meiotic DNA breakage and recombination. *Curr Biol*. Vol.18, No.11, pp.849-854, ISSN:0960-9822

de Massy, B., Rocco, V. & Nicolas, A. (1995). The nucleotide mapping of DNA double-strand breaks at the CYS3 initiation site of meiotic recombination in Saccharomyces cerevisiae. *EMBO J*. Vol.14, No.18, pp.4589-4598, ISSN:0261-4189

de Massy, B. (2003). Distribution of meiotic recombination sites. *Trends Genet*. Vol.19, No.9, pp.514-522, ISSN:0168-9525

Deardorff, M.A., Kaur, M., Yaeger, D., Rampuria, A., Korolev, S., Pie, J., Gil-Rodriguez, C., Arnedo, M., Loeys, B., Kline, A.D., Wilson, M., Lillquist, K., Siu, V., Ramos, F.J., Musio, A., Jackson, L.S., Dorsett, D. & Krantz, I.D. (2007). Mutations in cohesin complex members SMC3 and SMC1A cause a mild variant of cornelia de Lange syndrome with predominant mental retardation. *Am J Hum Genet*. Vol.80, No.3, pp.485-494, ISSN:0002-9297

Diaz-Martinez, L.A., Gimenez-Abian, J.F. & Clarke, D.J. (2007). Regulation of centromeric cohesion by sororin independently of the APC/C. *Cell Cycle*. Vol.6, No.6, pp.714-724, ISSN:1551-4005

Ding, D.Q., Sakurai, N., Katou, Y., Itoh, T., Shirahige, K., Haraguchi, T. & Hiraoka, Y. (2006). Meiotic cohesins modulate chromosome compaction during meiotic prophase in fission yeast. *J Cell Biol*. Vol.174, No.4, pp.499-508, ISSN:0021-9525

Dorsett, D. (2011). Cohesin: genomic insights into controlling gene transcription and development. *Curr Opin Genet Dev*. Vol.21, No.2, pp.199-206, ISSN:1879-0380

Eijpe, M., Heyting, C., Gross, B. & Jessberger, R. (2000). Association of mammalian SMC1 and SMC3 proteins with meiotic chromosomes and synaptonemal complexes. *J Cell Sci*. Vol.113 ( Pt 4), pp.673-682

Eijpe, M., Offenberg, H., Jessberger, R., Revenkova, E. & Heyting, C. (2003). Meiotic cohesin REC8 marks the axial elements of rat synaptonemal complexes before cohesins SMC1beta and SMC3. *J Cell Biol*. Vol.160, No.5, pp.657-670

Ellermeier, C. & Smith, G.R. (2005). Cohesins are required for meiotic DNA breakage and recombination in Schizosaccharomyces pombe. *Proc Natl Acad Sci U S A*. Vol.102, No.31, pp.10952-10957, ISSN:0027-8424

Fernandez-Capetillo, O., Mahadevaiah, S.K., Celeste, A., Romanienko, P.J., Camerini-Otero, R.D., Bonner, W.M., Manova, K., Burgoyne, P. & Nussenzweig, A. (2003). H2AX is required for chromatin remodeling and inactivation of sex chromosomes in male mouse meiosis. *Dev Cell*. Vol.4, No.4, pp.497-508,

Fernández-Capetillo, O., Lee, A., Nussenzweig, M. & Nussenzweig, A. (2004). H2AX: the histone guardian of the genome. *DNA Repair (Amst)*. Vol.3, No.8-9, pp.959-967

Gandhi, R., Gillespie, P.J. & Hirano, T. (2006). Human Wapl is a cohesin-binding protein that promotes sister-chromatid resolution in mitotic prophase. *Curr Biol*. Vol.16, No.24, pp.2406-2417, ISSN:0960-9822

Garcia-Cruz, R., Brieno, M.A., Roig, I., Grossmann, M., Velilla, E., Pujol, A., Cabero, L., Pessarrodona, A., Barbero, J.L. & Garcia Caldes, M. (2010). Dynamics of cohesin proteins REC8, STAG3, SMC1 beta and SMC3 are consistent with a role in sister chromatid cohesion during meiosis in human oocytes. *Hum Reprod.* Vol.25, No.9, pp.2316-2327, ISSN:1460-2350

Gerton, J.L., DeRisi, J., Shroff, R., Lichten, M., Brown, P.O. & Petes, T.D. (2000). Global mapping of meiotic recombination hotspots and coldspots in the yeast Saccharomyces cerevisiae. *Proc Natl Acad Sci U S A.* Vol.97, No.21, pp.11383-11390, ISSN:0027-8424

Gomez, R., Valdeolmillos, A., Parra, M.T., Viera, A., Carreiro, C., Roncal, F., Rufas, J.S., Barbero, J.L. & Suja, J.A. (2007). Mammalian SGO2 appears at the inner centromere domain and redistributes depending on tension across centromeres during meiosis II and mitosis. *EMBO Rep.* Vol.8, No.2, pp.173-180,

Gordillo, M., Vega, H., Trainer, A.H., Hou, F., Sakai, N., Luque, R., Kayserili, H., Basaran, S., Skovby, F., Hennekam, R.C., Uzielli, M.L., Schnur, R.E., Manouvrier, S., Chang, S., Blair, E., Hurst, J.A., Forzano, F., Meins, M., Simola, K.O., Raas-Rothschild, A., Schultz, R.A., McDaniel, L.D., Ozono, K., Inui, K., Zou, H. & Jabs, E.W. (2008). The molecular mechanism underlying Roberts syndrome involves loss of ESCO2 acetyltransferase activity. *Hum Mol Genet.* Vol.17, No.14, pp.2172-2180, ISSN:1460-2083

Grelon, M., Vezon, D., Gendrot, G. & Pelletier, G. (2001). AtSPO11-1 is necessary for efficient meiotic recombination in plants. *EMBO J.* Vol.20, No.3, pp.589-600, ISSN:0261-4189

Grey, C., Baudat, F. & de Massy, B. (2009). Genome-wide control of the distribution of meiotic recombination. *PLoS Biol.* Vol.7, No.2, pp.e35, ISSN:1545-7885

Gruber, S., Haering, C.H. & Nasmyth, K. (2003). Chromosomal cohesin forms a ring. *Cell.* Vol.112, No.6, pp.765-777, ISSN:0092-8674

Guacci, V. (2007). Sister chromatid cohesion: the cohesin cleavage model does not ring true. *Genes Cells.* Vol.12, No.6, pp.693-708, ISSN:1356-9597

Gutierrez-Caballero, C., Herran, Y., Sanchez-Martin, M., Suja, J.A., Barbero, J.L., Llano, E. & Pendas, A.M. (2011). Identification and molecular characterization of the mammalian alpha-kleisin RAD21L. *Cell Cycle.* Vol.10, No.9, pp.1477-1487, ISSN:1551-4005

Haering, C.H., Lowe, J., Hochwagen, A. & Nasmyth, K. (2002). Molecular architecture of SMC proteins and the yeast cohesin complex. *Mol Cell.* Vol.9, No.4, pp.773-788

Hauf, S., Roitinger, E., Koch, B., Dittrich, C.M., Mechtler, K. & Peters, J.M. (2005). Dissociation of cohesin from chromosome arms and loss of arm cohesion during early mitosis depends on phosphorylation of SA2. *PLoS Biol.* Vol.3, No.3, pp.e69

Hayashi, M., Chin, G.M. & Villeneuve, A.M. (2007). C. elegans germ cells switch between distinct modes of double-strand break repair during meiotic prophase progression. *PLoS Genet.* Vol.3, No.11, pp.e191, ISSN:1553-7404

Herran, Y., Gutierrez-Caballero, C., Sanchez-Martin, M., Hernandez, T., Viera, A., Barbero, J.L., de Alava, E., de Rooij, D.G., Suja, J.A., Llano, E. & Pendas, A.M. (2011). The cohesin subunit RAD21L functions in meiotic synapsis and exhibits sexual dimorphism in fertility. *EMBO J*:1460-2075

Heyer, W.D., Ehmsen, K.T. & Liu, J. (2010). Regulation of homologous recombination in eukaryotes. *Annu Rev Genet.* Vol.44, pp.113-139, ISSN:1545-2948

Hogarth, C.A., Mitchell, D., Evanoff, R., Small, C. & Griswold, M. (2011). Identification and expression of potential regulators of the mammalian mitotic-to-meiotic transition. *Biol Reprod.* Vol.84, No.1, pp.34-42, ISSN:1529-7268

Hou, F. & Zou, H. (2005). Two human orthologues of Eco1/Ctf7 acetyltransferases are both required for proper sister-chromatid cohesion. *Mol Biol Cell.* Vol.16, No.8, pp.3908-3918, ISSN:1059-1524

Hunter, N. & Borts, R.H. (1997). Mlh1 is unique among mismatch repair proteins in its ability to promote crossing-over during meiosis. *Genes Dev.* Vol.11, No.12, pp.1573-1582

Ishiguro, K., Kim, J., Fujiyama-Nakamura, S., Kato, S. & Watanabe, Y. (2011). A new meiosis-specific cohesin complex implicated in the cohesin code for homologous pairing. *EMBO Rep.* Vol.12, No.3, pp.267-275, ISSN:1469-3178

James, R.D., Schmiesing, J.A., Peters, A.H., Yokomori, K. & Disteche, C.M. (2002). Differential association of SMC1alpha and SMC3 proteins with meiotic chromosomes in wild-type and SPO11-deficient male mice. *Chromosome Res.* Vol.10, No.7, pp.549-560, ISSN:0967-3849

Jessberger, R., Riwar, B., Baechtold, H. & Akhmedov, A.T. (1996). SMC proteins constitute two subunits of the mammalian recombination complex RC-1. *EMBO J.* Vol.15, No.15, pp.4061-4068, ISSN:0261-4189

Jin, H., Guacci, V. & Yu, H.G. (2009). Pds5 is required for homologue pairing and inhibits synapsis of sister chromatids during yeast meiosis. *J Cell Biol.* Vol.186, No.5, pp.713-725, ISSN:1540-8140

Jones, G.H. (1973). Light and electron microscope studies of chromosome pairing in relation to chiasma localisation in Stethophyma grossum (Orthoptera: Acrididae). *Chromosoma.* Vol.42, No.2, pp.145-162

Keeney, S., Giroux, C.N. & Kleckner, N. (1997). Meiosis-specific DNA double-strand breaks are catalyzed by Spo11, a member of a widely conserved protein family. *Cell.* Vol.88, No.3, pp.375-384

Khalil, A.M., Boyar, F.Z. & Driscoll, D.J. (2004). Dynamic histone modifications mark sex chromosome inactivation and reactivation during mammalian spermatogenesis. *Proc Natl Acad Sci U S A.* Vol.101, No.47, pp.16583-16587

Kim, B.J., Kang, K.M., Jung, S.Y., Choi, H.K., Seo, J.H., Chae, J.H., Cho, E.J., Youn, H.D., Qin, J. & Kim, S.T. (2008). Esco2 is a novel corepressor that associates with various chromatin modifying enzymes. *Biochem Biophys Res Commun.* Vol.372, No.2, pp.298-304, ISSN:1090-2104

Kim, K.P., Weiner, B.M., Zhang, L., Jordan, A., Dekker, J. & Kleckner, N. (2010). Sister cohesion and structural axis components mediate homolog bias of meiotic recombination. *Cell.* Vol.143, No.6, pp.924-937:1097-4172

Kitajima, T.S., Kawashima, S.A. & Watanabe, Y. (2004). The conserved kinetochore protein shugoshin protects centromeric cohesion during meiosis. *Nature.* Vol.427, No.6974, pp.510-517

Kitajima, T.S., Sakuno, T., Ishiguro, K., Iemura, S., Natsume, T., Kawashima, S.A. & Watanabe, Y. (2006). Shugoshin collaborates with protein phosphatase 2A to protect cohesin. *Nature.* Vol.441, No.7089, pp.46-52, ISSN:1476-4687

Klein, F., Mahr, P., Galova, M., Buonomo, S.B., Michaelis, C., Nairz, K. & Nasmyth, K. (1999). A central role for cohesins in sister chromatid cohesion, formation of axial elements, and recombination during yeast meiosis. *Cell.* Vol.98, No.1, pp.91-103

Krantz, I.D., McCallum, J., DeScipio, C., Kaur, M., Gillis, L.A., Yaeger, D., Jukofsky, L., Wasserman, N., Bottani, A., Morris, C.A., Nowaczyk, M.J., Toriello, H., Bamshad,

M.J., Carey, J.C., Rappaport, E., Kawauchi, S., Lander, A.D., Calof, A.L., Li, H.H., Devoto, M. & Jackson, L.G. (2004). Cornelia de Lange syndrome is caused by mutations in NIPBL, the human homolog of Drosophila melanogaster Nipped-B. *Nat Genet*. Vol.36, No.6, pp.631-635, ISSN:1061-4036

Kugou, K., Fukuda, T., Yamada, S., Ito, M., Sasanuma, H., Mori, S., Katou, Y., Itoh, T., Matsumoto, K., Shibata, T., Shirahige, K. & Ohta, K. (2009). Rec8 guides canonical Spo11 distribution along yeast meiotic chromosomes. *Mol Biol Cell*. Vol.20, No.13, pp.3064-3076, ISSN:1939-4586

Kuroda, M., Oikawa, K., Ohbayashi, T., Yoshida, K., Yamada, K., Mimura, J., Matsuda, Y., Fujii-Kuriyama, Y. & Mukai, K. (2005). A dioxin sensitive gene, mammalian WAPL, is implicated in spermatogenesis. *FEBS Lett*. Vol.579, No.1, pp.167-172, ISSN:0014-5793

Lafont, A.L., Song, J. & Rankin, S. (2010). Sororin cooperates with the acetyltransferase Eco2 to ensure DNA replication-dependent sister chromatid cohesion. *Proc Natl Acad Sci U S A*. Vol.107, No.47, pp.20364-20369, ISSN:1091-6490

Lee, J. & Hirano, T. (2011). RAD21L, a novel cohesin subunit implicated in linking homologous chromosomes in mammalian meiosis. *J Cell Biol*. Vol.192, No.2, pp.263-276, ISSN:1540-8140

Lengauer, C., Kinzler, K.W. & Vogelstein, B. (1997). DNA methylation and genetic instability in colorectal cancer cells. *Proc Natl Acad Sci U S A*. Vol.94, No.6, pp.2545-2550, ISSN:0027-8424

Lengronne, A., Katou, Y., Mori, S., Yokobayashi, S., Kelly, G.P., Itoh, T., Watanabe, Y., Shirahige, K. & Uhlmann, F. (2004). Cohesin relocation from sites of chromosomal loading to places of convergent transcription. *Nature*. Vol.430, No.6999, pp.573-578, ISSN:1476-

Lichten, M. (2001). Meiotic recombination: breaking the genome to save it. *Curr Biol*. Vol.11, No.7, pp.R253-256

Lin, W., Jin, H., Liu, X., Hampton, K. & Yu, H.G. (2011). Scc2 regulates gene expression by recruiting cohesin to the chromosome as a transcriptional activator during yeast meiosis. *Mol Biol Cell*. Vol.22, No.12, pp.1985-1996, ISSN:1939-4586

Losada, A., Hirano, M. & Hirano, T. (1998). Identification of Xenopus SMC protein complexes required for sister chromatid cohesion. *Genes Dev*. Vol.12, No.13, pp.1986-1997

Losada, A., Yokochi, T., Kobayashi, R. & Hirano, T. (2000). Identification and characterization of SA/Scc3p subunits in the Xenopus and human cohesin complexes. *J Cell Biol*. Vol.150, No.3, pp.405-416

Losada, A., Yokochi, T. & Hirano, T. (2005). Functional contribution of Pds5 to cohesin-mediated cohesion in human cells and Xenopus egg extracts. *J Cell Sci*. Vol.118, No.Pt 10, pp.2133-2141, ISSN:0021-9533

Llano, E., Gomez, R., Gutierrez-Caballero, C., Herran, Y., Sanchez-Martin, M., Vazquez-Quinones, L., Hernandez, T., de Alava, E., Cuadrado, A., Barbero, J.L., Suja, J.A. & Pendas, A.M. (2008). Shugoshin-2 is essential for the completion of meiosis but not for mitotic cell division in mice. *Genes Dev*. Vol.22, No.17, pp.2400-2413, ISSN:0890-9369

MacQueen, A.J., Colaiacovo, M.P., McDonald, K. & Villeneuve, A.M. (2002). Synapsis-dependent and -independent mechanisms stabilize homolog pairing during meiotic prophase in C. elegans. *Genes Dev.* Vol.16, No.18, pp.2428-2442, ISSN:0890-9369

Madigan, J.P., Chotkowski, H.L. & Glaser, R.L. (2002). DNA double-strand break-induced phosphorylation of Drosophila histone variant H2Av helps prevent radiation-induced apoptosis. *Nucleic Acids Res.* Vol.30, No.17, pp.3698-3705

Maeshima, K. & Laemmli, U.K. (2003). A two-step scaffolding model for mitotic chromosome assembly. *Dev Cell.* Vol.4, No.4, pp.467-480

Mahadevaiah, S.K., Turner, J.M., Baudat, F., Rogakou, E.P., de Boer, P., Blanco-Rodriguez, J., Jasin, M., Keeney, S., Bonner, W.M. & Burgoyne, P.S. (2001). Recombinational DNA double-strand breaks in mice precede synapsis. *Nat Genet.* Vol.27, No.3, pp.271-276

Meuwissen, R.L., Offenberg, H.H., Dietrich, A.J., Riesewijk, A., van Iersel, M. & Heyting, C. (1992). A coiled-coil related protein specific for synapsed regions of meiotic prophase chromosomes. *EMBO J.* Vol.11, No.13, pp.5091-5100, ISSN:0261-4189

Michaelis, C., Ciosk, R. & Nasmyth, K. (1997). Cohesins: chromosomal proteins that prevent premature separation of sister chromatids. *Cell.* Vol.91, No.1, pp.35-45,

Miyazaki, W.Y. & Orr-Weaver, T.L. (1994). Sister-chromatid cohesion in mitosis and meiosis. *Annu Rev Genet.* Vol.28, pp.167-187

Moldovan, G.L., Pfander, B. & Jentsch, S. (2006). PCNA controls establishment of sister chromatid cohesion during S phase. *Mol Cell.* Vol.23, No.5, pp.723-732, ISSN:1097-2765

Molnar, M., Bahler, J., Sipiczki, M. & Kohli, J. (1995). The rec8 gene of Schizosaccharomyces pombe is involved in linear element formation, chromosome pairing and sister-chromatid cohesion during meiosis. *Genetics.* Vol.141, No.1, pp.61-73, ISSN:0016-6731

Musio, A., Selicorni, A., Focarelli, M.L., Gervasini, C., Milani, D., Russo, S., Vezzoni, P. & Larizza, L. (2006). X-linked Cornelia de Lange syndrome owing to SMC1L1 mutations. *Nat Genet.* Vol.38, No.5, pp.528-530, ISSN:1061-4036

Nabeshima, K., Villeneuve, A.M. & Colaiacovo, M.P. (2005). Crossing over is coupled to late meiotic prophase bivalent differentiation through asymmetric disassembly of the SC. *J Cell Biol.* Vol.168, No.5, pp.683-689, ISSN:0021-9525

Nagao, K., Adachi, Y. & Yanagida, M. (2004). Separase-mediated cleavage of cohesin at interphase is required for DNA repair. *Nature.* Vol.430, No.7003, pp.1044-1048, ISSN:1476-4687

Nasmyth, K. & Haering, C.H. (2005). The structure and function of SMC and kleisin complexes. *Annu Rev Biochem.* Vol.74, pp.595-648

Neale, M.J. & Keeney, S. (2006). Clarifying the mechanics of DNA strand exchange in meiotic recombination. *Nature.* Vol.442, No.7099, pp.153-158

Newman, J.J. & Young, R.A. (2010). Connecting transcriptional control to chromosome structure and human disease. *Cold Spring Harb Symp Quant Biol.* Vol.75, pp.227-235, ISSN:1943-4456

Nishiyama, T., Ladurner, R., Schmitz, J., Kreidl, E., Schleiffer, A., Bhaskara, V., Bando, M., Shirahige, K., Hyman, A.A., Mechtler, K. & Peters, J.M. (2010). Sororin mediates sister chromatid cohesion by antagonizing Wapl. *Cell.* Vol.143, No.5, pp.737-749, ISSN:1097-4172

Notaridou, M., Quaye, L., Dafou, D., Jones, C., Song, H., Hogdall, E., Kjaer, S.K., Christensen, L., Hogdall, C., Blaakaer, J., McGuire, V., Wu, A.H., Van Den Berg, D.J., Pike, M.C., Gentry-Maharaj, A., Wozniak, E., Sher, T., Jacobs, I.J., Tyrer, J., Schildkraut, J.M., Moorman, P.G., Iversen, E.S., Jakubowska, A., Medrek, K., Lubinski, J., Ness, R.B., Moysich, K.B., Lurie, G., Wilkens, L.R., Carney, M.E., Wang-Gohrke, S., Doherty, J.A., Rossing, M.A., Beckmann, M.W., Thiel, F.C., Ekici, A.B., Chen, X., Beesley, J., Gronwald, J., Fasching, P.A., Chang-Claude, J., Goodman, M.T., Chenevix-Trench, G., Berchuck, A., Pearce, C.L., Whittemore, A.S., Menon, U., Pharoah, P.D., Gayther, S.A. & Ramus, S.J. (2011). Common alleles in candidate susceptibility genes associated with risk and development of epithelial ovarian cancer. *Int J Cancer*. Vol.128, No.9, pp.2063-2074, ISSN:1097-0215

Novak, I., Wang, H., Revenkova, E., Jessberger, R., Scherthan, H. & Hoog, C. (2008). Cohesin Smc1beta determines meiotic chromatin axis loop organization. *J Cell Biol*. Vol.180, No.1, pp.83-90, ISSN:1540-8140

Ong, C.T. & Corces, V.G. (2011). Enhancer function: new insights into the regulation of tissue-specific gene expression. *Nat Rev Genet*. Vol.12, No.4, pp.283-293, ISSN:1471-0064

Page, J., Suja, J.A., Santos, J.L. & Rufas, J.S. (1998). Squash procedure for protein immunolocalization in meiotic cells. *Chromosome Res*. Vol.6, No.8, pp.639-642,

Page, S.L. & Hawley, R.S. (2004). The genetics and molecular biology of the synaptonemal complex. *Annu Rev Cell Dev Biol*. Vol.20, pp.525-558

Page, J., de la Fuente, R., Gomez, R., Calvente, A., Viera, A., Parra, M.T., Santos, J.L., Berrios, S., Fernandez-Donoso, R., Suja, J.A. & Rufas, J.S. (2006). Sex chromosomes, synapsis, and cohesins: a complex affair. *Chromosoma*. Vol.115, No.3, pp.250-259, ISSN:0009-5915

Panizza, S., Tanaka, T., Hochwagen, A., Eisenhaber, F. & Nasmyth, K. (2000). Pds5 cooperates with cohesin in maintaining sister chromatid cohesion. *Curr Biol*. Vol.10, No.24, pp.1557-1564, ISSN:0960-9822

Parra, M.T., Viera, A., Gomez, R., Page, J., Benavente, R., Santos, J.L., Rufas, J.S. & Suja, J.A. (2004). Involvement of the cohesin Rad21 and SCP3 in monopolar attachment of sister kinetochores during mouse meiosis I. *J Cell Sci*. Vol.117, No.Pt 7, pp.1221-1234

Pasierbek, P., Jantsch, M., Melcher, M., Schleiffer, A., Schweizer, D. & Loidl, J. (2001). A Caenorhabditis elegans cohesion protein with functions in meiotic chromosome pairing and disjunction. *Genes Dev*. Vol.15, No.11, pp.1349-1360, ISSN:0890-9369

Pelttari, J., Hoja, M.R., Yuan, L., Liu, J.G., Brundell, E., Moens, P., Santucci-Darmanin, S., Jessberger, R., Barbero, J.L., Heyting, C. & Hoog, C. (2001). A meiotic chromosomal core consisting of cohesin complex proteins recruits DNA recombination proteins and promotes synapsis in the absence of an axial element in mammalian meiotic cells. *Mol Cell Biol*. Vol.21, No.16, pp.5667-5677

Peters, A.H., Plug, A.W., van Vugt, M.J. & de Boer, P. (1997). A drying-down technique for the spreading of mammalian meiocytes from the male and female germline. *Chromosome Res*. Vol.5, No.1, pp.66-68

Pezzi, N., Prieto, I., Kremer, L., Perez Jurado, L.A., Valero, C., Del Mazo, J., Martinez, A.C. & Barbero, J.L. (2000). STAG3, a novel gene encoding a protein involved in meiotic chromosome pairing and location of STAG3-related genes flanking the Williams-Beuren syndrome deletion. *Faseb J*. Vol.14, No.3, pp.581-592

Plug, A.W., Peters, A.H., Keegan, K.S., Hoekstra, M.F., de Boer, P. & Ashley, T. (1998). Changes in protein composition of meiotic nodules during mammalian meiosis. *J Cell Sci*. Vol.111 ( Pt 4), pp.413-423, ISSN:0021-9533

Polakova, S., Cipak, L. & Gregan, J. (2011). RAD21L is a novel kleisin subunit of the cohesin complex. *Cell Cycle*. Vol.10, No.12, pp.1893, ISSN:1551-4005

Prieto, I., Suja, J.A., Pezzi, N., Kremer, L., Martinez, A.C., Rufas, J.S. & Barbero, J.L. (2001). Mammalian STAG3 is a cohesin specific to sister chromatid arms in meiosis I. *Nat Cell Biol*. Vol.3, No.8, pp.761-766

Prieto, I., Pezzi, N., Buesa, J.M., Kremer, L., Barthelemy, I., Carreiro, C., Roncal, F., Martinez, A., Gomez, L., Fernandez, R., Martinez, A.C. & Barbero, J.L. (2002). STAG2 and Rad21 mammalian mitotic cohesins are implicated in meiosis. *EMBO Rep*. Vol.3, No.6, pp.543-550, ISSN:1469-221X

Qiao, H., Lohmiller, L.D. & Anderson, L.K. (2011). Cohesin proteins load sequentially during prophase I in tomato primary microsporocytes. *Chromosome Res*. Vol.19, No.2, pp.193-207, ISSN:1573-6849

Rankin, S. (2005). Sororin, the cell cycle and sister chromatid cohesion. *Cell Cycle*. Vol.4, No.8, pp.1039-1042, ISSN:1551-4005

Redon, C., Pilch, D., Rogakou, E., Sedelnikova, O., Newrock, K. & Bonner, W. (2002). Histone H2A variants H2AX and H2AZ. *Curr Opin Genet Dev*. Vol.12, No.2, pp.162-169, ISSN:0959-437X

Revenkova, E., Eijpe, M., Heyting, C., Gross, B. & Jessberger, R. (2001). Novel meiosis-specific isoform of mammalian SMC1. *Mol Cell Biol*. Vol.21, No.20, pp.6984-6998

Revenkova, E., Eijpe, M., Heyting, C., Hodges, C.A., Hunt, P.A., Liebe, B., Scherthan, H. & Jessberger, R. (2004). Cohesin SMC1 beta is required for meiotic chromosome dynamics, sister chromatid cohesion and DNA recombination. *Nat Cell Biol*. Vol.6, No.6, pp.555-562, ISSN:1465-7392

Revenkova, E. & Jessberger, R. (2005). Keeping sister chromatids together: cohesins in meiosis. *Reproduction*. Vol.130, No.6, pp.783-790

Revenkova, E. & Jessberger, R. (2006). Shaping meiotic prophase chromosomes: cohesins and synaptonemal complex proteins. *Chromosoma*. Vol.115, No.3, pp.235-240, ISSN:0009-5915

Royo, H., Polikiewicz, G., Mahadevaiah, S.K., Prosser, H., Mitchell, M., Bradley, A., de Rooij, D.G., Burgoyne, P.S. & Turner, J.M. (2010). Evidence that meiotic sex chromosome inactivation is essential for male fertility. *Curr Biol*. Vol.20, No.23, pp.2117-2123, ISSN:1879-0445

Schalk, J.A., Dietrich, A.J., Vink, A.C., Offenberg, H.H., van Aalderen, M. & Heyting, C. (1998). Localization of SCP2 and SCP3 protein molecules within synaptonemal complexes of the rat. *Chromosoma*. Vol.107, No.8, pp.540-548

Schmitz, J., Watrin, E., Lenart, P., Mechtler, K. & Peters, J.M. (2007). Sororin is required for stable binding of cohesin to chromatin and for sister chromatid cohesion in interphase. *Curr Biol*. Vol.17, No.7, pp.630-636, ISSN:0960-9822

Shinohara, A. & Shinohara, M. (2004). Roles of RecA homologues Rad51 and Dmc1 during meiotic recombination. *Cytogenet Genome Res*. Vol.107, No.3-4, pp.201-207

Skibbens, R.V., Corson, L.B., Koshland, D. & Hieter, P. (1999). Ctf7p is essential for sister chromatid cohesion and links mitotic chromosome structure to the DNA replication machinery. *Genes Dev*. Vol.13, No.3, pp.307-319

Skibbens, R.V. (2009). Establishment of sister chromatid cohesion. *Curr Biol.* Vol.19, No.24, pp.R1126-1132, ISSN:1879-0445

Sonoda, E., Matsusaka, T., Morrison, C., Vagnarelli, P., Hoshi, O., Ushiki, T., Nojima, K., Fukagawa, T., Waizenegger, I.C., Peters, J.M., Earnshaw, W.C. & Takeda, S. (2001). Scc1/Rad21/Mcd1 is required for sister chromatid cohesion and kinetochore function in vertebrate cells. *Dev Cell.* Vol.1, No.6, pp.759-770

Stack, S.M. & Anderson, L.K. (2009). Electron microscopic immunogold localization of recombination-related proteins in spreads of synaptonemal complexes from tomato microsporocytes. *Methods Mol Biol.* Vol.558, pp.147-169, ISSN:1064-3745

Strom, L., Lindroos, H.B., Shirahige, K. & Sjogren, C. (2004). Postreplicative recruitment of cohesin to double-strand breaks is required for DNA repair. *Mol Cell.* Vol.16, No.6, pp.1003-1015

Strom, L. & Sjogren, C. (2005). DNA damage-induced cohesion. *Cell Cycle.* Vol.4, No.4, pp.536-539, ISSN:1551-4005

Strom, L. & Sjogren, C. (2007). Chromosome segregation and double-strand break repair - a complex connection. *Curr Opin Cell Biol.* Vol.19, No.3, pp.344-349, ISSN:0955-0674

Suja, J.A. & Barbero, J.L. (2009). Cohesin complexes and sister chromatid cohesion in mammalian meiosis. *Genome Dyn.* Vol.5, pp.94-116

Sumara, I., Vorlaufer, E., Gieffers, C., Peters, B.H. & Peters, J.M. (2000). Characterization of vertebrate cohesin complexes and their regulation in prophase. *J Cell Biol.* Vol.151, No.4, pp.749-762,

Szostak, J.W., Orr-Weaver, T.L., Rothstein, R.J. & Stahl, F.W. (1983). The double-strand-break repair model for recombination. *Cell.* Vol.33, No.1, pp.25-35, ISSN:0092-8674

Tanaka, T., Fuchs, J., Loidl, J. & Nasmyth, K. (2000). Cohesin ensures bipolar attachment of microtubules to sister centromeres and resists their precocious separation. *Nat Cell Biol.* Vol.2, No.8, pp.492-499

Tarsounas, M., Morita, T., Pearlman, R.E. & Moens, P.B. (1999). RAD51 and DMC1 form mixed complexes associated with mouse meiotic chromosome cores and synaptonemal complexes. *J Cell Biol.* Vol.147, No.2, pp.207-220, ISSN:0021-9525

Tonkin, E.T., Wang, T.J., Lisgo, S., Bamshad, M.J. & Strachan, T. (2004). NIPBL, encoding a homolog of fungal Scc2-type sister chromatid cohesion proteins and fly Nipped-B, is mutated in Cornelia de Lange syndrome. *Nat Genet.* Vol.36, No.6, pp.636-641, ISSN:1061-4036

Toth, A., Ciosk, R., Uhlmann, F., Galova, M., Schleiffer, A. & Nasmyth, K. (1999). Yeast cohesin complex requires a conserved protein, Eco1p(Ctf7), to establish cohesion between sister chromatids during DNA replication. *Genes Dev.* Vol.13, No.3, pp.320-333, ISSN:0890-9369

Uhlmann, F., Lottspeich, F. & Nasmyth, K. (1999). Sister-chromatid separation at anaphase onset is promoted by cleavage of the cohesin subunit Scc1. *Nature.* Vol.400, No.6739, pp.37-42, ISSN:0028-0836

Uhlmann, F., Wernic, D., Poupart, M.A., Koonin, E.V. & Nasmyth, K. (2000). Cleavage of cohesin by the CD clan protease separin triggers anaphase in yeast. *Cell.* Vol.103, No.3, pp.375-386, ISSN:0092-8674

Uhlmann, F. (2001). Chromosome cohesion and segregation in mitosis and meiosis. *Curr Opin Cell Biol.* Vol.13, No.6, pp.754-761

Uhlmann, F. (2011). Cohesin subunit Rad21L, the new kid on the block has new ideas. *EMBO Rep*. Vol.12, No.3, pp.183-184, ISSN:1469-3178

Unal, E., Heidinger-Pauli, J.M., Kim, W., Guacci, V., Onn, I., Gygi, S.P. & Koshland, D.E. (2008). A molecular determinant for the establishment of sister chromatid cohesion. *Science*. Vol.321, No.5888, pp.566-569, ISSN:1095-9203

Valdeolmillos, A.M., Viera, A., Page, J., Prieto, I., Santos, J.L., Parra, M.T., Heck, M.M., Martinez, A.C., Barbero, J.L., Suja, J.A. & Rufas, J.S. (2007). Sequential loading of cohesin subunits during the first meiotic prophase of grasshoppers. *PLoS Genet*. Vol.3, No.2, pp.e28

Van Den Berg, D.J. & Francke, U. (1993). Roberts syndrome: a review of 100 cases and a new rating system for severity. *Am J Med Genet*. Vol.47, No.7, pp.1104-1123, ISSN:0148-7299

Vega, H., Waisfisz, Q., Gordillo, M., Sakai, N., Yanagihara, I., Yamada, M., van Gosliga, D., Kayserili, H., Xu, C., Ozono, K., Jabs, E.W., Inui, K. & Joenje, H. (2005). Roberts syndrome is caused by mutations in ESCO2, a human homolog of yeast ECO1 that is essential for the establishment of sister chromatid cohesion. *Nat Genet*. Vol.37, No.5, pp.468-470, ISSN:1061-4036

Verni, F., Gandhi, R., Goldberg, M.L. & Gatti, M. (2000). Genetic and molecular analysis of wings apart-like (wapl), a gene controlling heterochromatin organization in Drosophila melanogaster. *Genetics*. Vol.154, No.4, pp.1693-1710, ISSN:0016-6731

Viera, A., Rufas, J.S., Martinez, I., Barbero, J.L., Ortega, S. & Suja, J.A. (2009a). CDK2 is required for proper homologous pairing, recombination and sex-body formation during male mouse meiosis. *J Cell Sci*. Vol.122, No.Pt 12, pp.2149-2159, ISSN:0021-9533

Viera, A., Santos, J.L. & Rufas, J.S. (2009b). Relationship between incomplete synapsis and chiasma localization. *Chromosoma*. Vol.118, No.3, pp.377-389

Waizenegger, I.C., Hauf, S., Meinke, A. & Peters, J.M. (2000). Two distinct pathways remove mammalian cohesin from chromosome arms in prophase and from centromeres in anaphase. *Cell*. Vol.103, No.3, pp.399-410, ISSN:0092-8674

Wallace, B.M.N. & Jones, G.H. (1978). Incomplete chromosome pairing and its relation to chiasma localisation in Stethophyma grossum spermatocytes. *Heredity*. Vol.40, pp.385-396

Wang, T.F., Kleckner, N. & Hunter, N. (1999). Functional specificity of MutL homologs in yeast: evidence for three Mlh1-based heterocomplexes with distinct roles during meiosis in recombination and mismatch correction. *Proc Natl Acad Sci U S A*. Vol.96, No.24, pp.13914-13919

Watanabe, Y. & Nurse, P. (1999). Cohesin Rec8 is required for reductional chromosome segregation at meiosis. *Nature*. Vol.400, No.6743, pp.461-464,

Watanabe, Y. (2004). Modifying sister chromatid cohesion for meiosis. *J Cell Sci*. Vol.117, No.Pt 18, pp.4017-4023

Watrin, E. & Peters, J.M. (2006). Cohesin and DNA damage repair. *Exp Cell Res*. Vol.312, No.14, pp.2687-2693, ISSN:0014-4827

Xu, H., Beasley, M., Verschoor, S., Inselman, A., Handel, M.A. & McKay, M.J. (2004). A new role for the mitotic RAD21/SCC1 cohesin in meiotic chromosome cohesion and segregation in the mouse. *EMBO Rep*. Vol.5, No.4, pp.378-384

Xu, H., Beasley, M.D., Warren, W.D., van der Horst, G.T. & McKay, M.J. (2005). Absence of mouse REC8 cohesin promotes synapsis of sister chromatids in meiosis. *Dev Cell.* Vol.8, No.6, pp.949-961, ISSN:1534-5807

Yuan, L., Liu, J.G., Zhao, J., Brundell, E., Daneholt, B. & Hoog, C. (2000). The murine SCP3 gene is required for synaptonemal complex assembly, chromosome synapsis, and male fertility. *Mol Cell.* Vol.5, No.1, pp.73-83

Zetka, M.C., Kawasaki, I., Strome, S. & Muller, F. (1999). Synapsis and chiasma formation in Caenorhabditis elegans require HIM-3, a meiotic chromosome core component that functions in chromosome segregation. *Genes Dev.* Vol.13, No.17, pp.2258-2270, ISSN:0890-9369

Zhang, L., Tao, J., Wang, S., Chong, K. & Wang, T. (2006). The rice OsRad21-4, an orthologue of yeast Rec8 protein, is required for efficient meiosis. *Plant Mol Biol.* Vol.60, No.4, pp.533-554, ISSN:0167-4412

Zhang, B., Jain, S., Song, H., Fu, M., Heuckeroth, R.O., Erlich, J.M., Jay, P.Y. & Milbrandt, J. (2007). Mice lacking sister chromatid cohesion protein PDS5B exhibit developmental abnormalities reminiscent of Cornelia de Lange syndrome. *Development.* Vol.134, No.17, pp.3191-3201, ISSN:0950-1991

Zhang, N., Kuznetsov, S.G., Sharan, S.K., Li, K., Rao, P.H. & Pati, D. (2008a). A handcuff model for the cohesin complex. *J Cell Biol.* Vol.183, No.6, pp.1019-1031, ISSN:1540-8140

Zhang, J., Shi, X., Li, Y., Kim, B.J., Jia, J., Huang, Z., Yang, T., Fu, X., Jung, S.Y., Wang, Y., Zhang, P., Kim, S.T., Pan, X. & Qin, J. (2008b). Acetylation of Smc3 by Eco1 is required for S phase sister chromatid cohesion in both human and yeast. *Mol Cell.* Vol.31, No.1, pp.143-151, ISSN:1097-4164

Zhang, J., Hakansson, H., Kuroda, M. & Yuan, L. (2008c). Wapl localization on the synaptonemal complex, a meiosis-specific proteinaceous structure that binds homologous chromosomes, in the female mouse. *Reprod Domest Anim.* Vol.43, No.1, pp.124-126, ISSN:0936-6768

# 4

# Dynamics of Cellular Components in Meiotic and Premeiotic Divisions in *Drosophila* Males

Yoshihiro H. Inoue, Chie Miyauchi, Tubasa Ogata and Daishi Kitazawa
*Insect Biomedical Research Center, Kyoto Institute of Technology, Japan*

## 1. Introduction

Meiosis in higher organisms is programmed as a part of gametogenesis. It should be discussed separately from a yeast meiosis that initiates in response to extracellular nutrient conditions. In this chapter, we would like to introduce current knowledge including our new findings about dynamics of meiosis in *Drosophila* males. At first, we will introduce general views of cell divisions and cell growth during *Drosophila* spermatogenesis as we illustrated in Fig. 1A. At the tip of the testis in adult *Drosophila* males, several germline stem cells (GSCs) are surrounding next to a cluster of smaller hub cells. The GSCs receive a signal to maintain their multi-potential stem cell characteristics secreted from the adjoining hub cells. A secreted protein encoded by the *unpaired* gene acts as a ligand of the maintenance signal (Kiger, *et al.*, 2001, Fuller & Spradling, 2007). The insulin-like peptides in hemolymph first induce the cell cycle progression of the male GSCs from G2 phase to M phase (Ueishi et al., 2009). Between two daughter cells derived from asymmetric division of the GSC, a proximal daughter cell exclusively receives the Unpaird signal and becomes a self-renewed GSC. The other distal daughter cell leaves the niche and begins to differentiate as a spermatogonium. The spermatogonium then undergoes four cell cycles and generates a 16 cell unit known as a cyst (as a review Fuller, 1993). In ever mitosis, all spermatogonia within a cyst undergo cell divisions synchronously. Cytokinesis in spermatogonia mitoses as well as in following meiotic divisions terminates incompletely. The cleavage furrow ingression is arrested at the middle of cytokinesis and then the contractile rings transform into cytoplasmic bridges called ring canals (Hime et al., 1996). These 16 spermatocytes synchronously enter a growth phase during which the cells remarkably increase in volume by up to 25 times. Following completion of the enormous cell growth, primary spermatocytes carry out two consecutive meiotic divisions. A cyst of 16 spermatocytes gives rise to 64 spermatids simultaneously as a consequence of meiotic divisions. Every spermatid in a cyst at onion stage contains equally sized nucleus and Nebenkern that is a single large aggregate derived from mitochondria. This should be achieved as a consequence of proper chromosome segregation and cytokinesis in germ line cells as well as equal partition of mitochondria (Castrillon et al., 1993, Ichihara et al., 2007).

Next, we describe that the meiotic cells perform dynamic alterations of their cellular components as meiosis progress. If one would like to examine alterations of intracellular structures such as cytoskeletons and organelles during cell division, *Drosophila* male meiotic

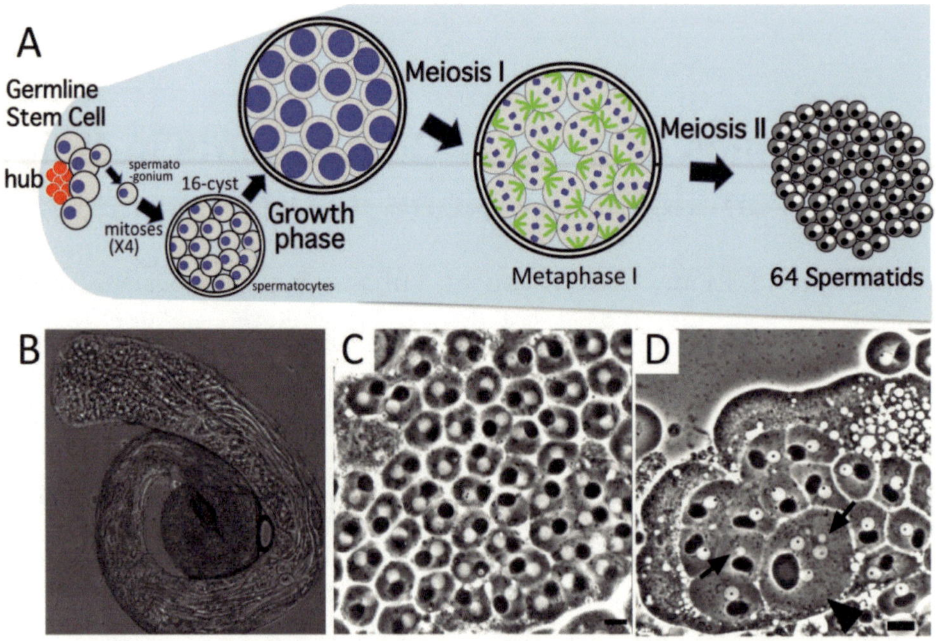


Fig. 1. A. Illustration of premeiotic cell division, cell growth of spermatocytes and meiotic divisions in testis. B. A micrograph of *Drosophila* testis. C, D. A phase contrast micrograph of spermatids at onion stage from wild-type (C) and *orbit*[7] mutant males. Each arrow indicates a smaller nucleus derived from unequal chromosome segregation. Arrowhead shows a larger spermatid containing a large Nebenkern and four nuclei, suggesting a failure of cytokinesis in both meiotic divisions. Bars, 10 µm. Panel C and D were reprinted from Inoue et al., (2004)

cells have several advantages. In *Drosophila*, good cultured cell lines that proliferate well in a standard culture condition are also available (Rogers & Rogers, 2008). However, their cell size, particularly cytoplasmic volume, is much smaller than that of mammalian cells. This is a disadvantage in examination of cellular components during cell division. Spermatocytes, on the other hand, achieve distinct cell growth before initiation of first meiotic division. The primary spermatocyte is the largest diploid cells among proliferative cells in *Drosophila* whole body. Thus, one can easily perform detailed observation of cellular structures in dividing cells using optical microscopes. In *Drosophila melanogaster*, well-advanced and sophisticated genetic techniques are available. Meiotic defects in chromosome segregation and in cytokinesis appear in cellular organization of spermatids just after completion of 2nd meiotic division. By observation of such early spermatids, one can easily find out even subtle meiotic abnormalities. Many of genes essential for cytokinesis have been identified by this method, as we discuss later. Furthermore, if a loss of microtubule integrity or its dynamics would have occurred in normal cultured cells, their cell cycle progression should be arrested before metaphase. Therefore, it is hard to examine how microtubules would influence later processes of cell divisions in the somatic cells. As spermatocytes, on the other hand, are less sensitive to microtubule abnormalities at microtubule assembly checkpoint before metaphase. A colchicine treatment of spermatocytes causes a delay of meiotic cell cycle but it does not make a cell cycle arrest (Rebollo & Gonzalez, 2000). One can, therefore, examine a role of microtubule-related genes in cytokinesis without arresting cell cycle. This is another great advantage of male meiotic cells in cell division studies.

We and other groups have established systems to facilitate dynamics of chromosomes or microtubules by expression of proteins with GFP fluorescence tag (Clarkson & Saint, 1999, Inoue et al., 2004). We describe behavior of chromosomes or chromatids in meiotic divisions and summarize about distribution of homologous chromosomes after premeiotic DNA replication to prophase I. And further, we can also observe other cellular components such as microtubules, actin filaments, endoplasmic reticulum, Golgi apparatuses or mitochondria during male meiosis by a simultaneous expression of proteins with different fluorescence tags. Not only chromosomes but these cellular components also perform dynamic distribution and are equally partitioned in *Drosophila* meiosis. In addition to meiotic divisions, we will also describe here on premeiotic mitoses to generate meiotic spermatocytes. As those cell division, growth and differentiation seen in *Drosophila* spermatogenesis are well conserved among higher eukaryotes, we believe that readers studying on other organisms should also be interested in dynamics of meiotic and premeiotic divisions in *Drosophila* males.

## 2. Chromosome dynamics in *Drosophila* male meiosis

### 2.1 Characteristics of chromosome behavior in male meiosis I

Unlike female meiosis, male meiosis in *Drosophila melanogaster* is unique in the following aspects. No chiasmata formation indicating crossing over is observed in male meiosis. Another consistent observation that synaptonemal complex is not formed at prophase I were also reported (Rasmussen, 1973). Thus, meiotic recombination does not occur in *D. melanogaster* males. Even so, the synapsis formation between homologous chromosomes, its maintenance until metaphase I and bivalent disjunction at anaphase I takes a place properly. In past studies, primary spermatocytes dissected from testis were incubated in a culture condition and living

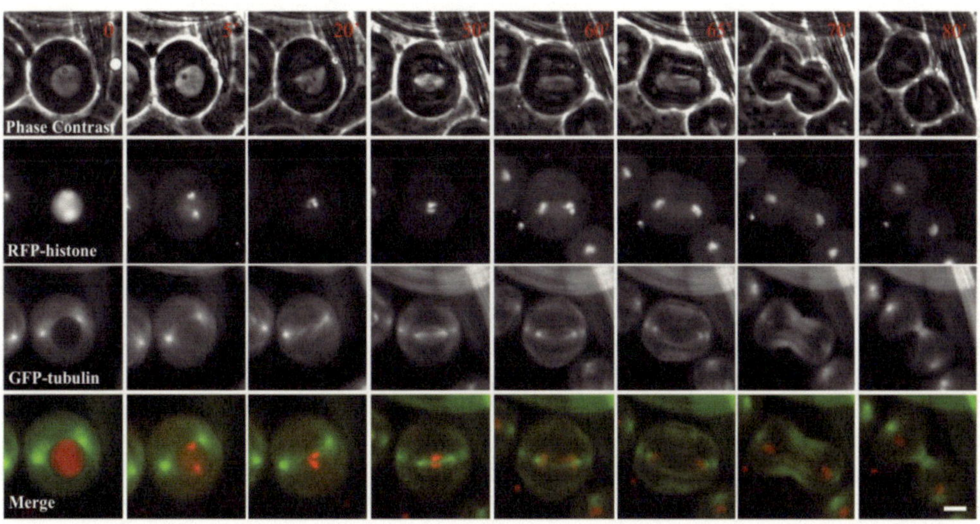


Fig. 2. Time-lapse observation of a living primary spermatocyte expressing GFP-βtubulin and mRFP-Histone2Av simultaneously. Selected fluorescence images of the primary spermatocyte showing chromosomes (red in bottom row, white in second row), microtubules (green in bottom, white in third) and the corresponding phase contrast images to observe cleavage furrow and ER-based cell organelles inside (top). Bar, 10 μm.

spermatocytes were observed under Phase contrast or Differential Interference Contrast (DIC) microscopy equipped video camera (Church & Lin, 1985). In order to trace chromosome behavior together with cell division apparatuses, we have induced simultaneous expression of histone 2Av and βtubulin fused with GFP and mRFP tag, respectively. Time-lapse observation of two kinds of fluorescence makes it possible to examine chromosome behavior such as condensation, congression and segregation as alteration of spindle microtubules (Fig.2).

### 2.1.1 Chromosome dynamics at meiotic prophase I

Vazquez and colleagues described the distribution of homologous chromosomes at premeiotic stage in primary spermatocytes (Vazquez, et al., 2002). They had established fly stocks in which *LacO* sequences from *E. coli* have been inserted into specific sites of *Drosophila* chromosomes. They then induced expression of GFP-LacI repressors to visualize a distribution of two homologous chromosomes within a nucleus. In spermatocytes at G1 phase just after a completion of 16-cell cyst, homologous chromosomes originally distribute closely each other. This is a characteristic known as a somatic pairing commonly observed in insect cells. This distribution of homologous chromosomes is maintained until meiotic prophase through premeiotic DNA replication. What is a molecular mechanism to fulfill the stable bivalent formation in male meiosis? It has been shown that the homologous chromosomes form a synapsis using specific chromosome regions so-called pairing sites. Church and Lin (1985) proposed that the pairing and separation of sex chromosome X-Y bivalents is controlled by a different mechanism from that of autosome bivalents. It was reported that X-Y pairing depends on a specific pairing site on heterochromatin region of sex chromosomes (Cooper, 1964, McKee and Karpen, 1990), while regions required for autosome pairing distribute across the euchromatin region (Ashburner et al., 2004). The X-Y pairing site seems to correspond to the rDNA gene localized in heterochromatin on X and Y chromosomes. The intergenic spacer regions of rDNA gene clusters play a role in X-Y pairing independent on nucleolus formation (McKee et al., 1992). On the other hand, there seems to be no pairing sites in heterochromatin regions of autosomes (Yamamoto, 1979, Ashburner et al., 2004). The autosome bivalents can be paired along entire chromosome regions. Trans-acting factors required for proper execution of meiotic chromosome pairing has also been identified. It was recently reported that a loss of a chromosomal passenger protein, Australin results in defects in chromosome segregation in *Drosophila* male meiosis (Gao et al., 2008). As the Australin is exclusively required for male meiosis, these genetic data is consistent with evidences that chromosome segregation in male meiotic divisions is regulated by different mechanisms from that in females. And further, mutations of *tef* gene encoding a chromatin binding protein with Zn finger disrupted autosomal pairing without affecting X-Y pairing and segregation in male meiosis I (Tomkiel et al., 2001). Common factors essential for the pairing of all chromosomes have been also identified. The *mod(mdg4)* encoding a chromosome binding protein required for segregation of all chromosomes in male meiosis (Soltani-Bejnood et al., 2007). These genetic data suggest that some of molecular mechanisms in meiotic chromosome segregation are different from each other in females and males but others are common in both sexes.

### 2.1.2 Chromosome movement in prometaphase I to telophase I

Church and Lin (1985) examined chromosome movement in meiosis I by time-lapse video microscopy. They observed unpredictable movement and frequent reorientation at prometaphase-like stage before the bivalents achieve a stable bipolar orientation. They described that *Drosophila* primary spermatocyte does not form a well-defined metaphase plate. We have observed four foci of GFP-Histone 2Av corresponding to bivalents between two major autosomes, X-Y chromosomes and tiny $4^{th}$ chromosomes in living primary spermatocytes at prometaphase I (Fig. 2). *Drosophila melanogaster* cells contain 3 major chromosomes and one small chromosome 4. Bivalents of smaller chromosomes are not usually observed because of overlapping with major chromosomes. Those three foci appear to congress into a single chromosome mass at the middle of the primary spermatocytes. Savoian and colleagues found that each chromosome carried out one or more rapid poleward movement with an average velocity of 11.2 ± 1.2 μm/min until bipolar kinetochore attachment (Savoian et. al., 2000, Savoian et al., 2004). However, it is not necessary for anaphase initiation to make all bivalents align at the cell equator. It was also revealed that state of microtubule assembly is surveyed at the M-phase checkpoint, although the checkpoint at male meiosis is less strict than that in somatic cells (Rebollo & Gonzalez, 2000). Past studies reported that chromosome movement at Anaphase I was highly irregular in velocity (Church and Lin, 1985). Savoian and colleagues described that Anaphase I takes 8 ± 1 min and that the chromosomes moved polewards at 1.9 ± 0.1 μm/min after dyad disjoining.

## 3. Dynamics of cytoskeletons and cell organelles as a progression of male meiosis

### 3.1 Dynamics of cytoskeletons in spermatocytes

It is well known that cytoskeletons perform dramatic changes in their structures during cell divisions. In *Drosophila* germline cysts, the most characteristic future concerning cytoskeletons in spermatocytes is a presence of fusome that is a germline specific cell organelle (Hime et al., 1996). This is the F-actin based branching structure containing alpha-Spectrin, ß-Spectrin, adducin-like protein (Hu-li tai shao) and Ankyrin. The fusome traverses cytoplasmic bridges to connect clonally related spermatogonia and premeiotic spermatocytes within a cyst. Male germline stem cells and early spermatogonia contain a spherical type of the fusome, called a spectrosome (Yamashita et al., 2003, Wilson, 2005). During the four rounds mitoses of spermatogonia, the fusome forms one large branched structure that extends though the ring canals into all the cells within a cyst. Before meiotic division I, the characteristic branched structure of fusome has disappeared and its fragmented remnants appear during meiotic divisions. And then similar branched structures devoid of F-actin appear to penetrate post-meiotic ring canals (Hime et al., 1996). It is possible to speculate that these fusome structures play a role in connecting individual spermatogonia with each other and in determination of their division axis as we discuss later.

#### 3.1.1 Actin cytoskeletons

At late anaphase, a contractile ring consisting of F-actin and myosin II is constructed on the middle of cell cortex in spermatocytes. Myosin II moves along the F-actin filaments by using the free energy of ATP hydrolysis. Shrinking of the ring constricts the cell membrane to form a cleavage furrow (Egger et al., 2006). Cytokinesis in spermatogonia mitoses as well as in meiotic divisions terminates incompletely. The cleavage furrow ingression is arrested at the middle of cytokinesis and then the contractile rings transform into cytoplasmic bridges called ring canals.

F-actin or Myosin II is no longer found in the ring canals of spermatocytes but instead large amount of phospho-tyrosin, anillin and septins are contained in the bridge architecture (Hime et al., 19996). It has been revealed that the position of contractile ring formation is determined by central spindles (as a review, Goldberg et al., 1998). The bundle of interdigitated microtubules emanating from both spindle poles formed between the separating homologous chromosomes (Inoue et al., 2004). Interestingly, the actin-based contractile ring shows a cooperative interaction with the central spindle microtubules. Both mutations of *chic* gene encoding a profillin homolog essential for actin polymerization and treatment of testis cells with cytochalasin B showed a similar cytokinesis phenotype. In both cases, not only a formation of the actin-based contractile ring but the central spindle microtubules also failed to be constructed (Giansanti et al., 1998). On the contrary, for example, mutations for *orbit* gene encoding a microtubule-associated protein caused a sever disruption of central spindle microtubules and they also resulted in a failure of cytokinesis devoid of the F-actin rings (Inoue et al., 2004). These results strongly suggest that the central spindle microtubules and the contractile ring consisting actomyosin are interdependent structures, at least during cytokinesis in male meiosis. A molecular mechanism to link these intracellular structures remains to be uncovered. It should be necessary to identify a key molecule(s) to interact directly with both the central spindle microtubules and components of the contractile ring.

### 3.1.2 Microtubule structures

*Drosophila* primary spermatocytes possess characteristic microtubule structures for a preparation of meiotic divisions. Particularly, well-developed astral microtubules become to be prominent as initiation of meiosis I in primary spermatocytes. The astral microtubules are easy to recognize from spindle microtubules that are formed in the nuclear space surrounded by multiple membrane layers known as parafusorial membranes (Tates, 1971, Fuller, 2004, Bonaccorsi et al., 2000). To visualize astral and spindle microtubules and to examine the dynamics of microtubule behaviour in living primary spermatocytes, Inoue and colleagues used a transgenic line ubiquitously expressing GFP-tagged β-tubulin (Inoue et al., 2004). They performed simultaneous observation of multiple cellular structures by DIC microscopy as well as fluorescence microscopy. We presented here several selected figures of a primary spermatocyte undergoing meiosis I simultaneously expressing mRFP-histone 2Av and GFP-βtubulin (Fig. 2). As chromatin inside of nucleus has unevenly distributed at late prophase (t=0 minute), microtubules around both spindle poles become to be prominent. At prometaphase I, four condensed bivalent chromosomes would be observed within a nucleus in which nuclear membrane seems to be intact (t=5, under phase contrast microscope). Only two dyads seem to be in focus in Fig. 2. Developing asters have moved around nuclear membrane as to reach at opposite poles. Then, at 20 minutes later, all chromosome complements congress at the centre of the bipolar spindle structure. At this stage, nuclear morphology has already disintegrated and spindle microtubules free to elongate into inside of nuclear space. The kinetochore microtubules seem to capture the chromosomes and put them in the centre. At onset of anaphase I (t=50), A multilayer of nuclear membrane see as phase-dark structure surrounding around nuclear space separate spindle microtubules including thick kinetochore microtubules from well developed astral microtubules nucleated around each spindle pole. Two populations of central spindle microtubules appear after disjunction of bivalents (t=60 to 70, Fig. 1). A peripheral set of the microtubules elongating from spindle pole regions become more dynamic as if they look for the cytoplasm towards the cell equator (Inoue et al., 2004). Another set of the microtubule bundles corresponding spindle microtubules is localised interiorly at the middle of the cell. The peripheral microtubules from opposite poles met together at equator and form bubble-like structures protruding outwards (t=60). The interior and most of the peripheral central spindles then are released from each pole and they formed independent bundles at the equator (Inoue et al., 2004, Savoian et al., 2004). Furrow ingression was observed soon after the peripheral microtubules from both poles contacted the cell cortex. Thus, we speculate that interaction between the peripheral microtubules and the cell cortex plays a role in determination where and when cleavage furrow ingression initiate in male meiosis.

### 3.2 Mitochondria

It had been believed that inheritance of cytoplasmic organelles such as mitochondria is achieved passively as a consequence of equal cytokinesis (Shima and Warren, 1998). However, it has been described that mitochondria are transmitted toward a daughter cell by the active transport system in fission yeast mitosis (Yaffe et al., 2003). In *Drosophila* male meiosis, the mitochondria line up along nuclear membranes and are equally divided to two daughter cells at each division of *Drosophila* male meiosis (Fuller, 1993). Ichihara and colleagues examined carefully distribution of mitochondria during meiotic divisions in *Drosophila* males (Fig. 3 from Ichihara et al., 2007). At a beginning of prophase (Fig. 3A),

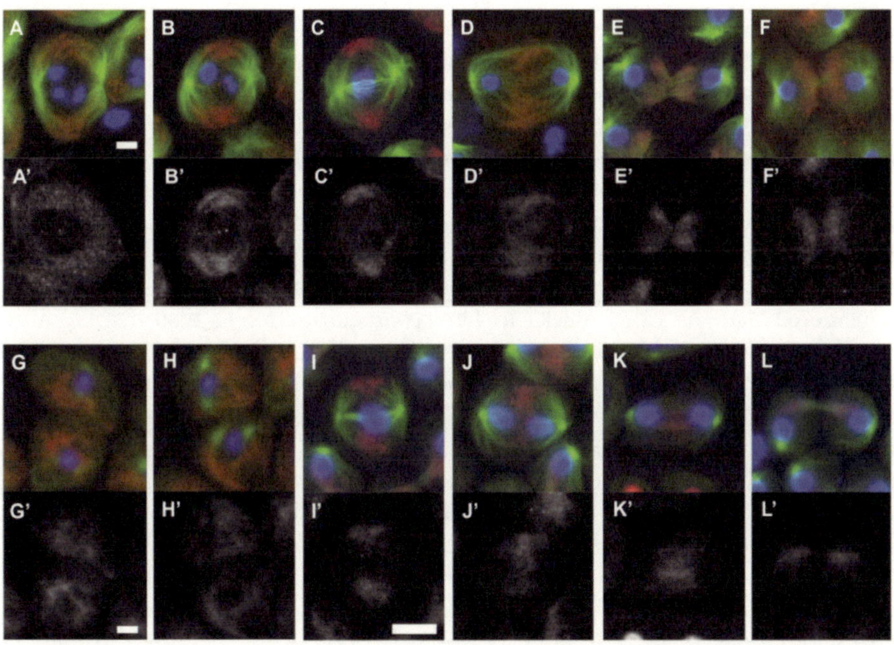


Fig. 3. Distribution of mitochondria with aster and spindle microtubules at meiotic stages in male meiosis I and II. Normal spermatocytes undergoing meiosis I (A-F) or II (G-L) were stained to visualize microtubules (green), mitochondria (red) and chromosomes (blue). Prophase (A, H), prometaphase (B), metaphase (C, I), anaphase A (D, J), anaphase B (E, K), telophase (F, L) and interphase (G), respectively. Bars, 10 μm. These all panels were reprinted from Ichihara et al., (2007).

mitochondria are homogenously distributed throughout cytoplasm. As aster microtubules are developing at prometaphase (Fig. 3B), mitochondria are expelled from inside of the asters and then assembled toward plus ends of aster microtubules. At metaphase, the mitochondria are clustered at the equator of a peripheral cytoplasmic region between facing two asters (Fig. 3C). As central spindle microtubules are formed between separating sister chromatids at anaphase (Fig. 3D), these mitochondria distribute along central spindles as if to decorate the microtubule structures. The mitochondria dispersed into cytoplasm (Fig. 3F), as the central spindles disintegrated. At the end of meiotic division II, mitochondria release from midbody microtubules and assemble to form single large aggregate called Nebenkern (Fig. 1). This transition of mitochondria is regulated by an ordered mode rather than a stochastic partitioning strategy. As spermatozoa require a consumption of higher amount of ATP for the motility, existence of regulation to facilitate equal inheritance of mitochondria in male meiosis may be of advantage that can produce a large number of spermatozoa with homogeneous quality at the same time.

### 3.3 Golgi stacks

During cell division, it was shown that some cell organelles lose their function and are fragmented by modification of their key components (Rabouille and Jokitalo, 2003; Rabouille and Klumperman, 2005). Golgi apparatus in mammalian cells is consisting of flattened membrane-bound compartments. The stacks interconnect each other and form a single large organelle so-called Golgi ribbon beside nucleus. The mammalian Golgi apparatus undergoes disassembly at onset of mitosis and reassembles into the ribbon structure at telophase (Misteli, 1997). A major difference in the Golgi organization between the mammalian and *Drosophila* cells is that a single Golgi ribbon as seen in mammals is not observed in *Drosophila*. Instead, multiple sets of smaller tER-Golgi unit that is a complex consisting of tER site and a piece of Golgi stacks dispersed throughout the cytoplasm (Kondylis & Rabouille, 2009). As membranous intracellular structures such as parafusorial membranes are well developed in spermatocytes (Tates 1971, Fuller, 2003), it is interesting to take up a dynamic behavior of membrane-based organelles in premeiotic and meiotic cells. It is considered that the Golgi stacks in *Drosophila* cultured cells also display a cycle of disassembly and reassembly during mitosis (Kondylis et al., 2007). We also observed carefully distribution of Golgi stack components visualized by immunostaining with antibody against a cis-Golgi protein, GM130 at several meiotic stages (Fig. 4). After spermatocytes initiate meiosis I, the Golgi-derived vesicles seem to increase in the number (compare Fig. 4A with B). The Golgi-derived vesicles were first uniformly distributed throughout the cytoplasm (Fig. 4A). They were then assembled into two groups containing similar amounts of Golgi vesicles prior to chromosome segregation (Fig. 4B). The Golgi vesicles were accumulated around each spindle pole until mid-telophase. At the end of cytokinesis after stage E in Fig. 4, the Golgi vesicles become to be redistributed throughout cytoplasm. These observations remind us equal partition of mitochondria in male meiosis described above. It might be possible to interpret that the Golgi-derived vesicles would be also partitioned equally between two daughter cells in male meiotic divisions. However, it was reported that vesicles containing another Golgi component, Rab11 was concentrated on the Golgi stacks and at the nuclear envelope from prophase to metaphase and that the Golgi-derived vesicles were subsequently accumulated at the cell poles (Giansanti, et al., 2007). At mid-telophase, the vesicles became to concentrate at cell equator possibly to contribute new membrane insertion in cytokinesis. Accumulation of Rab11-containing Golgi vesicles at each cell pole may be no more than storage of vesicles required at cleavage furrow site. Further examinations using other Golgi-related vesicles should be necessary to conclude significance of Golgi-derived vesicle distribution during male meiotic divisions.

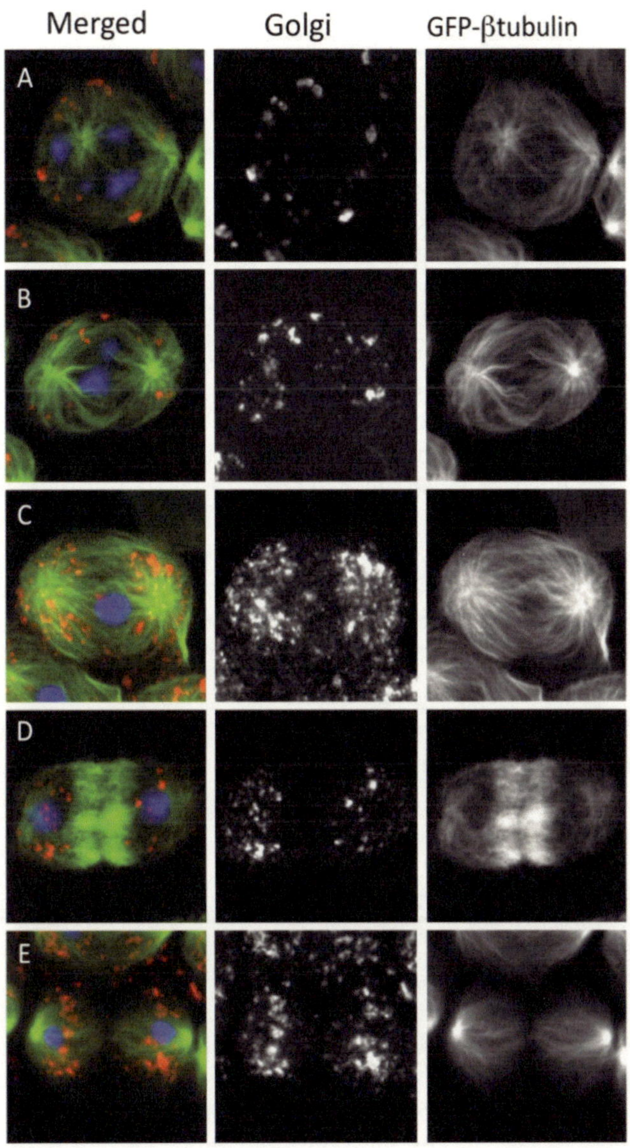


Fig. 4. Immunostainig of primary spermatocytes undergoing meiosis I with antibody against the cis-Golgi protein. Interphase or prophase I (A), prometaphase I (B), metaphase I (C), late anaphase I (D), telophase I (E). (Red) immunostaining with anti-GM130 antibody that recognizes a cis-Golgi protein. (Green) microtubules visualized by GFP-βtubulin, (blue) DNA staining. Prophase (A, H), prometaphase (B), metaphase (C, I), anaphase A (D, J), anaphase B (E, K), telophase (F, L) and interphase (G), respectively. Bars, 10μm

### 3.4 Endoplasmic Reticulum- based structures

Expression of Rtnl1 proteins residing predominantly in endoplasmic reticulum (ER) fused with GFP tag allowed us to observe its dynamics in primary spermatocytes. The ER-residing proteins are distributed on phase-dense structures observed around the nuclear space under phase contrast microscope (Miyauchi and Inoue, unpublished). This observation showed that the ER constructs distinct intracellular structures in spermatocytes during male meiotic divisions. Dorogova and colleagues have reported that ER network has distinctive reticular morphology immediately before initiation of male meiosis (Dorogova et al., 2009). The ER forms concentric circles on the outside of nuclear membrane at meiotic prophase. This ER network then dramatically changes as follows. As a progression of meiotic divisions, the ER networks form multi-layers of branchless membranous sheets appeared as phase-dense structure around nuclear space (Fig. 2 upper row). After prometaphase to telophase, the membranous structure develop very well around astral microtubules. This structure possibly corresponds to cellular organelles known as astral membrane in *Drosophila* embryos. This membranous organelles in embryo seem to be mainly consisted of ER sheets (Bobinnec et al., 2003). The reticular ER structure elongates along a direction of division axis and it transforms into multiple layers of membranes known as spindle envelopes, which surround the nuclear space. These two ER-based structures, astral membranes and spindle envelopes are especially characteristic in male meiotic cells. And they seem to be closely associated with astral microtubules and central spindle microtubules, respectively. These meiotic configurations restore to the reticular distribution around nucleus in next interphase. It is reasonable to speculate that these ER-based structures would interact with other cellular components and may have a role to facilitate dynamic changes of cellular components.

## 4. Identification of genes essential for proper execution of chromosome segregation and cytokinesis in male meiosis

*Drosophila* male meiosis provides us an advantage in examination of chromosome segregation and cytokinesis (Fuller, 1993; Maines and Wasserman, 1998). After a completion of meiotic divisions, every spermatid in a cyst consisting 64 cells contains equally sized single nucleus and a Nebenkern. This should be achieved as a consequence of proper chromosome segregation and cytokinesis in germ line cells. This is a quite convenient and sensitive method to find out those cell division defects in either or both meiotic divisions in living spermatids (Castrillon *et al.*, 1993). Mutants for either chromosome segregation or cytokinesis or even both in male meiotic divisions could easily be distinguished by the spermatid morphology at onion stage. The evidences that the volume of spermatid nuclei is proportional to numbers of chromosome complements allow us to find out defects in chromosome segregation on the base of a presence of different sized spermatids (Gonzalez et al., 1989). A failure of cytokinesis results in generation of spermatids carrying abnormally large Nebenkern and multiple nuclei. Another advantage of *Drosophila* male meiosis is its less strict checkpoint to monitor spindle assembly before metaphase. Even if meiotic cells carry spindle defects, they only delays anaphase onset rather than arresting the cell cycle before metaphase as observed in somatic cells. Therefore, one can examine influence of microtubules on later stages after microtubule assemble checkpoint such as chromosome segregation at anaphase or cytokinesis. After picking up mutant candidates by spermatid morphology, one can perform further careful examination in primary spermatocyte that is the largest proliferative cell. Using this convenient examination system, many of genes required for meiotic divisions have so far been identified. However, disadvantage of the cell type is that mutants for essential genes cannot usually be examined due to their earlier lethality. Hypomorphic mutations that can overcome the lethality at earlier developmental stages are useful for this purpose. And furthermore, we and other group have recently succeeded to perform knockdown experiments by induction of dsRNA for genes in premeiotic spermatocytes using the Gal4/UAS system (Goldbach et al., 2010 , Kitazawa et al., submitted). We put here a partial list of the genes required for meiotic cytokinesis in *Drosophila* male with especial focus on genes involved in a formation of central spindle microtubules and contractile ring (Table 1). The responsible genes for cytokinesis mutants includes genes encoding factors involved in dynamics of actin filaments, microtubules, motor proteins along cytoskeletons and so on. It is well known that spindle microtubules and contractile rings consisting actomyosin display mutual dependency in construction and function (Giansanti et al., 1998). To understand molecular mechanism of crosstalk between these two cytoskeletons, these *Drosophila* mutants and dsRNA stocks should be valuable genetic tools. These cytokinesis phenotypes appeared in *Drosophila* male meiosis, however, have not been completely confirmed by knockdown experiments in S2 cultured cells (Somma et al., 2002). For example, knockdown of *chic*, *fwd* and *klp3A* that have previously identified as essential genes for male meiosis did not impair cytokinesis of S2 cells treated with dsRNA. It is possible to speculate that a requirement of these gene products might differ from each cell type. It is important to continue comparative studies between somatic cells and meiotic cells for understanding general mechanisms to control cell divisions.

| Protein name | Symbol | Biochemical activity | Cell function | orthologue |
|---|---|---|---|---|
| abnormal spindle | asp | microtubule-associated protein (MAP) | microtubulesorganization & cytokinesis | ASPM(mammal) |
| Adenomatous polyposis coli homolog 2 | Apc2 | adenomatous polyposis coli homolog | centrosome localization in Germline Stem cells (GSCs) | Apc |
| Apc-like | Apc | adenomatous polyposis coli homolog | centrosome localization in GSCs | Apc |
| Anillin | scra | component of the contractile ring | cytokinesis | Anillin |
| arrest | aret | RNA-binding protein | regulation of mRNAs involved in gametogenesis | |
| asterless | asl | centriolar or PCM protein | centrosome organization | |
| aurora B | ial | Serine/Threonine kinase | chromosome condensation and cytokinesis | Aurora B |
| auxilin | aux | Serine/Threonine kinase | cytokinesis | cyclin G associated kinase |

Table 1. Proteins involved in organization of microtubules and actin filaments in *Drosophila* male meiosis.

| Protein name | Symbol | Biochemical activity | Cell function | orthologue |
|---|---|---|---|---|
| bag-of-marbles | bam | Serine/Threonine kinase | spermatogonia deivision | |
| james bond | bond | Serine/Threonine kinase | contractile ring assembly | GNS1/SUR4 (yeast) |
| Btk family kinase at 29A | Btk29A | protein-tyrosine kinase | maintaining the equilibrium between G- and F-actin | Btk |
| Bub1 | bub1 | Serine/Threonine kinase | microtubule assembly checkpoint | Bub1 |
| Centrosomin | cnn | pericentrosomal matrix protein | centrosome organization | CDK5 RAP2(mammal) |
| Chickadee | chic | profilin homolog | regulates polymerization of the actin cytoskeletone | Profilin |
| CIN85 and CD2AP orthologue | cindr | adaptor protein | links cell surface junctions and adhesion proteins | CIN85, CD2AP |
| Cortactin | cortactin | cytoskeletal component | stimulate actin polymerizationx | cortactin |
| courtless | crl | ubiquitin conjugating enzyme | male meiosis | Ubiquitin-conjugating enzyme, E2 |
| diaphanous | dia | Formin homology domain protein | cytokinesis | mDia(mammal) |
| Dynamin related protein 1 | drp1 | Dynamin family | mitochondrial fusion | Dynamin |
| effete | eff | UbcD1 | germline stem cell maintenance | |
| exo84 | exo84 | Cullin repeat | contractile ring constriction | exo8 |
| Fmr1 | Fmr1 | RNA binding | | FMR1 |
| four wheel drive | fwd | Phosholipid kinase | contractile ring constriction | 1-phosphatidylinositol 4-kinase |
| four way stop | fws | | contractile ring constriction | Cog5 |
| Fps oncogene analog | Fps85D | protein tyrosin kinase | protein tyrosin kinase cytoskeletal reorganization | Fps |
| sec8 | sec8 | exocyst complex component | contractile ring constriction | sec8 |
| gilgamesh | gish | Ser/Thr kinase sperm indivisualization | Ser/Thr kinase sperm indivisualization | casein kinase |
| Kinesin-like protein at 61F | klp61F | kinesin-5 family protein | microtubule crosslinking and sliding activities | Eg5 |
| Kinesin-like protein at 3A | klp3A | kinesin-4 family | cytokinesis | KIF4A |
| loquacious | loqs | RNA binding miRNA processing | germline stem cell maintenance | TARBP2 |
| mei-s332 | mei-s332 | Shugoshin related | sister chromatid cohesion | Shugoshin related |

Table 1. Proteins involved in organization of microtubules and actin filament in *Drosophila* male meiosis. (Continuation)

| Protein name | Symbol | Biochemical activity | Cell function | orthologue |
|---|---|---|---|---|
| Mytl | Mytl | protei kinase | meiosis and spermatid differentiation | Mytl |
| off-schedule | ofs | elF4G2 translation initiation | meiosis | elF |
| orientation disrupter | ord | unknown | meiotic sister chromatid cohesion | |
| parkin | park | E3 Ubiquichin ligase | mitochondria organization | parkin |
| pavarotti | pav | kinesin-6 family | spindle organization and cytokinesis | MKLP1 related |
| peanut | pnut | septin family | contractile ring formatioin | septin |
| pebble | pbl | RacGAP50C | cytokinesis | ECT2 |
| pelota | pelo | eRF1 domain protein | male meiosis progression | pelota homolog |
| pericentrin-like protein | cp309 | centriolar proetin | spindle pole organization | pericentrin |
| plk4 | plk4 | Ser/Thr kinase | centriole duplication | plk4 |
| polo | polo | Ser/Thr kinase | cytokinesis central spindle & contractile ring | plk |
| Rab-protein 11 | Rab11 | small GTPase | cytokinesis membrane traffic | Rab11 |
| Rac1 | Rac1 | small G protein | actin filament organization | Rac1 |
| rhomboid-7 | rho-7 | rhomboid family proteinase | mitochondrial fusion in spermatogenesis | PARL protease |
| shutdown | shu | FK506-binding protein domain | germline stem cell regulation | |
| Spageghetti squash | sqh | Myosin regulatory light chain | formation of central spindle & contractile ring | Myosin regulatory light chain |
| Spectrin a | aSpec | cytoskeletal protein | fusome organization | Spectrin a |
| spindle assembly abnormal 6 | sas-6 | centriolar proetin | centrosome duplication | Sas6 |
| sticky | sti | Rho effector kinase | cytokinesis | citron |
| subito | sub | kinesin-like protein | meiosis spindle organization | klp9 |
| Syntaxin 5 | Syx5 | t-SNARE homology | golgi traffic assembly | Syntaxin 5 |
| Transforming growth factor beta at 60A | gbb | TGF ligand | regulate germ line stem cells and other process | TGFb |
| twinstar | tsr | cofilin | meiosis and spermatid differentiation other process | cofillin |
| vibrator | vib | Phosphatidylinositol transfer protein | contractile ring constriction | |
| zipper | zip | myosin heavy chain II | cytokinesis formation of central spindle & contractile ring | Myosin II |

Table 1. Proteins involved in organization of microtubules and actin filament in *Drosophila* male meiosis. (Continuation)

Information about each *Drosophila* gene can be obtained from the flybase by linking to the following URL: http://flybase.org/.

## 5. Signaling pathways to control remarkable cell growth of spermatocytes before meiotic initiation

### 5.1 Cell growth of premeiotic spermatocytes

The *Drosophila* spermatocytes increase in size up to 25 times during 90 hours after premeiotic DNA replication. The cell growth of premeiotic spermatocytes is the largest cell growth among that seen in *Drosophila* proliferative cells. The growth phase of primary spermatocytes is clarified as S1 to S6 stages (Cenci et al., 1994, Bonaccorsi et al., 2000). After four rounds of spermatogonia mitosis to form a 16-cell cyst, premeiotic DNA replication takes a place at first S1 stage. S2 to S6 stage corresponds to extended G2 phase of cell cycle. The later S6 stage is possibly overlapping to meiotic prophase. In later S2 phase known as polar spermatocyte, mitochondria increase in number and form a cluster at opposite side of the nucleus, while nucleus is dislocated from central position. As the cell volume of spermatocytes has gradually increased after the S2 stage, a plenty of genes including testis-specific gene, βtub85D are highly transcribed at the growth stages. Male fertility factors such as KS-1 are highly expressed so that its transcripts become to be visible under phase contrast microscope (Bonaccorsi et al., 2000). Because chromosomes are highly condensed during meiosis and after later spermatogenesis, most of gene products required for meiotic divisions and later spermatogenesis should be expressed in primary spermatocytes before meiotic initiation. The extreme cell growth may be achieved in coordination with enhanced expression and accumulation of proteins required for later cell divisions and development.

### 5.2 Growth factors and signaling cascades to induce spermatocyte growth

As described above, the *Drosophila* spermatocytes have achieved most distinctive cell growth up to 25 times after premeiotic DNA replication. What is a molecular mechanism to induce such an enormous spermatocyte growth? Insulin-like peptides (ILPs) play an important role in induction of somatic cell growth (Brogiolo, et al., 2001, Ikeya et al., 2002). Ueishi and colleagues reported that a loss of ILPs by specific apoptosis induction to insulin-producing cells results in reduced growth of spermatocytes, suggesting that the spermatocyte cell growth is required for ILPs (Rulifson et al., 2000, Ueishi et al., 2009). They further showed that an accumulation of active Akt form phosphorylated by its upstream factor, PDK1 in the growing spermatocytes. A diameter of spermatocytes from mutant males for Insulin Receptor (InR) or IRS orthologue encoded by *chico* gene decreased to 70 % of normal size. These genetic data suggest that the insulin signaling plays an essential role in the remarkable cell growth of spermatocytes (Ueishi et al., 2009). We further examined whether $PI_3$ kinase acting upstream Akt is also involved in cell growth induction. The expression of constitutive active form of $PI_3$ kinase catalytic subunit was induced in spermatogonia to premeiotic spermatocyte stage (Ogata and Inoue unpublished). Such an induced expression results in 14% increase of spermatocytes in diameter. These genetic data strongly suggest that the ILPs and its signaling cascade through $PI_3$ kinase to Akt plays a role in induction of spermatocyte cell growth in *Drosophila*. As mammalian insulin can also activate the Ras-MAP kinase cascade after the Insulin receptor (as a review, Avruch, 1998), we further examine whether Ras signaling cascade acting downstream of Drosophila Insulin Receptor homologue (InR) is also involved in the cell growth of spermatocytes before male meiosis. Constitutively activated mutation for Ras85D, $Ras85D^{v12}$ (Kim et al., 2006) also induced approximately 10 % increase of cell diameter in length (Ogata and Inoue, unpublished). Therefore, these genetic data suggest that both $PI_3K$-

Akt cascade and Ras-MAP kinase cascades acting downstream of InR are essential for induction of the premeiotic spermatocyte growth.

## 6. Asymmetric division of germline stem cells and directional divisions of spermatogonia before meiosis

At the tip of the testis in adult *Drosophila* males, several germline stem cells (GSCs) can be observed. The GSCs receive a signal to maintain their stem cell characteristics secreted from the adjoining hub cells. A ligand protein encoded by the *unpaired* gene is used as the maintenance signal and the signal is transmitted through the JAK-STAT signaling cascade (Kiger, *et al.*, 2001, Tulina & Matunis, 2001). A proximal cell of the two daughter cells derived from an asymmetric division of the GSC exclusively receives the signal and becomes a self-renewed GSC. For self-renewal and differentiation of GSC daughters, it is crucial to set up cell division axis perpendicular to a cluster of the hub cells (Yamashita et al., 2003). What is a molecular mechanism to set up the spindle axis perpendicular? It was shown that mother centrosome in GSC remains to be positioned at the cell cortex contiguous to the hub cells and that daughter centrosome derived from duplication of the mother in GSCs is released from the cortex and migrates toward an opposite pole (Yamashita et al., 2007). The distal daughter cell derived from a GSC division leaves the niche and differentiates as a spermatogonium.

The spermatogonium then initiates four times of cell cycles to generate a cyst consisting of 16 cells. Every spermatogonium in a cyst undergoes these four rounds of cell division synchronously. The orientation of these spermatogonia divisions rotates at 90 degree in every mitosis. Like GSCs, it is possible to speculate that a daughter centrosome derived from the mother anchored to the fusome is free from a connection with the fusome extended over spamatogonia within a cyst and thus it could migrate toward an opposite pole until prometaphase. In this way, spermatogonia could alternate division orientation at 90 degree in every cell division. Such unusual mitoses may be advantageous to store a cyst containing constant numbers of spermatogonia within a limited space of testis.

## 7. Future researches

The primary spermatocyte is considered as one of the cells most thoroughly examined about cell division together with a S2 cultured cell. In addition to genetic analyses using hypomorphic mutants viable up to developmental stages in which male meiosis can be observed, targeted knockdown of all most of the *Drosophila* genes currently became to be possible in spermatocytes. We can expect that saturation genetic studies to examine variety of phenotypes should be frequently carried out near future. It should be fruitful for us to collect whole information about cell phenotypes appeared in primary spermatocytes from such large scale knock down experiments. These efforts would certainly increase value of male meiotic cell as a model cell for researches on cell proliferation and growth. As the primary spermatocytes have some specific futures in terms of intracellular structures or cell cycle regulation, it is necessary to perform comparative studies using common cultured cells for confirmation of genetic results obtained in male meiotic cells. For more detailed real-time observation to examine dynamics of multiple cellular components simultaneously during male meiosis, it is important to develop cultured system to make it possible to do longer observation from spermatogonial stage to onion stage of spermatid. We currently succeeded to carry out continuous observation from onset of meiosis to onion stage spermatids. It is also necessary to establish *Drosophila* stocks to induce simultaneous expression of several cellular components fused with different fluorescence tag, GFP, mRFP or CFP. They allow us to perform multi-color time lapse observation that would make it possible to trace alterations of chromosomes, microtubules or actin filaments and other cellular organelles in a single cell. Such a new observation system should stimulate understanding of dynamic feature of male meiosis in *Drosophila*. As a series of cellular events such as cell division, growth, elongation and differentiation in spermatogenesis is considerably conserved between *Drosophila* and mammals (Zhou and Griswold, 2008), we expect that *Drosophila* data would also bring us valuable information to help better understanding of mammalian spermatogenesis.

## 8. Conclusion

In this chapter, we conclude that *Drosophila* primary spermatocytes undergoing meiosis I is an excellent model cell to examine dynamics of chromosomes and other cellular components such as cell organelles and cytoskeletons. Although chiasmata formation and homologous recombination does not occur in *Drosophila* male meiosis, we can study on more simple chromosome pairing and segregation of homologous chromosomes. We showed a simultaneous observation of chromosomes, microtubules and cell organelles in living primary spermatocytes expressing proteins fused with different fluorescence tags. Microtubules and actin filaments display dynamic alterations as a progression of male meiotic divisions. Furthermore, our observation indicates cell organelles such as mitochondria or golgi foci are also transmitted equally toward two daughter cells dependent on microtubule structures. By examination of hypomorphic mutants or knockdown spermatocytes, it have been shown that a plenty of cell cycle related genes including many novel genes play a important role in male meiotic divisions. Before initiation of meiotic division I, the cells achieve largest extent of cell growth in *Drosophila*. We also discussed molecular mechanisms to induce the distinct cell growth of premeiotic spermatocytes by insulin-like peptides, their signaling pathways and other related pathways showing crosstalk with the insulin cascade. In addition to male meiotic divisions, we briefly referred four round premeiotic divisions of spermatogonia to generate a 16-cell cyst and discussed about its regulatory mechanism. These mitoses are synchronous cell divisions in which spindle axis rotate by 90 degree in every division. Animal meiosis is a part of development programs in gametogenesis. It is basically different from yeast meiosis that can be induced by environment cues. *Drosophila* male provides us a good model to understand common molecular mechanisms to control animal meiosis.

## 9. Acknowledgment

We would like to acknowledge L. Cooley, E. Mathe, R. Saint, and Bloomington stock center, Drosophila Genetic Resource Center, Vienna Drosophila RNAi Center, for providing fly stocks and This work was partially supported by Grants-in-Aid for Scientific Research on Priority Area and Grants-in-Aid for Scientific Research (C) to Y.H.I.

## 10. References

Ashburner, M., Golic, K. G. & Hawley R. S. (2004) Male meiosis, *Drosophila. A Laboratory Handbook, 2nd ed.* pp.827-860. Cold Spring Harbor Laboratory Press, ISBN0-87969-706-7, NewYork, USA

Avruch, J. (1998). *Insulin signal transduction through protein kinase cascades Mol.Cell. Biochem.* 182: pp.31–48, 1998. doi:10.1023/A:1006823109415

Bobinnec, Y., Marcaillou, C., Morin, X. & Debec. A. (2003). Dynamics of the endoplasmic reticulum during early development of *Drosophila* melanogaster. *Cell Motil Cytoskeleton.* 54: 217-225. doi: 10.1002/cm.10094

Bonaccorsi, S., Giansanti, M.G., Cenci, G., and Gatti, M. (2000). Cytological analysis of spermatocytes growth and male meiosis in *Drosophila melanogaster.* In: *Drosophila* Protocol. (W. Sullivan, M. Ashburner, R. S. Hawley, eds.) Cold Spring Harbor Laboratory Press, ISBN0-87969-584-4, Cold Spring Harbor, New York, pp 87-109.

Castrillon, D.H., Gonczy, P., Alexander, S., Rawson, R., Eberhart, C.G., Viswanathan, S., DiNardo, S., & Wasserman, S.A. (1993). Toward a molecular genetic analysis of spermatogenesis in Drosophila melanogaster: characterization of male-sterile mutants generated by single P element mutagenesis. *Genetics* 135: 489-505.

Cenci, G., Bonaccorsi, S., Pisano, C., Verni, F., and Gatti, M. (1994). Chromatin and microtubule organization during premeiotic, meiotic and early postmeiotic stages of *Drosophila melanogaster* spermatogenesis. *J. Cell Sci.* 107: 3521-3534.

Cooper, K. W. (1964). Meiotic conjunctive elements not involving chiasmata. *Proc. Natl. Acad. Sci.* 52:1248-1255. doi:10.1073/pnas.52.5.1248

Church, K. & Lin, H. P. (1985) Kinetochore microtubules and chromosome movement during prometaphase in *Drosophila melanogaster* spermatocytes studied in life and with the electron microscope. *Chromosoma* 92: 273-282. doi:10.1007/BF00329810

Drogova, N. V., Nerusheva, O. O. & Omelyanchuk, L. V. (2009). Structural organization and dynamics of the endoplasmic Reticulum during spermatogenesis of Drosophila melanogaster: Studies using PDI-GFP chimera protein. *Biochemistry (Moscow)* :55-61.

Duffy, J. B. GAL4 system in *Drosophila.* (2002) A fly geneticist's swiss army knife. *Genesis* 34:1–15. doi:10.1002/gene.10150.

Eggert, U. S., Kiger, A. A., Richter, C., Perlman, Z. E., Perrimon, N., Mitchison, T. J., & Field, C. M. (2004) Parallel Chemical Genetic and Genome-Wide RNAi Screens Identify Cytokinesis Inhibitors and Targets. *PLoS Biol.* 2: e379. doi:10.1371/journal.pbio.0020379

Fuller, M.T., & Spradling, A.C. (2007). Male and female *Drosophila* GSCs: two versions of immortality. *Science,* 316: 402-404. doi:10.1126/science.1140861

Fuller, M.T. (1993). Spermatogenesis, In The development of *Drosophila.* (M. Bate, and A. Martinez-Arias, eds.) Cold Harbor Laboratory Press, Cold Spring Harbor, New York, pp 71-147.

Gao, S., Giansanti, M.G., Buttrick, G.J., Ramasubramanyan, S., Auton, A., Gatti, M., & Wakefield, J.G. (2008). Australin: a chromosomal passenger protein required specifically for Drosophila melanogaster male meiosis. *J. Cell Biol.* 180: 521--535. doi:10.1083/jcb.200708072

Giansanti, M.G., Bonaccorsi, S., Williams, B., Williams, E.V., Santolamazza, C., Goldberg, M.L., & Gatti, M. (1998). Cooperative interactions between the central spindle and the contractile ring during *Drosophila* cytokinesis. *Genes Dev.* 12: 396-410. doi:10.1101/gad.12.3.396.

Giansanti, M. G., Belloni, G. & Gatti, M. (2007). Rab11 Is Required for Membrane Trafficking and Actomyosin Ring Constriction in Meiotic Cytokinesis of *Drosophila* Males. *Mol Biol Cell.* 18: 5034–5047. 2007. doi:10.1091/mbc.E07-05-0415

Goldbach, P., Wong, W., Beise, N., Sarpal, R., Trimble, W. S., & Brill, J. A. (2010). Stabilization of the actomyosin ring enables spermatocyte sytokinesis in *Drosophila*. *Mol. Biol. Cell,* 21, 1482-1493. doi: 10.1091/mbc.E09-08-0714.

Goldberg, M.L., K.C. Gunsalus, R.E. Karess, and F. Chang. (1998). Cytokinesis. In *Dynamics of Cell Division*. S.A. Endow and D.M. Glover, editors. Oxford University Press, Oxford. 270–316.

Gonzalez, C., Casal, J., & Ripol, P. 1989. Relationship between chromosome content and nuclear diameter in early spermatids of *Drosophila melanogaster*. Genet. Res.54: 205-212. doi: 10.1017/S0016672300028664.

Hime, G.R., Brill, J.A., & Fuller, M.T. (1996). Assembly of ring canals in the male germ line from structural components of the contractile ring. *J. Cell Sci.***109**: 2779--2788.

Ikeya, T., Galic, M., Belawat, P., Nairz,K., & Hafen, E. 2002. Nutrient-dependent expression of Insulin-like peptides from neuroendocrine cells in the CNS contributes to growth regulation in *Drosophila*. *Curr biol.*, 12: 1293-1300. doi:10.1016/S0960-9822(02)01043-6

Ichihara, K., Shimizu, H., Taguchi, O., Yamaguchi, M., & Inoue, Y. H. (2007). A *Drosophila* orthologue of Larp protein family is required for multiple processes in male meiosis. *Cell Struct. Funct.* 32: 89-100. doi:10.1247/csf.07027

Inoue, Y.H., Savoian, M. Suzuki, T. Yamamoto, M., & Glover, D.M.. (2004). Mutation in *orbit/mast*, reveal that the central spindle is comprised of two microtubule populations; those that initiate cleavage and those that propagate furrow ingression. *J. Cell Biol.* 116: 1-12. doi: 10.1083/jcb.200402052

Jean Maines, S.W., & Wasserman, S. (1998). Regulation and execution of meiosis in *Drosophila* males. *Curr. Top. Dev. Biol.* 37: 301-332.

Kondylis, V., tot Pannerden, H.E., Herpers, B., Friggi-Grelin, F. & Rabouille, C. (2007) The golgi comprises a paired stack that is separated at G2 by modulation of the actin cytoskeleton through Abi and Scar/WAVE. *Dev. Cell.* 12, 901–915. doi:10.1016/j.devcel.2007.03.008

Kondylis V and Rabouille C. (2009). The Golgi apparatus: Lessons from *Drosophila. FEBS Letters.* 3827-3838. doi:10.1016/j.febslet.2009.09.048

Kim, M., Lee, J.H., Koh, H., Lee, S.Y., Jang, C., Chung, C.J., Sung, J.H., Blenis, J., Chung, J. (2006). Inhibition of ERK-MAP kinase signaling by RSK during *Drosophila* development. EMBO J. 25(13): 3056--3067. doi:10.1038/sj.emboj.7601180

Kiger, A.A., Jones, D.L., Schulz, C., Rogers, M.B., and Fuller, M.T. (2001). Stem cell self-renewal specified by JAK-STAT activation in response to a support cell cue. *Science,* 294: 2542-2545. doi:10.1126/science.1066707

McKee B.D., Habera L, Vrana J.A. (1992). Evidence that intergenic spacer repeats of *Drosophila* melanogaster rRNA genes function as X-Y pairing sites in male meiosis, and a general model for achiasmatic pairing. *Genetics.* 132:529-544.

Mckee B.D., and G. Karpen, *Drosophila* ribosomal RNA genes function as an X-Y meiotic pairing site. *Cell* 61 (1990), pp. 61–72. doi:10.1016/0092-8674(90)90215-Z

Misteli, T. (1997). The mammalian Golgi apparatus during M-phase. *Prog. Cell Cycle Res.* 2: 267, pp.267-277, doi:0.1007/978-1-4615-5873-6_24

Pandey, R. Heidmann, S. Lehner, C.F. (2005). Epithelial re-organization and dynamics of progression through mitosis in *Drosophila* separase complex mutants. *J. Cell Sci.* 118: pp.733--742

Rabouille, C. Jokitalo, E. (2003). Golgi apparatus partitioning during cell division. *Mol. Membr. Biol.* 20: pp.117-27. doi:10.1080/0968768031000084163

Rabouille, C. & Klumperman, J. (2005). The maturing role of COPI vesicles in intra-Golgi transport. *Nat Rev Mol Cell Biol.* 6: 812-817. doi:10.1038/nrm1735

Rebollo, E., & Gonzalez, C. (2000). Visualising the spindle checkpoint in *Drosophila. EMBO Report.* 1: 65-70. doi:10.1093/embo-reports/kvd011

Rulifson, E.J., Kim, S.K., & Nusse, R. (2002). Ablation of insulin-producing neurons in flies: growth and diabetic phenotypes. *Science,* 296: 1118-1120. doi:10.1126/science.1070058

Rasmussen, S. W. (1973). Ultrastructural studies of spermatogenesis in *Drosophila* nelanogaster Meigen. Z. Zellforsch. 140, 125-144. doi:10.1007/BF00307062

Savoian, M.S., Goldberg, M.L., & Rieder, C.L. (2000). The rate of poleward chromosome motion is attenuated in *Drosophila zw10* and *rod* mutants. Nat. Cell Biol.2: 948—952. doi:10.1038/35046605

Somma, M. P. Fasulo, B. Cenci, G. Cundari, E. & Gatti, M. (2002). Molecular dissection of cytokinesis by RNA interference in *Drosophila* cultured cells. *Mol Biol Cell.* 13, pp.2448–2460. doi: 10.1091/mbc.01-12-0589

Soltani-Bejnood, M. Thomas, S. E. Villeneuve, L. Schwartz, K. Hong, C-S. & McKee, B. D. (2007). Role of the mod(mdg4) common region in homolog segregation in *Drosophila* male meiosis. *Genetics* 176(1): 161—180. doi:10.1534/genetics.106.063289

Shima, D.T., & Warren, G. (1998). Inheritance of the cytoplasm during cell division. In *Dynamics of cell division.* (S.A. Endow, and D.M. Glover eds.) Oxford Press, Oxford, pp 248-269.

Savoian, M.S. Gatt, M.K. Riparbelli, M.G. Callaini, G. & Glover, D.M. (2004). *Drosophila* KLP67A is required for proper chromosome congression and segregation during meiosis I. *J. Cell Sci.* 117: 3669-3677. doi:10.1242/jcs.01213

Tates, A.D. (1971). Cytodifferentiation during spermatogenesis in *Drosophila melanogaster.* An electron microscope study. Ph.D. thesis, Rijksuniversiteit, Leiden.

Ueishi S, Shimizu H, & Inoue Y. H. (2009). Male germline stem cell division and spermatocyte growth require insulin signaling in *Drosophila. Cell Struct Funct.* 34, 61-9. doi:10.1247/csf.08042

Tomkiel, J.E., Wakimoto, B.T., & Briscoe, A. (2001). The *teflon* gene is required for maintenance of autosomal homolog pairing at meiosis I in male *Drosophila melanogaster. Genetics* 157(1): 273--281.

Vazquez, J., Belmont, A. S., & Sedat, J. W. (2002). The dynamics of homologous chromosome pairing during Male *Drosophila* Meiosis. *Cur. Biol.,* 12, 1473-1483. doi:10.1016/S0960-9822(02)01090-4

White-Cooper, H. (2004). Spermatogenesis, Analysis of meiosis and morphogenesis. *Methods Mol.Biol.* 247: 45-75.

Wilson, P.G., (2005). Centrosome inheritance in the male germ line of *Drosophila* requires hu-li tai-shao function. *Cell Biol. Int.* 29, 360–369. doi:10.1016/j.cellbi.2005.03.002

Tulina, N., and Matunis, E. (2001). Control of stem cell self-renewal in *Drosophila* spermatogenesis by JAK-STAT signaling. *Science,* 294, 2546-2549. doi:10.1126/science.1066700

Yaffe, M.P., Stuurman, N., and Vale, R.D. (2003). Mitochondrial positioning in fission yeast is driven by association with dynamic microtubules and mitotic spindle poles. *Proc. Natl. Acad. Sci. U. S. A.* 100, 11424-11428.

Yamashita, Y.M. Jones, D. L. Fuller, M. T. (2003) Orientation of asymmetric stem cell division by the APC Tumor Suppressor and Centrosome. Science 301: pp. 1547-1550. DOI: 10.1126/science.1087795

Yamashita, Y.M., Mahowald, A/P. Perlin J.R. & Fuller, M.T. (2007). Asymmetric inheritance of mother versus daughter centrosome in stem cell division. *Science,* 315: 518-521. doi:10.1126/science.1134910

Yamamoto, M. (1979). Cytological studies of heterochromatin function in the *Drosophila melanogaster* male: Autosomal meiotic pairing. Chromosoma 72:293-328. doi:10.1007/BF00331091

Zhou, Q. & Griswold, M.D. (2008) Regulation of spermatogonia, StemBook, ed. The Stem Cell Research Community, StemBook, doi/10.3824/stembook.1.7.1

# 5

# Sex Chromosomes and Meiosis in Spiders: A Review

Douglas Araujo[1], Marielle Cristina Schneider[2], Emygdio Paula-Neto[3] and Doralice Maria Cella[3]
[1]*Universidade Estadual de Mato Grosso do Sul-UEMS, Unidade Universitária de Ivinhema,*
[2]*Universidade Federal de São Paulo-UNIFESP, Campus Diadema,*
[3]*Universidade Estadual Paulista-UNESP, Campus Rio Claro,*
*Brazil*

## 1. Introduction

According to Platnick (2011), the order Araneae possesses 110 families, 3,849 genera, and 42,473 species. It is divided into two suborders: Mesothelae, consisting of only one family (Liphistiidae), and Opisthothelae. The latter suborder is divided into two infra-orders: Mygalomorphae, consisting of spiders with paraxial chelicerae, and Araneomorphae, consisting of spiders with diaxial chelicerae. The latter infra-order is divided into the basal clades (Hypochilidae and Austrochiloidea), Haplogynae, and Entelegynae, which includes the majority of extant spiders (Coddington & Levi, 1991) (Fig. 1).

In the first cytogenetic studies in spiders performed by Carnoy (1885), gonads of male or female individuals were imbedded in paraffin, sectioned, and stained with Heidenhain's iron haematoxylin. Chromosome visualisation and interpretation of cytogenetic analyses were difficult to achieve with this method. Decades later, Sharma et al. (1959) and Beçak & Beçak (1960) were the first researchers to obtain spider chromosomes by the aceto-orcein or aceto-carmin squash methods.

Pinter & Walters (1971) introduced the use of colchicine solution for cytological preparations of spider testes and ovaries. This solution promotes an increase in the number of cells in mitotic and/or meiotic metaphase, the stage in which chromosomes are most easily visualised and identified. In the same decade, Brum-Zorrila & Cazenave (1974) applied 3:1 methanol:acetic acid as a fixative solution and Giemsa solution as a stain.

Matsumoto (1977) pioneered the observation of chromosomes in spider embryos. Embryos are a valuable source of mitotic metaphase cells due to the high rate of cellular division that occurs during embryonic development. There are a number of tissues that can be used in cytogenetic studies of spiders, such as gonads (testes and ovaries), cerebral ganglion, and cultured blood cells, as described by Wang & Yan (2001).

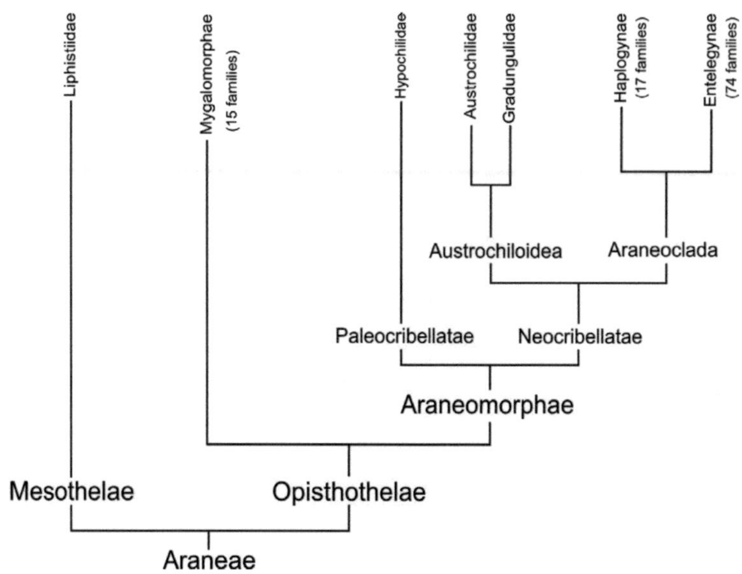


Fig. 1. Phylogenetic relationships within major clades of spiders according to Coddington & Levi (1991). The number of families was determined according to Platnick (2011).

The gonads, especially the testes, have been found to be more suitable than other tissues for karyotype analysis in the vast majority of cytogenetic investigations. Analysis of gonads allows both mitotic and meiotic chromosomes to be studied. In addition to data regarding the diploid number, length, and morphology of chromosomes, analyses of chromosomes during meiosis have contributed to the identification of types of sex chromosome systems (SCS) in spiders. This is very important in the case of Araneae due to the diversity of simple or multiple SCS that have been recorded in representatives of this order. Furthermore, in investigations of mitotic cells, it is not possible to recognise certain types of SCS, such as X0 and $X_1X_2Y$, by only taking into account the difference in the diploid number observed in male and female individuals. However, analysis of meiotic cells allows investigation of the behaviour of chromosomes in relation to association, synapsis, recombination, and segregation. These features are indispensable for understanding the origin and evolution of sex chromosomes.

## 2. Sex chromosome systems (SCS) in spiders

Currently, there are 678 cytogenetic records in spiders (www.arthropodacytogenetics.bio.br/spiderdatabase). Of these, 456 species (67.3%) have an SCS of the $X_1X_20$ type; 105 species (15.5%) have an X0 system; 59 species (8.7%) have an $X_1X_2X_30$ system; 10 species (1.5%) have an SCS of the $X_1X_2Y$ type; 5 species (0.7%) have an $X_1X_2X_3X_40$ system; 5 species (0.7%) have an XY SCS; 5 species (0.7%) have an SCS of the $X_1X_2X_3Y$ type; 1 species (0.1%) has an SCS of the $X_1X_2X_3X_4X_5Y$ type; and 1 species exhibits variations of a multiple $X_nY_n$ SCS. In 31 species (4.6%), the SCS has not been identified (Fig. 2). The number of cytogenetic records (678) in spiders is slightly higher than the number of spider species analysed chromosomally (665) because more than one type of SCS has been registered for some species.

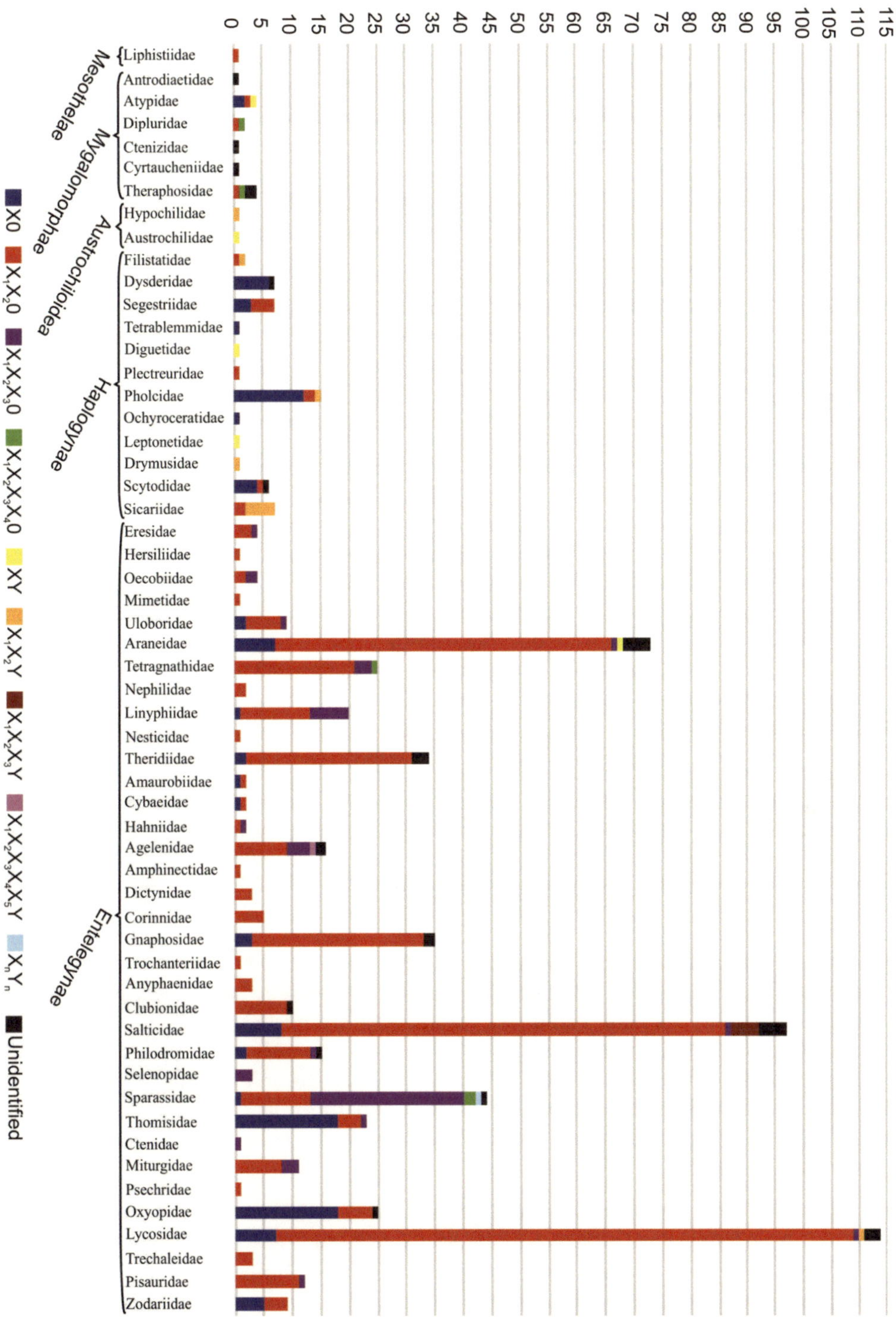


Fig. 2. Distribution of sex chromosome systems within cytogenetically characterised spider families.

### 2.1 Meiotic behaviour of sex chromosomes

The pioneering works describing the $X_1X_20$ and X0 SCS in spiders were those of Wallace (1900, 1905) and Berry (1906), respectively. These researchers identified the sex chromosomes based on the positive heteropycnotic behaviour of these elements during meiosis (Fig. 3). According to White (1940), the term heteropycnosis was introduced to describe the different levels of condensation and staining that certain chromosomes exhibit in the course of mitosis and/or meiosis. This heteropycnotic pattern can be positive or negative, and it is related to a high or low degree of chromosome condensation, respectively.

Manifestation of heteropycnosis is commonly visualised in the sex chromosomes, especially in male meiotic cells; the high level of chromosome condensation in these cells seems to prevent recombination between nonhomologous regions of heteromorphic sex chromosomes (McKee & Handel, 1993). However, the autosomes and female sex chromosomes can also exhibit chromatin differentiation in some stages of the cell cycle.

In spider spermatogenesis, a heteropycnotic pattern of the sex chromosomes has been recorded for roughly 25% of the species that have been cytogenetically examined, which belong to different suborders (Mygalomorphae and Araneomorphae) and families. Regardless of the type of SCS, 95% of these spider species showed positively heteropycnotic sex chromosomes in premeiotic interphase and prophase I nuclei (Fig. 3a-c, e-g, i-m) and, occasionally, also in metaphase II cells (Fig. 3d). In late meiotic stages, the sex chromosomes usually appeared to be isopycnotic (Fig. 3o-p). The heteropycnotic pattern of sex chromosomes can be used as an additional criterion to determine the type of SCS in spiders, as the number of positive heteropycnotic corpuscles frequently corresponds to the number of sex chromosomes.

It is of note that in some SCS that were originated through relatively recent rearrangements between autosomes and sex chromosomes, such as the $X_1X_2X_3Y$ system of *Evarcha hoyi* (under *Pellenes hoyi*) (Maddison, 1982), the $X_nY_n$ system observed in *Delena cancerides* (Rowell, 1985), and the $X_1X_2X_3X_4X_5Y$ system found in *Malthonica ferruginea* (Král, 2007), only the ancient sex chromosomes exhibit positive heteropycnosis in the course of male meiosis.

Recently, positive heteropycnotic behaviour of one autosomal bivalent was verified during male meiosis of some spiders belonging to the families Dipluridae, Theraphosidae (Mygalomorphae), Diguetidae, and Sicariidae (basal Araneomorphae). According to Král et al. (2006, 2011), this bivalent could represent sex chromosomes in an early stage of differentiation because in addition to positive heteropycnosis, this bivalent showed a recurrent association with the sex chromosomes during the initial prophase I substages. Conclusive proof of the relationship between this homomorphic chromosome pair and sex determination has been obtained through ultrastructural chromosome analysis of the synaptonemal complex.

The modes of sex chromosome association and segregation are interesting features to investigate in meiotic cells. In spiders with an XY SCS, the sex chromosomes can present associations that vary from chiasmatic, such as those found in *Leptoneta infuscata* (Leptonetidae), to terminal pairing, such as in *Diguetia albolineata* and *Diguetia canities* (Diguetidae) (Král et al. 2006). An achiasmatic terminal association of the sex chromosomes has been recorded in some basal Araneomorphae with $X_1X_2Y$ SCS. In representatives of the families Drymusidae, Filistatidae, Hypochilidae, Pholcidae, and Sicariidae, in which all sex chromosomes are biarmed, the arms of the metacentric X chromosomes showed end-to-end pairing (Fig. 3n) with arms of the tiny Y chromosome (Oliveira et al. 1997, Silva et al. 2002, Král et al. 2006). In contrast, in *Pholcus phalangioides* (Pholcidae), which carries a submetacentric $X_2$ chromosome, only one arm of this sex chromosome was terminally paired with the Y chromosome (Král et al. 2006).

In derivative araneomorphs that possess other types of multiple SCS, such as $X_1X_2X_3Y$ and $X_1X_2X_3X_4X_5Y$, in which the sex chromosomes do not show a high degree of morphological and/or structural differentiation due to their recent origin, the association of the sex chromosomes during meiosis can be chiasmatic between some elements and achiasmatic between others. In the $X_1X_2X_3Y$ SCS of *E. hoyi*, an interstitial or terminal chiasma was present between one arm of the large submetacentric Y chromosome and the long arm of the acrocentric $X_2$ chromosome (Maddison, 1982). In *M. ferruginea* (Agelenidae), the $X_1$, $X_2$, and $X_3$ sex chromosomes appeared as univalents that were terminally associated with the $X_4X_5Y$ trivalent; this trivalent was composed of one large-sized Y chromosome and two small-sized acrocentric X chromosomes. Although Král (2007) did not register the presence of chiasma between these sex chromosomes due to the precocious dissociation of these elements during prophase I, ultrastructural analysis revealed the occurrence of a recombination nodule in the $X_4X_5Y$ trivalent.

From the zygotene stage to metaphase I, the X chromosomes of multiple X SCS usually present a parallel disposition (Fig. 3 e-g, j-l), without evidence of chiasmata, and proximity between each X chromosome commonly involves the centromere region (Král et al. 2011). Occasionally, in some mygalomorph species of the family Theraphosidae, the sex chromosomes of the $X_1X_2X_3X_40$ system exhibit an end-to-end association ($X_1X_2Y$-like pairing), and in representatives of the family Dipluridae, the sex chromosomes can appear as univalent elements that are highly condensed and separated. In addition, an $X_1X_2Y$-like pairing of the sex chromosomes has been observed in *Stegodyphus lineatus* (Eresidae) and *Pax islamita* (Zodariidae), which are carriers of the $X_1X_2X_30$ and $X_1X_20$ SCS, respectively (Král et al. 2011).

Contrary to data revealed by conventional chromosome analyses, in which the sex chromosomes of multiple X systems appeared to exhibit a simple behaviour that involved only parallel pairing, more recent cytogenetic ultrastructural studies have supplied surprising information. Benavente and Wettstein (1980) were the first to describe the presence of junctional lamina between the $X_1$ and $X_2$ sex chromosomes of *Schizocosa malitiosa* (under *Lycosa malitiosa*); this junctional lamina was structurally similar to the synaptonemal complex, formed in the early substages of prophase I, and persisted to the late substages.

Wise (1983) also encountered evidence of a junctional lamina in prophase I in two carriers of the $X_1X_20$ system, *Allocosa georgicola* (under *Lycosa georgicola*) and *Rabidosa rabida* (under *Lycosa rabida*). Furthermore, a terminal association between sex chromosomes and one homomorphic bivalent was observed in *S. malitiosa* and *A. georgicola*. However, the association between sex chromosomes and a homomorphic bivalent was only explained in recent ultrastructural analyses of *Pardosa morosa* (Lycosidae) and the agelenids *Malthonica campestris* and *Malthonica silvestris* performed by Král (2007) and Král et al. (2011). These studies indicated that this homomorphic bivalent is an element that belongs to the SCS; that is, the system included one pair of homomorphic sex chromosomes in addition to the morphologically differentiated $X_1$ and $X_2$ or $X_1$, $X_2$ and $X_3$ sex chromosomes (Fig. 3h).

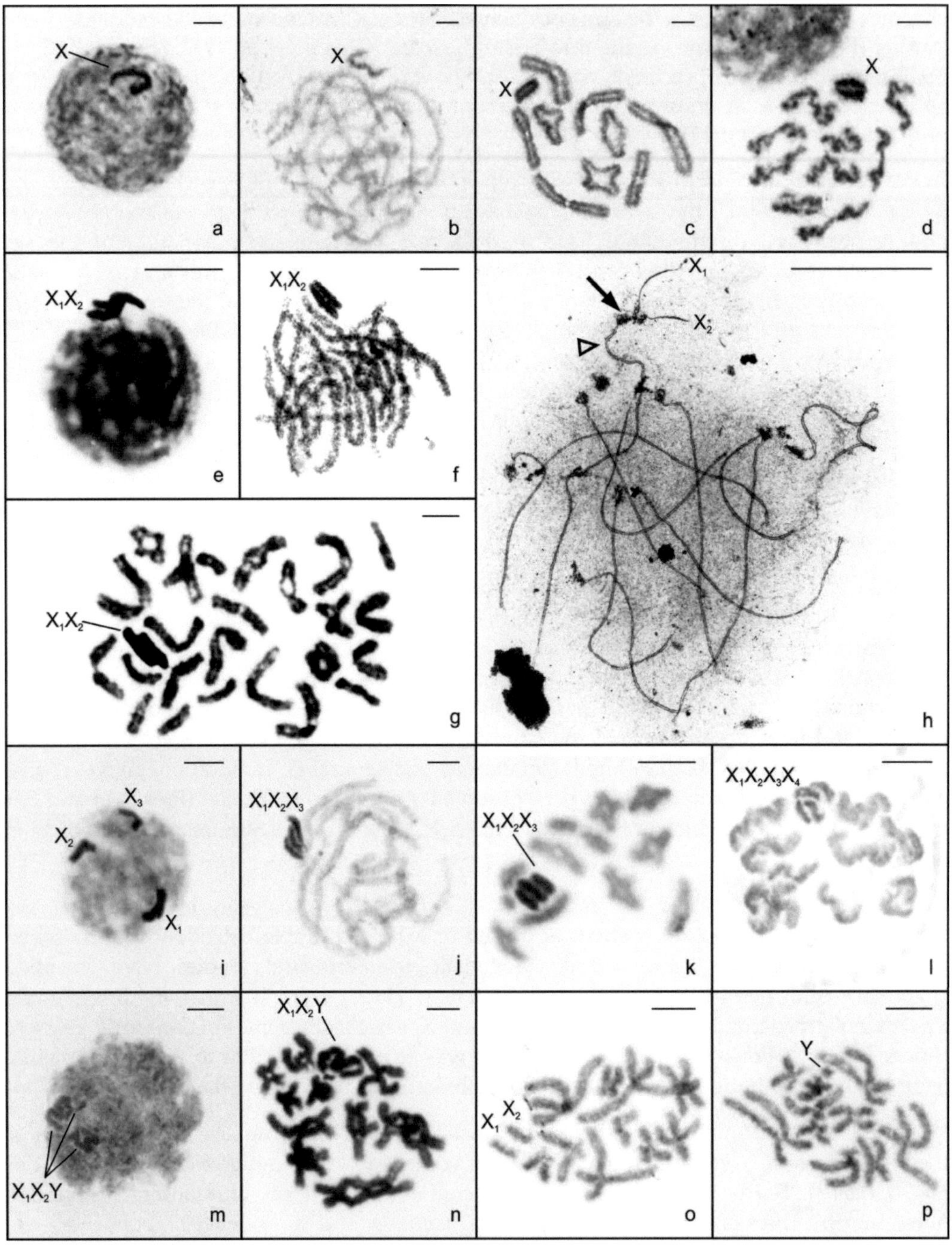


Fig. 3. Behaviour of the sex chromosomes during meiosis in male spiders. a – d. *Hogna sternalis* (X0); e. *Lycosa erythrognatha* ($X_1X_20$); f. *Falconina* sp. ($X_1X_20$); g. *Polybetes* sp. ($X_1X_20$); h. *Phoneutria* sp. ($X_1X_20$); i – k. *Trachelas* sp. ($X_1X_2X_30$); l. *Xeropigo* sp. ($X_1X_2X_3X_40$); m – p. *Loxosceles variegata* ($X_1X_2Y$). a, e, i, m. Premeiotic interphase nuclei. b, f, h, j. Pachytene cells. c, g, k, l, n. Diplotene cells. d, o, p. Metaphase II nuclei. In almost all cells, the sex

chromosomes can be easily recognised by their high degree of condensation and positive heteropycnosis (a-g, i-m) and/or association behaviour (e-h, j-l, n). Note the parallel pairing of the X chromosomes of the multiple sex chromosome system (e-f, j-l) and the end-to-end paring of the $X_1X_2Y$ chromosomes (n). In h, observe the probable junctional lamina (arrow) between the $X_1$ and $X_2$ chromosomes and the terminal association of these sex chromosomes with a homomorphic bivalent (arrowhead). Scale bar=10 μm.

Although employing cytogenetic techniques to identify specific chromosomal regions has provided relevant data on spider chromosomes, only approximately 50 and 30 species were characterised with respect to the constitutive heterochromatin and nucleolar organiser regions (NORs), respectively. In these species, constitutive heterochromatin exhibited a similar distribution among autosomes and sex chromosomes, occurring mainly in pericentromeric regions. However, in at least three representatives of the basal araneomorphs with an $X_1X_2Y$ SCS, *Pholcus phalangioides*, *Loxosceles intermedia*, and *Loxosceles laeta*, the Y chromosome was completely heterochromatic (Silva et al., 2002, Král et al. 2006). This reinforces the results obtained in analyses of the association behaviour of sex chromosomes during meiosis I; that is, the Y chromosome exhibits a high degree of differentiation and does not share homology with the $X_1$ and $X_2$ chromosomes. In mygalomorphs, basal and derived araneomorphs, the NORs are located predominantly on the terminal regions of one to three autosome pairs. Nevertheless, among basal araneomorph species with an X0 SCS, NORs can occur on autosomes and the X chromosome (Dysderidae, Pholcidae and Tetrablemmidae) or only on the X chromosome (Ochyroceratidae, Leptonetidae, and Scytodidae). Recently, Král et al. (2011) described the presence of NORs on the $X_2$ sex chromosome of derived araneomorph species belonging to the family Tetragnathidae. According to these authors, this unusual NOR localisation may be due to the translocation of rDNA cistrons from autosomes to sex chromosomes.

### 2.2 Early descriptions and discussions of nomenclature, function and origin

Carnoy (1885) presented the first, although inaccurate, chromosome numbers of some spider species. However, this study did not mention the existence of chromosomes that could be related to sex determination. Wallace (1900, 1909) was the first to describe double "accessory chromosomes" in a spider, *Agelenopsis naevia* (under *Agalena naevia*), and to associate the presence of these elements with sex determination. However, Wallace (1900, 1909) was not able to observe such chromosomes in females, thus concluding that male embryos were produced by fusion between a spermatozoon with accessory chromosomes and an egg without such elements, and female embryos were formed by fusion between a spermatozoon and an egg that both lack accessory chromosomes.

According to Wallace (1909), the accessory chromosomes corresponded to those that Wagner (1896) described as a "nucleolus". Subsequently, these chromosomes in spiders were also referred to as "heterochromosomes" (Montgomery, 1905) or "odd-chromosomes" (Berry, 1906). The nomenclature of "accessory chromosomes" was adopted by Painter (1914) and others. In a brief communication describing the X element in *Amaurobius* sp., King (1925) was the first to use the term "sex chromosome" in spiders. The designation of "accessory chromosomes" was still used by Hard (1939), but by the late 1940's, the nomenclature of "sex chromosomes" was definitively adopted in spiders.

An early explanation of the origin and evolution of sex chromosomes in spiders and other groups of organisms was elaborated by Montgomery (1905). According to this author, there were two types of so-called "heterochromosomes"; those that occurred in pairs in spermatogonia and then associated to form bivalents in spermatocytes (paired type), and those that were unpaired, or single, in spermatogonia and continued to be unpaired in the spermatocytes during the course of meiosis. According to this study, unpaired heterochromosomes could originate from those of the paired type through subsequent modifications. Furthermore, Montgomery (1905) stated that heterochromosomes of the paired type were derived from "ordinary chromosomes", but these heterochromosomes no longer carried out the same activities as the "ordinary chromosomes" and had the tendency to disappear. Thus, excessively minute heterochromosomes could represent the last stage before total deletion of these elements, instead of the first stage in the origin of this type of chromosome. Montgomery (1905) also suggested that heterochromosomes arose from "ordinary chromosomes" concomitantly with a change in chromosomal number, most likely from a higher to a lower number. However, the relationship between heterochromosomes and sex determination was only a hypothesis at that time because there was no record of such chromosomes in oocytes.

According to Painter (1914), the fact that accessory chromosomes were consistent with respect to their number, form, and behaviour in spider species belonging to 13 families suggested that these elements must have a very important and constant function in the life cycle of these spiders, in contrast to the autosomes, which were numerically variable among different species. Painter (1914) also noted that the accessory chromosomes were related to sex determination. The point of view of Painter (1914) was contrary to the conclusion presented by Wallace (1909), i.e., male embryos were produced by the fusion of one spermatozoon without accessory chromosomes and one egg with such elements, whereas female embryos were formed by the fusion of a spermatozoon and egg that both carried accessory chromosomes. The conclusion of Painter (1914) can be considered correct for all spider species without a Y chromosome.

### 2.3 Origin of the $X_1X_20$ sex chromosome system

The $X_1X_20$ SCS has been considered a plesiomorphic feature in spiders because it occurs in representatives of the phylogenetically basal family Liphistiidae (Mesothelae) (Suzuki, 1954). Various hypotheses concerning the origin of this system in spiders have been put forth.

Revell (1947) was the first to suggest that the $X_1X_20$ SCS most likely originated from an X0 system in spiders, considering the proposition of White (1940), who suggested that duplication of the X chromosome from an X0 system gave rise to the multiple X chromosome systems (Fig. 4). This hypothesis was based on the similarity of the sizes of X chromosomes and the probable homology between the X chromosomes during prophase I in a multiple sex chromosome system. However, Revell (1947) verified the presence of multiple X chromosomes of different sizes in *Tegenaria*, and he suggested that these X chromosomes had undergone evolutionary differentiation after originating from an X0 system (Fig. 5).

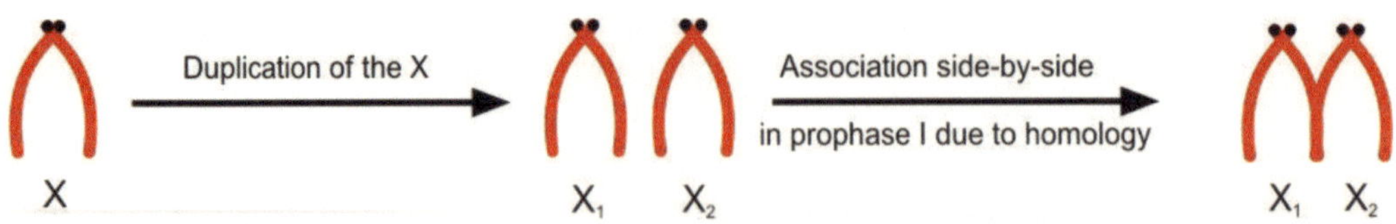


Fig. 4. Interpretive scheme of the origin of the $X_1X_20$ SCS based on descriptions of White (1940).

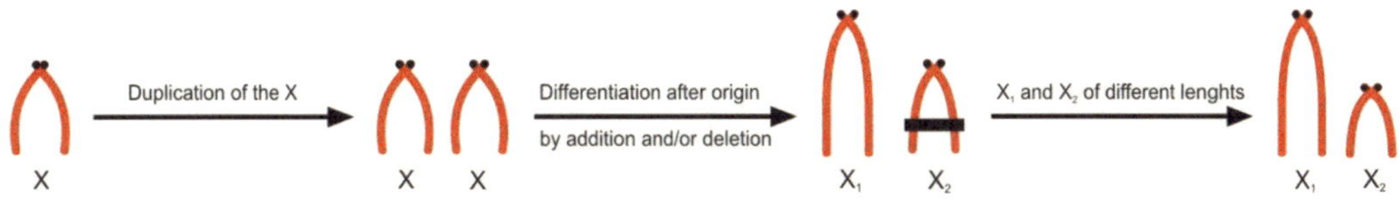


Fig. 5. Schematic representation of the origin of the $X_1X_20$ SCS based on descriptions of Revell (1947).

Studying the meiotic cells of *Araneus quadratus* (under *Aranea reaumuri*), Pätau (1948) suggested that there was no indication of homology between the $X_1$ and $X_2$ chromosomes; however, this author did not exclude the possibility of partial homology. Absence of homology between the $X_1$ and $X_2$ chromosomes was corroborated by Hackman (1948), Suzuki (1952) and Mittal (1964). Moreover, Pätau (1948) proposed that the $X_1X_20$ SCS was formed by centric fission of a large X chromosome in an X0 system.

Due to the fact that all X chromosomes of X0 systems that were registered at that time exhibited subterminal or terminal centromeres, Pätau (1948) suggested that the smaller $X_1$ and $X_2$ chromosomes had originated from the X0 system not only by simple centric fission, but through additional rearrangements such as 1) centric fragmentation and fission in the long arm terminal region followed by inversion of the long chromosome segment, resulting in a dicentric chromosome; 2) fission in the middle region of the dicentric chromosome, forming two acrocentric $X_1$ and $X_2$ chromosomes of similar size (Fig. 6).

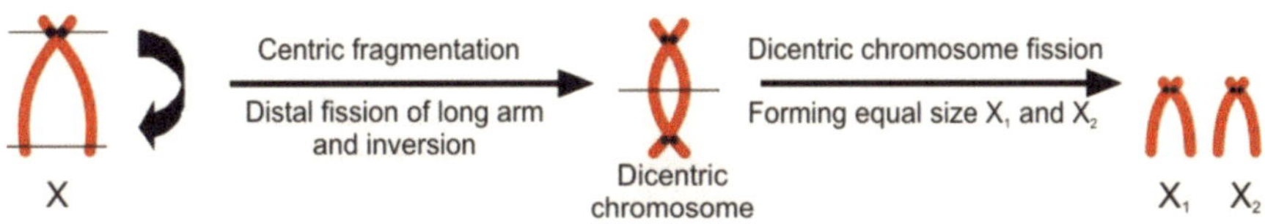


Fig. 6. Interpretive scheme of the origin of the $X_1X_20$ SCS based on descriptions of Pätau (1948).

Bole-Gowda (1950) asserted that the $X_1X_20$ SCS originated from an X0 system in the ancestor of spiders by fission in the middle of the X chromosome producing an acentric chromosome segment that then translocated to a supernumerary centric fragment. These rearrangements produced $X_1$ and $X_2$ chromosomes of similar sizes, one of which retained the original centromere of the X chromosome, while the other kept the supernumerary centromere (Fig. 7). Suzuki (1954) was in agreement with the hypothesis described by Pätau (1948) but disagreed with the assertion of Bole-Gowda (1950) regarding the origin of the $X_1X_20$ system in spiders because no explanation was provided for the origin of the supernumerary centric fragment involved in this hypothesis.

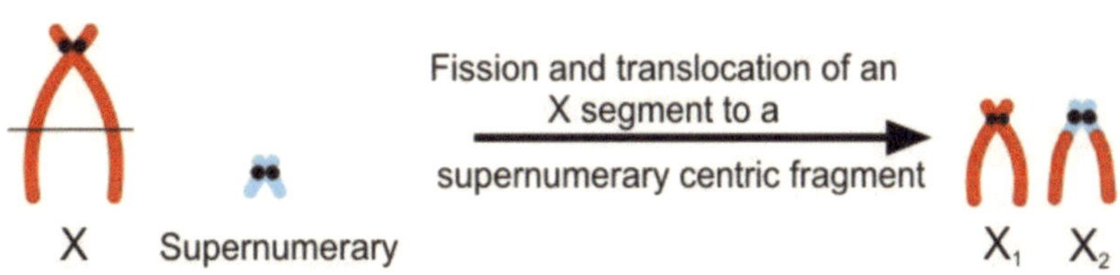


Fig. 7. Schematic representation of the origin of the $X_1X_20$ SCS based on the descriptions of Bole-Gowda (1950).

Considering the terminal position of the centromere and the size of the $X_1$ and $X_2$ chromosomes, Postiglioni & Brum-Zorrilla (1981) suggested that non-disjunction or duplication of a single telocentric X chromosome may have been responsible for the origin of the $X_1X_20$ SCS of *Lycosa* sp.3 (Fig. 8a). According to these researchers, the lack of homology between these chromosomes was most likely due to the occurrence of other rearrangements. However, the authors did not exclude the possibility that the origin of the $X_1X_20$ system of *Lycosa* sp.3. could have occurred by centric fission of a metacentric X chromosome (Fig. 8b).

Although previous authors reported that female X chromosomes form normal bivalents during meiosis (Hackman, 1948; Pätau, 1948; Sharma et al., 1959), Král (2007) and Král et al. (2011) found that the female X chromosomes of entelegyne and mygalomorph spiders paired during meiosis and also exhibited heterochromatinisation similar to that observed in male meiosis. This event could prevent recombination between the X chromosomes and accelerate their differentiation, a process that is consistent with the hypothesis of Postiglioni & Brum-Zorrilla (1981).

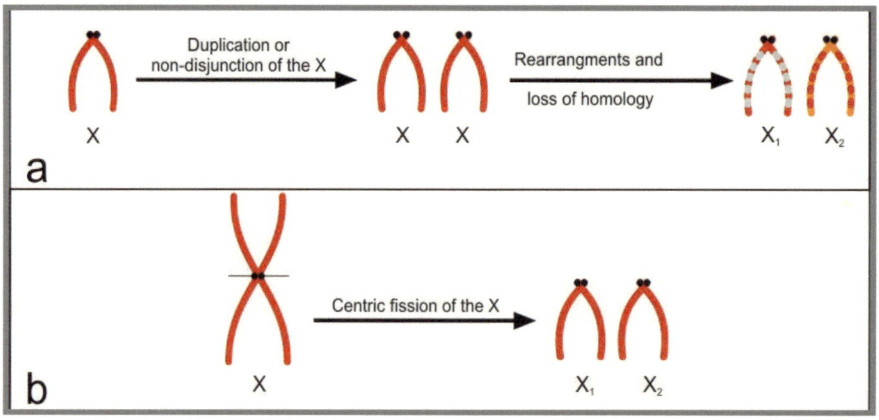


Fig. 8. Interpretive scheme of the origin of the $X_1X_20$ SCS based on descriptions of Postiglioni & Brum-Zorrilla (1981).

In addition to these hypotheses, some researchers have considered the $X_1X_20$ SCS to have originated secondarily from other multiple SCS. Oliveira et al. (2007) proposed that the $X_1X_20$ system could have arisen by gradual heterochromatinisation and erosion of the Y chromosome (Fig. 9). This hypothesis was based on the fact that the pholcid *Spermophora senoculata*, which exhibits an $X_1X_2Y$ system, was considered phylogenetically basal (Bruvo-Mararic et al., 2005) in relation to *Crossopriza lyoni*, which shows an $X_1X_20$ SCS.

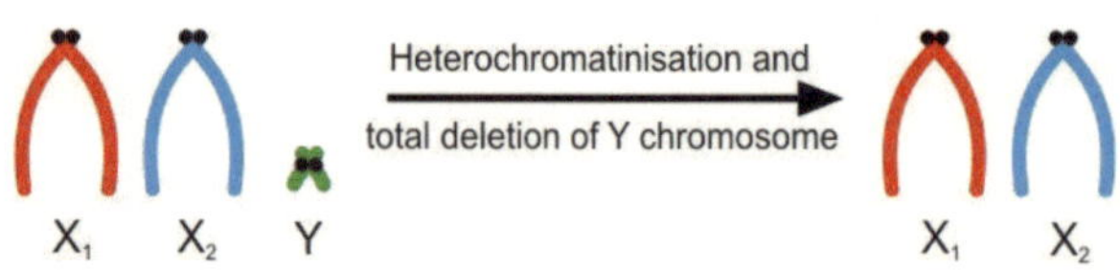


Fig. 9. Schematic representation of the origin of the $X_1X_20$ SCS based on the descriptions of Oliveira et al. (2007).

In some species of the genus *Malthonica* (Agelenidae), Král (2007) encountered three types of SCS, $X_1X_20$, $X_1X_2X_30$, and $X_1X_2X_3X_4X_5Y$, and therefore suggested that in this genus, the $X_1X_2X_30$ condition was ancestral and gave rise to the $X_1X_20$ system through a tandem fusion between two X chromosomes (Fig. 10). This proposition was based on the peculiar meiotic behaviour of the X chromosomes belonging to the $X_1X_2X_30$ SCS, the great difference in sizes between the X chromosomes of the $X_1X_20$ SCS, and the presence of the $X_1X_2X_30$ system in *Tegenaria parietina*, which is morphologically closely related to *Malthonica*.

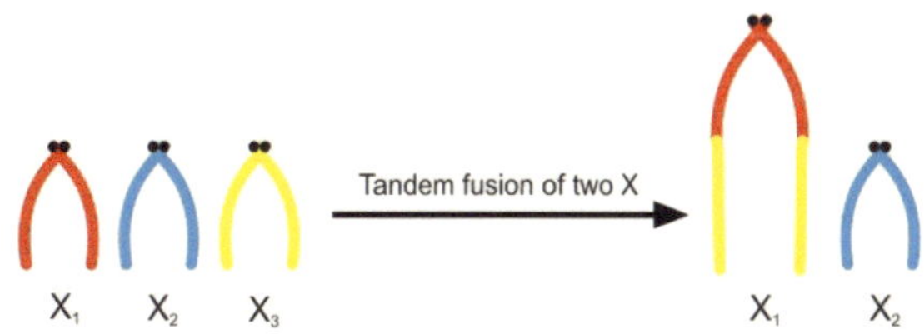


Fig. 10. Interpretive scheme of the origin of the $X_1X_20$ SCS based on descriptions presented by Král (2007).

### 2.4 Origin of the $X_1X_2X_30$ sex chromosome system

Revell (1947) found 2n♂=40+$X_1X_20$ in *Tegenaria atrica* and 2n♂=40+$X_1X_2X_30$ in *Tegenaria domestica*. Considering that the number of autosomes was constant (40 autosomes) in these two *Tegenaria* species, the author suggested that the X1X2X30 SCS originated from the $X_1X_20$ system, which was derived from an X0 system. However, this author did not state the chromosome rearrangements that were responsible for the origin of the $X_1X_2X_30$ system. The existence of X chromosomes of different lengths in species with an $X_1X_2X_30$ system was considered by Revell (1947) as evidence that the multiple X chromosomes of the $X_1X_2X_30$ system were modified after the origination of this SCS.

According to Pätau (1948), in the *Tegenaria* species studied by Revell (1947), the largest X chromosome found in *T. atrica* ($X_1X_20$) was equivalent to the sum of the lengths of the two smallest X chromosomes observed in *T. domestica* ($X_1X_2X_30$). In this case, an $X_1X_20$ SCS could give rise to an $X_1X_2X_30$ system through rearrangements similar to those proposed by Pätau (1948) for the origin of the $X_1X_20$ SCS (Fig. 11, 6). This explanation was supported by Suzuki (1954) and Sharma et al. (1959). However, these authors analysed *Selenops radiatus*, which showed three X chromosomes of equal size, and proposed that the similarity in the length of the sex chromosomes in some species with the $X_1X_2X_30$ system could be the result of additional rearrangements after their origin from an $X_1X_20$ system.

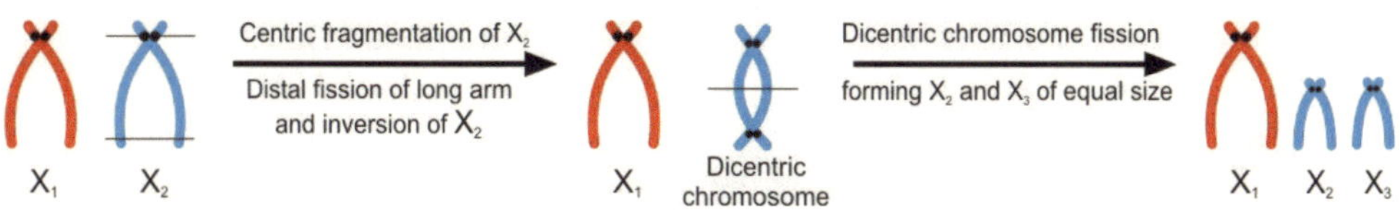


Fig. 11. Schematic representation of the origin of the $X_1X_2X_30$ SCS based on the descriptions of Pätau (1948).

Sharma et al. (1959) demonstrated that the six X chromosomes in the zygotene and pachytene stages in *Selenops radiatus* females (males were $X_1X_2X_30$) did not show any positive heteropycnosis and formed only normal bivalents but did not form multivalents; similar meiotic behaviour of chromosomes was observed in female meiotic cells of a species with four X chromosomes (males were $X_1X_20$) by Hackman (1948), Pätau (1948) and Suzuki (1954), reinforcing the suggestion that there was no homology between the X chromosomes of the $X_1X_20$ and $X_1X_2X_30$ SCS.

Bole-Gowda (1952) proposed that the $X_1X_2X_30$ system found in *Heteropoda venatoria* arose from an ancestor with an $X_1X_20$ system by translocation of a segment of one X chromosome of the $X_1X_20$ system and one supernumerary centric fragment (Fig. 12). This is similar to this author's hypothesis for the origin of the $X_1X_20$ system from the X0 system.

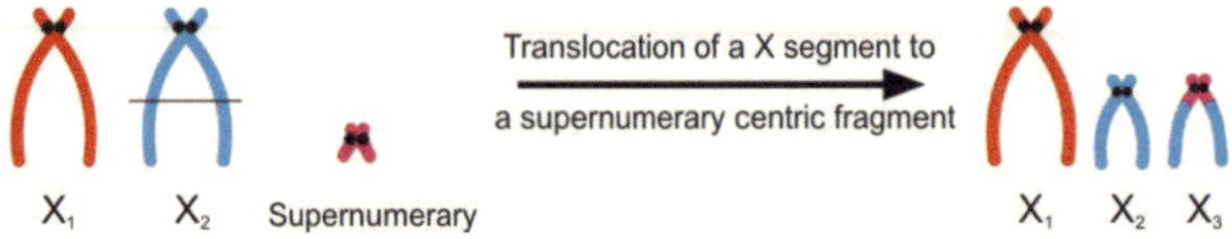


Fig. 12. Interpretive scheme of the origin of the $X_1X_2X_30$ SCS based on descriptions of Bole-Gowda (1952).

To explain the origin of the $X_1X_2X_30$ SCS found in *Lycosa* sp. (*thorelli* group), Postiglioni & Brum-Zorrilla (1981) hypothesised that non-disjunction of one X chromosome of the $X_1X_20$ system, followed by loss of homology between the X chromosomes had occurred (Fig. 13). To corroborate the hypothesis of non-disjunction, the authors cited the observation of a particular behaviour involving early condensation and isolation of one X chromosome at the pachytene stage. Taking into account that the $X_1X_20$ system could be ancestral in spiders, Postiglioni & Brum-Zorrilla (1981) suggested that each sex chromosome would undergo independent mutations during the course of evolution; however, if one of the X chromosomes had suffered a recent non-disjunction, these last two elements would present similar behaviour during meiotic prophase I, and the X chromosome not involved in the event would conserve its individuality and would appear condensed in early stages.

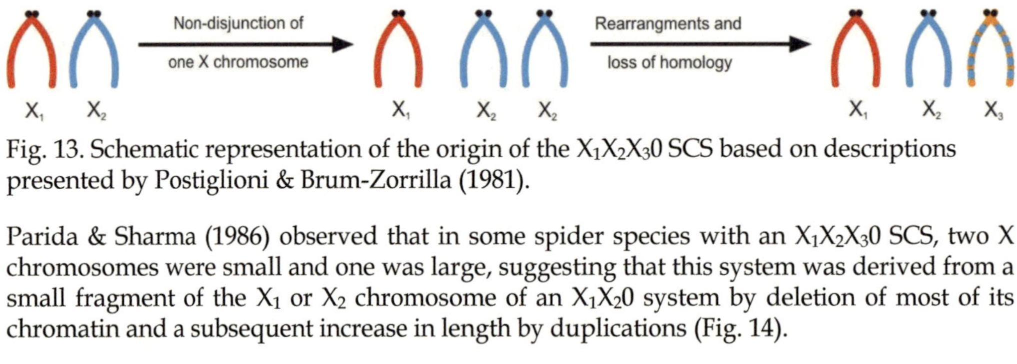


Fig. 13. Schematic representation of the origin of the $X_1X_2X_30$ SCS based on descriptions presented by Postiglioni & Brum-Zorrilla (1981).

Parida & Sharma (1986) observed that in some spider species with an $X_1X_2X_30$ SCS, two X chromosomes were small and one was large, suggesting that this system was derived from a small fragment of the $X_1$ or $X_2$ chromosome of an $X_1X_20$ system by deletion of most of its chromatin and a subsequent increase in length by duplications (Fig. 14).

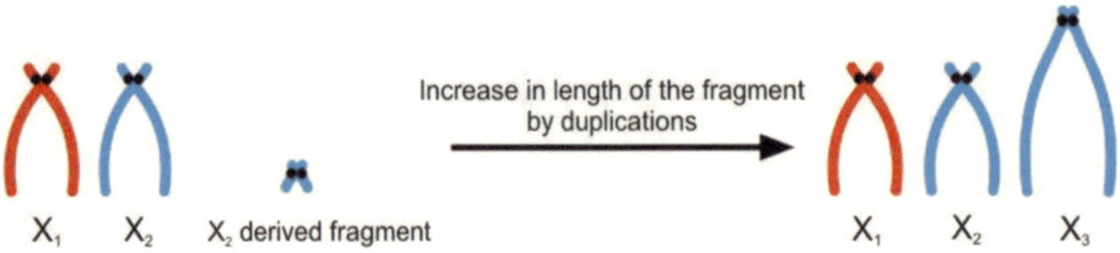


Fig. 14. Interpretive scheme of the origin of the $X_1X_2X_30$ SCS based on descriptions of Parida & Sharma (1986).

### 2.5 Origin of the $X_1X_2X_3X_40$ sex chromosome system

Data & Chatterjee (1983, 1988) were the first to record an $X_1X_2X_3X_40$ SCS in spiders. This SCS was found in *Metellina segmentata* (*Meta segmentata*) (Tetragnathidae) and *Bhutaniella sikkimensis* (*Heteropoda sikkimensis*) (Sparassidae). In 1988, these researchers presented a proposal for the origin of the $X_1X_2X_3X_40$ system: duplication or non-disjunction of one X chromosome of the $X_1X_2X_30$ SCS, with subsequent loss of homology (Fig. 15). This proposition was similar to that formulated by Postiglioni & Brum-Zorrilla (1981) to explain the origin of the $X_1X_20$ and $X_1X_2X_30$ systems.

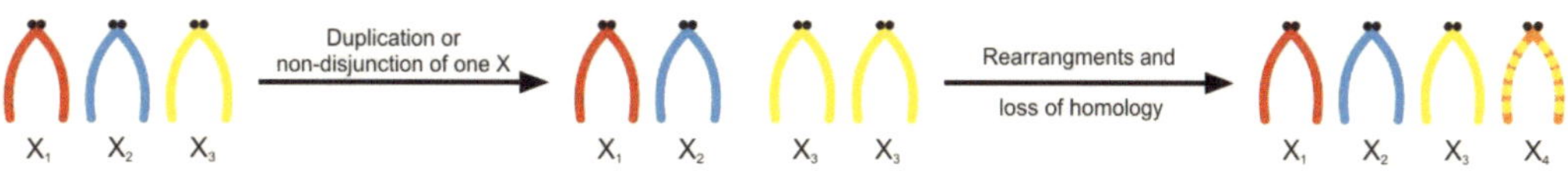


Fig. 15. Interpretive scheme of the origin of the $X_1X_2X_3X_40$ SCS based on descriptions of Datta & Chatterjee (1988).

In *Diplura* species, which employ an $X_1X_2X_3X_40$ system, Král et al. (2011) found that one heteropycnotic and one isopycnotic portion could be distinguished in the $X_1$ and $X_2$ chromosomes, most likely corresponding to the original $X_1$ and $X_2$ chromosomes and the original autosomes, respectively, indicating that the $X_1$ and $X_2$ sex chromosomes originated by sex chromosome/autosome translocation. Additionally, Král et al. (2011), suggested that this system probably originated by duplication of the $X_1X_20$ system via non-disjunctions or polyploidisation (Fig. 16) based on the chromomere pattern and size of the sex chromosomes observed in the $X_1X_2X_3X_40$ *Diplura*.

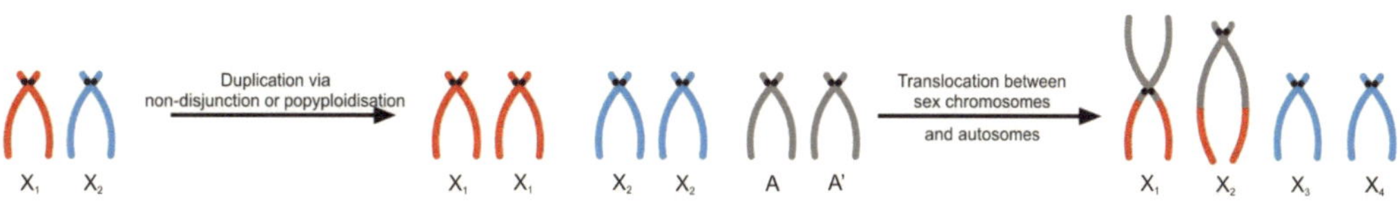


Fig. 16. Schematic representation of the origin of the $X_1X_2X_3X_40$ SCS based on the descriptions of Král et al. (2011).

### 2.6 Origin of the X0 sex chromosome system

Hackman (1948) found the supposed first case of a metacentric X chromosome in spiders in *Oxyopes ramosus* and noted that the X0 SCS verified in *Oxyopes* (metacentric), *Myrmarachne*, *Misumena*, and *Xysticus* (acrocentric) had most likely been derived from the $X_1X_20$ system in two ways:

1. The metacentric X of the X0 system could have been derived by centric fusion between $X_1$ and $X_2$ chromosomes (Fig. 17). This mechanism was also employed by several authors (Bole-Gowda, 1952; Suzuki, 1954; Postiglioni & Brum-Zorrilla, 1981; Řezáč et al., 2006; Král et al., 2011; Stávale et al. 2011) to explain the origin of the X0 SCS, which involves a metacentric X, in many spider groups.
2. The acrocentric X of the X0 system could have originated through gradual elimination of one X chromosome of the $X_1X_20$ SCS, as suggested by Suzuki (1952, 1954). This author put forth this proposition based on the fact that some thomisid species with an $X_1X_20$ system presented gradual differences between the lengths of $X_1$ and $X_2$ chromosomes (with both showing the same, slightly different or markedly different sizes). Furthermore, some species even exhibited an X0 system, suggesting that elimination of one X of the $X_1X_20$ system had taken place in the course of evolution (Fig. 18).

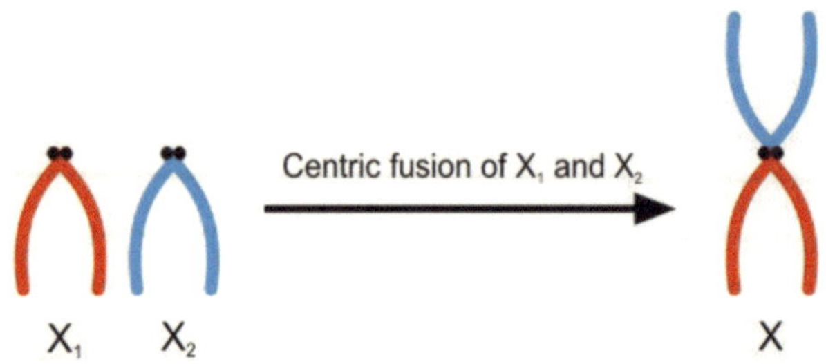


Fig. 17. Schematic representation of the origin of the X0 SCS based on descriptions presented by Hackman (1948).

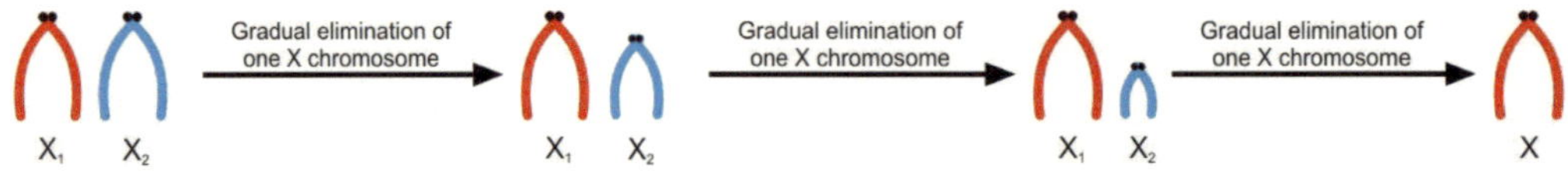


Fig. 18. Interpretive scheme of the origin of the X0 SCS based on descriptions of Hackman (1948).

Bole-Gowda (1950) proposed that the X0 system found in several spider species could have evolved by reciprocal translocation between the $X_1$ and $X_2$ chromosomes, preceded by distal fission in one sex chromosome and proximal fission in the other X, giving rise to a large acrocentric X chromosome, as found in *Oxyopes hindostanicus*; the centric fragment produced in this process was lost (Fig. 19).

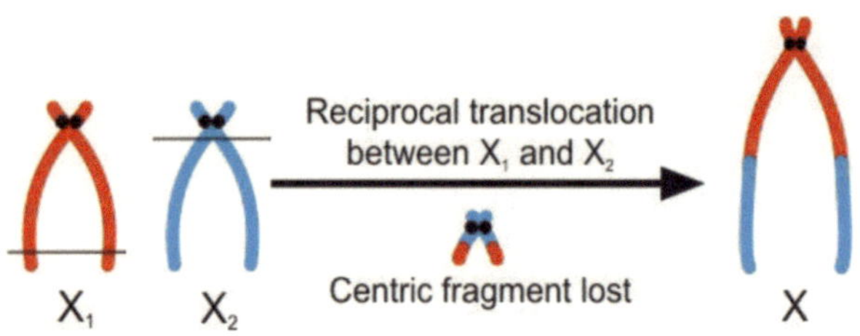


Fig. 19. Schematic representation of the origin of the X0 SCS based on descriptions presented by Bole-Gowda (1950).

Datta & Chatterjee (1989, 1992) proposed that the X0 system found in lycosid and uloborid spiders originated from the $X_1X_20$ SCS by centric fusion of the $X_1$ and $X_2$ chromosomes, followed by pericentric inversion (Fig. 20a) or partial deletion (Fig. 20b) in one of the X chromosome arms, giving rise to an acrocentric element. Alternatively, the acrocentric X chromosome could have originated from tandem fusion between the $X_1$ and $X_2$ chromosomes (Fig. 20c).

Tandem fusion was postulated as the mechanism involved in the derivation of the acrocentric X chromosome (X0 system) of *Zodarion* from the acrocentric $X_1$ and $X_2$ chromosomes ($X_1X_20$ system) present in species of the same genus (Pekár & Král, 2001). Pekár et al. (2005) proposed that two positive heteropycnotic bodies observed in the premeiotic interphase nuclei of two *Zodarion* species with the X0 SCS were segments of the X chromosome that corresponded to the original $X_1$ and $X_2$.

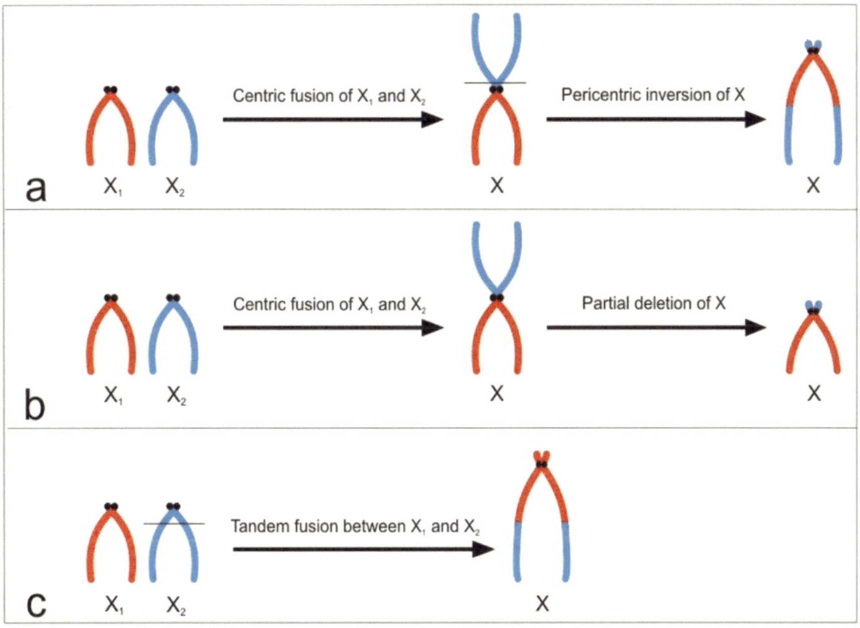


Fig. 20. Interpretive scheme of the origin of the X0 SCS based on descriptions of Datta & Chatterjee (1989, 1992).

According to Král et al. (2006), the XY SCS, which was originated from the $X_1X_2Y$ system, gave rise to an X0 SCS through loss of the Y chromosome (Fig. 21). The SCS of the X0 type was found in many pholcids and Scytodes (Scytodidae).The evidence for this degeneration and complete elimination of the Y chromosome was the high level of constitutive heterochromatin detected in this chromosome in *Pholcus phalangioides*.

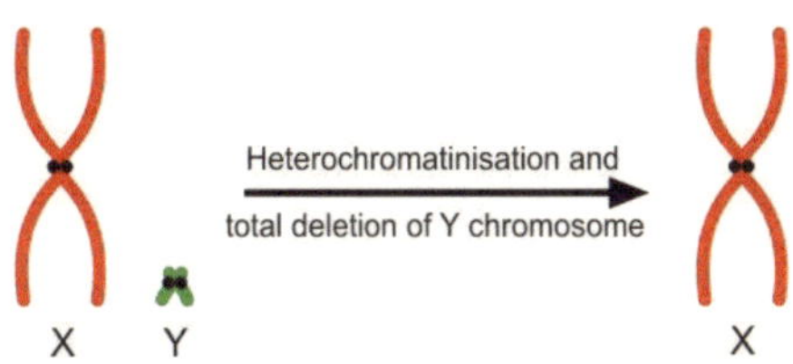


Fig. 21. Schematic representation of the origin of the X0 SCS based on descriptions of Král et al. (2006).

### 2.7 Origin of the XY sex chromosome system

Řezáč et al. (2006) described the first XY SCS in a spider of the genus *Atypus* (Mygalomorphae). According to these authors, this neo-XY system was formed from an X0 system, which was recorded in other species of this genus and involved rearrangements between the X chromosome and autosomes.

Král et al. (2006) studied the evolution of the chromosomes in several basal araneomorphs and formulated some hypotheses about SCS evolution. These authors discovered that SCS that include a Y chromosome are more common in spiders than previously believed, at least in basal araneomorphs. Several species with XY and $X_1X_2Y$ SCS were described in many families, and the authors highlighted the fact that in some species previously described as carriers of the $X_1X_20$ system, the tiny Y chromosome could have been neglected. Based on the diversity of SCS in basal araneomorphs, specifically in pholcids, Král et al. (2006) proposed that the $X_1X_2Y$ SCS involving metacentric chromosomes in this group of spiders was similar to that found in Filistatidae and *Loxosceles* and was converted into an XY SCS. First, by pericentric inversion transforming one of the metacentric X chromosomes into a subtelo- or acrocentric form, the $X_1X_2Y$ became similar to that described in *Pholcus phalangioides* (Pholcidae). Subsequently, the other X chromosome of the $X_1X_2Y$ system was also pericentrically inverted, forming a hypothetical configuration in which both X chromosomes of the $X_1X_2Y$ system exhibit acrocentric morphology. In the next step, centric fusion between the acrocentric X chromosomes of the hypothetical $X_1X_2Y$ SCS occurred, generating an XY system, as found in *Smeringopus pallidus* (Pholcidae) and *Diguetia* (Diguetidae). In *Diguetia albolineata*, which exhibits an XY SCS, both arms of the metacentric Y chromosome paired with only one arm of the metacentric X during meiosis. In *Diguetia canities*, the metacentric X chromosome was supposedly pericentrically inverted, resulting an acrocentric element (Fig. 22).

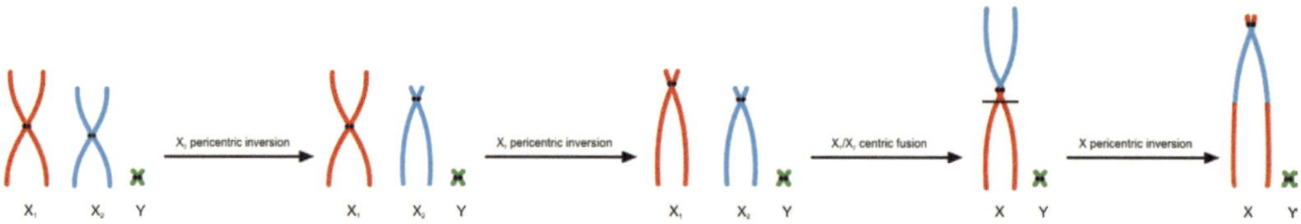


Fig. 22. Interpretive scheme of the origin of the XY SCS of Pholcidae and Diguetidae based on the descriptions of Král et al. (2006).

The proposed origin of the XY SCS observed in *Leptoneta* (Leptonetidae) was quite different. The XY system was believed to have originated from the X0 system, not from the $X_1X_2Y$ system, in a mechanism involving translocation between the X and one autosome constituting the neo X chromosome; the homolog of the autosome involved in the rearrangement formed the Y chromosome (Fig. 23). This hypothesis put forth by Král et al. (2006) was based on the fact that the distal part of the X chromosome in *Leptoneta*, which has an XY SCS (probably corresponding to the translocated autosome), presented a different pattern of condensation during meiosis I. This last characteristic was not detected in the sex chromosomes of *Diguetia* species.

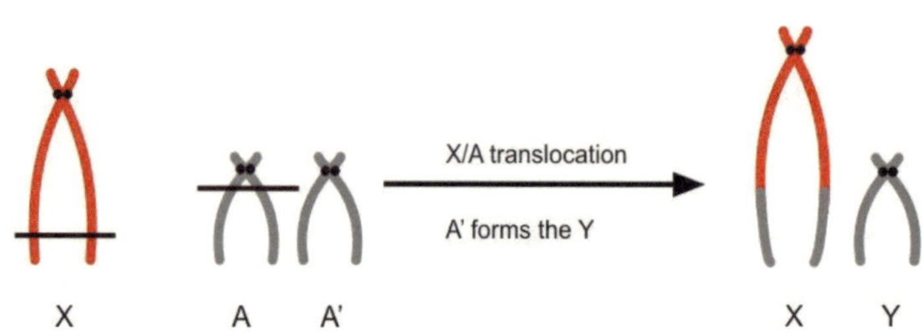


Fig. 23. Schematic representation of the origin of the XY SCS of Leptonetidae based on the descriptions of Král et al. (2006).

### 2.8 Origin of the $X_1X_2Y$ sex chromosome system

Silva (1988) was the first to record an $X_1X_2Y$ SCS in spiders. Although the author noted the possibility that the small acrocentric chromosome found in *Loxosceles laeta* was a supernumerary chromosome, she concluded that this element could correspond to the Y chromosome of the $X_1X_2Y$ SCS. A very general citation of many types of rearrangements that could be involved in the origin of the $X_1X_2Y$ system was presented, though without explaining the sequence of steps involved in the evolution of this SCS in spiders. Subsequently, Silva et al. (2002) proposed that the $X_1X_2Y$ system found in *Loxosceles* (Sicariidae) was derived from an $X_1X_20$ SCS through a mechanism involving translocations between X chromosomes and autosomes; however, they did not provide details associated with this process.

### 2.9 Origin of the $X_1X_2X_3Y$ sex chromosome system

Maddison (1982) described an SCS of the $X_1X_2X_3Y$ type in five species of Salticidae and, surprisingly, verified that in *Evarcha hoyi* (under *Pellenes hoyi*), some individuals presented the $X_1X_2X_3Y$ system, whereas others showed the $X_1X_20$ system.

According to Maddison (1982), during the process of arising from the $X_1X_20$ system, the $X_1$ chromosome of the $X_1X_2X_3Y$ system remained unaltered, while the $X_2$ chromosome became tandemly fused (or centrically fused followed by pericentric inversion) with an autosome that then constituted the distal portion of the neo $X_2$ long arm. The homolog of this autosome involved in the autosome/$X_2$ fusion became centrically fused with other autosome, forming the Y chromosome (short and long arms, respectively); the homolog of this last autosome (the Y long arm) became the $X_3$ chromosome without undergoing modifications (Fig. 24). This hypothesis was based on the difference in diploid number detected in salticid species (i.e., individuals with the $X_1X_20$ system had two additional autosomal pairs when compared with individuals with the $X_1X_2X_3Y$ system). These two autosomal pairs could be the pairs involved in fusions with the original $X_1X_20$ system. Furthermore, the meiotic features of the sex chromosomes, such as pycnosis, achiasmatic and chiasmatic pairing, and segregation, were considered to represent additional supporting evidence of this mode of origin of the $X_1X_2X_3Y$ SCS.

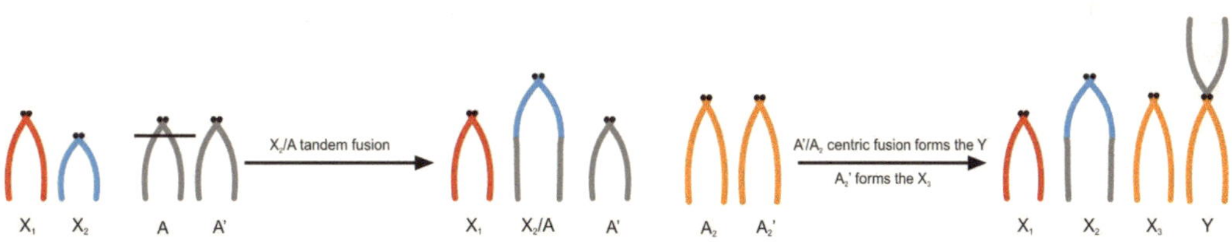


Fig. 24. Interpretive scheme of the origin of the $X_1X_2X_3Y$ SCS based on descriptions of Maddison (1982).

### 2.10 Origin of the $X_1X_2X_3X_4X_5Y$ sex chromosome system

The $X_1X_2X_3X_4X_5Y$ SCS verified in *Malthonica ferruginea* by Král (2007) formed a multivalent association in the pachytene stage, which was constituted by three univalents ($X_1X_2X_3$) and one trivalent ($X_4X_5Y$). In the trivalent, a synaptonemal complex was observed between the metacentric Y and the $X_4X_5$ chromosomes. Pairing between the univalents and the trivalent occurred end-to-end and involved only the X chromosomes. This mode of pairing was not visualised at the end of the diplotene stage. Observation of end-to-end pairing between the X chromosomes and a specific bivalent during meiosis of related species (Král, 2007), as well as in other spider groups (Benavente & Wettstein, 1977; Wise, 1983), compelled Král (2007) to hypothesise that the $X_1X_2X_3X_4X_5Y$ SCS originated from the $X_1X_2X_30$ system. First, the three univalents ($X_1X_2X_3$) paired with a proto-X proto-Y bivalent or homomorphic sex chromosome pair (a bivalent that did not present morphological peculiarities but probably exhibited molecular differentiation into new sex chromosomes). Subsequently, the proto-Y chromosome underwent centric fusion with an autosomal element, forming a neo Y (metacentric) that maintained the pairing with the protoX (newly denominated $X_4$). The homolog of the autosome element involved in centric fusion with the protoY was designated the $X_5$ chromosome, which paired with its homologous arm in the neo Y (Fig. 25). According to Král (2007), these proto-X and proto-Y chromosomes probably represented ancestral chromosomes involved in the origin of the multiple X chromosomes by nondisjunction.

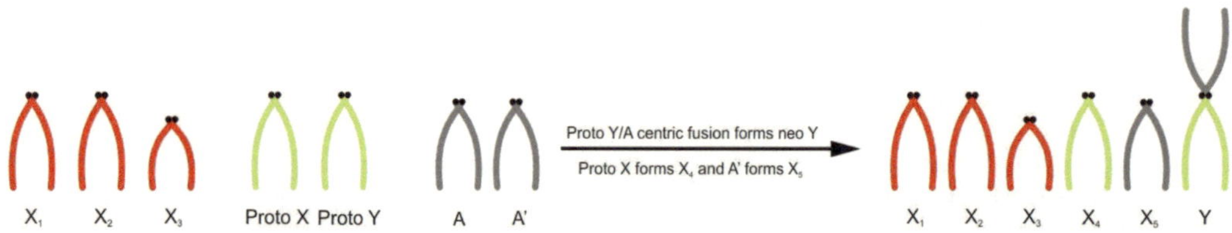


Fig. 25. Schematic representation of the origin of the $X_1X_2X_3X_4X_5Y$ SCS based on the descriptions of Král (2007).

## 2.11 Origin of multiple $X_nY_n$ sex chromosome systems

Rowell (1985, 1988, 1990, 1991), Hancock & Rowell (1995), and Sharp & Rowell (2007) described a range of multiple $X_nY_n$ SCS in populations of the social spider *Delena cancerides* (Sparassidae). Considering that some populations of this species presented an $X_1X_2X_30$ SCS, the authors provided an explanation for the origin of the multiple X and multiple Y chromosomes from the $X_1X_2X_30$ SCS, which is a system also found in other sparassid species. The first step in this process was centric fusion between two X chromosomes of the original $X_1X_2X_30$ SCS, giving rise to one metacentric X chromosome, while one X chromosome was unchanged. Subsequently, the telocentric X underwent centric fusion with one telocentric autosome, and the homolog of this autosome became part of the SCS. Subsequently, a series of centric fusions between the newly formed sex chromosome and telocentric autosomes gave rise to populations with $X_1X_2X_3Y$, $X_1X_2X_3X_4Y_1Y_2$ (Fig. 26), and multiple X and Y chromosome systems. In all of these populations, the metacentric X formed by the fusion of two original X chromosomes was a univalent, and the neoX and neoY chromosomes, which had originated through centric fusions between autosomes, formed chromosomal chains with different numbers of elements involved (from 3 to 19 elements) during meiosis.

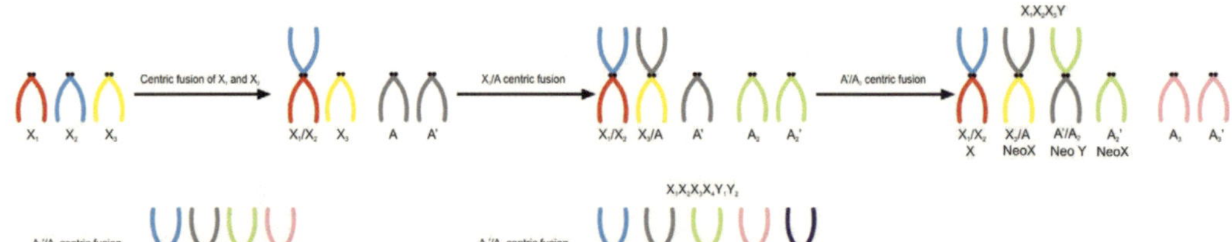


Fig. 26. Interpretive scheme of the origin of the $X_nY_n$ SCS based on descriptions of Rowell (1985, 1988, 1990, 1991), Hancock & Rowell (1995), and Sharp & Rowell (2007).

## 3. Conclusion

Despite the fact that spider meiosis analyses have been carried out for more than 100 years, relatively little has been learned about sex chromosome origin and evolution in this group. The vast majority of studies on this topic have been based solely on assumptions or on basic chromosomal characteristics (chromosome length, number, meiotic condensation, and meiotic segregation). Recent advances in spider cytogenetics, such as ultrastructural analysis of cells during meiosis and examination of female meiosis, have added new insights into SCS evolution. However, only 665 (~1.6%) of the 42,423 known spider species (110 families) have been chromosomally characterised. Fifty-four families have not been studied cytogenetically, resulting in several gaps in the existing hypotheses on sex chromosome evolution.

To provide a broader knowledge base leading to better inferences regarding the origin and evolution of sex chromosomes, further efforts involving spider meiosis analysis should include a broader range of species and use conventional, ultrastructural (synaptonemal complex), and molecular (rDNA and telomere FISH and chromosome painting) cytogenetic techniques.

## 4. Acknowledgments

Financial support was provided by the Conselho Nacional de Desenvolvimento Científico e Tecnológico (CNPq - 471821/2008-0) and the Fundação de Amparo à Pesquisa do Estado de São Paulo (FAPESP - 2008/055633-0 and 2010/14193-7).

## 5. References

Araujo, D.; Schneider, M.C.; Paula-Neto, E. & Cella, D.M. (October 2011). The spider cytogenetic database. In: *Arthropoda cytogenetics website*, 07.10.2011, Available from www.arthropodacytogenetics.bio.br/spiderdatabase

Carnoy, J.B. (1885). La cytodiérèse chez les arthropodes. *La Cellule*, Vol.1, pp. 191-440, ISSN 0008-8757

Beçak, W. & Beçak, M.L. (1960). Constituição cromossômica de duas espécies de aranhas do gênero "*Loxosceles*". *Revista Brasileira de Biologia*, Vol.20, No.4 (December 1960), pp. 425-427, ISSN 0034-7108

Benavente, R. & Wettstein, R. (1977). An ultrastructural cytogenetic study on the evolution of sex chromosomes during the spermatogenesis of *Lycosa malitiosa* (Arachnida). *Chromosoma*, Vol.64, No.3, (September 1977), pp. 255-277, ISSN 0009-5915

Benavente, R. & Wettstein, R. (1980). Ultrastructural characterization of the sex chromosomes during spermatogenesis of spider having holocentric chromosomes and a long diffuse stage. *Chromosoma*, Vol.77, No.1, (February 1980), pp. 69-81, ISSN 0009-5915

Berry, E.H. (1906). The "acessory chromosome" in *Epeira*. *Biological Bulletin*, Vol.11, No.4, (September 1906), pp. 193-201, ISSN 0006-3185

Bole-Gowda, B.N. (1950). The chromosome study in the spermatogenesis of two lynx-spiders (Oxyopidae). *Proceedings of the Zoological Society of Bengal*, Vol.3, No.2, (September 1950), pp. 95-107, ISSN 0373-5893

Bole-Gowda, B.N. (1952). Studies on the chromosomes and the sex-determining mechanism in four hunting spiders (Sparassidae). *Proceedings of the Zoological Society of Bengal*, Vol.5, No.1, (March 1952), pp. 51-70, ISSN 0373-5893

Brum-Zorrilla, N. & Cazenave, A.M. (1974). Heterochromatin localization in the chromosomes of *Lycosa malitiosa* (Arachnida). *Experientia*, Vol.30, No.1, (January 1974) pp. 94-95, ISSN 0014-4754

Bruvo-Mađarić, B.; Huber, B.A.; Steinacher, A. & Pass, G. Phylogeny of pholcid spiders (Araneae: Pholcidae): Combined analysis using morphology and molecules. *Molecular Phylogenetics and Evolution*, Vol.37, No.3, (December 2005), pp. 661-673, ISSN 1055-7903

Coddington, J.A. & Levi, H.W. (1991). Systematics and evolution of spiders (Araneae). *Annual Review of Ecology and Systematics*, Vol.22, (November 1991), pp. 565-592, ISSN 0066-4162

Datta, S.N. & Chatterjee, K. (1983). Chromosome number and sex-determining system in fifty-two species of spiders from North-East India. *Chromosome Information Service*, Vol.35, pp. 6-8, ISSN 0574-9549

Datta, S.N. & Chatterjee, K. (1988) Chromosomes and sex determination in 13 araneid spiders of North-Eastern India. *Genetica*, Vol.76, No.2, (March 1988), pp. 91-99, ISSN 0016-6707

Datta, S.N. & Chatterjee, K. (1989). Study of meiotic chromosomes of four hunting spiders of north eastern India. *Perspectives in Cytology and Genetics*, Vol.6, pp. 414-424, ISSN 0970-4507

Datta, S.N. & Chatterjee, K. (1992). Chromosomes and sex determination in three species of spinner spiders from northeastern India. *Cell and Chromosome Research*, Vol.15, No.2, pp. 64-69

Hackman, W. (1948). Chromosomenstudien an Araneen mit besonderer berücksichtigung der geschlechtschromosomen. *Acta Zoologica Fennica*, Vol.54, pp. 1-101, ISSN 0001-7299

Hancock, A.J. & Rowell, D.M. (1995). A chromosomal hybrid zone in the Australian huntsman spider, *Delena cancerides* (Araneae: Sparassidae). Evidence for a hybrid zone near Canberra, Australia. *Australian Journal of Zoology*, Vol.43, No.2, pp. 173-180, ISSN 0004-959X

Hard, W.L. (1939). The spermatogenesis of the lycosid spider *Schizocosa crassipes* (Walckenaer). *Journal of Morphology*, Vol.65, No.1, (July 1939), pp. 121-153, ISSN 0362-2525

King, S.D. (1925). Spermatogenesis in a spider (*Amaurobius* sp.). *Nature*, Vol.116, (October 1925), pp. 574-575, ISSN 0028-0836

Král, J.; Musilová, J.; Šťálavský, F.; Řezáč, M.; Akan, Z.; Edwards, R.L.; Coyle, F.A. & Almerje, C.R. (2006). Evolution of the karyotype and sex chromosome systems in basal clades of araneomorph spiders (Araneae: Araneomorphae). *Chromosome Research*, Vol.14, No.8, (December 2006), pp. 859-880, ISSN 0967-3849

Král, J. (2007). Evolution of multiple sex chromosomes in the spider genus *Malthonica* (Araneae: Agelenidae) indicates unique structure of the spider sex chromosome systems. *Chromosome Research*, Vol.15, No.7 (November 2007), pp. 863-879, ISSN 0967-3849

Král, J.; Kořínková, T.; Forman, M. & Krkavcová, L. (2011). Insights into the meiotic behavior and evolution of multiple sex chromosome systems in spiders. *Cytogenetic and Genome Research*, Vol.133, No.1, (March 2011), pp. 43-66, ISSN 1424-8581

Maddison, W.P. (1982). XXXY sex chromosomes in males of the jumping spider genus *Pellenes* (Araneae: Salticidae). *Chromosoma*, Vol.85, No.1 (April 1982), pp. 23-37, ISSN 0009-5915

Matsumoto, S. (1977). An observation of somatic chromosomes from spider embryo-cells. *Acta Arachnologica*, Vol.27, pp. 167-172, ISSN 0001-5202

McKee, B.D. & Handel, M.A. (1993). Sex chromosomes, recombination and chromatin conformation. *Chromosoma*, Vol. 102, No.2, (January 1993), pp. 71-80, ISSN 0009-5915

Mittal, O.P. (1964). Karyological studies on the Indian spiders II. An analysis of the chromosomes during spermatogenesis in five species of spiders belonging to the family Salticidae. *Research Bulletin (N.S.) of the Panjab University*, Vol.15, No.3-4, (December 1964), pp. 315-326, ISSN 0555-7631

Montgomery, T.H. (1905). The spermatogenesis of *Syrbula* and *Lycosa*, with general considerations upon chromosome reduction and the heterochromosomes. *Proceedings of the Academy of Natural Sciences of Philadelphia*, Vol.57, (February 1905), pp. 162-205, ISSN 0097-3157

Oliveira, E.G.; Cella, D.M. & Brescovit, A.D. (1997). Karyotype of *Loxosceles intermedia* and *Loxosceles laeta* (Arachnida, Araneae, Sicariidae): Neo$X_1$ Neo$X_2$ Y sex determination mechanism and NORs. *Revista Brasileira de Genética*, Vol.20, pp.77, ISSN 0100-8455

Oliveira, R.M.; Jesus, A.C.; Brescovit, A.D. & Cella, D.M. (2007) Chromosomes of *Crossopriza lyoni* (Blackwall 1867), intraindividual numerical chromosome variation in *Physocyclus globosus* (Taczanowski 1874), and the distribution pattern of NORs (Araneomorphae, Haplogynae, Pholcidae). *Journal of Arachnology*, Vol.35, No.2, pp. 293-306, ISSN 0161-8202

Painter, T.S. (1914). Spermatogenesis in spiders. *Zoologische Jahrbuecher Abteilung fuer Anatomie und Ontogenie der Tiere*, Vol.38, pp. 509-576, ISSN 0044-5177

Parida, B.B. & Sharma, N.N. (1986). Karyotype and spermatogenesis in an Indian hunting spider, *Sparassus* sp. (Sparassidae: Arachnida) with multiple sex chromosomes. *Chromosome Information Service*, Vol.40, pp. 28-30, ISSN 0574-9549

Pätau, K. (1948). X-segregation and heterochromasy in the spider *Aranea reaumuri*. *Heredity*, Vol.2, No.1, (June 1948), pp. 77-100, ISSN 0018-067X

Pekár, S. & Král, J. (2001). A comparative study of the biology and karyotypes of two central European Zoodariid spiders (Araneae, Zodariidae). *Journal of Arachnology*, Vol.29, No.3, pp. 345-353, ISSN 0161-8202

Pekár, S.; Král, J.; Malten, A. & Komposch, C. (2005). Comparison of natural history and karyotypes of two closely related ant-eating spiders, *Zodarion hamatum* and *Z.italicum* (Araneae, Zodariidae). *Journal of Natural History*, Vol.39, No.19, pp. 1583-1596, ISSN 0022-2933

Pinter, L.J. & Walters, D.M. (1971). Karyological studies I. A study of the chromosome numbers and sex-determining mechanism of three species of the genus *Phidippus* (Aranea: Salticidae, Dendryphantinae). *Cytologia*, Vol.36, No.1, pp. 183-189, ISSN 0011-4545

Platnick, N.I. (July 2011). The world spider catalog version 12.0, In: *American Museum of Natural History*, 07.08.2011, Available from http://research.amnh.org/entomology/spiders/catalog/index.html

Postiglioni, A. & Brum-Zorrilla, N. (1981). Karyological studies on Uruguayan spiders II. Sex chromosomes in spiders of the genus *Lycosa* (Araneae-Lycosidae). *Genetica*, Vol.56, No.1, (July 1981), pp. 47-53, ISSN 0016-6707

Revell, S.H. (1947). Controlled X-segregation at meiosis in *Tegenaria*. *Heredity*, Vol.1, No.3, (December 1947), pp. 337-347, ISSN 0018-067X

Řezáč, M.; Král, J.; Musilová, J. & Pekár, S. (2006). Unusual karyotype diversity in the European spiders of the genus *Atypus* (Araneae: Atypidae). *Hereditas*, Vol.143, (December 2006), pp. 123-129, ISSN 0018-0661

Rowell, D.M. (1985). Complex sex-linked fusion heterozygosity in the Australian huntsman spider *Delena cancerides* (Araneae: Sparassidae). *Chromosoma*, Vol.93, No.2, (November 1985), pp. 169-176, ISSN 0009-5915

Rowell, D.M. (1988). The chromosomal constitution of *Delena cancerides* Walck. (Araneae: Sparassidae) and its role in the maintenance of social behaviour. *The Australian Entomological Society Miscellaneous Publication*, Vol.5, pp. 107-111

Rowell, D.M. (1990). Fixed fusion heterozigosity in *Delena cancerides* Walck. (Araneae: Sparassidae): an alternative to speciation by monobrachial fusion. *Genetica*, Vol.80, No.2, (February 1990), pp. 139-157, ISSN 0016-6707

Rowell, D.M. (1991). Chromosomal fusion and meiotic behavior in *Delena cancerides* (Araneae: Sparassidae). I. Chromosome pairing and X-chromosome segregation. *Genome*, Vol.34, No.4, (August 1991), pp. 561-566, ISSN 0831-2796

Sharma, G.P.; Jande, S.S. & Tandon, K.K. (1959). Cytological studies on the Indian spiders IV. Chromosome complement and meiosis in *Selenops radiatus* Latreille (Selenopidae) and *Leucauge decorata* (Blackwall) (Tetragnathidae) with special reference to XXX0-type of male sex determining mechanism. *Research Bulletin (N.S.) of the Panjab University*, Vol.10, No.1, (March 1959), pp. 73-80, ISSN 0555-7631

Sharp, H.E. & Rowell, D.M. (2007). Unprecedent chromosomal diversity and behaviour modify linkage patterns and speciation potential: structural heterozigosity in an Australian spider. *Journal of Evolutionary Biology*, Vol.20, No.6, (November 2007), pp. 2427-2439, ISSN 1010-061X

Silva, D. (1988). Estudio cariotípico de *Loxosceles laeta* (Araneae: Loxoscelidae). *Revista Peruana de Entomologia*, Vol.31, (December 1988), pp. 9-12, ISSN 0080-2425

Silva, R.W.; Klisiowicz, D.R.; Cella, D.M.; Mangili, O.C. & Sbalqueiro, I.J. (2002). Differential distribution of constitutive heterochromatin in two species of brown spider: *Loxosceles intermedia* and *L. Laeta* (Araneae, Sicariidae), from the metropolitan region of Curitiba, PR (Brazil). *Acta Biologica Paranaense*, Vol.31, No.1-4, pp. 123-136, ISSN 0301-2123

Stávale, L.M.; Schneider, M.C.; Brescovit, A.D. & Cella, D.M. (2011). Chromosomal characteristics and karyotype of Oxyopidae spiders (Araneae, Entelegynae). *Genetics and Molecular Research*, Vol.10, No.2, (May 2011), pp. 752-763, ISSN 1676-5680

Suzuki, S. (1952). Cytological studies in spiders II. Chromosomal investigation in twenty two species of spiders belonging to the four families, Clubionidae, Sparassidae, Thomisidae and Oxyopidae, which constitute Clubionoidea, with special reference to sex chromosomes. *Journal of Science of the Hiroshima University, Series B, Division 1*, Vol.13, pp. 1-52, ISSN 0368-4113

Suzuki, S. (1954). Cytological studies in spiders III. Studies on the chromosomes of fifty-seven species of spiders belonging to seventeen families, with general considerations on chromosomal evolution. *Journal of Science of the Hiroshima University, Series B, Division 1*, Vol.15, pp. 23-136, ISSN 0368-4113

Wagner, J. (1896). Einige Beobachtungen über die spermatogenese bei den spinnen. *Zoologischer Anzeiger*, Vol.19, pp. 180-190, ISSN 0044-5231

Wallace, L.B. (1900). The acessory chromosome in the spider. *Anatomischer Anzeiger*, Vol.18, pp. 327-329, ISSN 0003-2786

Wallace, L.B. (1905). The spermatogenesis of the spider. *Biological Bulletin*, Vol.8, No.3, (February 1905), pp. 169-184, ISSN 0006-3185

Wallace, L.B. (1909). The spermatogenesis of *Agalena naevia*. *Biological Bulletin*, Vol.17, No.2, (July 1909), pp. 120-161, ISSN 0006-3185

Wang, Z. & Yan, H.M. (2001). Technique of chromosome on spider blood cell. *Chinese Journal of Zoology*, Vol.36, pp. 45-46, ISSN 0250-3263

White, M.J.D. (1940). The origin and evolution of multiple sex-chromosome mechanisms. *Journal of Genetics*, Vol.40, No.1-2, (May 1940), pp. 303-336, ISSN 0022-1333

Wise, D. (1983). An electron microscope study of the karyotypes of two wolf spiders. *Canadian Journal of Genetics and Cytology*, Vol.25, pp. 161-168, ISSN 0008-4093

# 6

# How Does the Alteration of Meiosis Evolve to Parthenogenesis? - Case Study in a Water Flea, *Daphnia pulex* -

Chizue Hiruta[1] and Shin Tochinai[1,2]
[1]*Department of Natural History Sciences, Graduate School of Science, Hokkaido University,*
[2]*Department of Natural History Sciences, Faculty of Science, Hokkaido University, Japan*

## 1. Introduction

This chapter reviews progress in our understanding of two different reproductive modes in *Daphnia pulex* and discusses the interesting modifications found in meiosis during parthenogenesis.

Most daphnid species reproduce parthenogenetically as well as sexually, resulting in the production of diploid progenies in both cases. In natural populations, parthenogenesis is the common mode of reproduction, and parthenogenetic offspring are all female. However, in response to certain environmental conditions, such as crowding or seasonal change, male offspring are also produced parthenogenetically, and sexual reproduction occurs (Hebert, 1978). Although they switch between parthenogenesis and sexual reproduction in response to environmental conditions, little is known about the molecular and cytological mechanisms switching and governing each reproductive mode. It can be interpreted that *D. pulex* develops a reproductive strategy utilizing 'parthenogenesis', which has high reproductive power, and 'sexual reproduction', which generates genetic diversity, in response to different environments. These theoretical studies have been made on evolutionary mechanism of reproductive modes (Decaestecker *et al.*, 2009); however, practically no study analyzing the evolutionary mechanism while taking the developmental constraints into consideration has so far been conducted. Our understanding of the evolution of reproductive strategy would increase once we precisely clarify the developmental gene programs operating there. We have recently started to develop *D. pulex* as an experimental model for studying oogenesis and developmental mechanisms during evolution.

### 1.1 Chapter contents

- At first, we explain why we are interested in the comparative research of two reproductive modes: parthenogenesis and sexual reproduction, and why we chose *D. pulex* as an experimental animal.

- From our experiments, it was concluded that diploid progeny are produced by non-reductional division in parthenogenetic *D. pulex*. We found that, when a parthenogenetic egg entered the first meiosis, division was arrested in the early first anaphase. Then, two half-bivalents, which were dismembered from each bivalent, moved back to the equatorial plate and assembled to form a diploid equatorial plate. Finally, the sister chromatids were separated and moved to opposite poles in the same manner as the second meiotic division.
- We hypothesized that *D. pulex* switches reproductive mode by controlling the maturation division of oocytes (arrest or progress), depending on whether the egg is fertilized or not.
- We use *D. pulex* as an example of the evolutionary process of parthenogenesis which arose from sexual reproduction. Suggestions for future research are also presented.

## 2. A water flea, *Daphnia pulex*

Water fleas of the genus *Daphnia* are members of the order Cladocera, which are small crustaceans that live in various aquatic environments varying from temporary ponds to large lakes as a cosmopolitan species. They occupy a key position (food chain) in aquatic communities, both as important herbivores eating algae and bacteria and as major prey items of fish, aquatic insects and other predators. Moreover, they have a value as environmental indicator organisms because of their high sensitivity to water quality. Thus, many previous studies have concentrated on ecology, taxonomy and toxicology. Recently however, the spotlight has been on the phenotypic plasticity of *D. pulex*. One example of this phenomenon is that they express morphological, life history, and behavioral defenses in response to chemical cues released by predators (Tollrian & Dodson, 1999).

### 2.1 General feature

#### 2.1.1 Anatomical characteristics

The carapace is transparent and encloses the whole trunk, except the head and the apical spine. The trunk appendages are flattened, leaf-like structures that serve for suspension feeding and for locomotion. There is a single central compound eye in the head. The large, paired appendages used for swimming are second antennae.

**Female**: The body length of the female is about 1-3 mm. The first antennae are small and short, not extending beyond the rostrum. The ovaries are a pair of elongated organs lying on either side of the gut. In the posterior part of the each ovary, the oviduct opens into the brood chamber. As shown in Fig. 1C, oogonia and smaller oocytes are located in the most-posterior part of the ovary, and move anteriorly as development progresses. The number of eggs spawned in a clutch depends on the nutritional state and the size of the female. The space between the body and the carapace is used as a brood chamber.

**Male**: The males are smaller than the females. The rostrum is generally indistinct and the first antennae are large and long. The male has a copulatory hook, which is used for holding on to the female during mating, on the first thoracic leg. The testes are a pair of elongated organs lying on either side of the gut. The two gonopores open near the anus. As shown in Fig. 1F, the mature testis has spermatozoa in the lumen. Spermatogenesis begins at the walls and proceeds into the innermost part (lumen).

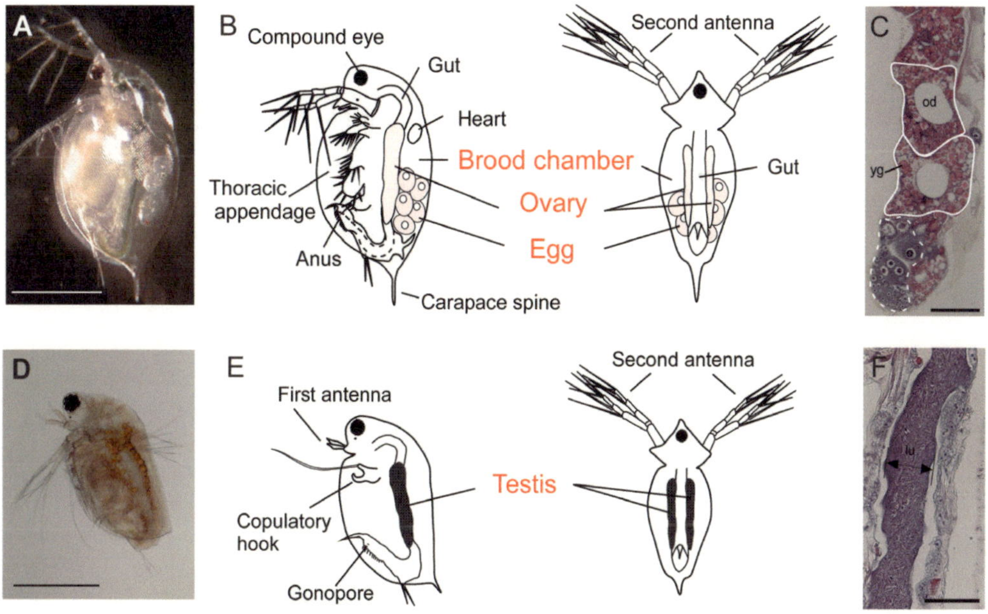


Fig. 1. *Daphnia pulex*. Anatomical characteristics of an adult female (top row) and male (bottom row). (A,D) Photo. Scale bars = 1 mm in A; 0.5 mm in D. (B,E) Lateral (left) and frontal (right) view of anatomy. (C) Sagittal section of the ovary. The largest eggs (solid white line) contain a large amount of yolk granules and oil droplets. Oogonia and smaller oocytes are located in the most-posterior part of the ovary (dashed white line). Scale bar = 50 µm. yg, yolk granule; od, oil droplet. (F) Sagittal section of the testis. Sperms are located in the lumen. Scale bar = 100 µm. lu, lumen.

### 2.1.2 Life cycle

*Daphnia pulex* reproduce either by parthenogenesis or sexual reproduction and populations are almost exclusively female. Under favorable conditions, eggs are produced in clutches of one to several dozen, and one female may produce several clutches, which is linked with the molting process. The eggs are laid in the brood chamber shortly after molting. Embryonic development occurs in the brood chamber and the larvae are miniature versions of the adults. The neonates are released from the brood chamber just before the mother molts. In this way, the parthenogenetic individual repeats the cycle of molting, egg laying and releasing during her life (Fig. 2, Non-resting cycle).

Unfavorable conditions, such as changes in water temperature or food deprivation as a result of population increase, may induce the production of males. In other words, a single parthenogenetic female can produce either parthenogenetic female offspring and/or males for sexual reproduction. The male clasps the female and display copulatory behavior. Then the resting eggs are produced (Fig. 2, Resting cycle). Only two large eggs produced in a single clutch (one from each ovary) are enclosed in an ephippium which used to be a part of the dorsal exoskeleton and is darkly pigmented with melanin. The resting eggs are resistant to desiccation and freezing during winter, playing an important role in colonizing new habitats or in the re-establishment of an extinguished population after unfavorable conditions.

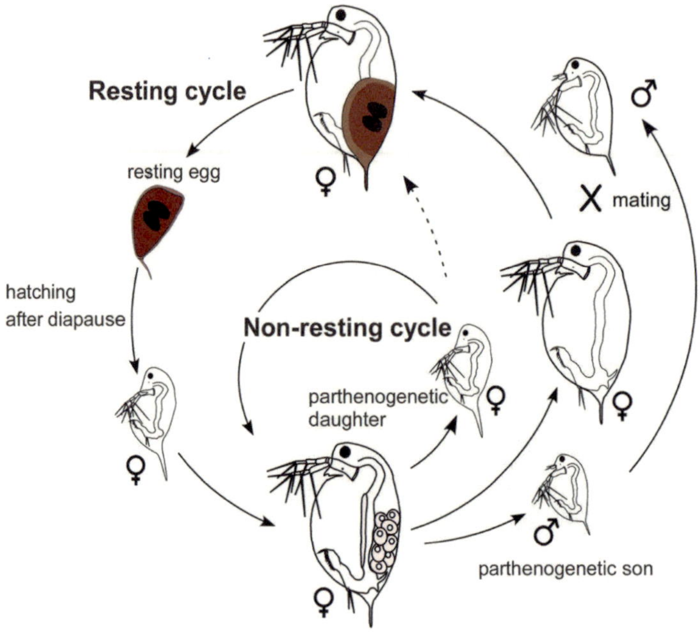


Fig. 2. Life cycle of *D. pulex*. Life cycle can be divided into 'resting cycle' and 'non-resting cycle'. In natural populations, parthenogenesis is the common mode of reproduction, and parthenogenetic offspring are normally female (parthenogenetic non-resting cycle). However, in response to unfavorable conditions, such as crowding or seasonal change, male offspring are also produced parthenogenetically, and then sexual reproduction occurs (sexual resting cycle). Although a female usually produces resting eggs requiring fertilization by sperm, it sometimes happens that a female produces parthenogenetic resting eggs (parthenogenetic resting cycle, dashed arrow).

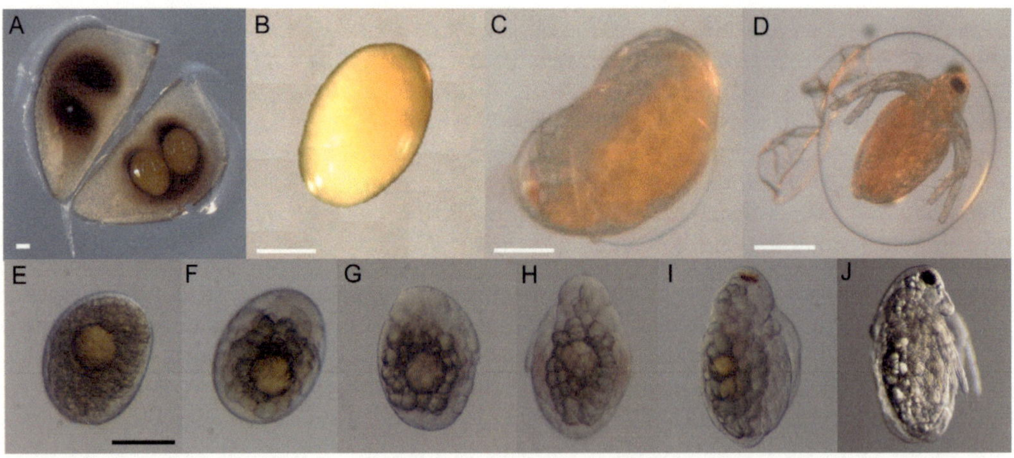


Fig. 3. Embryogenesis of resting egg (top row) and non-resting egg (bottom row). (A-D) The resting egg was produced by parthenogenesis. There was no difference in the manner of development between a parthenogenetic resting egg and a sexual resting egg. Scale bars = 100 µm. (E-J) Embryonic development was completed in about 3 days at 18°C. Scale bar = 100 µm.

There are two types of eggs, i) **resting egg**, also termed 'winter egg', 'diapause egg', 'dormant egg' or 'ephippial egg', ii) **non-resting egg**, also known as 'summer egg' or 'subitaneous egg', as mentioned above (Figs. 2 and 3). In any maturation stage they are easily distinguishable from each other in the ovary of the living animal. Although the non-resting eggs produce both female and male neonates, the resting eggs produce female offspring without exception.

Examination of the literature on reproduction of this species reveals a great deal of confusion regarding the relationship between the types of egg and reproductive modes. Interestingly, Hobæk & Larsson (1990) reported that the formation of male offspring and resting eggs are independently controlled, possibly by distinct sets of environmental cues. We have also observed parthenogenetic resting eggs in *D. pulex* (Fig. 2, dashed arrow) and confirmed that the eggs have the potential to develop normally (Fig. 3A-D). Most daphnids are believed to switch to sexual reproduction resulting in the production of resting eggs; however, several daphnid species, not forgetting *D. pulex*, can produce them without fertilization. Moreover, the switch to sexual reproduction involves a commitment by the mother to produce a resting egg case (ephippium) and to produce eggs capable of diapause. Thus, the decision to produce a non-resting or a resting egg must be made long before the point at which the egg is fertilized. So far, it is clear that 1) both non-resting and resting eggs are produced by parthenogenesis, 2) resting eggs are also produced by sexual reproduction. Whether non-resting eggs can be produced by sexual reproduction or not has never been studied.

### 2.2 *Daphnia pulex* as an evolutionary developmental biology (evo-devo) model

*Daphnia pulex* is an ideally suited laboratory animal for workers in the fields of development and genetic research: It is easy to raise under laboratory conditions, propagates quickly because of its short reproductive cycle, and can induce male offspring by a juvenile hormone, methyl farnesoate (Olmstead & Leblanc, 2002). In addition, new experimental techniques (e.g., *in situ* hybridization, immunofluorescence, microinjection, RNAi) were established in daphnid species over the past several years (Sagawa *et al.*, 2005; Tsuchiya *et al.*, 2009; Kato *et al.*, 2011). Moreover, a recent description of the complete genome sequence for *Daphnia pulex* (Colbourne *et al.*, 2011) and genetic linkage map (Cristescu *et al.*, 2006) will provide us with a powerful tool for analyzing the molecular mechanism of any aspect in this species, including enigmatic meiotic processes. *Daphnia pulex* has only a 200-megabase genome and as many as about 31,000 genes. Thirty-six percent of *Daphnia pulex* genes have no detectable homologs with other animal species and about 13,000 genes have been identified as paralogs. There will be a good chance to find novel genes which enable the evolution of a unique reproductive strategy in this species. For these reasons, *D. pulex* started to garner attention as an evo-devo model animal (Jenner & Wills, 2007).

## 3. Reproductive mode of *D. pulex*

*Daphnia pulex* adopt parthenogenesis and sexual reproduction differentially in response to varied environmental cues as mentioned above. The production of diploid progenies is a common finding in both reproductive modes.

### 3.1 Parthenogenesis

The reproductive modes of *D. pulex* were studied over the past century. Previous studies suggested that *D. pulex* produces parthenogenetic eggs via apomixis; the nuclear division of mature oocytes should be an equational division equal to somatic mitosis (Kühn, 1908; Ojima, 1954, 1958; Zaffagnini & Sabelli, 1972). However, due to the presence of a large amount of yolk and the minute size of chromosomes, it was not easy to observe the nucleus during the process of oogenesis and therefore the behavior of chromosomes in the ovarian egg remained undescribed. In spite of previous reports that suggested the occurrence of mitosis in parthenogenetic oocytes, we found "abortive meiosis" instead during the oogenesis of parthenogenetic *D. pulex*, as mentioned below (see section 5). This finding suggests that parthenogenetic *D. pulex* may switch to sexual reproduction by progressing the maturation division of oocytes from arrest. Moreover, it would give parthenogenetic *D. pulex* a mechanism making recombination possible even under parthenogenesis. In other words, it can lead to offspring with genetic variability because chromosomal recombination can take place between homologous chromosomes, while there is no introduction of new genes from another individual.

### 3.2 Sexual reproduction

At present very little is known about the process of meiosis and fertilization during sexual reproduction in this species. Although it still is a matter of debate, Ojima (1958) reported that sperm seemed to penetrate into the ovarian egg. The structure of the spermatozoa is very atypical in daphnid species. The mature sperm of *D. pulex* lacks a flagellum and is therefore not actively mobile. Indeed, during mating, the male deposits sperm near the openings of the female gonopore. Studies are needed to clarify the timing of fertilization and the process of meiosis. It will provide us not only with insight into the switching mechanism of reproductive modes, but also with the differences between normal meiosis and abortive meiosis.

## 4. Oogenesis of parthenogenetic *D. pulex*

In this section, we offer a close overview of the growth and maturation of the parthenogenetic eggs. Mature and spawned eggs in the same brood were the same size and mostly synchronized in the maturation stage (cell cycle). It takes approximately 60 h for oocytes to grow in the ovary (from 0 to 60 h, Fig. 4). Inclusions such as yolk granules and oil droplets increased in size and number until the fully-grown egg is formed. The nuclear division apparatus appears just after molting (at 0 min after molting (0 AM): Fig. 4). We observed the precise states of nuclei in the eggs with the following timing during the course of parthenogenesis (from egg maturation to early development): 1) the time of molting of the female (Fig. 4, 0 AM), 2) the interval between molting and 13 min after molting. The parthenogenetic eggs began to migrate from the ovary to the brood chamber and this process was completed within about 3 min, 3) the time when oviposition was completed (Fig. 4, 0 min post oviposition (0 PO)), and 4) the time during which the parthenogenetic eggs in the brood chamber began to develop.

At the stage of 0 h of egg maturation, the oocyte was at first morphologically indistinguishable from the nurse cell (Fig. 5A). In early stages, the development of both oocytes and nurse cells proceeds in a similar manner, but only the egg cells developed to form yolk granules and oil droplets during maturation, whereas the nurse cells became smaller in size and finally degenerated (Fig. 5B-D). With the passage of time, the yolk granules and oil droplets increased in number in the oocytes. Soon after grown juveniles were discharged from the brood chamber, the nuclear membrane of the fully-matured ovarian egg to be spawned gradually disappeared, and finally the breakdown of the germinal vesicle took place just before molting of the mother (Fig. 5E).

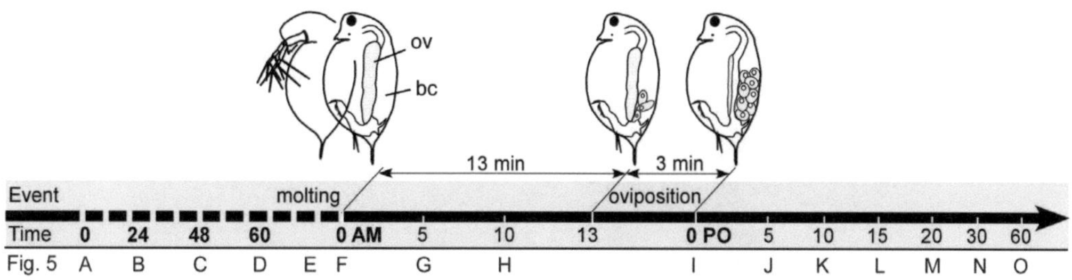


Fig. 4. The time course of parthenogenesis in *D. pulex*. The oviposition cycle is about 3 days at 18°C. The broken line of the time axis (from 0 to 60) indicates the time scale in hours, and the solid line of time axis (from 0 AM to 60 PO) indicates the time scale in minutes. Usually, after releasing all neonates that developed in the dorsal brood chamber, females molt. After this molt occurs at 0 AM (minutes after molting), a strict time course proceeds. The female begins extruding eggs into the brood chamber at 13 AM and this process is completed within about 3 min. The point of 0 PO (minutes post oviposition) indicates the time when the female extruded the last egg. Then, the parthenogenetic eggs in the brood chamber develop into juveniles. Ovarian and spawned eggs in a clutch are approximately the same size and mostly synchronized in the cell cycle. In the lower part of Fig. 4, the capital letters show the point of time when the specimens were observed in Fig. 5. ov, ovary; bc, brood chamber. Modified from Hiruta *et al.*, 2010.

The chromosomes co-oriented in a position midway between the poles, and then each bivalent started to separate into two half-bivalents, one moving to each pole of the spindle by 5 AM (Fig. 5F, G). However, the movement of chromosomes from the metaphase plate to the poles was arrested at an early stage of anaphase before 10 AM (Fig. 5H). Egg laying (oviposition) began at 13 AM. The migration of all eggs from the ovary to the brood chamber was completed within about 3 min (= 0 PO). At 0 PO, the chromosomes moved back and assembled as a diploid equatorial plate around the equator of the spindle in the spawned egg (Fig. 5I). By 5 PO, the division apparatus migrated to the periphery and the cell division cycle restarted. Then the sister chromatids moved apart, one going to each pole of the spindle through metaphase and anaphase by 10 PO (Fig. 5J, K). The complete set of chromosomes was lifted above the egg surface and eventually one polar body-like small daughter cell was extruded at around 20 PO (Fig. 5L, M).

After the completion of oogenesis, the chromosomes left in the egg moved deeper inside the egg (Fig. 5N) and mitosis occurred without cytokinesis, resulting in a polynuclear syncytial embryo (Fig. 5O). Then, the nuclei migrated to the periphery, and a typical superficial cleavage proceeded.

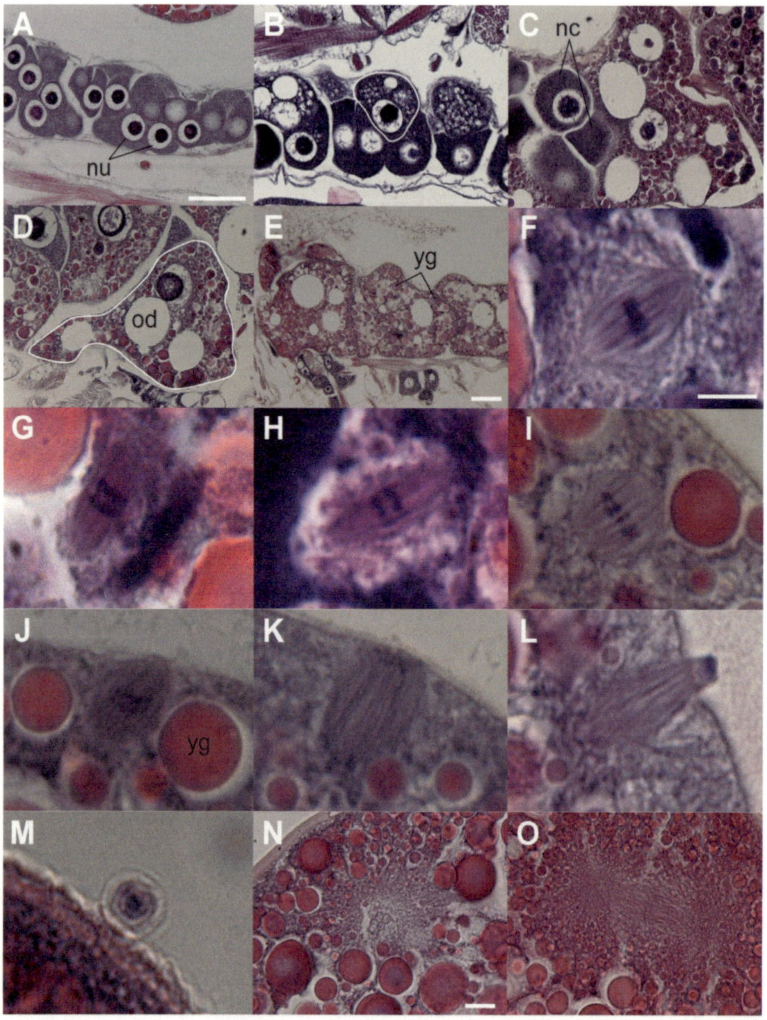


Fig. 5. Oogenesis of parthenogenetic *D. pulex*. (A-E) Oocytes and nurse cells in the ovary. (F-H) The division apparatus in ovarian eggs. (I-O) The division apparatus in eggs spawned to the brood chamber. (A) 0 h. The oocytes and nurse cells were indistinguishable. (B) 24 h. Yolk and oil droplet formation took place only in oocytes. (C) 48 h. The yolk granules and oil droplets increased. (D) 60 h. The degeneration of nurse cells proceeded. (E) Just before molting. The breakdown of the germinal vesicle (GVBD) took place. (F) 0 AM. Division apparatus appeared and chromosomes aligned at the metaphase plate. (G) 5 AM. Each bivalent is separated into two half-bivalents. (H) 10 AM. The division seemed to stop at early anaphase. (I) 0 PO. The chromosomes moved back and rearranged around the equator of the spindle. (J) 5 PO. The chromosomes started to separate. (K) 10 PO. The division proceeded to anaphase. (L) 15 PO. One complete set of chromosomes was lifted above the egg surface. (M) 20 PO. A polar body-like small daughter cell was extruded. (N) 30 PO. The swelled chromosomes left in the egg moved to a deeper part. (O) 60 PO. The first cleavage proceeded without cytokinesis. Scale bars = 100 µm in A-E; 5 µm in F-M; 10 µm in N and O. nc, nurse cell; nu, nucleus; od, oil droplet; yg, yolk granule. Solid white circle indicates an oocyte. Modified from Hiruta *et al.*, 2010 and unpublished data.

## 5. Abortive meiosis found in parthenogenetic *D. pulex*

Parthenogenetic eggs achieve two successive divisions like normal meiosis while the first division is abortive (see section 4). In the first meiosis, bivalents align at the equatorial plate (Fig. 6A) and begin to separate into two half-bivalents (Fig. 6B). Then, each half-bivalent moves back and sister chromatids rearrange as a diploid equatorial plate around the equator of the spindle (Fig. 6C). Finally, the second meiosis-like division takes place normally, producing a single polar body-like extremely small daughter cell (Fig. 6D). Compared with meiosis, it is known that the first meiotic division is skipped there.

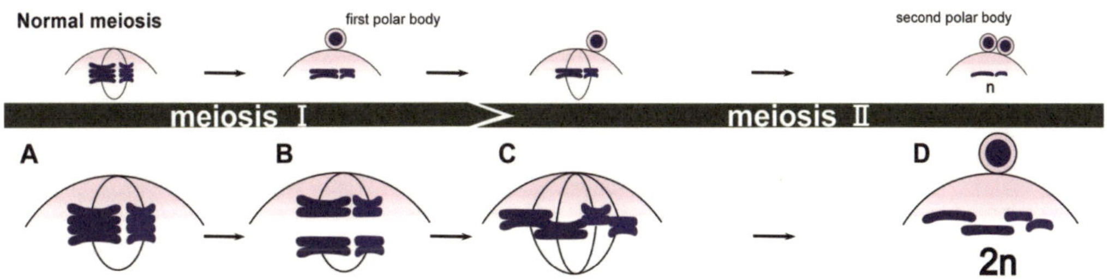


Fig. 6. Schematic illustration of parthenogenesis in *D. pulex*. The top row shows the process of meiosis. In the first meiosis, bivalents aligned at the metaphase plate and separate into two half-bivalents, producing the first polar body. Then, the second meiosis takes place, producing the second polar body. As a result, a haploid egg is produced. By contrast, a diploid egg is produced by parthenogenesis in *D. pulex*. (A) In the first meiosis, bivalents align at the equatorial plate and begin to separate into two half-bivalents. (B) However, the division is arrested at early anaphase. (C) Then each half-bivalent moves back and sister chromatids rearrange as a diploid equatorial plate around the equator of the spindle. (D) Finally, the second meiosis-like division takes place normally, producing a single polar body-like extremely small daughter cell. Illustration adopted from Hiruta *et al.*, 2010.

### 5.1 Hypothetical model for reproductive strategy in *D. pulex*

We hypothesized that *D. pulex* switches its reproductive mode (sexual or parthenogenetic) depending on whether the egg is fertilized or not. It is highly plausible that, if the egg is not fertilized, the first meiosis is aborted and, subsequently, a second meiosis-like division takes place as observed in our study. On the other hand, normal meiosis may well occur if the ovarian egg is fertilized. If this is true, it seems appropriate to assume that fertilization occurs at the stage between first metaphase and anaphase in the ovarian egg.

Since the two reproductive modes (sexual reproduction or parthenognesis) are not strictly associated with the two types of egg (resting or non-resting egg) as mentioned in section 2.1.2, a study will need to be conducted to verify the hypothesis including whether the non-resting egg is produced by sexual reproduction. If this hypothesis is true, daphnid species adopt the least waste system in the production of eggs, because eggs are able to develop regardless of fertilization. In order to verify this hypothesis, we are currently trying to establish the methods for *in vitro* maturation of ovarian eggs and artificial insemination.

## 6. Spindle assembly and spatial distribution of γ-tubulin during abortive meiosis in parthenogenetic *D. pulex*

During the analysis of nuclear maturation division, which resulted in either parthenogenetic or sexual development of the egg, we found that the spindle in abortive meiosis was barrel-shaped, anastral, and organized without centrosomes (Fig. 7, Hiruta C., unpublished). Corresponding to our results, a barrel-shaped meiotic spindle without centrosomes has been reported in several animal species including parthenogenetic pea aphid (Riparbelli *et al.*, 2005). The centrosomes are present in cleavage division (mitosis) of both reproductive modes. In the case of sexual reproduction in various animals, the sperm supplies the centriole after fertilization. On the other hand, in the case of parthenogenesis in insects, centrosomes are spontaneously assembled in mitotic spindle microtubules. We suspect that *de novo* assembled centrosomes could be an evolutionary conserved process leading to parthenogenetic development.

Even more surprisingly, gamma (γ)-tubulin is localized along spindle microtubules for the duration of abortive meiosis, while it is present only on the centrosomes in parthenogens' cleavage division (Fig. 7, Hiruta C., unpublished). The results from *D. pulex* are identical with those from pig oocytes, but not universal among animals (Lee *et al.*, 2000). Incidentally, the localization of γ-tubulin to centrosomes corresponds to a typical spindle formation which is highly conserved in animals. Comparative research needs to be conducted to reveal whether sperm entry affects the localization of γ-tubulin in *D. pulex* or not.

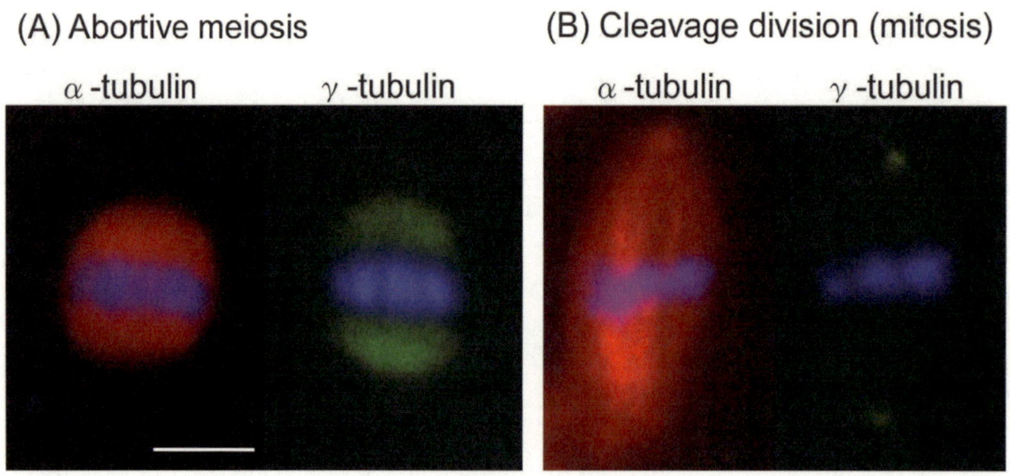


Fig. 7. Immunofluorescence localization of α- and γ-tubulin during abortive meiosis and cleavage division (mitosis). Scale bar = 5 μm. Chromosomes were counter-stained with DAPI (blue). (A) Spindle formation was barrel-shaped, anastral, and organized without centrosomes. Gamma-tubulin was distributed along spindle microtubules during abortive meiosis. (B) Spindle formation was spindle-shaped, astral, and had organized centrosomes. Gamma-tubulin was present only the spindle poles. Hiruta C., unpublished.

## 7. Molecular basis of the transition from sexual reproduction to parthenogenesis

There are variations of the meiotic program that would produce diploid oocytes by skipping a division, by fusion of a haploid oocyte with a polar body, or by premeiotic endoreplication of chromosomes (Suomalainen *et al.*, 1987; Schön *et al.*, 2009). At any rate, it is thought that parthenogenesis evolved from sexual reproduction by changing the meiotic program. It seems likely that a relatively simple deviation from the established program of oogenesis, *i.e.*, meiosis, is sufficient to permit parthenogenesis. Schurko *et al.* (2009) reported that expression patterns of meiosis-related and meiosis-specific genes (*e.g.*, SMCs, REC8) during sexual reproduction of *D. pulex* are similar to that during parthenogenesis. Some of these genes are present in multiple copies and might be expressed differently in sexual reproduction and parthenogenesis. To cite one example, there are seven RECQ2 copies, which limit crossing over, which could have evolved novel roles in parthenogenesis. In fact, as if to correspond to the expectation, we have so far failed to observe chiasmata where crossing over occurred. In addition, it is suggested that PLK1, which is involved in orienting kinetochores during mitosis and meiosis, controls the localization within the spindle of γ-tubulin for mitotic spindle formation through the augmin complex in human and *drosophila* cells (Goshima *et al.*, 2008; Uehara *et al.*, 2009). As mentioned in section 6, the γ-tubulin is localized along the spindle in abortive meiosis. There is a possibility that a PLK copy is expressed in parthenogenesis specifically to operate the localization of γ-tubulin. We expect to reveal how the meiotic program is altered resulting in parthenogenesis. On the other hand, the absence of meiosis-specific DMC1 suggests that innovations for recombination in meiosis and parthenogenesis in *D. pulex* may have evolved. In the last paragraph, we stated factors associated with regulation of chromosomal organization. The following discussion is about the cell cycle control factors. There are several copies of cell cycle proteins, such as cyclins, cdks and polo kinases in *D. pulex*. In particular, the Mos-MAPK (mitogen-activated protein kinase) pathway, which is responsible for metaphase arrest in meiosis I or II before fertilization in many animal species (Sagata, 1996), might be a candidate for cell cycle arrest in parthenogenetic *D. pulex*. We have preliminary data that MAP kinase is expressed in *D. pulex* oocyte in metaphase of meiosis I.

Consequently, a precise description of the reproductive modes in *D. pulex* allows us to understand the mechanism which is widely preserved in eukaryotes and in the *Daphnia*-specific mechanism, namely, commonality and diversity of the pattern of division.

## 8. How does the transition from sexual reproduction to parthenogenesis occur during evolution?

Parthenogenesis, which is thought to arise from the alteration of meiosis, has been found in various animal species (Suomalainen *et al.*, 1987; Schön *et al.*, 2009). In many taxonomic groups, parthenogenesis was independently acquired during evolution. By comparing those cases, we could gain insight into the transition from sexual reproduction to parthenogenesis, many of which resulted from the change made during meiosis. According to Suomalainen *et al.* (1987), the following cases have been categorized as the type of 'skipped the first meiosis' (Fig. 8).

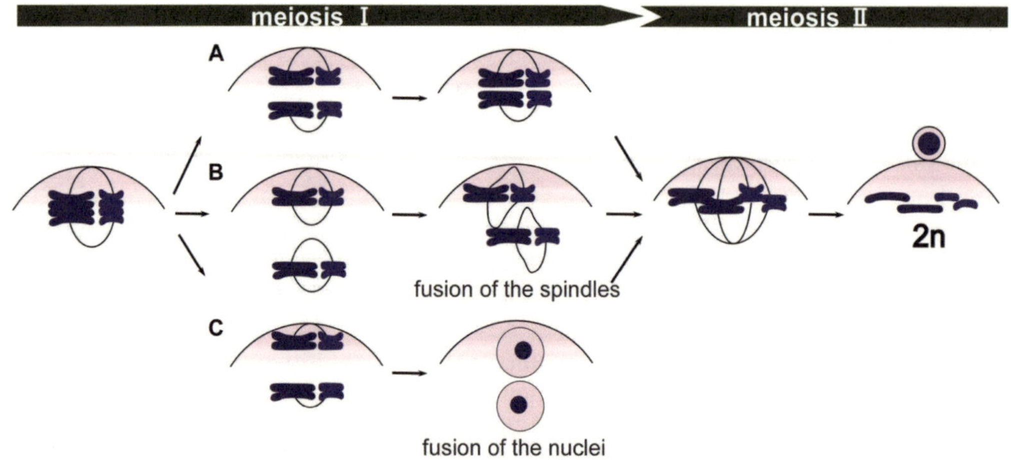


Fig. 8. Different types of abortive meiosis. These are categorized as 'skipped the first meiosis'. (A) *Daphnia pulex*. Two half-bivalents move back to the equatorial plate. (B) *Apterona helix*. Two spindles, an inner and outer, come together side by side and fuse. (C) *Fasciola hepatica*. Two haploid nuclei fuse.

In Lepidoptera *Apterona helix* (Fig. 8B), the first meiosis is aborted at the end of anaphase and two metaphase plates, an inner and outer, are formed. Both of these contain the haploid number of chromosomes and have separate spindles. Before the second meiosis, the inner metaphase spindle with its chromosome plate moves to the side of the outer spindle. Finally, the two spindles and the metaphase plates lie side by side and fuse (Narbel, 1946). In Crustacea *Artemia salina,* Lepidoptera *Solenobia lichenella, Luffia ferchaultella* and *L. lapidella,* meiosis is interrupted at some stage between the end of the first anaphase and the second metaphase (Narbel-Hofstetter, 1950, 1963, 1965; Stefani, 1960). Then the two haploid plates reunite, forming a new metaphase spindle, and the second diploid meiosis is accomplished. In Trematoda *Fasciola hepatica* (Fig. 8C), the first meiosis occurs without cytokinesis, giving rise to two haploid nuclei. These nuclei fuse and form a diploid cleavage nucleus (Sanderson, 1952).

There are differences at the stage of division arrest and restoration or maintenance of diploidy even in the same division that skipped the first meiosis. At any rate, if first meiosis is completely skipped, parthenogenetic division becomes congruent with mitosis and finally turns out to be obligate parthenogenesis. A comparative and detailed study of the parthenogenetic mechanism will bring us to a better understanding of the possible alteration of meiosis during evolution.

## 9. Conclusion

In conclusion, *D. pulex* is suitable for experimentation to understand the evolution of reproductive modes from a viewpoint of evolutionary developmental biology. The case study in *D. pulex* will contribute to a discussion of challenges such as how does parthenogenesis work and how evolution of sexual reproduction and parthenogenesis occurs.

## 10. Acknowledgments

We are grateful to the members of the Tochinai laboratory for their helpful advice and discussion. We also thank a great number of *D. pulex* that made a sacrifice for our research. CH was supported by a JSPS Research Fellowships for Young Scientists (No. 09J01653). This work was supported by a Grant-in-Aid for Exploratory Research, financed by the Ministry of Education, Culture, Sports, Science and Technology, Japan to ST (No. 21657054).

## 11. References

Colbourne, JK., Pfrender, ME., Gilbert, D., Thomas, WK., Tucker, A., Oakley, TH., Tokishita, S., Aerts, A., Arnold, GJ., Basu, MK., Bauer, DJ., Cáceres, CE., Carmel, L., Casola, C., Choi, JH., Detter, JC., Dong, Q., Dusheyko, S., Eads, BD., Fröhlich, T., Geiler-Samerotte, KA., Gerlach, D., Hatcher, P., Jogdeo, S., Krijgsveld, J., Kriventseva, EV., Kültz, D., Laforsch, C., Lindquist, E., Lopez, J., Manak, JR., Muller, J., Pangilinan, J., Patwardhan, RP., Pitluck, S., Pritham, EJ., Rechtsteiner, A., Rho, M., Rogozin, IB., Sakarya, O., Salamov, A., Schaack, S., Shapiro, H., Shiga, Y., Skalitzky, C., Smith, Z., Souvorov, A., Sung, W., Tang, Z., Tsuchiya, D., Tu, H., Vos, H., Wang, M., Wolf, YI., Yamagata, H., Yamada, T., Ye, Y., Shaw, JR., Andrews, J., Crease, TJ., Tang, H., Lucas, SM., Robertson, HM., Bork, P., Koonin, EV., Zdobnov, EM., Grigoriev, IV., Lynch, M. & Boore, JL. (2011). The ecoresponsive genome of *Daphnia pulex*. *Science*, Vol.331, No.6017, pp.555-561

Cristescu, MEA., Colbourne, JK., Radivojac, J. & Lynch, M. (2006). A microsatellite-based genetic linkage map of the waterflea, *Daphnia pulex*: On the prospect of crustacean genomics. *Genomics*, Vol.88, No.4, pp.415-430

Decaestecker, E., Meester, LD. & Mergeay, J. (2009). Cyclical parthenogenesis in *Daphnia*: Sexual versus asexual reproduction, In: *Lost sex: The evolutionary biology of parthenogenesis*, Schön, I., Martens, K. & Dijk, PV., pp.295-316, Springer, ISBN 978-90-481-2769-6

Goshima, G., Mayer, M., Zhang, N., Stuurman, N. & Vale, RD. (2008). Augmin: a protein complex required for centrosome-independent microtubule generation within the spindle. *J Cell Biol.*, Vol.181, No.3, pp.421-429

Hebert, PDN. (1978). The population biology of *Daphnia* (Cruatacea, Daphnidae). *Biol. Rev.*, Vol.53, pp.387-426

Hiruta, C., Nishida, C. & Tochinai, S. (2010). Abortive meiosis in the oogenesis of parthenogenetic *Daphnia pulex*. *Chromosome Res.*, Vol.18, No.7, pp.833-840

Hobæk, A. & Larsson, P. (1990). Sex determination in *Daphnia magna*. *Ecology*, Vol.71, No.6, pp.2255-2268

Jenner, RA. & Wills, MA. (2007). The choice of model organisms in evo-devo. *Nat Rev Genet*, Vol.8, No.4, pp.311-319

Kato, Y., Shiga, Y., Kobayashi, K., Tokishita, S., Yamagata, H., Iguchi, T. & Watanabe, H. (2011). Development of an RNA interference method in the cladoceran crustacean *Daphnia magna*. *Dev Genes Evol*, Vol.220, pp.337-345

Kühn, A. (1908). Die Entwicklung der Keimzellen in den parthenogenetischen Generationen der Cladoceren *Daphnia pulex* de Geer und *Polyphemus pediculus* de Geer. *Arch Zellforsch*, Vol.1, pp.538-586

Lee, J., Miyano, T. & Moor, RM. (2000). Spindle formation and dynamics of γ-tubulin and nuclear mitotic apparatus protein distribution during meiosis in pig and mouse oocytes. *Biol Reprod*, Vol.62, No.5, pp.1184-1192

Narbel, M. (1946). La cytologie de la parthénogenèse chez *Apterona helix* Sieb. (Lepid, Psychides). *Rev. Suisse Zool*, Vol.53, pp.625–681

Narbel-Hofstetter, M. (1950). La cytologie de la parthénogenèse chez *Solinobia* sp. (*lichenella* L.?) (Lépidoptères, Psychides). *Chromosoma*, Vol.4, pp.56–90

Narbel-Hofstetter, M. (1963). Cytologie de la pseudogamie chez *Luffia lapidella* Goeze (Lepidoptera, Psychidae). *Chromosoma*, Vol.13, pp.623-645

Narbel-Hofstetter, M. (1965). La variabilité cytologique dans la descendance des femelles de *Luffia ferchaultella* Steph. (Lepidoptera, Psychidae). *Chromosoma*, Vol.16, pp.345–350.

Ojima, Y. (1954). Some cytological observations on parthenogenesis in *Daphnia pulex* (de Geer). *Jour Fac Sci Hokkaido Univ, Ser.VI, Zool.12*, pp.230-241

Ojima, Y. (1958). A cytological study on the development and maturation of the parthenogenetic and sexual eggs of *Daphnia pulex* (Crustacea, Cladocera). *Kwansei Gakuin Univ*, Annual Studies 6, pp.123-176

Olmstead, AW. & Leblanc, GA. (2002). Juvenoid hormone methyl farnesoate is a sex determinant in the crustacean *Daphnia magna*. *J Exp Zool*, Vol.293, No.7, pp.736-739

Riparbelli, MG., Tagu, D., Bonhomme, J. & Callaini, G. (2005). Aster self-organization at meiosis: a conserved mechanism in insect parthenogenesis?. *Dev Biol*, Vol.278, No.1, pp.220-230

Sagata, N. (1996). Meiotic metaphase arrest in animal oocytes: its mechanisms and biological significance. *Trends Cell Biol*, Vol.6, No.1, pp.22-28

Sagawa, K., Yamagata, H. & Shiga, Y. (2005). Exploring embryonic germ line development in the water flea, *Daphnia magna*, by zinc-finger-containing VASA as a marker. *Gene Expr Patterns*, Vol.5, pp.669-678

Sanderson, AR. (1952). Maturation and probable gynogenesis in the liver fluke, *Fasciola hepatica* L.. *Nature*, Vol.172, pp.110-112

Schön, I., Martens, K. & Dijk, PV. (2009). *Lost sex: The evolutionary biology of parthenogenesis*. Springer, ISBN 978-90-481-2769-6

Schurko, AM., Logsdon, JM Jr. & Eads, BD. (2009). Meiosis genes in *Daphnia pulex* and the role of parthenogenesis in genome evolution. *BMC Evol Biol*, Vol.9, No.78

Stefani, R. (1960). L'*Artemia salina* parthenogenetica a Cagliari. *Riv Biol*, Vol.52, pp.463-490

Suomalainen, E., Saura, A. & Lokki, J. (1987). *Cytology and evolution in parthenogenesis*. CRC Press, ISBN 0-8493-5981-3, Boca Raton, FL

Tollrian, R. & Dodson, SI. (1999). Inducible defenses in Cladocera: Constraints, costs, and multipredator environments, In: *The ecology and evolution of inducible defenses*, Tollrian, R. & Harvell, CD., pp.177-202, Princeton, ISBN 0-691-00494-3, UK

Tsuchiya, D., Eads, BD. & Zolan, ME. (2009). Methods for meiotic chromosome preparation, immunofluorescence, and fluorescence *in situ* hybridization in *Daphnia pulex*, In: *Meiosis, Volume 2: Cytological Methods, vol. 558*, Keeney, S., pp.235-249, Springer, ISBN 978-1-60761-103-5, USA

Uehara, R., Nozawa, RS., Tomioka, A., Petry, S., Vale, RD., Obuse, C. & Goshima, G. (2009). The augmin complex plays a critical role in spindle microtubule generation for mitotic progression and cytokinesis in human cells. *Proc Natl Acad Sci*, Vol.106, No.17, pp.6998-7003

Zaffagnini, F. & Sabelli, B. (1972). Karyologic observations on the maturation of the summer and winter eggs of *Daphnia pulex* and *Daphnia middendorffiana*. *Chromosoma*, Vol.36, No.2, pp.193-203

# Avian Meiotic Chromosomes as Model Objects in Cytogenetics

Katarzyna Andraszek and Elżbieta Smalec
*Siedlce University of Natural Sciences and Humanities, Poland*

## 1. Introduction

The beginning of the new millennium proved critical for life sciences. The team of scientists working on the Human Genome Mapping Project published and made available on the website of *Nature* a complete set of information on the human genome. Almost simultaneously an independent private company, Celera Genomics, published the results of its study of human DNA sequence in *Science*. The dream of scientists trying to read the human genome sequence for the last ten years was fulfilled. The end of the related rivalry was the beginning of a new epoch and a new field in genetics - genomics.

At present, genomics and cytogenetics are the two fastest-developing genetic disciplines. Genome mapping and karyotype standardization projects involve an increasingly greater number of animal and plant species. Genome exploration by physical mapping requires a knowledge of the karyotype of a given species for which the map is being created. The gene/chromosome interdependence is investigated through cooperation between international mapping projects and international karyotype standardization programs. A particularly dynamic rate of progress is observed in mapping the genomes of higher vertebrates. The most numerous group of vertebrates is constituted by birds and, as a paradox, it is their genome that is least well-known. Although they guard the secrets of their karyotype with the high diploid number and microchromosomes, birds have meiotic chromosomes of easy access and the intriguing lampbrush chromosomes.

The high number of chromosomes and the presence of microchromosomes in the avian karyotype have made cytogeneticists look for other sources of information on chromosomes. The extension of cytogenetic investigations over a greater number of chromosomes required the use of chemical agents, such as amethopterin or thymidine that inhibit chromosome condensation. Such experiments were undertaken on hens and produced poorly condensed chromosomes with bands in fine resolution. This made it possible to identify sixteen chromosome pairs.

Meiotic chromosomes are a valuable object for avian karyotype analyses. Meiosis is normally observed in males, as spermatocytes are relatively small, numerous and readily available. The most often analysed meiotic chromosomes are those contained in cells in the pachytene and diplotene of the first meiotic division. The experiments have predominantly concerned samples of testes. The observation of female meiotic chromosomes is limited by the large size of the egg cell, technical difficulty in sampling chromosomes from the egg cell and low numbers of the cells as compared with spermatocytes. Nevertheless, female meiotic chromosomes are worth paying attention to. The maturing oocytes isolated form the ovaries constitute the material for this type of experiments. Meiosis guarantees the stability of the chromosome number in the consecutive generations of sexually reproducing organisms. Generally, meiosis is represented as a process during which the cell passes through totally different stages that correspond with particular structure and behaviour of chromosomes. The observation of the changes occurring in the structure of meiotic chromosomes leads to an understanding of the nature of meiosis. The first prophase of meiosis, in which the crossing-over takes place, should be paid particular attention.

## 2. Lampbrush chromosomes

Oocytes - female reproductive cells are formed in oogenesis in ovaries. After the mitoses cease, the oogonia (primary sex cells) become first-order or primary oocytes. Next, they quickly enter the S phase, the preleptotene during which DNA is replicated for the last time. The oocyte grows during the meiotic prophase and, in most animals, stops expanding in the metaphase of the first meiotic division. Most of this cell growth takes place in the diplotene stage. In that stage, diplotene chromosomes of some vertebrates, e.g. birds assume the form of lampbrush chromosomes and generate thousands of loops along their axis, interpreted as sites of transcriptional activity (Macgregor & Varley, 1988; Morgan, 2002).

Lampbrush chromosomes still need to be fully explored. It is still unknown how they form out of the small mitotic structures, nor how they function in the oocyte. What is known is that they are intermediary structures present in the first meiotic division in the prolonged diplotene stage. They originate from a small telophase form at the end of the last oogonium mitosis. As they enter the diplotene stage of the first meiotic division, they undergo rapid decondensation that generates very large chromosome structures (Macgregor & Varley, 1988; Schmid et al., 2005).

Lampbrush chromosomes were discovered in 1882 by Flemming who observed salamander egg cells (*Ambystoma mexicanum*). Ten years on, LBCs were identified in shark egg cells and described by Rückert. It was Rückert who introduced the term "lampbrush chromosome" into biological nomenclature. The chromosomes take their name from 19th century brushes for cleaning street lamps to which Rückert likened them. The modern version of the item are bottle or test-tube brushes (Fig. 1) (Callan, 1986; Macgregor, 1977, 1980, 1987; Macgregor & Varley, 1988).

Lampbrush chromosomes are intermediate structures present during the first meiotic division. In the prolonged diplotene stage, they undergo decondensation that produces very large chromosomal structures. LBC length ranges (depending on the species) from 400 to 800 μm, which makes them up to 30 times larger than their mitotic counterparts (Callan, 1986; Callan et al., 1987; Rodionov, 1996). The basic profile of LBCs is performed with a 20x zoom of the microscope. In the case of avian mitotic chromosomes, a 20x zoom only makes it possible to identify the metaphase plate, not always enabling the determination of the number of chromosomes.

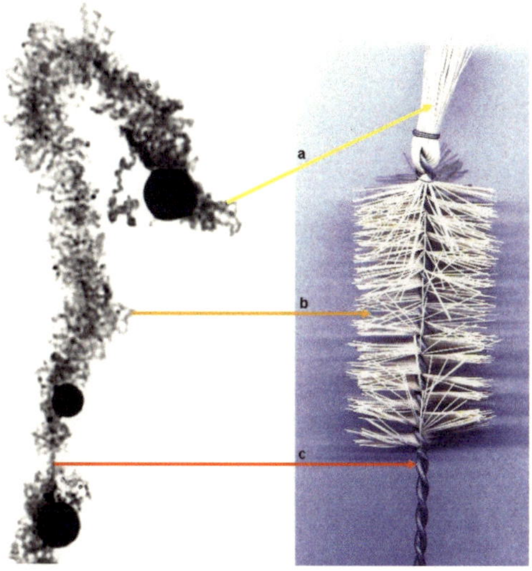


Fig. 1. A lampbrush chromosome and the "original item". The arrows indicate analogous structures; a- telomeric loop, b- side loops, c- a chromatid without loops (Katarzyna Andraszek).

Figure 2 shows a 20-fold microscopic magnification of the metaphase plate (a) compared in size with (b) 100-fold magnification of the second-pair mitotic chromosome) a 20-fold magnification of the second lampbrush bivalent (c). The arrow shows the second-pair mitotic chromosome on the metaphase plate.

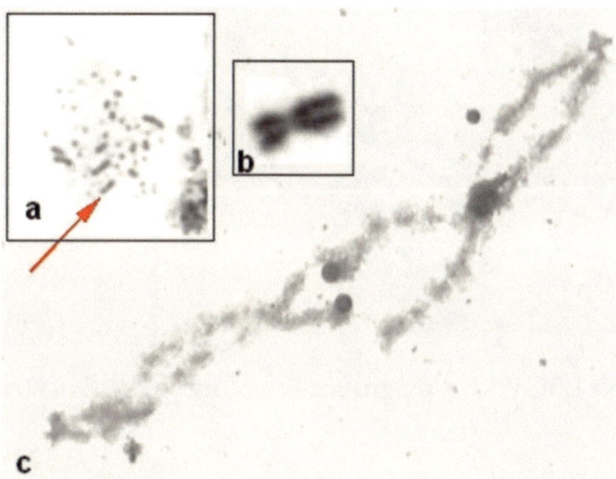


Fig. 2. A comparison of the size of LBC and mitotic chromosomes (Katarzyna Andraszek).

In the early prophase, a lampbrush chromosome is a bivalent that consists of two conjugating homologues ultimately becoming a tetrad. The axis of each of the homologue chromosomes is constituted by sister chromatids. Each chromatid is composed of alternately positioned regions of condensed inactive chromatin (chromomeres visible as dark irregular structures and also observed in the interphase nucleus) and side loops of decondensed chromatin. In the homologous sections of the bivalent, chromatin is condensed (spirally twisted) or decondensed in the form of side loops - two per each chromosome and four at the level of the bivalent. The loop constitutes a part of the chromosome axis. It is both extensible and contractible. The contractibility of the loop results in the contraction and dilation of the chromomere (Angelier et al., 1984, 1990, 1996; Chelysheva et al., 1990; Macgregor, 1987; Morgan, 2002).

The use of a 100x zoom to analyse LBC structure made it possible to observe chromomeres, chiasmata and sister chromatids of each bivalent homologue. The identical zoom used for the analysis of avian mitotic chromosomes enables only the identification of their morphological structure in relation to the first couple of macrochromosome pairs. Figure 3 shows a 20-fold magnification of the second goose bivalent (a) and its distinctive structures visible with a 100x zoom (b, f - telomeres, c - centromere, d - chiasm, e - sister chromatids). In the case of the structural analysis of male meiotic chromosomes it is not possible to observe these crucial meiotic cytogenetic features.

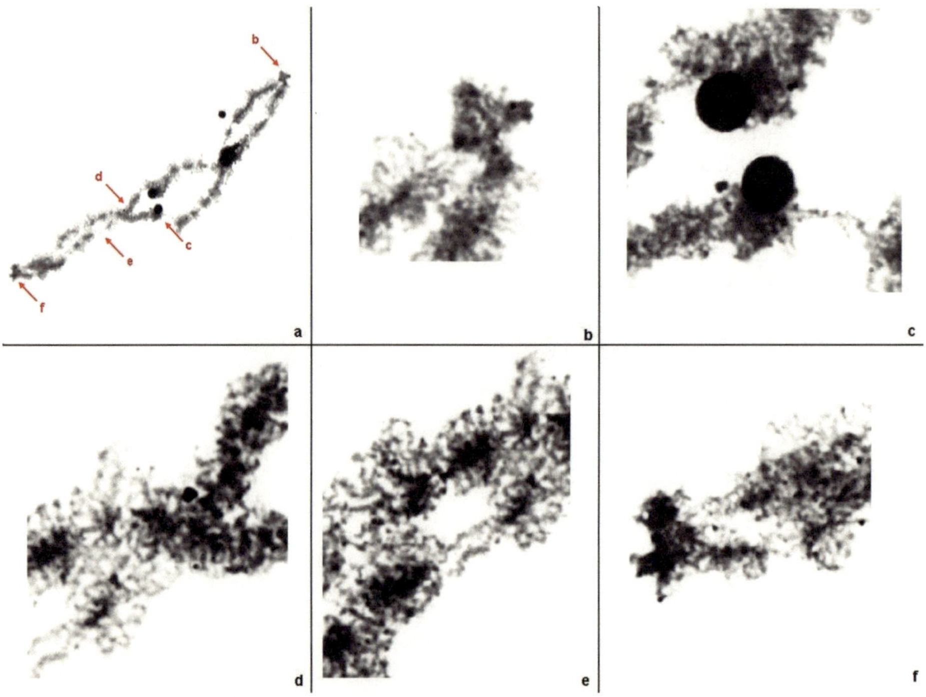


Fig. 3. The second goose LBC with a magnification of its distinctive structures (Katarzyna Andraszek).

As a tool, lampbrush chromosomes were introduced into poultry cytogenetics by Kropotova and Gaginskaya (1984), and by Hutchison (1987). The former authors support a thesis that chromosomes provide valuable information on bird gene expression, and are irreplaceable in cytogenetic research on animals with small genomes in which a large number of small-sized mitotic chromosomes makes it impossible for scientists to carry out microchromosome analysis. Just like in the case of banded patterns of mitotic chromosomes, LBCs are characterised by a special arrangement of active and inactive chromomeres visible as a pattern of side loops and regions without loops. In the Second Report on Chicken Genes and Chromosomes LBCs have been recognised as a new model in avian cytogenetics (Schmid et al., 2005).

Lampbrush chromosomes represent a new model in avian cytogenetics and are increasingly more often used in poultry chromosome analyses. Additionally, lampbrush chromosomes are considered as model structures in the study of transcription regulation. Changes in transcription activity are reflected as modifications of LBC morphological structure and are associated with physiological processes of the organism. The transcription activity analysis is carried out according to the concept assuming that it takes place in LBC side loops.

The aim of the present study (Andraszek et al., 2009; Andraszek & Smalec, 2011) was to compare the structure of the first five lampbrush macrochromosomes and ZW sex lampbrush bivalents, sampled from the oocytes of geese prior to and after the reproductive period and compare the transcription activity of lampbrush chromosomes and the G band pattern of corresponding mitotic chromosomes of the European domestic goose Anser anser.

The pre-reproduction bivalents were marked with lowercase "a", the post-reproduction ones with lowercase "b". The marker structures of the bivalents were successively numbered. The structure of the lampbrush chromosomes was analysed paying special attention to the comparison of the transcription-active parts and the GTG pattern on the corresponding mitotic chromosomes. The following marker structures were identified in the LBCs under analysis: GLLs - giant lumpy loops, MLs - marker loops, DBLs - distal boundary loops, PBLs - proximal boundary loops, TLs - telomeric loops, TBLs - telomeric bow-like loops, TLLs - telomeric lumpy loops, DBs - double bridges, Chs - chiasmata, PBs - protein bodies.

The respective bivalents sampled prior to and after reproduction have similar sizes but differ in morphological structure. The lampbrush chromosomes sampled after reproduction have reduced side loops - sites of intensive transcription activity. On the other hand, inactive chromomeres become prominent in the chromosomes. Marker loops are those structures that are degraded last after the end of reproduction. Consequently, they are used as the basis for identifying particular bivalents at different stages of transcriptional activity of the cell. The dark blocks correspond to the location of transcription active regions.

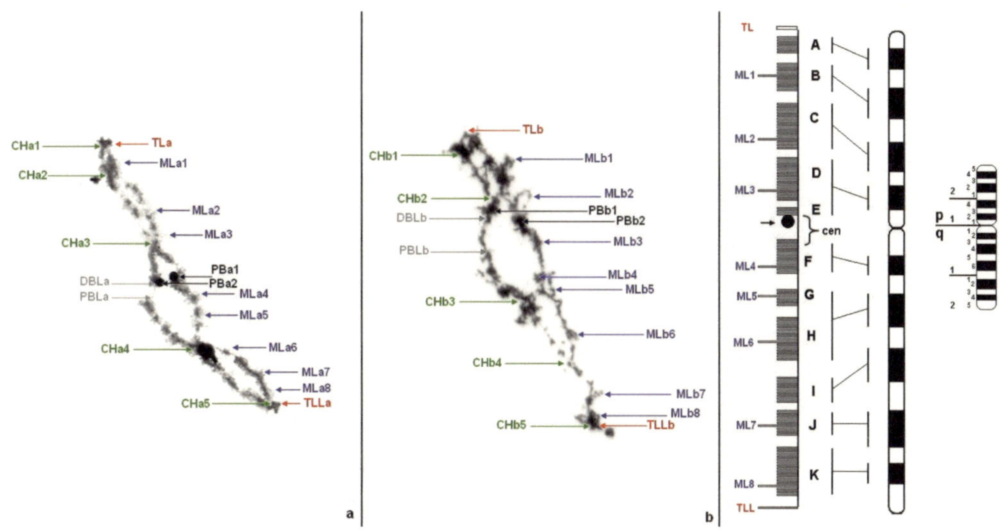


Fig. 4. Comparison of the structure of LBC 2 prior to (a), after (b) the reproductive period and graphic comparison of transcription activity of the second LBC and G bands on the second mitotic chromosome (c). Arrows indicate marker structures of bivalents.

The comparison of the location of regions with and without loops of the analysed lampbrush chromosomes with the GTG pattern of the corresponding mitotic chromosomes revealed that the arrangement of regions with side loops on LBCs which are transcription active corresponded to the GTG pattern on the mitotic chromosomes.

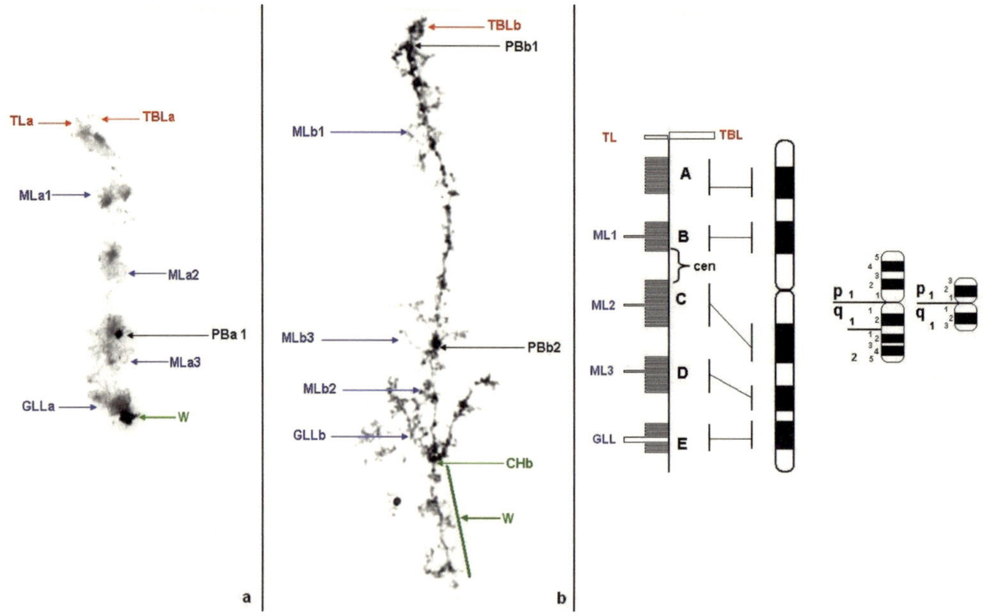


Fig. 5. Comparison of the structure of sex LBC prior to (a), after (b) the reproductive period and graphic comparison of transcription activity of the sex LBC and G bands on the sex mitotic chromosome (c). Arrows indicate marker structures of bivalents.

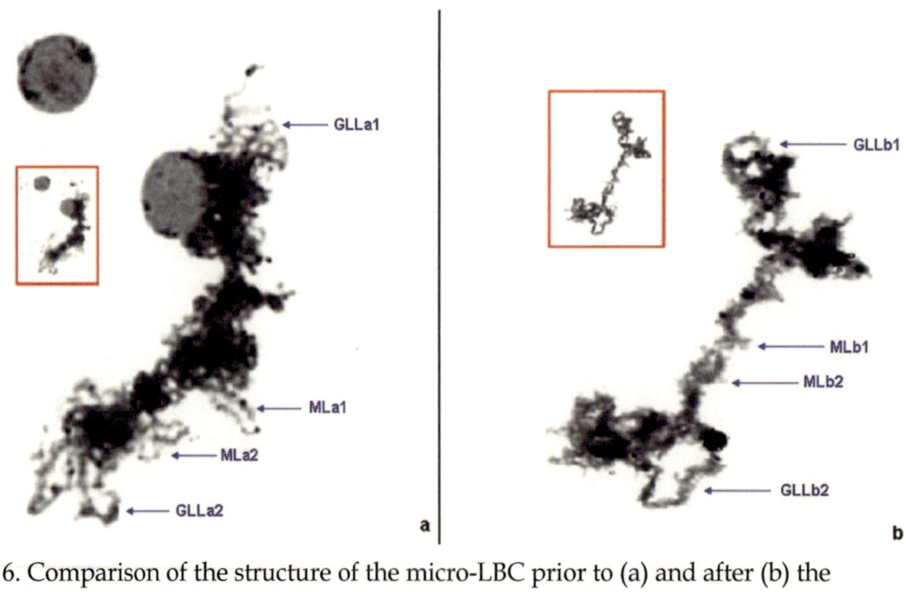


Fig. 6. Comparison of the structure of the micro-LBC prior to (a) and after (b) the reproductive period. Arrows indicate marker structures of bivalents.

Particular interest in recent years has been devoted to possibilities of using lampbrush chromosomes in genome mapping. This strategy can combine chromosome marker mapping and physical gene mapping using the in situ hybridisation technique with genetic maps constructed on the basis of chiasm incidence in the analysed bivalents. Equally important is also the possibility of using lampbrush chromosomes in analyses of the interaction of genes with other cellular structures. Particularly promising seem to be the possibilities of using lampbrush chromosomes in the mapping of avian genomes. This strategy can combine chromosome marker mapping and physical gene mapping using the FISH technique with genetic maps constructed on the basis of chiasm incidence in the analysed bivalents.

## 3. Meiosis during spermatogenesis

The cytogenetic analysis of breeding animals is problematic in the case of birds. The reason for the stalemate in research are the specific characteristics of the avian karyotype. A typical avian karyotype consists of several or a dozen or so macrochromosomes and about sixty microchromosomes. (Christidis, 1989; 1990). The only systematic description of avian chromosomes is the karyotype of the domestic hen (Smith et al., 2000).

A high number of chromosomes and the presence of microchromosomes in the bird karyotype made cytogeneticists look for other sources of information on the chromosomes. An important material for the analysis of the avian karyotype are meiotic chromosomes. The earliest studies of meiotic chromosome structure were conducted in the United States. The first investigations provided information on the huge variability of meiotic chromosomes, even within one genus. Among Batrachoseps salamanders, some species were unique in having a specific stage of chromosome dispersal between pachytene and diplotene, whereas no such phase was observed in other species (Macgregor & Varley, 1988).

Meiosis is usually observed in males, as spermatocytes are relatively small, numerous and easily accessible. The observation of meiotic chromosomes in females is impeded by the large size of the egg cell, technical difficulty in acquiring chromosomes from the egg cell and the fact that, compared with spermatocytes, oocytes are so few. Meiotic chromosomes are most often analysed in pachytene and diplotene cells during the first meiotic division. Cells typical of the 2nd meiotic division are few. Therefore, colchicine and vinblastine sulphate are applied to increase the number of the cells (Fechheimer, 1990).

In contrast to mitotic chromosome analyses, the number of studies of avian meiotic chromosomes is limited. Miller was the first to analyse meiosis in Gallus domesticus in 1938. He used primary spermatocytes of cocks as the experimental material. He identified 39 or 40 bivalents in metaphase I (Ford & Woollam, 1964). Similar experiments were performed by Ohno (1961). He identified 39 bivalents in Gallus. Moreover, he concluded that micro- and macrochromosomes follow identical behaviour during meiosis. The abovementioned studies concerned only diakinesis and the pre-meiotic phase and were conducted on a small number of cells sampled from several animals. Comprehensive information on meiotic chromosomes and the process of meiosis in hens was provided by Pollock & Fechheimer (1978). They analysed chromosomes at every stage of meiosis. Additionally, the number of chiasmata in the bivalents was determined. A separate group of studies of meiotic chromosomes in Gallus is constituted by analyses of synaptonemal complex structure both in spermatocytes (Kaelbing and Fechheimer, 1983, 1985) and oocytes (Solari, 1977; Rahn & Solari, 1986; Solari et al., 1988).

A paper by Andraszek and Smalec (2008) presents the course of meiosis in goose spermatocytes, with particular emphasis on the first meiotic prophase, the stage at which crossing over takes place, a process that guarantees recombination variability of organisms.

The results provided in the publication represent the only available study of avian meiosis in the relevant literature. They can be treated not only as practical reference data on the cytogenetics and biology of bird reproduction but also as didactic material.

Figure 7a shows the early prophase of the first meiotic division - leptotene. At this stage, chromosomes have the form of thin and long chromatin threads within which the chromatids cannot be distinguished. It is impossible to distinguish particular chromosomes which resemble an entangled wool-ball. In Figure 7b, early prophase chromosomes are also visible. Gradual chromatin condensation that occurs during the entire prophase causes the chromosome looping to become looser offering the possibility to distinguish particular chromatin threads. At this stage it is still impossible to distinguish particular chromosomes.

Figure 7c shows an image of late-zygotene bivalents. Due to progressive chromatin condensation particular chromosomes become separated. They are still long, while the chromatids remain indistinguishable. At this stage in the prophase, it is already possible to discern macro- and microchromosomes. However, it still remains impossible to identify particular homologous chromosomes, as they conjugate over their entire length. At this stage, synaptonemal complexes are observable only with an electron microscope. Figure 7d shows late-pachytene bivalents. Due to progressive chromatin condensation, particular bivalents are already distinguishable. It is possible to discern particular bivalents. Meiosis is not a strictly synchronous process. In some cells it is still impossible to recognise the homologues of the bivalent, since they conjugate over their entire length. Arrows in Figure 7e show the initiation sites of synaptonemal complex degradation . Figure 7f shows typical early-diplotene chromosomes. The cell is preparing for crossing over. The bivalents begin to divide into chromatids. At some points in the chromosome it is possible to observe chiasmata (indicated with arrows). The next Figure 7g depicts meiotic chromosomes in early diakinesis. Arrows indicate the prominent chiasmata, discernible due to gradual chromosome condensation. At this stage, the chromosomes are already after recombination. During the entire prophase, the nucleoli disintegrate. However, they remain observable until the end of the first meiotic prophase. Different numbers of bivalent-specific nucleoli (indicated with arrows) (Figure 7h) of different sizes (figure 7i) were observed in the analysed preparations. Figure 7j shows an image of a cell in late diakinesis, after the terminalisation of chiasmata. The chromosomes, with discernible micro- and macrochromosomes, contain condensed chromatin. A cell with such organisation enters the metaphase of the first meiotic division.

The work did not attempt to profile the cells in the remaining meiotic stages. Cells that are observed during the second meiotic division are the rarest category of reproductive cells in cytogenetic analysis. Even if they are visible under the microscope, the quality of definition is not satisfactory enough to enable description. Apart from that, the authors intended to focus on the prophase of the first meiotic division, the stage at which the recombination of the genetic material occurs.

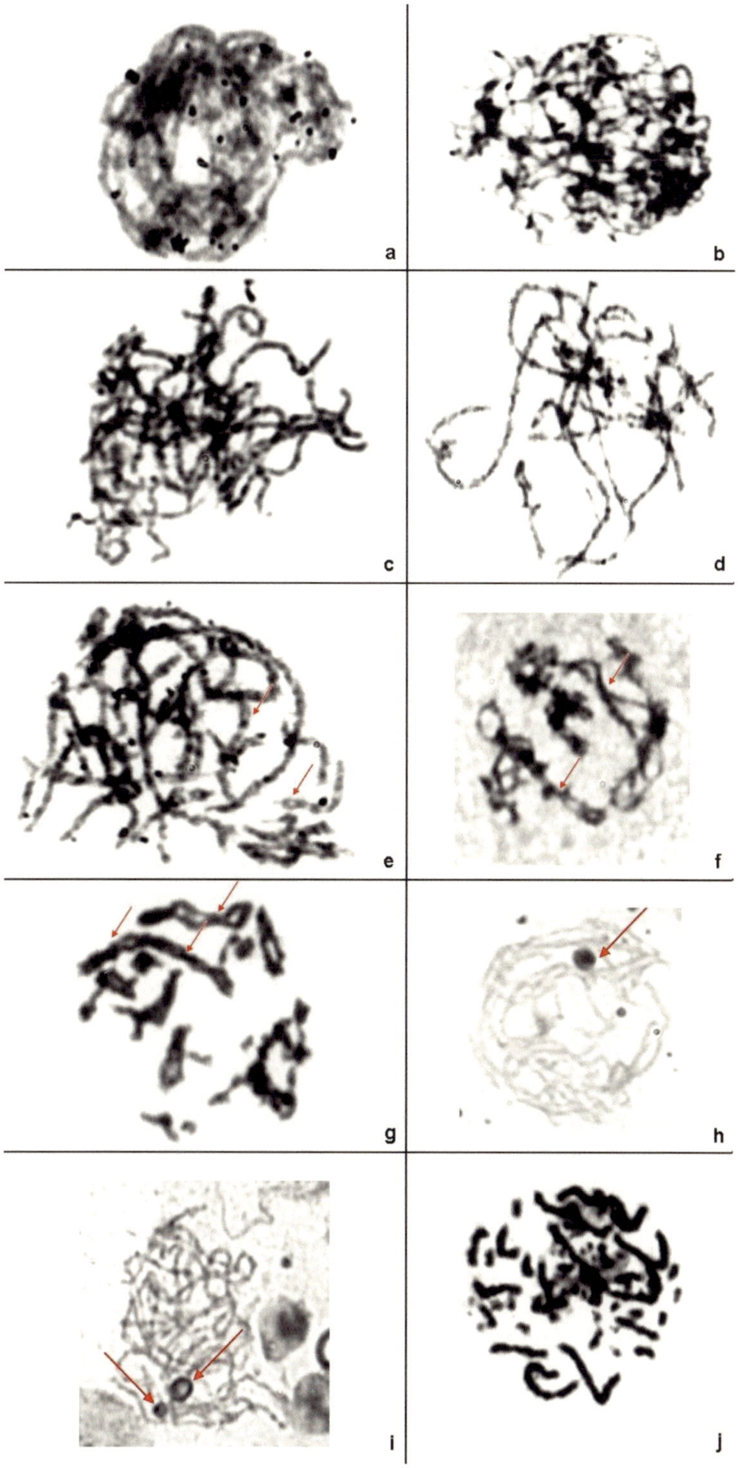


Fig. 7. The prophase of the first meiotic division in domestic goose spermatocytes.

## 4. Synaptonemal complex

A structure that is inextricably associated with the meiotic division of the cell is the synaptonemal complex (SC) - a proteinic structure which binds homologous chromosomes during the prophase of the 1st meiotic division and ensures correct genetic recombination. Apart form mutative variability, recombination variability is the reason for the huge diversity of organisms. Recombination occurs within the two homologous chromosomes that mutually exchange fragments of chromatids. This produces unique combinations of alleles of maternal and paternal origin in the genome. Due to crossing-over and DNA content reduction to the level of 1C, diploid organisms generate gametes, thus being able to create a new organism, different from the parental one.

An immense role in this process is played by the synaptonemal complex that "clasps" together two parallel homologous chromosomes and enables their conjugation (synapsis) (Turner et al., 2004). The synaptonemal complex was first observed more than fifty years ago in the spermatocytes of crayfish (Moses, 1956) and, subsequently, the dove, cat and man (Fawcett, 1956). The name of this unique nuclear structure was coined slightly later on. This meiotic structure is evolutively conservative in the bulk of sexually reproducing eukaryota, including the nonnucleated Protozoa, Fungi and algae, as well as vertebrates (Marec, 1996; Penkina et al., 2001)

A fully formed synaptonemal complex is situated between two prophase homologous chromosomes, binding them along their entire lengths into a pair that constitutes the bivalent. This is a three-tier proteinic structure that consists of two lateral elements (LE) and a central element (CE) located between them. Between the lateral elements there are recombination nodules (RN). They are ellipsoid, highly electron-absorbing protein complexes which are present only in euchromatinic regions of the chromosome (Holm & Rasmussen, 1980; Schmekel & Daneholt, 1998). At the centre of the complex it is possible to notice the so-called ladder structure produced by the linking of lateral elements with the central element using microfilaments (TFs) (Marec, 1996; Penkina et al., 2002).

The molecular structure of the synaptonemal complex can only be analysed using an electron or scanning microscope. An optical microscope, even with a high resolution and zoom, makes it possible to make out only the bivalent structure with clear-cut synaptic chromosomes. The available sources equate bivalent presence with the synaptonemal complex due to the fact that bivalent existence directly results from the presence of the synaptonemal complex. However, the bivalent and the synaptonemal complex are two separate structures. Figure shows prophase, meiotic chromosomes of a European domestic goose male (a), the ladder-like structure of the bivalents indicates that the synaptonemal complexes have fully developed (ringed in the photo). Alongside: a schematic structure of the synaptonemal complex (b).

The synaptonemal complex begins to form during the first meiotic prophase. At that time chromatin organisation undergoes dramatic changes. Starting with leptotene, chromatid DNA (present as chromatin loops) begins to connect to proteinic elements that constitute the matrix for emergent LEs. Homologous chromosomes have to be positioned in the distance of approx. 300nm for synapsis to occur (Marec, 1996). In zygotene, the homologues start to approach each other and connect using SC elements (Penkina et al., 2002).

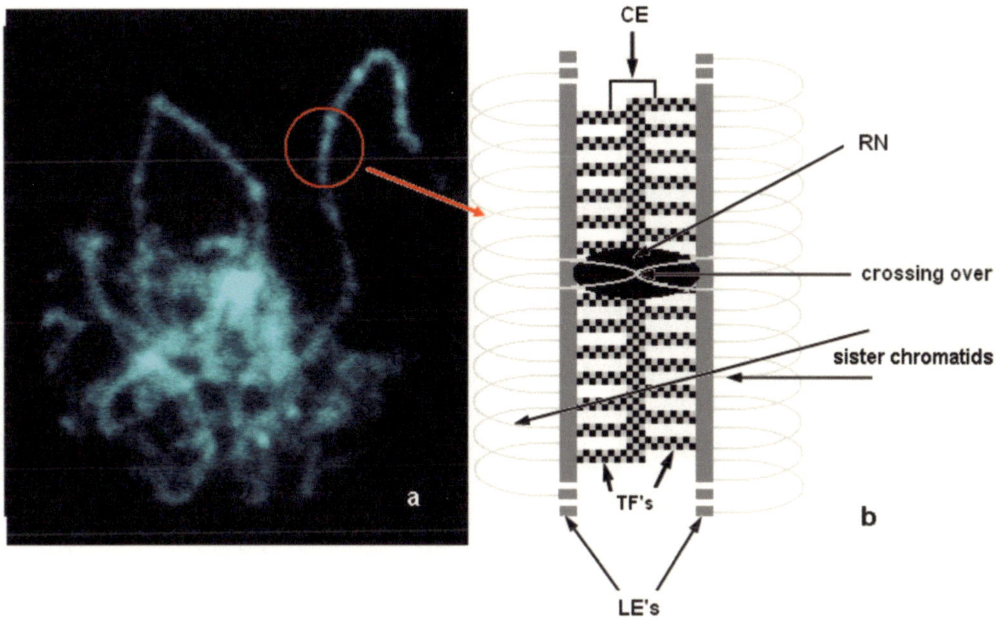


Fig. 8. The structure of the synaptonemal complex, Anser anser meiotic chromosomes, DAPI staining - (a); an outline of the synaptonemal complex – (b).

Chromatin loops depart radially from SC lateral elements. Most of the SC-bound chromatin is inactive – it is not transcribed (Marec, 1996). During the early prophase, LEs appear as proteinic axes (axial elements), each connected with two sister chromatids. Lateral elements are always built out of newly synthetised proteins, never as a result of the reorganisation of already existing components (Heyting et al., 1989). At first, LEs are visible as single, short fragments entangled in chromatin. Next, they become anchored to the inner side of the nuclear membrane with the aid of telomeres. The anchoring site of SCs is always situated in the region of the nucleus that is located opposite to the nucleolus, close to the diplosome. Lateral elements become continuous in mid-zygotene, when first complete bivalents appear and telomeres enter the distinctive bouquet stage at SC-anchoring sites of the nuclear membrane. LEs then stretch from one telomere to another in each chromosome. After LE formation, the CE begins to appear, connecting the homologues in a "zipper" fashion over their entire length, except for the sites at which the process has been inhibited by interlocking (Marec, 1996).

In early pachytene, all the homologues are in full-blown synapsis. Fragments of chromosomes that form the nucleolar organizer region are the latest to attain complete synapsis (Rasmussen, 1986; Marec, 1996). The formation of the complex in yeast and higher plants is initiated at many points in the bivalent, whereas in animals it always starts from the telomeric regions and and progresses lengthwise. Interstitial synapsis also occurs, if homologue mobility is impeded due to interengaging with other homologues – interlocking (Rasmussen, 1986; Penkina et al., 2002). SC formation is initiated in subterminal regions of the chromosome and progresses towards the nearest telomere. The above observations show that chromosome conjugation is caused by the existence of two identification sites in each chromosome, not by absolute homology of chromosome regions. The SC retains its structure until late diplotene. The first to disintegrate are CEs. Next, LEs crack along their longitudinal axis. They are decondensed in a number of stages and the SC is removed from the bivalents (Penkina et al., 2002).

### 4.1 Heterochromosomal synapsis

In the cells of homogametic organisms sex chromosome pairing does not differ from autosome pairing. In species whose sex is determined by the XY or ZW pair a considerable morphological and genetic variability of these chromosomes is observed. What is problematic is the length and the gene composition of the chromosomes. In the majority of such cases chromosome behaviour during conjugation seems to be forced and slightly unnatural. Despite the abovementioned impediments, the process runs correctly, which testifies to a huge adaptative potential and dynamics of the complex (Marec, 1996; Page et al., 2006).

All of the karyologically studied birds (about 10% of the living species) have a heterogametic system of sex determination in females in the form of the ZW pair. Avian sex chromosomes are rich in euchromatin, with the exception of centromeric regions and the short arm of the W chromosome. The W chromosome is often metacentric and entirely consists of heterochromatin. During pachytene, the axes of the Z and W chromosomes form a bivalent bound by a synaptonemal complex. The length of the SC corresponds to the length of the W chromosome axis. Next, from late to mid-pachytene, the unpaired section of the Z arm shortens into a streamer-like structure so as to assume the length of fully developed SC lateral elements. In this way, the Z arm twists and forms a loop around the straight W arm. The size of this loop corresponds to the size of the non-homologous pairing region in this bivalent (Pigozzi & Solari, 1999).

The synaptonemal complex in higher organisms begins to form starting from the telomeric regions. It might seem that also in birds shorter microchromosomes would be the first to form synapsis. In preparations sampled from one-day-old Anser anser goslings it was observed that macrobivalents were the first to accomplish synapsis (Andraszek et al., 2008). Figure9a shows a cell with the developed first macrobivalent (closed arrow). The dark structures in the subproximal area of the bivalents and the dark structures on the background of chromatin are kinetochores which become intensely hued after silver nitrate staining (open arrows). Kinetochores in the subproximal regions of macrochromosomes (open arrows) evidence the submetacentric forms of the first two goose macrobivalents (Figure 9b). Figure 9c shows a cell with developed synaptonemal complexes within the first four macrobivalents and the ZW univalent, as well as within the acrocentric bivalents differing successively in size.

The phenomenon provides an explanation to the specific character of the bird genome which, unlike in mammals, possesses a marked number of telomeric sequences in the interstitial parts of chromosome arms (Solovei et al., 1994; Nanda et al., 2002). The occurrence of interstitially located telomeric sequences on macrochromosomes is connected with an increase in the number of places where the formation of SCs is initiated, which explains why synapsis is achieved quicker. Santos et al. (1993) observed that in submetacentric bivalents synaptonemal complex formation begins from subtelomeric regions of chromosomes. In acrocentric bivalents there exist two potential initiation sites which are in the distal and proximal parts of the q arm. Short p arms pair much later.

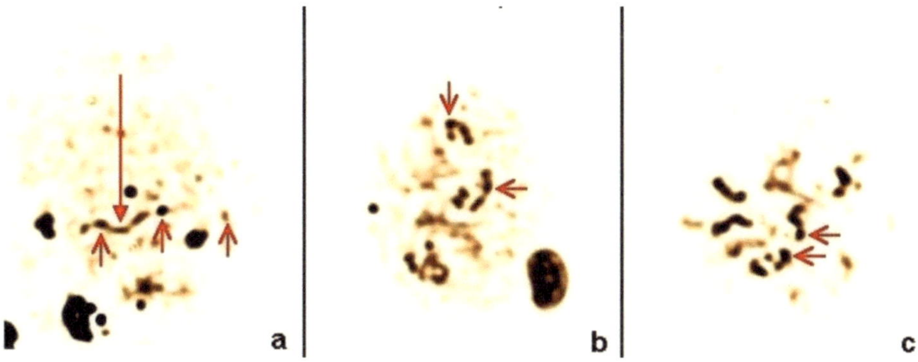


Fig. 9. Chromatin organisation in one-day-old gosling cells; isolation - Counce & Meyer (1973), staining - Howell & Black (1980)

In geese the largest macrochromosomes are submetacentric whereas the largest microchromosomes are acrocentric, so the theory of Santos et al. (1993) and the presence of interstitial telomeric sequences in chromosomes may explain why it is macrochromosomes and not microchromosomes that are the first to undergo synapsis. Moreover, compared with macrochromosomes, microchromosomes are characterised by a lower adenine-thymine content which is accompanied by a higher guanine-cytosine content (Fillon et al., 1998; Gregory, 2002). G-C-rich sequences constitute about 60% of Zyg DNA which is responsible for the linkage with SC. Zyg DNA undergoes replication not during the pre-meiotic S-phase but as late as in zygotene (Marec, 1996) so synapsis formation is delayed in those places.

It remains unexplained whether non-simultaneous synapsis is intended or coincidental, a consequence of the occurrence of interstitial telomeric sequences or Zyg DNA sequences, considering that most genes are concentrated in delayed microchromosomes (Fillon et al., 1998; Gregory, 2002). Perhaps, this is connected with the loop repair mechanism of chromosomes stuck due to interlocking. Later synapsis makes it possible for the repair mechanism to thoroughly verify whether the bivalent structure is correct, which is a way of preventing the loss of a valuable chromosome fragment. Unfortunately, this hypothesis cannot be testes as, apart from birds, no animal group has micro- and macrochromosomes in such a form.

The distinctive morphology of the ZW pair, in the form of a univalent in which chromosome W is bound to the distal part of chromosome Z, is also a consequence of synaptonemal complex formation starting from subtelomeric sequences. Moreover, as all the chromosomes start to connect and form a bivalent from telomeric sequences, the risk of losing their distal endings is reduced to a minimum. This would not be possible, if the complex formation proceeded from the centromere towards the chromosomal endings. One can think that the role of the SC is to stabilise the bivalent structure, in parallel to the role of telomeres that stabilise the chromosome structure.

The application of conventional techniques of synaptonemal complex identification and preparation staining does not make it possible to identify and analyse syn-aptonemal complex molecular structure. The presence of SCs on the preparations obtained from one-day-old goslings can be inferred from the presence of macrobivalents and darkly stained kinetochores and subtelomeric regions. In preparations obtained from 17-week-old ganders, the presence of the complexes was once again deduced from the presence of a complete set of bivalents as well as the number of kinetochores typical of the haploid set of chromosomes.

Figure 10a shows a cell with all the bivalents already visible. This is evidenced in the number of kinetochores. In the macrobivalents, kinetochores in the subproximal regions of the bivalents (open arrow) and dark-hued subtelomeric regions (closed arrow) are identifiable Figure 10b shows all the bivalents fully developed. The macrobivalents are long and well identifiable. It is possible to distinguish kinetochores and telomeric regions within them. It is also possible to observe the different lengths of the bivalents, ranging from the longest first one (closed arrow) to the very short acrocentric microbivalents (open arrow).

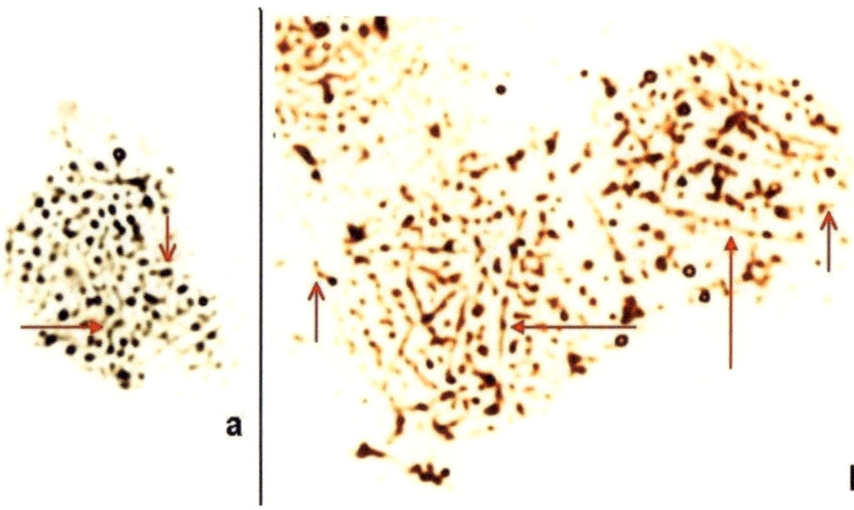


Fig. 10. Bivalent structure in 17-day-old gander cells; isolation - Counce & Meyer (1973), staining - Howell & Black (1980)

The standard technique for synaptonemal complex identification is the Counce and Meyer method (1973). The preparations for which it was used are presented above, in photograph 11a and 11b. On the other hand, promising results were obtained using the technique of meiotic chromosome isolation described by Pollock and Fehcheimer (1978), followed by silver nitrate staining and DAPI fluorochrome staining tentatively used in the experiment. After the application of the above techniques the homologues and bivalents were easily discernible. Additionally, the distinctive, ladder-like structure of synaptonemal complexes resulting from a different protein composition of the lateral elements was observed. Moreover, in the DAPI-stained preparations unique structures were identified during the basic cytogenetic analysis - two parallel homologous chromosomes just before synaptic union (Andraszek et al., 2008).

Figure 11a shows a cell with developed synaptonemal complexes within the bivalents. The structure of the complex is well visible both in the macrobivalents (closed arrow) and microbivalents (open arrow). Figure 11b shows a cell at the onset of synaptonemal complex degradation. It is possible to distinguish particular homologues of the bivalent (arrows). The distinctive synaptonemal complex structure can still be observed as alternating dark and light chromatin regions (circled) similar to the high-fidelity banding pattern of mitotic chromosomes. Such cells are typical of late pachytene and the onset of diplotene. Figure 11c shows a cell in zygotene. The homologues of the bivalents are already connected by synapsis (open arrow). In turn, the closed arrows indicate the bivalent homologues before the complete stabilisation of the SC. In Figure 11d , the bivalents have the typically synaptic ladder-like structure and prominent light fluorescent telomeres and kinetochores (open arrow) over their entire length . It is also possible to see the onset of synaptonemal complex disintegration (closed arrow) and two clear bivalent homologues after the break-up of synapsis.

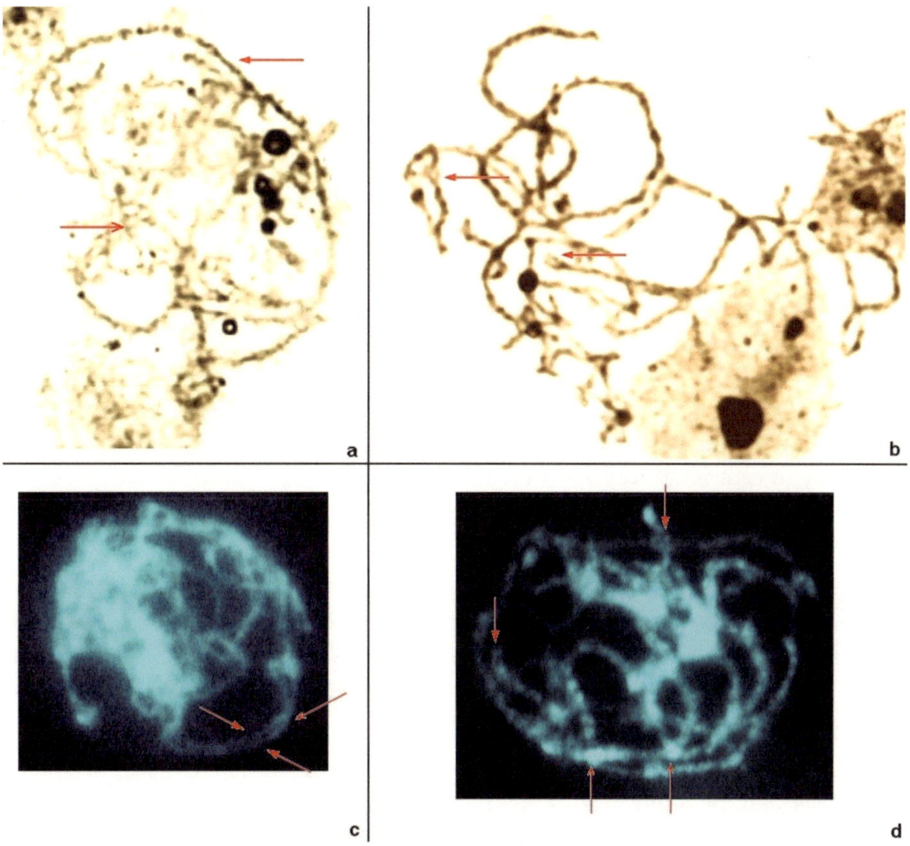


Fig. 11. Bivalent structure in 17-day-old gander cells; isolation – Pollock & Fehcheimer (1978), staining a, b – Howell & Black, c, d - Schweizer et al. (1978).

Paired or unpaired chromosome regions may indicate the chromosomal position of such marker structures as centromeres, nucleolar organizers, nucleoli, telomeres or even heterochromatin regions.

Such preparations may be very useful for analysing prophase chromosomes, and generating the so-called SC karyotypes. The karyotypes would make it possible to observe pairing initiations, sequences participating in pairing, the frequency of recombination occurrence, as well as potential meiotic chromosome structure anomalies. What follows is the fact that the complex lateral elements connect to DNA in strictly determined sequences. Thus, by convention, the ladder-like SC structure can be treated as a bivalent banding pattern indicating, similarly to banded staining, the location of specific sequences in the chromosome.

## 5. Nucleolus

The nucleolus is the largest and best known functional constituent of the cell nucleus. It is formed by original products of ribosomal RNA genes contained in the nucleolar organiser, related proteins and various enzymes, including RNA polymerase, RNA methylase and RNA endonuclease (Shaw & Jordan, 1995; Scheer & Hock, 1999; Hernandez-Verdun, 2006). The nucleolus is the site of synthesis and maturation of ribosomal RNA (rRNA) molecules. The molecules also bond with proteins in the nucleolus. rRNA genes are situated in particular chromosomes, in nucleolar organizer regions (NORs) that participate in the formation of nucleoli (Olson, 2004; Raška et al., 2004, 2006; Lam et al., 2005; Prieto & McStay, 2005; Derenzini et al., 2006). Nucleoli are present in the nuclei of almost all eukaryotic cells since they contain elementary metabolic genes, with the exception of spermatozoa and mature avian erythrocytes (Kłyszejko-Stefanowicz, 2002; Raška et al., 2006).

The weight of nucleoli is higher than that of the nucleoplasm in which the nucleoli are suspended. On account of its distinctive density, compact structure and low water content (10%) the nucleolus is an organelle that can be readily distinguished. Due to its characteristics, following cell nucleus fragmentation, the nucleolus remains intact in the saline solution even after the destruction of most nuclear structures, thereby allowing its isolation through centrifugation. The isolated nucleolus is identical to the one present in the nucleus of a living cell, and even retains its transcriptional activity in some cases (Olson, 2004; Hernandez-Verdun, 2006; Raška et al., 2006).

The number of nucleoli in a cell nucleus is determined by the number of active nucleolar organiser regions (NORs). It may be equal to the number of those NOR-chromosomes. Yet, normally, it is lower. This can be explained either with the fusion of nucleoli in the interphase nucleus or the suppression of activity of certain rDNA loci (Kłyszejko-Stefanowicz, 2002; Raška et al., 2006).

Nucleoli are very dynamic structures. This may be reflected in their cyclical disappearance during mitosis and reappearance at its end (Scheer & Benavente, 1990). The nucleolus disappears during cytokinesis and is reproduced in the reconstructed nuclei as a result of NOR activity (Kłyszejko-Stefanowicz, 2002; Olson, 2004) Nucleolar material appears between the chromosomes during the reconstruction of the NOR-associated telophase nucleus. Next, rRNA synthesis is resumed causing the nucleoli to become more visible. During the interphase, the nucleolus is spherical in shape. In the prophase, when the chromosomes become visible, it is evident that the nucleoli are associated with particular nucleolus organising chromosomes (Raška et al., 2006)

Both nucleoli and nucleolar organiser regions have chemical affinity for heavy metals and can be identified through staining with silver nitrate in a protective colloidal solution of formalin or gelatine (Howell & Black, 1980). Since nucleolar organiser regions (NORs) determine the structure of nucleoli, an alternative source of information on the activity of avian rRNA-encoding genes can be found in the analysis of the numbers and sizes of nucleoli in the prophase of the first meiotic division. Throughout the prophase, nucleoli are not degraded. As opposed to mitotic NORs, they are large structures (Andraszek & Smalec, 2007; Andraszek et al., 2009a; Andraszek et al., 2010a, 2010b).

The nucleoli disintegrate throughout the entire prophase of the first meiotic division. The way in which they decay is probably typical of particular vertebrate groups, this being possibly a species-specific characteristic. In the spermatocytes of domestic cattle, the nucleoli gradually become fragmented and "disintegrate" into tiny structures whose number corresponds with the number of NOR regions (Andraszek, unpublished). The studies which analysed the number and size of nucleoli in avian spermatocytes (Andraszek & Smalec, 2007; Andraszek et al., 2010b) reported a different mechanism of disappearance of nucleoli. In birds, chromatin reorganisation during the prophase of the first meiotic division and the related change in the cell nucleus size is correlated with decreasing sizes of the nucleoli. At the beginning of the prophase, in the early leptotene, the nucleoli are visible as large oval structures. In turn, at the end of the prophase they are observed as tiny points associated with specific bivalents. The figure 12 shows the different sizes of nucleoli at the beginning and end of the first meiotic prophase.

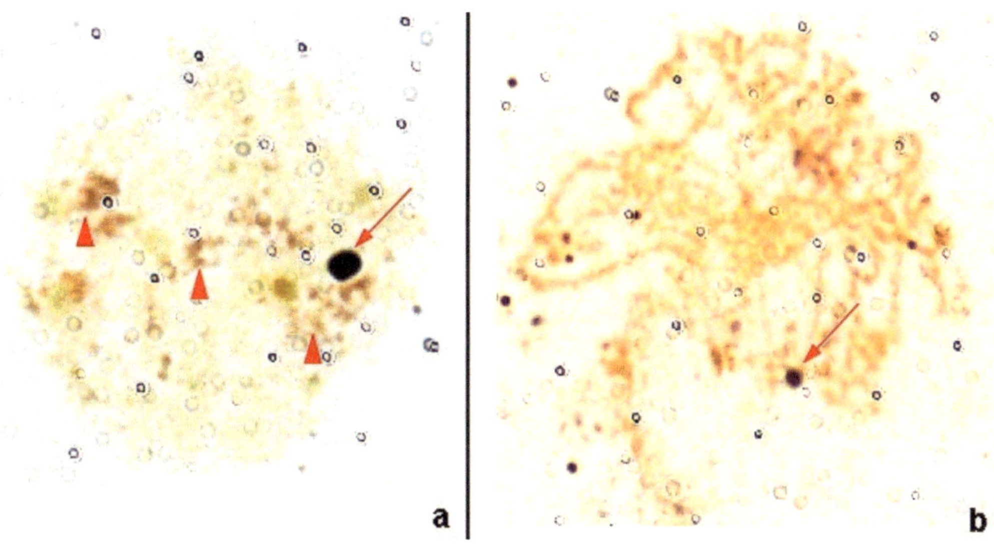


Fig. 12. Meiotic chromosomes of quail - early prophase (a), late prophase (b). The nucleoli indicated with arrows, kinetochores - arrow points.

Another distinctive characteristic of nucleoli in avian cells are the variations of their sizes unrelated with the prophase stage. Different sizes of nucleoli can be observed in cells that are at the same stage of meiosis. Figure 13 shows different sizes of nucleoli in goose (a), chicken (b) and quail spermatocytes (c).

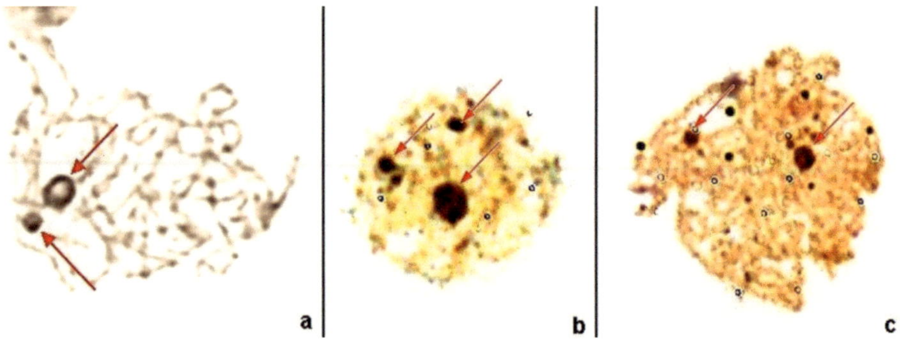


Fig. 13. Variability of the sizes of nucleoli in cells. The nucleoli indicated with arrows.

Avian cells also have variable numbers of nucleoli. This variability occurs at the individual, cellular and interindividual level. The number of nucleoli in the spermatocytes of geese and hens ranges from 1 to 4, and from 1 to 2 in quail cells. Next figures shows different numbers of nucleoli in goose (figure 14), chicken (figure 15) and quail spermatocytes (figure 16)

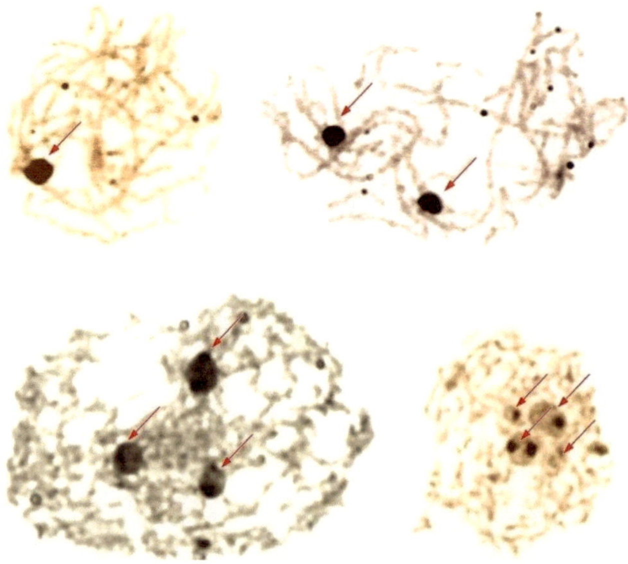

Fig. 14. Variability of the number of nucleoli in goose cells. The nucleoli indicated with arrows.

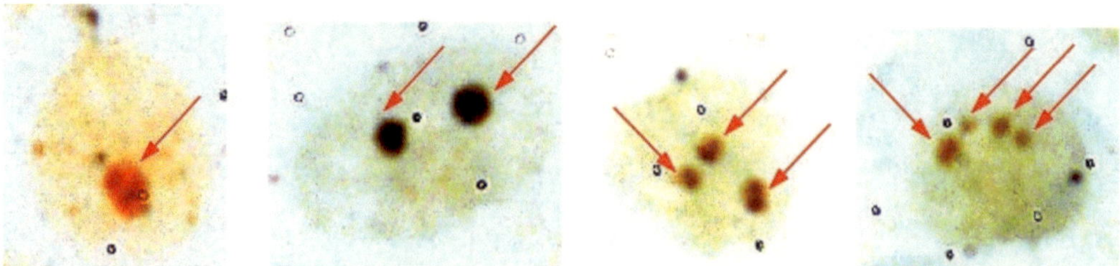

Fig. 15. Variability of the number of nucleoli in chicken cells. The nucleoli indicated with arrows.

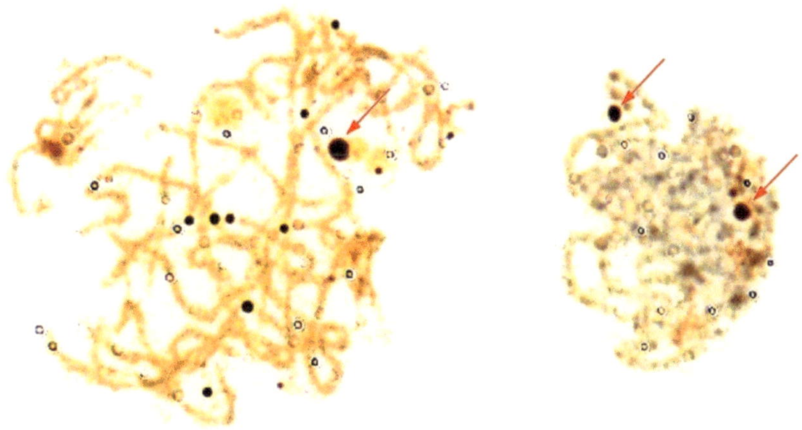

Fig. 16. Variability of the number of nucleoli in quail cells. The nucleoli indicated with arrows.

Apart from its functions being directly connected with ribosome biogenesis, the nucleolus is associated or involved in other cellular processes (Pederson, 1998; Santoro & Grummt, 2001; Olson et al., 2002; Gerbi et al., 2003; Raška et al., 2006). At present, it is not possible to determine whether these unconventional roles are the main functions of the nucleolus or adaptations of individual species or species groups. As regards the functions discussed further on, there is now a rich and still expanding body of literature available that deals with the relationship between the nucleolus and viral infections (Hiscox, 2002, 2003; Olson et al., 2002), including DNA, RNA and retroviruses.

Nucleolar morphology was one of the key criteria of neoplasm classification. The morphometric parameters of nucleoli are: the number, size and distance from the nuclear membrane (Nafe & Schlote, 2004; Smetana et al., 2005, 2006; Raška et al., 2006). Taking advantage of previous observations of Montgomery (1895), biologists dealing with neoplasms quickly tracked down the connection between AgNOR stains and cell proliferation (Derenzini et al., 1990; 2006; Raška et al., 2006).

Most studies during the last few years exploited the potential offered by the newly discovered nuclear oncogenes connected with the promotion and inhibition of tumours by cytogenetically diagnosed nucleolar mechanisms. c-Myc proteins (the product of the c-myc proto-oncogene) are located in the nucleolus and control rRNA synthesis (Oskarsson & Trumpp, 2005; Raška et al., 2006). It has also been shown that c-Myc is capable of controlling the activity of all the three polymerases in mammalian cells and coordinating the entire ribosome synthesis and cell growth (Arabi et al., 2005). These observations point at the crucial role of c-Myc in the development of promotional neoplastic actions via ribosome biogenesis control.

pRb (the protein of malignant retinoblastoma) and p53 proteins play a major role in the control of the cell cycle progress, as well as ensuring the correct development of daughter cells. These are oncosuppressive proteins, concentrated in the nucleolus (Ryan et al., 2001; Trere et al., 2004). The ARF/p16INK4a encoding gene is the second most common inactive human neoplastic gene (Ruas & Peters, 1998). ARF is situated at the nucleolus where it is associated with p53 (Kashuba et al., 2003). It has also been observed that there is a direct functional link between the nucleolus and p53 control (Ryan et al., 2001; Olson 2004). Most stress treatments activating p53 also cause the breakdown of nucleolar structure.

A considerable number of somatic cells do not have active telomerase. This puts a limit to the number of cell division cycles and suggests that telomerase is a factor in the processes of aging and carcinogenesis (Maser & DePinho, 2002; Raška et al., 2006). Telomerase has been found to be present in the nucleolus. Its function is connected with nucleolus activity control (Raška et al., 2006). Together with a class of snoRNA, telomerase locates RNA telomerase within the nucleolus (Lukowiak et al., 2001). hTERT - the reverse transcriptase of the catalytic subunit of human telomerase also has a nucleolar location (Khurts et al., 2004). Evidence of a functional relationship between telomerase and nucleoli has been provided by studies of human cell lines (Wong et al., 2002). In tumours and transmuted cell lines hTERT was eliminated from the nucleolus (Wong et al., 2002). The nucleolar phosphoproteinic nucleoid reacts with hTERT, the interaction being affected by RNA telomerase. This interaction is probably connected with dynamic telomerase anchoring. The TRF2 binding agent of the telomere is located in certain nucleolar modifications during the cell cycle (Khurts, 2004; Raška et al., 2006).

## 6. Conclusion

Meiosis guarantees the stability of the chromosome number in the consecutive generations of sexually reproducing organisms. Generally, meiosis is represented as a process during which the cell passes through totally different stages that correspond with particular structure and behaviour of chromosomes. The observation of the changes occurring in the structure of meiotic chromosomes leads to an understanding of the nature of meiosis. The first prophase of meiosis, in which the crossing-over takes place, should be paid particular attention. Moreover, meiotic chromosome research makes it possible to analyse the structure of nucleoli. In the meiotic prophase, they can be an alternative source of information on the activity of rRNA-encoding genes. In addition, synaptonemal complexes, which are extraordinary structures that guarantee recombination variability of organisms, are formed during meiosis. Summing up, meiotic chromosomes can not only be successfully used in applications in reproductive cytogenetics and biology but also as didactic aids.

## 7. References

Andraszek, K. & Smalec E. (2007). Number and size of nucleoli in the spermatocytes of European domestic goose (*Anser anser*). *Archiv für Geflügelkunde*, Vol. 71, No. 5, pp. (237-240), ISSN 0003-9098

Andraszek, K. & Smalec E. (2008). Spermatogenesis process as exemplified by meiosis in European domestic goose (*Anser anser*). *Archiv für Geflügelkunde*, Vol. 72, No. 3, pp. (110-115), ISSN 0003-9098

Andraszek, K. & Smalec E. (2011). Comparison of active transcription regions of lampbrush chromosomes with the mitotic chromosome G pattern in the

European domestic goose *Anser anser*. *Archiv Tierzucht*, Vol. 54, No. 1, pp. (69-82), ISSN 0003-9438

Andraszek, K.; Smalec, E. & Czyżewska, D. (2008). The structure of the synaptonemal complexes in meiocytes of European domestic goose (*Anser anser*). *Folia Biologica (Krakow)*, Vol. 56, No. 3-4, pp. (139-147), ISSN 0015-5497

Andraszek, K.; Horoszewicz, E. & Smalec, E. (2009a). Nucleolar organizer regions, satellite associations and nucleoli of goat cells (*Capra hircus*). *Archiv Tierzucht*, Vol. 52, No. 2, pp. (177-186), ISSN 0003-9438

Andraszek, K.; Smalec, E. & Tokarska, W. (2009b). Identification and structure of lampbrush sex bivalents prior to and after the reproduction period of the European domestic goose *Anser anser*. *Folia Biologica (Krakow)*, Vol. 57, No. 3-4, pp. (143-148), ISSN 0015-5497

Andraszek, K.; Danielewicz, A.; Smalec, E. & Kaproń, M. (2010a). Identification of the nucleoli in domestic horse spermatocytes - preliminary investigations. *Roczniki Naukowe PTZ*, Vol. 6, No. 4, pp. (13-21), ISSN 0003-9438

Andraszek, K.; Gryzińska, M.; Knaga, S.; Wójcik, E. & Smalec, E. (2010b).Number and size of nucleoli in the spermatocytes of chicken and Japanese quail. *Proceedings of 51*, Olsztyn, Poland, September 2010. ISBN

Angelier, N.; Paintraud, M.; Lavaud, A. & Lechaire, J.P. (1984). Scanning electron microscopy of amphibian lampbrush chromosomes. *Chromosoma*, Vol. 89, No. 4, pp. (243-253), ISSN 0009-5915

Angelier, N.; Bonnanfant-Jais, M.L.; Herberts, C.; Lautredou, N.; Moreau, N.; N'Da, E.; Penrad-Mobayed, M.; Rodriguez-Martin, M.L. & Sourrouille P. (1990). Chromosomes of amphibian oocytes as a model for gene expression: significance of lampbrush loops. *The International Journal of Developmental Biology*, Vol. 34, No. 1, pp. (69-80), ISSN 0214-6282

Angelier, N.; Penrad-Mobayed, M.; Billoud, B.; Bonnanfant-Jais, M.L. & Coumailleau P. (1996). What role might lampbrush chromosomes play in maternal gene expression? *The International Journal of Developmental Biology*, Vol. 40, No. 4, pp. (645-652), ISSN 0214-6282

Arabi, A.; Wu, S.; Ridderstrale, K.; Bierho, V.H.; Shiue, C.; Fatyol, K.; Fahlen, S.; Hydbring, P.; Soderberg, O.; Grummt I.; Larson, L.G. & Wright A.P. (2005): c-Myc associates with ribosomal DNA and activates RNA polymerase I transcription. *Nature Cell Biology*, Vol. 7, No. 3, pp. (303-310), ISSN 1465-7392

Callan, H.G. (1986). *Lampbrush chromosomes*. Springer-Verlag New York, Incorporated, ISBN - 10:0387164308, Berlin, Heidelberg, New York, Toronto

Callan H.G.; Gall J.G. & Berg C.A. (1987). The lampbrush chromosomes of *Xenopus laevis*: preparation, identification, and distribution of 5S DNA sequences. *Chromosoma*, Vol. 95, No. 4, pp. (236-250), ISSN 0009-5915

Chelysheva, L.A.; Solovei, I.V.; Rodionov, A.V.; Yakovlev, A.F. & Gaginskaya, E.R. (1990). Lampbrush chromosoms of the chicken: the cytological map of the macrobivalents. *Tsitologiia*, Vol. 32, No. 4, pp. (303-316), ISSN 0041-3771

Counce, S.J. & Meyer, G.F. (1973). Differentation of the synsptonemal complex and the kinetochore in Locusta spermatocytes studied by whole mount electron microscopy. *Chromosoma*, Vol. 44, No. 2, pp. (231-253), ISSN 0009-5915

Derenzini, M.; Pession, A. & Trere, D. (1990). Quantity of nucleolar silver-stained proteins is related to proliferating activity in cancer cells. *Laboratory Investigation*, Vol. 63, No. 1, pp. (137-140), ISSN 0023-6837

Derenzini, M.; Pasquinelli, G.; O'Donohue, M.F.; Ploton, D. & Thiry, M. (2006). Structural and functional organization of ribosoma, genes within the mammalian cell nucleolus. *The journal of histochemistry and cytochemistry*, Vol. 54, No. 2, pp. (131-145), ISSN 0022-1554

Fawcett D.W. (1956): The fine structure of chromosomes in the meiotic prophase of vertebrate spermatocytes. *The Journal of Biophysical and Biochemical Cytology*, Vol. 2, No. 4, pp. (403-406), ISSN 0095-9901

Fechheimer, N.S. (1990) Chromosomes of Chickens, In: *Domestic Animal Cytogenetics*, McFeely R.A., pp (169-207), Academic Press, ISBN 0120392348, New York

Fillon, V.; Morisson, M.; Zoorob, R.; Auffray, C.; Douaire, M.; Gellin, J. & Vignal, A. (1998). Identification of sixteen chicken microchromosomes by molecular markers using two color fluorescent in situ hybridization (FISH). *Chromosome Research*, Vol. 4, No. 6, pp. (307-313), ISSN 0967-3849

Ford, E.H.R. & Woollam, D.H.M. (1964). Testicular chromosomes of *Gallus domesticus*. *Chromosoma*, Vol. 15, pp. (568-578), ISSN 0009-5915

Gerbi, S.A.; Borovjagin, A.V. & Lange, T.S. (2003). The nucleolus: A site of ribonucleoprotein maturation. *Current Opinion in Cell Biology*, Vol. 15, No. 3, pp. (318-325), ISSN 0955-0674

Gregory, T.R. (2002): A bird's-eye view of the C-value enigma: genome size, cell size, and metabolic rate in the class aves. *Evolution*, Vol. 56, No. 1, pp. (121-130), ISSN 0014-3820

Hernandez-Verdun, D. (2006). Nucleolus: From structure to dynamics. *Histochemistry and Cell Biology*, Vol. 125, No. 1-2, pp. (127-137), ISSN 0948-6143

Heyting, C.A.; Dietrich, J.J.; Moens, P.B.; Dettemers, R.J.; Offenberg, H.H.; Redeker, E.J.W. & Vink, A.C.G. (1989). Synaptonemal complex proteins. *Genome*, Vol. 31, No. 1, pp. (81-87), ISSN 0831-2796

Hiscox, J.A. (2002). The nucleolus-a gateway to viral infection? *Archives of Virology*, Vol. 147, No. 6, pp. (1077–1089), ISSN 0304-8608

Hiscox, J.A. (2003). The interaction of animal cytoplasmic RNA viruses with the nucleus to facilitate replication. *Virus Research*, Vol. 95, No. 1-2, pp. (13-22), ISSN 0168-1702

Holm, P.B. & Rasmussen, S.W. (1980). Chromosome pairing, recombination nodules and chiasma formation in diploid Bombyx males. *Carlsberg Research Communications*, Vol. 45, No. 6, pp. (483-548), ISSN 0105-1938

Howell, W.M. & Black, D.A. (1980). Controlled silver-staining of nucleolus organizer regions with a protective colloidal developer a 1-step method. *Experientia*, Vol. 36, No. 8, pp. (1014-1015), ISSN 0014-4754

Hutchison, N. (1987). Lampbrush chromosomes of the chicken *Gallus domesticus*. *The Journal of Cell Biology*, Vol. 105, No. 4, pp. (1493-1500), ISSN 0021-9525

Kaelbling, M. & Fechheimer, N.S. (1983). Synaptonemal complexes and the chromosome complement of domestic fowl *Gallus domesticus*. *Cytogenetics and Cell Genetics*, Vol. 35, No. 2, pp. (87-92), ISSN 0301-0171

Kaelbling, M. & Fechheimer, N.S. (1985) Synaptonemal complex analysis of a pericentric inversion in chromosome 2 of domestic fowl *Gallus domesticus*. *Cytogenetics and Cell Genetics*, Vol. 39, No. 2, pp. (82-86), ISSN 0301-0171

Kashuba, E.; Mattsson, K.; Klein, G. & Szekely, L. (2003). p14ARF induces the relocation of HDM2 and p53 to extranucleolar sites that are targeted by PML bodies and proteasomes. *Molecular Cancer*, Vol. 2, No. 18, ISSN 1476-4598, < doi:10.1186/1476-4598-2-18>

Khurts, S.; Masutomi, K.; Delgermaa, L.; Arai, K.; Oishi, N.; Mizuno, H.; Hayashi, N.; Hahn, W.C. & Murakami, S. (2004). Nucleolin interacts with telomerase. *The Journal of Biological Chemistry*, Vol. 279, No. 49, pp. (51508-51515), ISSN 0021-9258

Kłyszejko-Stefanowicz, L. (2002). *Cytobiochemia*, (three edition), PWN, ISBN: 83-01-13824-6, Warsaw, Poland

Lam, Y.W.; Trinkle-Mulcahy, L. & Lamond, A.L. (2005). The nucleolus. *Journal of Cell Science*, Vol. 118, No. 7, pp. (1335-1337), ISSN 0021-9533

Lukowiak, A.A.; Narayanan, A.; Li, Z.H.; Terns, R.M. & Terns, M.P. (2001). The snoRNA domain of vertebrate telomerase RNA functions to localize the RNA within the nucleus. *RNA*, Vol. 7, No. 12, pp. (1833-1844), ISSN 1355-8382

Macgregor, H.C. (1977). Lampbrush chromosomes, In: *Chromatin and Chromosome Structure*, Eckhardt, R. A., and Hsueh-jei, Li., pp. (339-357), Academic Press, ISBN: 0124505503, New York and London

Macgregor, H.C. (1980). Recent developments in the study of lampbrush chromosomes. Heredity, Vol. 44, pp. (3-35), ISSN 0018-067X

Macgregor, H.C. (1987). Lampbrush chromosomes. *Journal of Cell Science*, Vol. 88, No. 1, pp. (7-9), ISSN 0021-9533

Macgregor, H.C, Varley J., „Working with Animal Chromosomes". John Wiley & Sons. London, New York, Brisbane, Toronto, Singapore, 1988.

Marec, F. (1996). Synaptonemal complexes in insects. International Journal of Insect Morphology and Embryology, Vol. 25, No. 3, pp. (205-233), ISSN 0020-7322

Maser, R.S. & DePinho, R.A. (2002). Keeping telomerase in its place. *Nature Medicine*, Vol. 8, No. 9, pp. (934-936), ISSN 1078-8956

Morgan, G.T. (2002). Lampbrush chromosomes and associated bodies: new insights into principles of nuclear structure and function. *Chromosome Research*, Vol. 10, No. 3, pp. (177-200), ISSN 0967-3849

Moses, M.J. (1956). Chromosomal structures in crayfish spermatocytes. *The Journal of Biophysical and Biochemical Cytology*, Vol. 2, No. 2, pp. (215-218), ISSN 0095-9901

Nafe, R. & Schlote, W. (2004). Histomorphometry of brain tumours. *Neuropathology and Applied Neurobiology*, Vol. 30, No. 4, pp. (315–328), ISSN 0305-1846

Nanda, I.; Schrama, D.; Feichtinger, W.; Haaf, T.; Schartl, M. & Schmid, M. (2002). Distribution of telomeric (TTAGGG)n sequences in avian chromosomes. *Chromosoma*, Vol. 111, No. 4, pp. (215-227), ISSN 0009-5915

Ohno, S. (1961). Sex chromosomes and microchromosomes of *Gallus domesticus*. *Chromosoma*, Vol. 11, pp. (484-498), ISSN 0009-5915

Olson, M.O. (2004). *The nucleolus*. Kluwer Academic Plenum Publisher, ISBN 0306478730, 9780306478734, London

Olson, M.O.; Hingorani, K. & Szebeni, A. (2002). Conventional and nonconventional roles of the nucleolus. *International Review of Cytology*, Vol. 219, pp. (199–266), ISSN 0074-7696

Oskarsson, T. & Trumpp, A. (2005). The Myc trilogy: Lord of RNA polymerases. *Nature Cell Biology*, Vol. 7, No. 3, pp. (215-217), ISSN 1465-7392

Pederson, T. (1998). The plurifunctional nucleolus. *Nucleic Acids Research*, Vol. 26, No. 17, pp. (3871–3876), ISSN 0305-1048

Penkina, M.V.; Karpowa, O.I. & Bogdanov, F.Y. (2002). Synaptonemal Complex Proteins: Specific Proteins of Meiotic Chromosomes. Molekuliarnaia Biologiia, Vol. 36, No. 3, pp. (397-407), ISSN 0026-8984

Pigozzi, M.I. & Solari, A.J. (1999). The ZW pairs of two paleognath birds from two orders show transitional stages of sex chromosome differentiation. *Chromosome Research*, Vol. 7, No. 7, pp. (541-551), ISSN 0967-3849

Pollock, D.L. & Fechheimer, N.S. (1978). The chromosomes of cockerels (*Gallus domesticus*) during meiosis. *Cytogenetics and Cell Genetics*, Vol. 21, No. 5, pp. (267-281), ISSN 0301-0171

Prieto, J.L. & McStay, B. (2005). Nucleolar biogenesis: the first small steps. Biochemical Society Transactions, Vol. 33, No. 6, pp. (1441-1443), ISSN 0300-5127

Rahn, M.I. & Solari, A.J. (1986). Recombination nodules in the oocytes of the chicken Gallus domesticus. *Cytogenetics and Cell Genetics*, Vol. 43, No. 3-4, pp. (187-193), ISSN 0301-0171

Raška, I.; Koberna, K.; Malinsk, J.; Fodlerova, H. & Masata, M. (2004). The nucleolus and transcription of ribosomal genes. *Biology of the Cell*, Vol. 96, No. 8, pp. (579–594), ISSN 0248-4900

Raška, I.; Shaw, P.J. & Cmarko, D. (2006). New Insights into Nucleolar Architecture and Activity. *International Review of Cytology*, Vol. 255, pp. (177-235), ISSN 0074-7696

Rodionov, A.V. (1996). Micro vs. macro: structural-functional organization of avian micro- and macrochromosomes. Genetika, Vol. 32, No. 5, pp. (597-608), ISSN 0016-6758

Ruas, M. & Peters, G. (1998): The p16INK4a/CDKN2A tumor suppressor and its relatives. Biochimica et Biophysica Acta, Vol. 1378, No. 2, pp. (F115-F177), ISSN 0006-3002

Ryan, K.M.; Philips, A.C. & Vousden, K.H. (2001). Regulation and function of the p53 tumor suppressor protein. *Current opinion in cell biology*, Vol. 13, No. 3, pp. (332–337), ISSN 0955-0674

Santoro, R. & Grummt, I. (2001). Molecular mechanisms mediating methylation dependent silencing of ribosomal gene transcription. *Molecular Cell*, Vol. 8, No. 3, pp. (719–725), ISSN 1097-2765

Santos, J.L.; del Cerro, A.L. & Díez, M. (1993): Spreading synaptonemal complexes from the grasshopper Chorthippus jacopsi: pachytene and zygotene obserwations. *Hereditas*, Vol. 118, No. 3, pp. (235-241), ISSN 0018-0661

Scheer, U. & Benavente, R. (1990). Functional and dynamic aspects of the mammalian nucleolus. *BioEssays*, Vol. 12, No. 1, pp. (14-21), ISSN 0265-9247

Scheer, U. & Hock, R. (1999). Structure and function of the nucleolus. *Current opinion in cell biology*, Vol. 11, No. 3, pp. (385–390), ISSN 0955-0674

Schmekel, K. & Daneholt, B. (1998). Evidence for close contact between recombination nodules and the central element of the synaptonemal complex. *Chromosome Research*, Vol. 6, No. 3, pp. (155-159), ISSN 0967-3849

Schmid, M.; Nanda, I.; Hoehn, H.; Schartl, M.; Haaf, T.; Buerstedde, J.M.; Arakawa, H., Caldwell, R.B.; Weigend, S.; Burt, D.W.; Smith, J.; Griffin, D.K.; Masabanda, J.S.; Groenen, M.A.M.; Crooijmans, R.P.M.A.; Vignal, A.; Fillon, V.; Morisson, M.; Pitel, F.; Vignoles, M.; Garrigues, A.; Gellin, J.; Rodionov, A.V.; Galkina, S.A.; Lukina, N.A.; Ben-Ari, G.; Blum, S.; Hillel, J.; Twito, T.; Lavi, U.; David, L.; Feldman, M.W.; Delany, M.E.; Conley, C.A.; Fowler, V.M.; Hedges, S.B.; Godbout, R.; Katyal, S.; Smith, C.; Hudson, Q.; Sinclair, A. & Mizuno, S. (2005). Second Report on Chicken Genes and Chromosomes 2005. *Cytogenetics and Genome Research*, Vol. 109, No. 4, pp. (415-479), ISSN 1424-8581

Shaw, P.J. & Jordan, E.G. (1995). The nucleolus. *Annual Review of Cell and Developmental Biology*, Vol. 11, pp. (93–121), ISSN 1081-0706

Smetana, K.; Klamova, H.; Pluskalova, M.; Stockbauer, P.; Jiraskova, I. & Hrkal, Z. (2005). Intranucleolar translocation of AgNORs in early granulocytic precursors in chronic myeloid leukaemia and K 562 cells. *Folia Biologica (Praha)*, Vol. 51, No. 4, pp. (89-92), ISSN 0015-5500

Smetana, K.; Klamova, H.; Pluskalova, M.; Stockbauer, P. & Hrkal, Z. (2006). To the intranucleolar translocation of AgNORs in leukemic early granulocytic and plasmacytic precursors. *Histochemistry and Cell Biology*, Vol. 125, No. 1-2, pp. (165-170), ISSN 0948-6143

Smith, J.; Paton, I.R.; Bruley, C.K.; Windsor, D.; Burke, D.; Ponce de Leon, F.A. & Burt, D.W. (2000). Integration of the genetic and physical maps of the chicken macrochromosomes. *Animal Genetics*, Vol. 31, No. 1, pp. (20-27), ISSN 0268-9146

Solari, A.J. (1977). Ultrastructure of the synaptic autosomes and ZW biwalent in chicken oocytes. *Chromosoma*, Vol. 64, No. 2, pp. (155-165), ISSN 0009-5915

Solari, A.J.; Fechheimer, N.S. & Bitgood, J.J. (1988). Pairing of ZW gonosomes and the localized recombination nodule in two Z-autosome translocation in *Gallus domesticus*. *Cytogenetics and Cell Genetics*, Vol. 48, No. 3, pp. (130-136), ISSN 0301-0171

Solovei, I.V; Gaginskya, E.R. & Macgregor, H.C. (1994). The arrangement and transcription of telomere DNA seqences at the ends of lampbrush chromosomes of birds. *Chromosome Research*, Vol. 2, No. 6, pp. (460-470), ISSN 0967-3849

Trere, D.; Ceccarelli, C.; Montanaro, L.; Tosti, E. & Derenzini, M. (2004). Nucleolar size and activity are related to pRb and p53 status in human breast cancer. *The journal of histochemistry and cytochemistry*, Vol. 52, No. 12, pp. (1601–1607), ISSN 0022-1554

Turner, P.C.; McLennan, A.G.; Bates, A.D. & White, M.R.H. (2004). *Biologia molekularna* (two edition), PWN, ISBN: 978-83-01-14146-2, Warsaw, Poland.

Wong, J.M.; Kusdra, L. & Collins, K. (2002). Subnuclear shuttling of human telomerase induced by transformation and DNA damage. *Nature Cell Biology*, Vol. 4, No. 9, pp. (731–736), ISSN 1465-7392

# Part 2

# Molecular Biology of Mammalian Meiosis

# 8

# The Control of Meiotic Arrest and Resumption in Mammalian Oocytes

Sylvie Bilodeau-Goeseels and Nora Magyara
*Agriculture and Agri-Food Canada, Lethbridge Research Centre, Canada*

## 1. Introduction

In mammals, following implantation of the embryo, a small number of cells from the epiblast eventually become the precursors of primordial germ cells (reviewed by Edson et al., 2009). After mitotic proliferation of the primordial germ cells, migration to the genital ridges and rapid proliferation again, meiosis is initiated in the oogonia at about day 13 of development in mice, at day 82 in bovine and during the 3rd month in humans. A last round of DNA synthesis occurs after which the oocytes enter a long meiotic prophase which consists of different stages (leptotene, zygotene, pachytene). By the time of birth, oocytes of most mammals have reached the diplotene stage, meiosis is arrested and the nucleus is referred to as a germinal vesicle (GV). The timing of progression of oocytes through meiosis in relation to birth varies in different mammals and in a few species meiotic prophase is initiated only after birth (i.e., rabbits and cats). At about the time of birth, oocytes become surrounded by follicle cells and these primordial follicles and oocytes represent a large stockpile from which, at any given time, a few are selected to grow and develop. The gradual depletion of primordial follicles through either growth or degeneration (atresia) continues until menopause.

As oocytes grow, they also acquire the competence to re-initiate meiosis. In mammals, re-initiation of meiosis in the pre-ovulatory follicle is induced by the luteinizing hormone (LH) surge. The germinal vesicle membrane breaks down [this stage is called germinal vesicle breakdown (GVBD)] and chromosomes separate from one another: one set is extruded into the first polar body, whereas the other set aligns at the second metaphase (MII) plate. In most mammals, meiosis is arrested again at this stage until activation by a spermatozoon. When mammalian oocytes that are competent to re-initiate meiosis are removed from their follicles and cultured, they undergo spontaneous resumption of meiosis with progression to MII in the absence of gonadotropins, demonstrating that a signal(s) from the follicle holds oocytes in prophase arrest. Spontaneous resumption of meiosis was first observed by Pincus & Enzmann (1935) in rabbit oocytes and was subsequently observed in oocytes from other mammalian species (Edwards, 1965). Spontaneous oocyte maturation allowed the development of *in vitro* maturation (IVM), a reproductive technology which involves artificial removal of cumulus-oocyte complexes (COC) from antral follicles and culturing them in standard cell culture conditions for 24-48 h until they reach metaphase II. A proportion of these oocytes are then competent to develop following *in vitro* fertilization (IVF).

The cellular and molecular mechanisms involved in maintaining oocyte meiotic arrest for prolonged intervals in the ovary are not fully understood. Similarly, the chain of molecular and cellular events that leads to meiotic resumption, either *in vivo* in response to the gonadotropin surge, or spontaneously *in vitro*, has not been completely elucidated even though dramatic advances have been made in recent years in understanding the control of meiosis in rodent oocytes. Research aimed at understanding the mechanisms that control meiosis has relevance for practical applications as the oocyte, in addition to its important role in determining fertility, is a major player in reproductive biotechnologies such as IVM, IVF, cloning and transgenesis. For example, in livestock species, the efficiency of *in vitro* embryo production remains low as only approximately 40% of the fertilized oocytes develop to the blastocyst stage. One reason for this inefficiency is that although the oocytes are at the correct nuclear maturation stage (MII) after IVM, several of them did not have sufficient time to complete cytoplasmic maturation; i.e., they did not have time to accumulate all the mRNAs and proteins required for early development as RNA synthesis ceased when meiosis resumed. Physiological inhibition of spontaneous nuclear maturation *in vitro* for a period of time sufficient to complete cytoplasmic maturation, will be required to improve developmental competence. Similarly, the cornerstone of any wild animal fertility preservation approach is the capacity for successful *in vitro* culture of gametes and embryos (Comizzoli et al., 2010). Moreover, IVM has the potential to exploit the large supply of oocytes available within ovaries in the case of ovariectomy or death of a wild female donor. In 2009, the International Committee for Monitoring Assisted Reproductive Technologies reported that over 200,000 babies are born annually from assisted reproductive technologies (de Mouzon et al., 2009). Currently, the use of IVM for the treatment of human infertility is not widespread due to its low efficiency (Suikkari, 2008); however, IVM represents an attractive alternative as it would reduce the use of gonadotropins for ovarian stimulation, thereby reducing side effects and costs for patients. This chapter reviews research aimed at understanding the signalling pathways involved in the control of meiotic cell cycle arrest at the diplotene (GV) stage as well as in the control of meiotic resumption (GVBD) in oocytes from selected mammalian species.

## 2. The control of meiosis in rodent oocytes

### 2.1 Early data on the role of cAMP

Cyclic adenosine monophosphate (cAMP) is a second messenger which is responsible for the transduction of hormonal signals in a wide range of organisms. Cyclic AMP is synthesized from ATP by the enzyme adenylate cyclase (AC) which is located on the inner side of the plasma membrane. Adenylate cyclase is activated by a range of signalling molecules through the activation of adenylate cyclase stimulatory G (Gs)-protein-coupled receptors and inhibited by agonists of adenylate cyclase inhibitory G (Gi)-protein-coupled receptors. Cyclic AMP is degraded to 5′-AMP by phosphodiesterase (PDE) enzymes.

Cyclic AMP was thought early on to play a critical role in the control of meiotic maturation as LH, human chorionic gonadotropin (hCG), follicle-stimulating hormone (FSH) and prostaglandin $E_2$ ($PGE_2$) were effective in inducing meiotic resumption in rat oocytes cultured in intact follicles (Tsafriri et al., 1972). Additionally, injection of dibutyryl cyclic AMP (dbcAMP) into the follicular antrum also induced GVBD while LH and $PGE_2$ increased cAMP levels over 20-folds in follicles suggesting that the stimulatory effect of the hormones on maturation was mediated by cAMP (Tsafriri et al., 1972). Subsequently, several other studies, performed with cumulus-oocyte complexes cultured without follicles, provided evidence that cAMP levels within the oocyte determine meiotic status such that high levels result in meiotic arrest while low levels lead to re-initiation of meiotic maturation (Aberdam et al., 1987; Dekel et al., 1984; Schultz et al., 1983a). Therefore, cAMP appeared to have a dual role in the control of meiosis: mediation of the stimulatory action of gonadotropins on the follicle cells (oocytes do not have gonadotropin receptors) and an inhibitory effect on the oocyte itself. Challenging questions being addressed were: whether or not the oocyte itself could synthesize cAMP and whether the amount of cAMP synthesized by the oocyte was sufficient for meiotic arrest. Several studies with rodent oocytes suggested that cAMP derived from follicle cells was responsible for maintaining meiotic arrest as cAMP-elevating agents such as AC stimulators, PDE inhibitors and membrane-permeable cAMP derivatives did not inhibit meiosis in oocytes denuded of their cumulus cells [DO, (Dekel & Beers, 1978, 1980; Dekel et al., 1984; Racowsky, 1984)] and cAMP transfer from the cumulus cells to the oocyte was demonstrated (Bornslaeger & Schultz, 1985). However, other studies showed that the oocyte could synthesize cAMP and that cAMP-elevating agents could prevent GVBD in DO (Cho et al., 1974; Olsiewski & Beers, 1983; Urner et al., 1983).

### 2.2 Events downstream of cAMP and the control of maturation promoting factor

Maturation promoting factor (MPF) is a key regulator of the mitotic and meiotic cell cycle and integrates the signals from several pathways to control mitosis and meiosis. It is a serine-threonine kinase protein heterodimer composed of a catalytic subunit, cyclin-dependent kinase 1 (CDK1, also known as $p34^{cdc2}$), and a regulatory subunit, cyclin B. The activated form of MPF involves dephosphorylation at Thr14 and Tyr15 of CDK1 and its association with cyclin B (Clarke & Karsenti, 1991). For meiotic arrest to be maintained at prophase I, MPF must be kept inactive. How do high levels of cAMP in the oocyte maintain MPF inactive? In general, cAMP acts via protein kinase A (PKA). Recent studies [reviewed by Han & Conti (2006)] in mouse and Xenopus oocytes indicate that PKA directly regulates the activities of a kinase (Wee1B) and a phosphatase (Cdc25) for CDK1. High cAMP levels in oocytes result in active PKA, active Wee1B, and the phosphorylation and inactivation of CDK1 while a decrease in oocyte cAMP levels leads to PKA inactivation, Cdc25 activation, dephosphorylation of CDK1 and MPF activation. Regulation of the level of cyclin B by synthesis and degradation is also involved in the control of MPF activity (Ledan et al., 2001).

### 2.3 New findings on the control of meiosis in rodent oocytes

It is no longer believed that cAMP from follicle cells contributes significantly to mouse oocyte meiotic arrest. Horner et al. (2003) showed that mRNA and protein for the adenylate cyclase 3 (AC3) isoform were detected in rat and mouse oocytes and that the regulation of cAMP levels in oocytes indicated that the main AC from rat oocytes possessed properties similar to AC3 of somatic cells. Moreover, more than 50% of early antral follicles from AC3-deficient mice contained oocytes that had resumed meiosis (10-15% in wild-type oocytes), providing evidence that rodent oocytes contain a functional AC involved in meiotic arrest (Horner et al., 2003).

The development of a method to inject mouse oocytes within antral follicles allowed experiments to be performed that would shed more light on the mechanisms involved in the control of meiosis. Microinjection of a Gs antibody caused resumption of meiosis in follicle-enclosed oocytes indicating that inhibition of Gs in the oocyte leads to meiotic resumption and conversely, Gs activity in the oocyte is required to maintain meiotic arrest in the follicle (Mehlmann et al., 2002). Similarly, microinjection of a dominant negative form of Gs into mouse oocytes (also in Xenopus oocytes) caused resumption of meiosis (Kalinowski et al., 2004). Since Gs by itself has no constitutive activity, it was suspected that a receptor is required to activate Gs. A potential receptor, the orphan receptor GPR3, was identified through searching an expressed sequence tag database derived from a cDNA library obtained from mouse oocytes (Mehlmann et al., 2004). This receptor was of interest because it elevated cAMP when expressed in various cell lines. *In situ* hybridization showed that GPR3 RNA was localized in oocytes and 82% of the oocytes in antral follicles of ovaries from prepubertal GPR3 knockout mice had resumed meiosis (0% in wild-type, Mehlmann et al., 2004). Injection of GPR3 RNA into $GPR3^{-/-}$ oocytes reversed the knockout phenotype indicating that the GPR3 of the oocyte itself maintained meiotic arrest rather than the GPR3 of the follicle cells (Mehlmann et al., 2004). From these results, it appeared that the meiosis inhibitory signal was a GPR3 agonist which activated Gs and AC3; however, removal of oocytes from their follicles did not decrease Gs activation by GPR3 (Freudzon et al., 2005). Therefore, although GPR3 and Gs are required to maintain meiotic arrest, the signal from follicle cells acts by a mechanism other than providing a GPR3-activating ligand to maintain meiotic arrest.

If the signal from follicle cells to inhibit meiosis is not a GPR3-activating ligand then what are the other potential signals? The signal may act via gap junctions as initially believed, since gap junction inhibitors caused a decrease in oocyte cAMP and meiotic resumption (Norris et al., 2008; Sela-Abramovich et al., 2006). This brings us back to the original hypothesis that cAMP from somatic cells is transferred to the oocyte and inhibits meiosis. However, because the major oocyte phosphodiesterase is PDE3A (Masciarelli et al., 2004) which is inhibited by cyclic guanosine monophosphate (cGMP), and various studies showed that cGMP could be involved in meiotic arrest (Sela-Abramovich et al., 2008; Törnell et al., 1990), it was hypothesized that cGMP from the somatic cells could reach the oocyte through gap junctions, inhibit PDE3A and maintain meiotic arrest. Using Förster resonance energy transfer-based cyclic nucleotide sensors in follicle-enclosed oocytes, Norris et al. (2009) showed that cGMP does pass through gap junctions into the oocyte to contribute to the maintenance of high cAMP levels by inhibiting PDE3A.

How does LH stimulation of follicles lead to oocyte meiotic resumption? In the study from Norris et al. (2009), LH stimulation lowered cGMP levels in follicle cells and closed gap junctions. As a result, cGMP levels in the oocyte also decreased, PDE3A activity increased approximately 5-folds, oocyte cAMP decreased also approximately 5-folds and meiosis resumed (Norris et al., 2009). It is possible that LH could regulate oocyte cAMP via other mechanisms; for example, activation of Gi family G protein can inhibit AC or stimulate PDE thereby lowering cAMP. However, injection of pertussis toxin (a Gi inhibitor) into follicle-enclosed mouse oocytes did not prevent LH-induced meiotic resumption (Mehlmann et al., 2006). Similarly, the LH response was not prevented by inhibition of a $Ca^{2+}$ elevation by injection of EGTA into follicle-enclosed mouse oocytes (Mehlmann et al., 2006) indicating that LH does not regulate cAMP in the oocytes via a Gi family G protein or calcium. Further studies also showed that LH does not act by terminating receptor-G(s) signalling (Norris et al., 2007).

There are still a number of questions remaining to answer to complete this exciting story such as: whether there is a direct role for somatic cell cAMP in meiotic inhibition. What maintains high cGMP levels? How does LH decrease cGMP in somatic cells: through inhibition of a guanylate cyclase or stimulation of a cGMP-specific phosphodiesterase? Further studies showed that the epidermal growth factor (EGF) pathway is required for LH-induced gap junction closure and a portion or all of the cGMP decrease (Norris et al., 2010; Vaccari et al., 2009). Another important question is how do other signalling pathways that can affect meiosis fit into this model? For example, several studies demonstrated that the energy sensor adenosine monophosphate-activated protein kinase (AMPK) plays a role in controlling the resumption of nuclear maturation in mouse oocytes. Pharmacological activation of AMPK induced nuclear maturation in cumulus-enclosed and denuded oocytes that had been arrested with dibutyryl cAMP or hypoxanthine (Downs et al., 2002). Moreover, oocyte AMPK was also activated by hormones and stress; this activation preceded GVBD, and inhibiting AMPK activity blocked the effects of these stimuli (Chen et al., 2006; Chen & Downs, 2008; LaRosa & Downs, 2006, 2007). A recent study provided evidence that AMPK is also involved after GVBD to promote the completion of meiosis and to prevent premature activation (Downs et al., 2010). In conclusion, these studies show that the control of oocyte meiosis probably involves a complex network of cross-talk between several signalling pathways in the oocyte and also in cumulus cells.

## 3. The control of meiosis in bovine oocytes

Research on the control of meiosis in livestock species has to accommodate a number of variables not encountered in laboratory animals. For example, the majority of studies were performed with oocytes recovered from ovaries collected from slaughtered animals. Although most researchers collect oocytes from a narrow range of follicle sizes and further select the oocytes based on morphological criteria, it remains that the selected oocytes represent a mixed population originating from follicles at varying stages of development, dominance and/or atresia. Moreover, contrary to laboratory animals for which all animals in an experiment are synchronized and treated the same way, the livestock females from which the oocytes are recovered are at different stages of the estrus cycle and are exposed to different environments such as nutrition, temperature or stress level, all of which can potentially affect reproductive cells. In addition, the generation of knockout animals to study molecules of interest is currently not possible in livestock species; therefore, definitive conclusions on the role of a specific enzyme isoform in a biological process can sometimes not be reached. Our understanding of the control of oocyte meiosis in livestock species has relied on the study of the presence of mRNA and proteins, the study of protein phosphorylation and, to a large extent, on pharmacological studies.

### 3.1 Role of cAMP in the control of bovine oocyte meiosis

As in rodent oocytes, several early studies showed that cAMP-elevating agents could decrease meiotic maturation of bovine cumulus-enclosed oocytes (Jagiello et al., 1975, 1981). However, higher concentrations of the cAMP-elevating agents were necessary to transiently increase the percentage of bovine oocytes remaining at the GV stage after *in vitro* culture

(Jagiello et al., 1981, Sirard & First, 1988) compared to concentrations that were effective in rodent oocytes. Since AC was detected on their plasma membrane (Kuyt et al., 1988), it was concluded that bovine oocytes could possibly generate sufficient amount of cAMP for meiotic arrest. In support of this hypothesis, the AC stimulator forskolin (FSK) transiently inhibited GVBD in oocytes denuded of cumulus cells (Homa, 1988), or denuded of both cumulus cells and zona pellucida thereby eliminating the possibility that the AC in the cumulus cell projections embedded in the zona pellucida was contributing to the FSK effect (Bilodeau et al., 1993). However, transfer of cAMP from cumulus cells to the oocyte was indirectly demonstrated in a few studies. For example, the culture of COCs with FSK led to ~20 to 90-fold increases in intra-oocyte cAMP compared to oocytes from complexes cultured in control conditions, whereas the culture of denuded oocytes with FSK resulted in only 2 to 6-fold increases in cAMP levels (Bilodeau et al., 1993; Thomas et al., 2004).

The enzyme AC possesses two metal ion-binding sites in its active site and $Mn^{2+}$ is an AC activator (Tesmer et al., 1999). Moreover, a $Mn^{2+}$-dependent soluble AC is present in sperm cells (Braun & Dods, 1975). Culture of bovine oocytes in the presence of $MnCl_2$ resulted in an increase in the percentage of cumulus-enclosed oocytes (CEO) remaining at the GV stage after 7 h of culture, a decrease in the percentage of oocytes reaching the MII stage after 22 h of culture, and a six fold cAMP increase in complexes (Bilodeau-Goeseels, 2001, 2003a). An increase in cAMP in oocytes from complexes in response to $MnCl_2$ was detected in the presence of FSK only. In contrast to CEO, $Mn^{2+}$ increased the percentage of denuded oocytes resuming meiosis, but also increased cAMP in the presence of FSK only (Bilodeau-Goeseels, 2003a). These results could be explained by the fact that $Mn^{2+}$ is an activator of AC; however, $Mn^{2+}$ is also a cofactor for many enzymes and the addition of $MnCl_2$ to the culture medium could possibly alter the activity of other enzymes involved in meiotic progression. The fact that inhibition of protein kinase A (PKA) activity abrogated the inhibitory effect of $MnCl_2$ in bovine CEO (Bilodeau-Goeseels, 2003a) supports the former possibility. Moreover, stimulation of protein kinase C (PKC) also abrogated the inhibitory effect of $Mn^{2+}$ on meiosis (Bilodeau-Goeseels, 2003a) suggesting that the inhibitory effect of $Mn^{2+}$ can be due to activation of AC4, 6, or 9 as these isoforms are inhibited by PKC (Sadana & Dessauer, 2009). Taken together, these results indicate that bovine oocytes and cumulus cells may contain AC isoforms with different sensitivities to $Mn^{2+}$. Lastro et al., (2006) determined that bovine cumulus cells obtained from follicles 2-8 mm contained mRNA for AC isoforms 1, 3, 4, 6, and 9 and were enriched in PKC-inhibited isoforms 4 and 6 and the $Ca^{2+}$-stimulated isoform 1. However, the AC isoforms of bovine oocytes have not yet been determined.

### 3.2 Role of phosphodiesterases in the regulation of bovine oocyte meiosis

As was the case with dbcAMP, the non-specific PDE inhibitor 3-isobutyl-1-methylxanthine (IBMX) inhibited bovine oocyte meiotic resumption partially and transiently (Sirard, 1990; Sirard & First, 1988) when used at much higher concentrations than concentrations that were inhibitory in rodent oocytes (Dekel et al., 1988; Schultz et al., 1983b; Vivarelli et al., 1983). In bovine oocytes, specific inhibition of PDE3 *in vitro* delayed spontaneous meiotic maturation and increased cAMP levels in cumulus cells and in denuded oocytes (Bilodeau-Goeseels, 2003b; Mayes & Sirard, 2002; Thomas et al., 2002). A study of PDE isoforms present in bovine follicle components showed that PDE3 accounted for 80% of the PDE activity in the oocyte, while PDE8 activity accounted for the remaining 20 and 60% of PDE activity in oocytes and cumulus cells, respectively. Inhibition of PDE8 in bovine COCs increased cAMP levels in oocytes and delayed meiosis (Sasseville et al., 2009). Collectively, these results suggest that cAMP and PDE enzymes are involved in the control of meiosis in bovine oocytes. However, even when cAMP levels were increased substantially and/or PDE inhibitors specific for the isoforms present in oocytes were used; meiosis was generally delayed and not totally inhibited as in rodent oocytes. It is suspected that other pathways acting in synergy with cAMP are probably important for the control of meiotic arrest in bovine oocytes.

### 3.3 Role of AMPK in the control of bovine oocyte meiosis

Contrary to results obtained with mouse oocytes where AMPK activation led to meiotic resumption (see section 2.3), meiosis was inhibited when bovine oocytes were cultured with the AMPK activator 5′-aminoimidazole-4-carboxamide 1-β-D-ribofuranoside (AICAR, Bilodeau-Goeseels et al., 2007). The inhibitory effect of AICAR was observed in cumulus-enclosed and denuded oocytes, was reversible, increased the inhibitory effect of the AC activator FSK, was dependent on its phosphorylation by adenosine kinase and was not due to increased cAMP levels or to increased purine nucleotide synthesis (Bilodeau-Goeseels et al., 2007). Metformin [MET, one of the most widely used drugs for the treatment of type 2 diabetes and an AMPK activator (Zhou et al., 2001)], was also reported to inhibit GVBD in bovine CEO and DO by Bilodeau-Goeseels et al. (2007). In a subsequent study, however, the AMPK inhibitor Compound C (CC) did not reverse the effect of AICAR and MET and even had a significant inhibitory effect itself on bovine oocyte meiosis (Bilodeau-Goeseels et al., 2011). In mouse oocytes, CC prevented AICAR-induced maturation and on its own had a slight inhibitory effect on GVBD (Chen et al., 2006).

No changes in the ratio of Thr172 phosphorylation (phosphorylation of Thr172 of the α subunit of AMPK is required for activation) to total AMPK were detected in extracts of cumulus cells, CEO or DO that had been treated with AICAR or MET at concentrations that inhibited meiosis (Bilodeau-Goeseels et al., 2011) suggesting that the inhibitory effect of AICAR and MET on bovine oocyte meiosis was not due to AMPK activation in cumulus cells or the oocyte. Different results were obtained in another laboratory where MET inhibited meiosis in CEO but not in DO, CC accelerated GVBD and culture with 5 or 10 mM MET [2 mM was used by Bilodeau-Goeseels et al. (2007)] resulted in increased Thr172 phosphorylation in cumulus cells and oocytes from complexes (Tosca et al., 2007). The different results were likely due to the different MET concentrations used and/or the different culture conditions. In both studies, but especially in the Bilodeau-Goeseels et al. 2011 study, there was already a certain level of Thr172 phosphorylation at the onset of culture ($t = 0$) and this could have made small changes in Thr172 phosphorylation in response to MET (and also AICAR) difficult to detect. In conclusion, more studies are needed to determine the extent of AMPK involvement in the control of meiosis in bovine oocytes. More specifically, the determination of the effects of culture conditions on basal AMPK activation and on the effects of activators and inhibitors, as well as the identification of the upstream kinase(s) that phosphorylates Thr172 will be the next steps.

### 3.4 Other signalling pathways involved in the control of bovine oocyte meiosis

As mentioned above, AICAR and MET may not inhibit bovine oocyte meiosis through AMPK activation and therefore, may act through other inhibitory signalling molecules. Additionally, since the inhibitory effect of cAMP is transient and high concentrations are required, it is possible that cAMP acts in synergy with another signalling pathway(s) to inhibit meiosis in bovine oocytes. Is the cGMP pathway as involved in the control of bovine oocyte meiosis as it is in rodent oocytes? The cGMP analog 8-bromo-cGMP as well as the guanylate cyclase stimulators atrial natriuretic peptide and protoporphyrin 1X did not have any effect on bovine oocyte meiosis after 7h of culture (Bilodeau-Goeseels, 2007), while cGMP derivatives inhibited spontaneous nuclear maturation in rat denuded oocytes (Törnell et al., 1990). The cGMP pathway can also be activated by nitric oxide (NO), which is synthesized by NO synthase (NOS) and activates soluble cytoplasmic guanylate cyclase. Inducible NOS (iNOS) inhibition studies suggested that endogenous NO is necessary for spontaneous nuclear maturation (Bilodeau-Goeseels, 2007) and/or the MI to MII transition (Matta et al., 2009; Schwarz et al., 2010). Yet, NO donors also inhibited GVBD (Bilodeau-Goeseels, 2007; Schwarz et al., 2008; Viana et al., 2007) but the inhibitory effect of the NO donor sodium nitroprusside was not through the cGMP/protein kinase G (PKG) pathway (Bilodeau-Goeseels, 2007). In mouse oocytes, NO donors reversed the inhibitory effect of NOS inhibitor on meiosis (Bu et al., 2003), demonstrating yet again differences in the control of meiosis between bovine and rodent oocytes.

There are even fewer studies on the role of other signalling pathways in the control of bovine oocyte meiosis, and meiotic resumption has not been studied as extensively as meiotic arrest in oocytes from livestock species. The role of $Ca^{2+}$ in bovine oocyte fertilization and activation of development has been studied extensively (Tosti et al., 2002) and it appears to also be necessary for GVBD and progression of meiosis (He et al., 1997; Homa, 1995). Similarly, few studies have examined the role of PKC in bovine oocytes. Protein kinase C activation accelerated GVBD (Mondadori et al., 2008; Rose-Hellekant & Bavister, 1996) while PKC inhibition prevented GVBD (Homa, 1991). Using *in vivo* and *in vitro* experiments, Barreta et al. (2008) provided evidence that angiotensin II mediates LH-induced meiotic resumption in bovine oocytes and this event is dependent on prostaglandin $E_2$ or $F_{2\alpha}$ from follicular cells.

## 4. The control of meiosis in porcine oocytes

### 4.1 Role of cAMP, phosphodiesterases and AMPK

As in rodent and bovine oocytes, cAMP-elevating agents such as dbcAMP, the AC activator forskolin and non-specific and specific PDE isoform inhibitors can prevent or delay GVBD in porcine oocytes (Fan et al., 2002; Kim et al., 2008; Kren et al., 2004; Laforest et al., 2005; Racowsky, 1985). Phosphodiesterase activity in DO was almost completely inhibited by cilostamide (a PDE3 inhibitor) and PDE3A mRNA was detected by RT-PCR, suggesting that PDE3 is the main PDE in porcine oocytes (Sasseville et al., 2006). Although PDE3 activity represented only 19% of the total PDE activity in porcine COC, it potentially has a functional role in meiotic resumption as its mRNA level and activity were upregulated in COC but not in oocytes (therefore, upregulation was in cumulus cells) after 4 h of IVM. The up-regulation was gonadotropin- and cAMP-dependent (Sasseville et al., 2007). Similarly, cGMP-specific PDE activity also increased in a gonadotropin-dependent manner in porcine cumulus cells after 24 and 48 h of IVM (Sasseville et al., 2008). This PDE activity increase could potentially be responsible for a cGMP decrease leading to meiotic resumption as described in mouse follicles (see section 2.3). Although the presence and roles of AC3 or other AC isoforms and the GPR3 receptor have not yet been determined in porcine oocytes, an inhibitory role of

Gsalpha for meiotic resumption has been demonstrated as injection of an anti-Gsalpha antibody into porcine oocytes maintained in meiotic arrest with IBMX promoted cyclin B synthesis, MPF activation and GVBD (Morikawa et al., 2007). Similarly, as in mouse and Xenopus oocytes, Wee1B, the kinase which catalyzes the inhibitory phosphorylation of CDK1, is involved in meiotic arrest of porcine oocytes (Shimaoka et al., 2009).

Porcine oocytes and cumulus cells contained transcripts for at least one isoform of each of the three AMPK subunits. Moreover, AMPK activators alone or in combination with PDE inhibitors maintained porcine cumulus-enclosed oocytes in meiotic arrest (Mayes et al., 2007). As in bovine oocytes, the AMPK inhibitor CC did not reverse the effect of AMPK activators on meiosis and was itself inhibitory to oocyte nuclear maturation (Bilodeau-Goeseels et al., unpublished). Therefore, the effects of AMPK modulators on porcine oocyte meiosis are more similar to their effects on bovine oocytes compared to mouse oocytes indicating that the level of involvement of AMPK (and/or other signalling pathways affected by the AMPK modulators) is probably similar in bovine and porcine oocytes and different from rodent oocytes.

### 4.2 The role of mitogen-activated protein kinase in the control of porcine oocyte meiosis

#### 4.2.1 MAPK in oocytes

Mitogen-activated protein kinase (MAPK) is universally activated in oocytes during maturation in all vertebrates studied so far. However, several studies suggested that MAPK activation in porcine oocytes is not implicated in meiotic resumption as spontaneous meiotic resumption occurred normally in porcine DO cultured with the MAPK inhibitor U0126 (Fan et al., 2003) and MAPK activation in pig oocytes occurred after GVBD (Liang et al., 2005). Moreover, microinjection of porcine oocytes with c-mos antisense RNA (c-mos is an upstream activator of MAPK) completely inhibited phosphorylation and activation of MAPK but did not have an effect on spontaneous meiotic resumption (Ohashi et al., 2003). Studies of the timing of MAPK activation and studies using inhibitors suggested that MAPK is probably involved in the regulation of meiosis after GVBD or during the MI/MII transition (Inoue et al., 1995; Lee et al., 2000; Ye et al., 2003). Similar conclusions were obtained in rodent and bovine oocytes (reviewed by Liang et al., 2007).

#### 4.2.2 MAPK in follicular cells

Contrary to the situation in oocytes where MAPK is not necessary for GVBD, MAPK in follicular somatic cells is required for gonadotropin-induced meiotic resumption. Gonadotropins induced early and rapid MAPK activation in cumulus cells, MAPK activation in oocytes then occurred later at around the time of GVBD (Ebeling et al., 2007). The selective MEK inhibitors PD98059 and U0126 blocked FSH-induced meiotic resumption in mouse and porcine CEO but not spontaneous meiotic resumption in DO (Liang et al., 2005; Meinecke & Krischek, 2003; Su et al., 2002).

The mediator(s) between LH stimulation and MAPK activation in follicular cells as well as the mechanisms for inducing oocyte meiotic resumption following MAPK activation in follicle cells are not completely elucidated. Activation of MAPK could potentially lead to the production of a putative meiosis-inducing factor (Downs et al., 1988). However, LH stimulation closed gap junctions (Norris et al., 2009) and inhibition of MAPK activation blocked oocyte GVBD (Liang et al., 2005) as well as LH-induced inhibition of gap junction protein Cx43 translation in rat follicle cells (Kalma et al., 2004), suggesting that a MAPK-dependent pathway mediates LH-induced breakdown of gap junction communication and thus leads to oocyte maturation. The mediator of LH-stimulated MAPK activation could potentially be PKA as increased cAMP levels in porcine cumulus cells (resulting from inhibition of cumulus cell-specific PDE) activated MAPK (Liang et al., 2005). Protein kinase C also stimulated MAPK and oocyte meiotic resumption. The epidermal growth factor (EGF) network has an important role to play in mediating LH function during oocyte meiotic resumption; therefore, EGF could potentially be a mediator of LH-stimulated MAPK activation. In porcine granulosa cells, MAPK can be activated after a transient treatment with EGF (Keel & Davis, 1999) and EGF can induce meiotic maturation in porcine oocytes (Ding & Foxcroft, 1994). Studies in other species also suggested that activation of EGF receptor triggers signalling via the MAPK pathway (reviewed by Liang et al., 2007).

In conclusion, several questions remain unanswered about the role of MAPK in oocyte meiosis. For example, if PKA and PKC activate MAPK, are there other proteins in the signalling cascade between PKA/PKC and MAPK? Similarly, what is the mediator(s) between EGF receptor and MAPK?

## 5. The control of meiosis in equine oocytes

An increase in follicle diameter has been positively linked with increased nuclear and cytoplasmic maturation rates in the horse; however, oocyte diameter is not directly linked to oocyte competence (Goudet et al., 1997). Similar to other domestic species such as bovine and porcine, equine oocytes used for research tend to be recovered from slaughtered animals; however, due to the large size of follicles, ultrasound guided follicular puncture is often performed on mares. Follicular punctures are not nearly as efficient as follicle scraping of slaughterhouse ovaries with only approximately 8-9 COC being recovered every 22 days (Goudet et al., 1997); however, it allows for repeated harvesting of oocytes from the same mare when its reproductive cycle is known, thereby increasing the repeatability of results.

Equine oocytes have the lowest *in vitro* nuclear maturation rates of all of the domestic species discussed in the present review (Del Campo et al., 1995); therefore, the majority of studies on equine oocyte meiosis have focused on how to improve meiosis *in vitro* rather than on how to inhibit it. The low maturation rates may be related to the fact that the LH surge that triggers *in vivo* maturation lasts 4-6 days versus a 6-8 hour period observed in ewes (Alexander & Irvine, 1987; Irvine & Alexander, 1994); therefore, equine oocytes probably have different requirements and culture conditions still need to be optimized.

### 5.1 The role of follicular cells in the control of equine oocyte meiosis

Follicular cells play a key role in the control of meiosis since removal of oocytes from their follicle environment leads to spontaneous meiotic resumption (Pincus & Enzmann, 1935). Equine ovaries are especially suitable for the study of the role of follicular cells due to the follicles' large size which allows the different cell types to be easily isolated. Equine oocytes cultured while still attached to the membrana granulosa resumed meiosis. However, in the presence of theca cells or in theca cell-conditioned medium, more oocytes (attached to membrana granulosa) remained at the GV stage indicating that theca cells secrete a meiosis-inhibiting factor (Tremolada et al., 2003). These results are similar to results obtained with bovine oocytes as theca cells but not granulosa cell monolayers maintained meiotic arrest *in vitro* (Richard & Sirard, 1996).

### 5.2 Role of MPF, MAPK and other signalling molecules in the control of equine oocyte meiosis

The two subunits of MPF, $p34^{cdc2}$ and cyclin B protein, are present in both immature and mature oocytes before and after *in vitro* culture (Goudet et al., 1998). Therefore, equine oocytes have all the key components required for MPF formation, suggesting a lack of MPF regulators in incompetent oocytes. Mitogen-activated protein kinase (MAPK) is present at all nuclear stages after *in vitro* culture (Goudet et al., 1998). Of the two forms of MAPK, ERK1 and ERK2, only ERK2 is detected in equine oocytes during the GV stage with decreased electrophoretic mobility due to modification by phosphorylation in Metaphase I and Metaphase II. Thus MAPK remains non-phosphorylated (inactive) in incompetent and immature oocytes but becomes phosphorylated (activated) after GVBD in competent and preovulatory oocytes (Goudet et al., 1998). The reasons for the inability to phosphorylate MAPK in incompetent equine oocytes are unknown. An extracellular calcium sensing receptor agonist, NPS R-467, increased the activity of MAPK in equine cumulus cells and oocytes (De Santis et al., 2009).

Epidermal growth factor (EGF), insulin-like growth factor-I (IGF-I) and growth hormone had a positive effect on *in vitro* nuclear maturation of equine oocytes (Carneiro et al., 2001; Lorenzo et al., 2002; Pereira et al., 2011). Receptors for EGF have been localized in equine follicles particularly in cumulus cells and to some extent in mural granulosa cells. The addition of A-47, a specific tyrosine kinase inhibitor, inhibited maturation, suggesting that EGF has a physiological role in the regulation of equine oocyte maturation (Lorenzo et al., 2002). Contrary to other mammalian species discussed above, we are not aware of any studies on the role of cAMP in the control of equine oocyte meiosis, except for a preliminary study which concluded that the positive effect of growth hormone on equine oocyte meiosis was mediated by the PKA pathway (Lorenzo et al., 2005).

## 6. The control of meiosis in ovine oocytes

### 6.1 The role of cumulus cells in the control of ovine oocyte meiosis

The presence of cumulus cells during ovine oocyte culture may have more importance in the promotion of nuclear maturation compared to bovine oocytes: only 3.6% of ovine DO reached MII (81.3% for CEO) after 24 h of culture in a complex medium containing serum, pyruvate and hormones (Shi et al., 2009). In contrast, 40-80% of bovine DO reached the mature stage after culture without hormones (Bilodeau-Goeseels, 2001, 2003b).

A study of paracrine factors released by gonadotropin-stimulated ovine COC also highlighted some differences in the control of meiosis between rodent and ovine (and potentially other species) oocytes. Meiosis-inducing signals from gonadotropin-stimulated cumulus cells from competent oocytes acted on cumulus cells from incompetent oocytes to induce meiosis but they did not have any effect on incompetent DO (Cecconi et al., 2008). In contrast, meiosis-stimulating factors from cumulus cells can act directly on mouse denuded oocytes (Downs, 2001). Additionally, cumulus expansion appears to be regulated by the cumulus cells themselves rather than by the oocyte as in mice (Cecconi et al., 2008; Su et al., 2003).

### 6.2 Role of cAMP, MAPK in the control of meiosis in ovine oocytes

Similar to bovine oocytes, meiotic resumption was only partially inhibited by cAMP-elevating agents in ovine oocytes (Jagiello et al., 1981). Ovine oocytes possess an AC enzyme as cholera toxin, a Gs activator, stimulated cAMP synthesis in isolated sheep oocytes (Crosby et al., 1985). As in other mammals, MAPK is activated at the time of GVBD in ovine cumulus cells from competent oocytes in response to gonadotropins, then later in the oocyte (Cecconi et al., 2008). Cumulus cells from incompetent oocytes (from small follicles) did not show MAPK activation even after exposure to gonadotropins. However, when co-cultured with competent complexes (and gonadotropins), more oocytes from small follicles could resume meiosis and MAPK was activated in these oocytes but not in their cumulus showing that meiotic arrest in oocytes from small follicles could be due to the inability of their surrounding cumulus cells to respond to gonadotropins (Cecconi et al., 2008).

## 7. Conclusion

The results obtained in rodent models suggest that, similarly to several other biological processes, oocyte nuclear maturation involves a complex network of cross-talk between several signalling pathways in oocytes and follicular cells. This review highlighted some differences between rodent and livestock species and it is anticipated that more differences will be discovered in the mechanisms controlling meiotic arrest and meiotic resumption as research progresses in non-rodent species.

## 8. References

Aberdam, E., Hanski, E. & Dekel, N. (1987). Maintenance of meiotic arrest in isolated rat oocytes by the invasive adenylate cyclase of *Bordetella Pertussis*. *Biology of Reproduction*, Vol.36, No.3, (April 1987), pp. 530-535, ISSN 0006-3363

Alexander, S.L. & Irvine, C.H.G. (1987). Secretion rates and short-term patterns of gonadotrophin-releasing hormone, FSH and LH throughout the periovulatory period in the mare. *Journal of Endocrinology*, Vol.114, No.3, (September 1987), pp. 351-362, ISSN 0022-0795

Barreta, M.H., Oliveira, J.F.C., Ferreira, R., Antoniazzi, A.Q., Gasperin, B.G., Sandri, L. & Gonçalves, B.D. (2008). Evidence that the effect of angiotensin II on bovine oocyte nuclear maturation is mediated by prostaglandins $E_2$ and $F_{2\alpha}$. *Reproduction*, Vol.136, No.6, (December 2008), pp. 733-740, ISSN 1470-1626

Bilodeau, S., Fortier, M.A. & Sirard, M.A. (1993). Effect of adenylate cyclase stimulation on meiotic resumption and cyclic AMP content of zona-free and cumulus-enclosed bovine oocytes in vitro. *Journal of Reproduction and Fertility*, Vol.97, No.1, (January 1993), pp. 5-11, ISSN 0022-4251

Bilodeau-Goeseels, S. (2001). Manganese inhibits spontaneous nuclear maturation in bovine cumulus-enclosed oocytes. *Canadian Journal of Animal Science,* Vol.81, No.2, (June 2001), pp.223-228, ISSN 0008-3984

Bilodeau-Goeseels, S. (2003a). Manganese inhibits spontaneous nuclear maturation via the cAMP/protein kinase A pathway in bovine cumulus-enclosed oocytes. *Journal of Animal and Veterinary Advance,* Vol.2, No.1, (January 2003), pp. 12-21, ISSN 1680-5593

Bilodeau-Goeseels, S. (2003b). Effects of phosphodiesterase inhibitors on spontaneous nuclear maturation and cAMP concentrations in bovine oocytes. *Theriogenology,* Vol.60, No.9, (December 2003), pp. 1679-1690, ISSN 0093-691X

Bilodeau-Goeseels, S. (2007). Effects of manipulating the nitric oxide/cyclic GMP pathway on bovine oocyte meiotic resumption *in vitro*. *Theriogenology,* Vol.68, No.5, (September 2007), pp. 693-701, ISSN 0093-691X

Bilodeau-Goeseels, S., Panich, P.L. & Kastelic, J.P. (2011). Activation of AMP-activated protein kinase may not be involved in AICAR- and metformin-mediated meiotic arrest in bovine denuded and cumulus-enclosed oocytes *in vitro*. *Zygote,* Vol.19, No.2, (May 2011), pp. 97-106, ISSN 0967-1994

Bilodeau-Goeseels, S., Sasseville, M., Guillemette, C. & Richard, F.J. (2007). Effects of adenosine monophosphate-activated kinase activators on bovine oocyte nuclear maturation *in vitro*. *Molecular Reproduction and Development,* Vol.74, No.8, (August 2007), pp. 1021-1034, ISSN 1040-452X

Bornslaeger, E.A. & Schultz, R.M. (1985). Regulation of oocyte maturation: effect of elevating cumulus cell cAMP on oocyte cAMP levels. *Biology of Reproduction,* Vol.33, No.3, (October 1985), pp. 698-704, ISSN 0006-3363

Braun, T. & Dods, R.S. (1975). Development of a Mn-2+-sensitive, "soluble" adenylate cyclase in rat testis. *Proceedings of the National Academy of Science of the USA,* Vol.72, No.3, (March 1975), pp. 1097-1101, ISSN 0027-8424

Bu, S., Xia, G., Tao, Y., Lei, L. & Zhou, B. (2003). Dual effects of nitric oxide on meiotic maturation of mouse cumulus cell-enclosed oocytes in vitro. *Molecular and Cellular Endocrinology,* Vol.207, No.1-2, (September 2003), pp. 21-30, ISSN 0303-7207

Carneiro, G., Lorenzo, P., Pimentel, C., Pegoraro, M., Ball, B., Anderson, G. & Liu, I. (2001). Influence of insulin-like growth factor-I and its interaction with gonadotropins, estradiol, and fetal calf serum on *in vitro* maturation and parthenogenic development in equine oocytes. *Biology of Reproduction,* Vol.65, No.3, (September 2001), pp. 899-905, ISSN 0003-3363.

Cecconi, S., Mauro, A., Capacchietti, G., Berardinelli, P., Bernabò, N., Di Vincenzo, A.R., Mattiolo, M. & Barboni, B. (2008). Meiotic maturation of incompetent prepubertal oocytes is induced by paracrine factor(s) released by gonadotropin-stimulated oocyte-cumulus cell complexes and involves mitogen-activated protein kinase activation. *Endocrinology,* Vol.149, No.1, (January 2008), pp. 100-107, ISSN 0013-7227

Chen, J. & Downs, S.M. (2008). AMP-activated protein kinase is involved in hormone-induced mouse oocyte meiotic maturation in vitro. *Developmental Biology,* Vol.313, No.1, (January 2008), pp. 47-57, ISSN 0012-1606

Chen, J., Hudson, E., Chi, M.M., Chang, A.S., Moley, K.H., Hardie, D.G. & Downs, S.M. (2006). AMPK regulation of mouse oocyte meiotic resumption *in vitro*. *Developmental Biology*, Vol.291, No.2, (March 2006), pp. 227-238, ISSN 0012-1606

Cho, W.K., Stern, S. & Biggers, J.D. (1974). Inhibitory effect of dibutyryl cAMP on mouse oocyte maturation in vitro. *Journal of Experimental Zoology*, Vol.187, No.3, (March 1974), pp. 383-386, ISSN 0022-104X

Clarke, P.R. & Karsenti, E. (1991). Regulation of p34cdc2 protein kinase: new insights into protein phosphorylation and the cell cycle. *Journal of Cell Science*, Vol.100, No.Pt3, (November 1991), pp. 403-414, ISSN 0021-9533

Comizzoli, P., Songsasen, N. & Wildt, D.E. (2010). Protecting and extending fertility for females of wild and endangered mammals. *Cancer Treatment and Research*, Vol.156, pp. 87-100.

Crosby, I.M., Moor, R.M., Heslop, J.P. & Osborn, J.C. (1985). cAMP in ovine oocytes: localization of synthesis and its action on protein synthesis, phosphorylation, and meiosis. *Journal of Experimental Zoology*, Vol.234, No.2, (May 1985), pp. 307-318, ISSN 0022-104X

Dekel, N., Aberdam, E. & Sherizly, I. (1984). Spontaneous maturation *in vitro* of cumulus-enclosed rat oocytes is inhibited by forskolin. *Biology of Reproduction*, Vol.31, No.2, (September 1984), pp. 244-250, ISSN 0006-3363

Dekel, N. & Beers, W.H. (1978). Rat oocyte maturation in vitro: relief of cyclic AMP inhibition by gonadotropins. *Proceedings of the National Academy of Science of the USA*, Vol.75, No.9, (September 1978), pp. 4369-4373, ISSN 0027-8424

Dekel, N. & Beers, W.H. (1980). Development of the rat oocyte in vitro: inhibition and induction of maturation in the presence or absence of the cumulus oophorus. *Developmental Biology*, Vol.75, No.2, (March 1980), pp. 247-254, ISSN 0012-1606

Dekel, N., Galiani, D. & Sherizly, I. (1988). Dissociation between the inhibitory and stimulatory action of cAMP on maturation of rat oocytes. *Molecular and Cellular Endocrinology*, Vol.56, No.1-2, (March 1988), pp. 115-121, ISSN 0303-7207

Del Campo, M.R., Donoso, X., Parrish, J.J. & Ginther, O.J. (1995). Selection of follicles, preculture oocyte evaluation, and duration of culture for *in vitro* maturation of equine oocytes. *Theriogenology*, Vol. 43, No. 7, (May 1995), pp. 1141-1153, ISSN 0093-691X

De Mouzon, J., Lancaster, P., Nygren, K.G., Sulliva, E., Zegers-Hochschild, F., Mansour, R., Ishihara, O. & Adamson, D. (2009). World collaborative report on assisted reproductive technology, 2002. *Human Reproduction*, Vol.24, No.9, (September 2009), pp. 2310-2320, ISSN 0268-1161

De Santis, T., Casavola, V., Reshkin, S.J., Guerra, L., Ambruosi, B., Fiandanese, N., Dalbies-Tran, R., Goudet, G. & Dell'Aquila, M.E. (2009). The extracellular calcium-sensing receptor is expressed in the cumulus-oocyte complex in mammals and modulates oocyte meiotic maturation. *Reproduction*, Vol.138, No.3, (September 2009), pp. 439-452, ISSN 1470-1626

Ding, J. & Foxcroft, G.R. (1994). Epidermal growth factor enhances oocyte maturation in pigs. *Molecular Reproduction and Development*, Vol.39, No.1, (September 1994), pp. 30-40, ISSN 1040-452X

Downs, S.M. (2001). A gap-junction-mediated signal, rather than an external paracrine factor, predominates during meiotic induction in isolated mouse oocytes. *Zygote*, Vol.9, No.1, (February 2001), pp. 71-82, ISSN 0967-1994

Downs, S.M., Daniel, S.A. & Eppig, J.J. (1988). Induction of maturation in cumulus cell-enclosed mouse oocytes by follicle-stimulating hormone and epidermal growth factor: evidence for a positive stimulus of somatic cell origin. *Journal of Experimental Zoology*, Vol. 245, No.1, (January 1988), pp. 86-96, ISSN 0022-104X

Downs, S.M., Hudson, E.R. & Hardie, D.G. (2002). A potential role for AMP-activated protein kinase in meiotic induction in mouse oocytes. *Developmental Biology*, Vol. 245, No.1, (May 2002), pp.200-212, ISSN 0012-1606

Downs, S.M., Ya, R. & Davis, C.C. (2010). Role of AMPK throughout meiotic maturation in the mouse oocyte: evidence for promotion of polar body formation and suppression of premature activation. *Molecular Reproduction and Development*, Vol.77, No.10, (October 2010), pp. 888-899, ISSN 1040-452X

Ebeling, S., Schuon, C. & Meinecke, B. (2007). Mitogen-activated protein kinase phosphorylation patterns in pig oocytes and cumulus cells during gonadotropin-induced resumption of meiosis in vitro. *Zygote,* Vol.15, No.3, (August 2007), pp. 139-147, ISSN 0967-1994

Edson, M.A., Nagaraja, A.K. & Matzuk, M.M. (2009). The mammalian ovary from genesis to revelation. *Endocrine Reviews*, Vol.30, No.6, (August 2009), pp. 624-712, ISSN 0163-769X

Edwards, R.G. (1965). Maturation in vitro of mouse, sheep, cow, pig, rhesus monkey and human ovarian oocytes. *Nature*, Vol.208, No.5008, (October 1965), pp. 349-351, ISSN 0028-0836

Fan, H.Y., Li, M.Y., Tong, C., Chen, D.Y., Xia, G.L., Song, X.F., Schatten, H. & Sun, Q.Y. (2002). Inhibitory effects of cAMP and protein kinase C on meiotic maturation and MAP kinase phosphorylation in porcine oocytes. *Molecular Reproduction and Development*, Vol.63, No.4 (December 2002), pp. 480-487, ISSN 1040-452X

Fan, H.Y., Tong, C., Lian, L., Li, S.W., Gao, W.X., Cheng, Y., Chen, D.Y., Schatten, H. & Sun, Q.Y. (2003). Characterization of ribosomal S6 protein kinase p90rsk during meiotic maturation and fertilization in pig oocytes: mitogen-activated protein kinase-associated activation and localization. *Biology of Reproduction*, Vol.68, No.3, (March 2003), pp. 968-977, ISSN 0006-3363

Freudzon, L., Norris, R.P., Hand, A.R., Tanaka, S., Saeki, Y., Jones, T.L., Rasenick, M.M., Berlot, C.H., Mehlmann, L.M. & Jaffe, L.A. (2005). Regulation of meiotic prophase arrest in mouse oocytes by GPR3, a constitutive activator of the Gs G protein. *Journal of Cell Biology*, Vol.24, No.2 (October 2005), pp. 255-265, ISSN 0895-2388

Goudet, G., Belin, F., Bézard, J. & Gérard, N. (1998). Maturation-promoting factor (MPF) and mitogen activated protein kinase (MAPK) expression in relation to oocyte competence for *in-vitro* maturation in the mare. *Molecular Human Reproduction*, Vol. 4, No.6, (June 1998), pp. 563-570, ISSN 1360-9947

Goudet, G., Bézard, J., Duchamp, G., Gérard, N. & Palmer, E. (1997). Equine oocyte competence for nuclear and cytoplasmic *in vitro* maturation: effect of follicle size and hormonal environment. *Biology of Reproduction*. Vol.57, No.2, (August 1997), pp. 232-245, ISSN 0006-3363

Han, S.J. & Conti, M. (2006). New pathways from PKA to the Cdc2/cyclin B complex in oocytes. *Cell Cycle*, Vol.5, No.3, (February 2006), pp. 227-232, ISSN 1538-4101

He, L.C., Damiani, P., Parys, J.B. & Fissore, R.A. (1997). Calcium, calcium release receptors, and meiotic resumption in bovine oocytes. *Biology of Reproduction*, Vol.57, No.5, (November 1997), pp. 1245-1255, ISSN 0006-3363

Homa, S.T. (1988). Effects of cyclic AMP on the spontaneous meiotic maturation of cumulus-free bovine oocytes cultured in chemically defined medium. *Journal of Experimental Zoology*, Vol.248, No.2, (November 1988), pp. 222-231 ISSN 0022-104X

Homa, S.T. (1991). Neomycin, an inhibitor of phosphoinositide hydrolysis, inhibits the resumption of bovine oocyte spontaneous meiotic maturation. *Journal of Experimental Zoology*, Vol.258, No.1, (April 1991), pp. 95-103, ISSN 0022-104X

Homa, S.T. (1995). Calcium and meiotic maturation of the mammalian oocyte. *Molecular Reproduction and Development*,Vol.40, No.1, (January 1995), pp. 122-134, ISSN 1040-452X

Horner, K., Livera, G., Hinckley, M., Trinh, K., Storm, D. & Conti, M. (2003). Rodent oocytes express an active adenylyl cyclase required for meiotic arrest. *Developmental Biology*, Vol.258, No.2 (June 2003), pp. 385-396, ISSN 0012-1606

Inoue, M., Naito, K., Aoki, F., Toyoda, Y. & Sato, E. (1995). Activation of mitogen-activated protein kinase during meiotic maturation in porcine oocytes. *Zygote*, Vol.3, No.3, (August 1995), pp. 265-271, ISSN 0967-1994

Irvine, C.H.G. & Alexander, S.L. (1994). The dynamics of gonadotrophin-releasing hormone, LH and FSH secretion during the spontaneous ovulatory surge of the mare as revealed by intensive sampling of pituitary venous blood. *Journal of Endocrinology*,Vol.140, No.2, (February 1994), pp. 283-295, ISSN 0022-0795

Jagiello, G., Ducayen, M.B. & Goonan, W.D. (1981). A note on the inhibition of *in vitro* meiotic maturation of mammalian oocytes by dibutyryl cyclic AMP. *Journal of Experimental Zoology*, Vol.218, No.2, (November 1981), pp. 309-311, ISSN 0022-104X

Jagiello, G., Ducayen, M., Miller, W., Graffeo, J. & Fang, J.S. (1975). Stimulation and inhibition with LH and other hormones of female mammalian meiosis *in vitro*. *Journal of Reproduction and Fertility*, Vol.43, No.1, (April 1975), pp. 9-22, ISSN 0022-4251

Kalinowski, R.R., Berlot, C.H., Jones T.L., Ross, L.F., Jaffe, L.A. & Mehlmann, L.M. (2004). Maintenance of meiotic prophase arrest in vertebrate oocytes by a Gs protein-mediated pathway. *Developmental Biology*, Vol.267, No.1, (March 2004), pp. 1-13, ISSN 0012-1606

Kalma, Y., Granot, I., Galiani, D., Barash, A. & Dekel, N. (2004). Luteinizing hormone-induced connexin 43 downregulation: inhibition of translation. *Endocrinology*, Vol. 145, No.4, (April 2004), pp. 1617-1624, ISSN 0013-7227

Keel, B.A. & Davis, J.S. (1999). Epidermal growth factor activates extracellular signal-regulated protein kinases (ERK) in freshly isolated porcine granulosa cells. *Steroids*, Vol.64, No.9, (September 1999), pp. 654-658, ISSN 0039-128X

Kim, J.S., Cho, Y.S., Song, B.S., Wee, G., Park, J.S., Choo, Y.K., Yu, K., Lee, K.K., Han, Y.M. & Koo, D.B. (2008). Exogenous dibutyryl cAMP affects meiotic maturation via protein kinase A activation; it stimulates further embryonic development including blastocyst quality in pigs. *Theriogenology*, Vol.69, No.3, (February 2008), pp. 290-301, ISSN 0093-691X

Kren, R., Ogushi, S. & Miyano, T. (2004). Effect of caffeine on meiotic maturation of porcine oocytes. *Zygote*, Vol.12, No.1, (February 2004), pp. 31-38, ISSN 0967-1994

Kuyt, J.R., Kruip, T.A. & de Jong-Brink, M. (1988). Cytochemical localization of adenylate cyclase in bovine cumulus-oocyte complexes. *Experimental Cell Research*, Vol.174, No.1, (January 1988), pp. 139-145, ISSN 0014-4827

Laforest, M.F., Pouliot, E., Guéguen, L. & Richard, F.J. (2005). Fundamental significance of specific phosphodiesterases in the control of spontaneous meiotic resumption in porcine oocytes. *Molecular Reproduction and Development*, Vol.70, No.3, (March 2005), pp. 361-372, ISSN 1040-452X

LaRosa, C. & Downs, S.M. (2006). Stress stimulates AMP-activated kinase and meiotic resumption in mouse oocytes. *Biology of Reproduction*, Vol.74, No.3, (March 2006), pp. 585-592, ISSN 0006-3363

LaRosa, C. & Downs, S.M. (2007). Meiotic induction by heat stress in mouse oocytes: involvement of AMP-activated protein kinase and MAPK family members. *Biology of Reproduction*, Vol.76, No.3, (March 2007), pp.476-486, ISSN 0006-3363

Lastro, M., Collins, S. & Currie, W.B. (2006). Adenylyl cyclases in oocyte maturation: a characterization of AC isoforms in bovine cumulus cells. *Molecular Reproduction and Development*, Vol.73, No.9, (September 2006), pp. 1202-1210, ISSN 1040-452X

Ledan E., Polanski, Z., Terret, M.E. & Maro, B. (2001). Meiotic maturation of the mouse oocyte requires equilibrium between cyclin B synthesis and degradation. *Developmental Biology*, Vol.232, No.2, (April 2001), pp. 400-413, ISSN 0012-1606

Lee, J., Miyano, T. & Moor, R.M. (2000). Localisation of phosphorylated MAP kinase during the transition from meiosis I to meiosis II in pig oocytes. *Zygote*, Vol.8, No.2, (May 2000), pp. 119-125, ISSN 0967-1994

Liang, C.G., Huo, L.J., Zhong, Z.S., Chen, D.Y., Schatten, H. & Sun, Q.Y. (2005). Cyclic adenosine 3′,5′-monophosphate-dependent activation of mitogen-activated protein kinase in cumulus cells is essential for germinal vesicle breakdown of porcine cumulus-enclosed oocytes. *Endocrinology*, Vol.146, No.10, (October 2005), pp. 4437-4444, ISSN 0013-7227

Liang, C.G., Su, Y.Q., Fan, H.Y., Schatten, H. & Sun, Q.Y. (2007). Mechanisms regulating oocyte meiotic resumption: roles of mitogen-activated protein kinase. *Molecular Endocrinology*, Vol.21, No.9, (September 2007), pp. 2037-2055, ISSN 0888-8809

Lorenzo, P.L., Liu, I.K., Carneiro, G.F., Conley, A.J. & Enders, A.C. (2002). Equine oocyte maturation with epidermal growth factor. *Equine Veterinary Journal*. Vol.34, No.4, (July 2002), pp. 378-382, ISSN 2042-3306

Lorenzo, P.L., Pereira, G.R., Bilodeau-Goeseels, S., Carneiro, G.F., Kastelic, J.P. & Liu, I.K.M. (2005). Effect of growth hormone and inhibitors on the *in vitro* maturation of equine oocytes. *Reproduction in Domestic Animal*, Vol.40, No.4, (August 2005), p. 378, ISSN 0936-6768

Masciarelli, S., Horner, K., Liu, C., Park, S.H., Hinckley, M., Hockman, S., Nedachi, T., Jin, C., Conti, M. & Manganiello, V. (2004). Cyclic nucleotide phosphodiesterase 3A-deficient mice as a model for female infertility. *Journal of Clinical Investigation*, Vol.114, No.2, (July 2004), pp. 196-205, ISSN 0021-9738

Matta, S.G., Caldas-Bussière, M.C., Viana, K.S., Faes, M.R., Paes de Carvalho, C.S., Dias, B.L. & Quirino, C.R. (2009). Effect of inhibition of synthesis of inducible nitric oxide synthase-derived nitric oxide by aminoguanidine on the *in vitro* maturation of oocyte-cumulus complexes of cattle. *Animal Reproduction Science,* Vol.111, No.2-4, (April 2009), pp. 189-201, ISSN 0378-4320

Mayes, M.A., Laforest, M.F., Guillemette, C., Gilchrist, R.B. & Richard, F.J. (2007). Adenosine 5'-monophosphate kinase-activated protein kinase (PRKA) activators delay meiotic resumption in porcine oocytes. *Biology of Reproduction,* Vol.76, No.4, (April 2007), pp. 589-597, ISSN 0006-3363

Mayes, M.A. & Sirard, M.A. (2002). Effect of type 3 and type 4 phosphodiesterase inhibitors on the maintenance of bovine oocytes in meiotic arrest. *Biology of Reproduction,* Vol.66, No.1, (January 2002), pp. 180-184, ISSN 0006-3363

Mehlmann, L.M., Jones, T.L.Z. & Jaffe, L.A. (2002). Meiotic arrest in the mouse follicle maintained by a Gs protein in the oocyte. *Science,* Vol.297, No.5585, (August 2002), pp. 1343-1345, ISSN 0036-8075

Mehlmann, L.M., Kalinowski, R.R., Ross, L.F., Parlow, A.F., Hewlett, E.L. & Jaffe, L.A. (2006). Meiotic resumption in response to luteinizing hormone is independent of a Gi family protein or calcium in the mouse oocyte. *Developmental Biology,* Vol.299, No.2, (November 2006), pp. 345-355, ISSN 0012-1606

Mehlmann, L.M., Saeki, Y., Tanaka, S., Brennan, T.J., Evsikov, A.V., Pendola, F.L., Knowles, B.B., Eppig, J.J. & Jaffe, L.A. (2004). The Gs-linked receptor GPR3 maintains meiotic arrest in mammalian oocytes. *Science,* Vol.306, No.5703, (December 2004), pp. 1947-1950, ISSN 0036-8075

Meinecke, B. & Krischek, C. (2003). MAPK/ERK kinase (MEK) signalling is required for resumption of meiosis in cultured cumulus-enclosed pig oocytes. *Zygote,* Vol.11, No.1, (February 2003), pp. 7-16, ISSN 0967-1994

Mondadori, R.G., Neves, J.P. & Gonçalves, P.B.D. (2008). Protein kinase C (PKC) role in bovine oocyte maturation and early embryo development. *Animal Reproduction Science,* Vol.107, No.1-2, (August 2008), pp. 20-29, ISSN 0378-4320

Morikawa, M., Seki, M., Kume, S., Endo, T., Nishimura, Y., Kano, K. & Naito, K. (2007). Meiotic resumption of porcine immature oocytes is prevented by ooplasmic Gsalpha functions. *Journal of Reproduction and Development,* Vol.53, No.6, (December 2007), pp. 1151-1157, ISSN 0916-8818

Norris, R.P., Freudzon, L., Freudzon, M., Hand, A.R., Mehlmann, L.M. & Jaffe, L.A. (2007). A G(s)-linked receptor maintains meiotic arrest in mouse oocytes, but luteinizing hormone does not cause meiotic resumption by terminating receptor-G(s) signaling. *Developmental Biology,* Vol.310, No.2, (October 2007), pp. 240-249, ISSN 0012-1606

Norris, R.P., Freudzon, M., Mehlmann, L.M., Cowan, A.E., Simon, A.M., Paul, D.L., Lampe, P.D. & Jaffe, L.A. (2008). Luteinizing hormone causes MAP kinase-dependent phosphorylation and closure of connexin 43 gap junctions in mouse ovarian follicles: one of two paths to meiotic resumption. *Development,* Vol.135, No.19, (October 2008), pp. 3229-3238, ISSN 0950-1991

Norris, R.P., Freudzon, M., Nikolaev, V.O. & Jaffe, L.A. (2010). Epidermal growth factor receptor kinase activity is required for gap junction closure and for part of the decrease in ovarian follicle cGMP in response to luteinizing hormone. *Reproduction,* Vol.140, No.5, (November 2010), pp. 655-662, ISSN 1470-1626

Norris, R.P., Ratzan, W.J., Freudzon, M., Mehlmann, L.M., Krall, J., Movsesian, M.A., Wang, H., Ke, H., Nikolaev, V.O. & Jaffe, L.A. (2009). Cyclic GMP from the surrounding somatic cells regulates cyclic AMP and meiosis in the mouse oocyte. *Development*, Vol.136, No.11, (June 2009), pp. 1869-1878, ISSN 0950-1991

Ohashi, S., Naito, K., Sugiura, K., Iwamori, N., Goto, S., Naruoka, H. & Tojo, H. (2003). Analysis of mitogen-activated protein kinase function in the maturation of porcine oocytes. *Biology of Reproduction*, Vol.68, No.2, (February 2003), pp. 604-609, ISSN 0006-3363

Olsiewski, P.J. & Beers, W.H. (1983). cAMP synthesis in the rat oocyte. *Developmental Biology*, Vol.100, No.2, (December 1983), pp. 287-293, ISSN 0012-1606

Pereira, G.R., Lorenzo, P.L., Carneiro, G.F., Ball, B.A., Gonçalves, P.B.D., Cantarelli Pegoraro, L.M., Bilodeau-Goeseels, S., Kastelic, J.P., Casey, P.J. & Liu, I.K.M. (2011).The effect of growth hormone (GH) and insulin-like growth factor-I (IGF-I) on *in vitro* maturation of equine oocytes. *Zygote*, Available on CJO 2011doi:10.1017/S0967199411000335

Pincus, G. & Enzmann, E.V. (1935). The comparative behaviour of mammalian eggs *in vivo* and *in vitro*. I. The activation of ovarian eggs. *Journal of Experimental Medicine*, Vol.62, No.5, (October 1935), pp. 665-677, ISSN 0022-1007

Rose-Hellekant, T.A. & Bavister, B.D. (1996). Roles of protein kinase A and C in spontaneous maturation and in forskolin or 3-isobutyl-1-methylxanthine maintained meiotic arrest of bovine oocytes. *Molecular Reproduction and Development*, Vol.44, No.2, (June 1996), pp. 241-249, ISSN 1040-452X

Racowsky, C. (1984). Effect of forskolin on the spontaneous maturation and cyclic AMP content of rat oocyte-cumulus complexes. *Journal of Reproduction and Fertility*, Vol.72, No.1, (September 1984), pp. 107-116, ISSN 0022-4251

Racowsky, C. (1985). Effect of forskolin on maintenance of meiotic arrest and stimulation of cumulus expansion, progesterone and cyclic AMP production by pig oocyte-cumulus complexes. *Journal of Reproduction and Fertility*, Vol.74, No.1, (May 1985), pp. 9-21, ISSN 0022-4251

Richard, F.J. & Sirard, M.A. (1996). Effects of follicular cells on oocyte maturation. II: Theca cell inhibition of bovine oocyte maturation *in vitro*. *Biology of Reproduction*, Vol.54, No.1, (January 1996), pp. 22-28, ISSN 0006-3363

Sadana, R. & Dessauer, C.W. (2009). Physiological roles for G protein-regulated adenylyl cyclase isoforms: insights from knockout and overexpression studies. *Neurosignals*, Vol.17, No.1, (October 2009), pp. 5-22, ISSN 1424-862X

Sasseville, M., Albuz, F.K., Côté, N., Guillemette, C., Gilchrist, R.B. & Richard, F.J. (2009). Characterization of novel phosphodiesterases in the bovine ovarian follicle. *Biology of Reproduction*, Vol.81, No.2, (August 2009), pp. 415-425, ISSN 0006-3363

Sasseville, M., Côté, N., Gagnon, M.C. & Richard, F.J. (2008). Up-regulation of 3′5′-cyclic guanosine monophosphate-specific phosphodiesterase in the porcine cumulus-oocyte complex affects steroidogenesis during *in vitro* maturation. *Endocrinology*, Vol.149, No.11, (November 2008), pp. 5568-5576, ISSN 0013-7227

Sasseville, M., Côté, N., Guillemette, C. & Richard, F.J. (2006). New insight into the role of phosphodiesterase 3A in porcine oocyte maturation. *BMC Developmental Biology*, Vol.6, No.6, (October 2006), p. 47, ISSN 1471-213X

Sasseville, M., Côté, N., Vigneault, C., Guillemette, C. & Richard, F.J. (2007). 3'5'-cyclic adenosine monophosphate-dependent up-regulation of phosphodiesterase type 3A in porcine cumulus cells. *Endocrinology,* Vol.148, No.4, (April 2007), pp. 1858-1867, ISSN 0013-7227

Schultz, R.M., Montgomery, R.R. & Belanoff, J.R. (1983a). Regulation of mouse oocyte meiotic maturation: implication of a decrease in oocyte cAMP and protein dephosphorylation in commitment to resume meiosis. *Developmental Biology,* Vol.97, No.2, (June 1983), pp. 264-273, ISSN 0012-1606

Schultz, R.M., Montgomery, R.R., Ward-Bailey, P.F. & Eppig, J.J. (1983b). Regulation of oocyte maturation in the mouse: possible roles of intercellular communication, cAMP, and testosterone. *Developmental Biology,* Vol.95, No.2, (February 1983), pp. 294-304, ISSN 0012-1606

Schwarz, K.R., Pires, P.R., Adona, P.R., Câmana de Bem, T.H. & Leal, C.L. (2008). Influence of nitric oxide during maturation on bovine oocyte meiosis and embryo development *in vitro. Reproduction Fertility and Development,* Vol.20, No.4, (April 2008), pp. 529-536, ISSN 1031-3613

Schwarz, K.R., Pires, P.R., de Bem, T.H., Adona, P.R. & Leal, C.L. (2010). Consequences of nitric oxide synthase inhibition during bovine oocyte maturation on meiosis and embryo development. *Reproduction in Domestic Animal,* Vol.45, No.1, (February 2010), pp. 75-80, ISSN 0936-6768

Sela-Abramovich, S., Edry, I., Galiani, D., Nevo, N. & Dekel, N. (2006). Disruption of gap junctional communication within the ovarian follicle induces oocyte maturation. *Endocrinology,* Vol. 147, No.5, (May 2006), pp. 2280-2286, ISSN 0013-7227

Sela-Abramovich, S., Galiani, D., Nevo, N. & Dekel, N. (2008). Inhibition of rat oocyte maturation and ovulation by nitric oxide: mechanism of action. *Biology of Reproduction,* Vol.78, No.6, (June 2008), pp. 1111-1118, ISSN 0006-3363

Shi, L., Yue, W., Zhang, J., Lv, L., Ren, Y. & Yan, P. (2009). Effect of ovarian cortex cells on nuclear maturation of sheep oocytes during in vitro maturation. *Animal Reproduction Science,* Vol.113, No.1-4, (July 2009), pp.299-304, ISSN 0378-4320

Shimaoka, T., Nishimura, T., Kano, K. & Naito, K. (2009). Critical effect of pig Wee1B on the regulation of meiotic resumption in porcine immature oocytes. *Cell Cycle,* Vol.8, No.15, (August 2009), pp. 2375-2384, ISSN 1538-4101

Sirard, M.A. (1990). Temporary inhibition of *in vitro* meiotic maturation by adenylate cyclase stimulation in immature bovine oocytes. *Theriogenology,* Vol.33, No.4, (April 1990), pp. 757-767, ISSN 0093-691X

Sirard, M.A. & First, N.L. (1988). *In vitro* inhibition of oocyte nuclear maturation in the bovine. *Biology of Reproduction,* Vol.39, No.2, (September 1988), pp. 229-234, ISSN 0006-3363

Su, Y.Q., Denegre, J.M., Wigglesworth, K.I., Pendola, F.L., O'Brien, M.J. & Eppig, J.J. (2003). Oocyte-dependent activation of mitogen-activated protein kinase (ERK1/2) in cumulus cells is required for the maturation of the mouse oocyte-cumulus cell complex. *Developmental Biology,* Vol.263, No.1, (November 2003), pp. 126-138, ISSN 0012 1606

Su, Y.Q., Wigglesworth, K., Pendola, F.L., O'Brien, M.J. & Eppig, J.J. (2002). Mitogen-activated protein kinase activity in cumulus cells is essential for gonadotropin-induced oocyte meiotic resumption and cumulus expansion in the mouse. *Endocrinology,* Vol.143, No.6, (June 2002), pp. 2221-2232, ISSN 0013-7227

Suikkari, A.M. (2008). *In vitro* maturation: its role in fertility treatment. *Current Opinion in Obstetrics & Gynecology,* Vol.20, No.3, (June 2008), pp. 242-248, ISSN 1040-872X

Tesmer, J.J.G., Sunahara, R.K., Johnson, R.A., Gosselin, G., Gilman, A.G. & Sprang, S.R. (1999). Two-metal-ion catalysis in adenylyl cyclase. *Science,* Vol.285, No.5428, (July 1999), pp. 756-760, ISSN 0036-8075

Thomas, R.E., Armstrong, D.T. & Gilchrist, R.B. (2002). Differential effects of specific phosphodiesterase isoenzyme inhibitors on bovine oocyte meiotic maturation. *Developmental Biology,* Vol.244, No.2, (April 2002), pp. 215-225, ISSN 0012-1606

Thomas, R.E., Armstrong, D.T. & Gilchrist, R.B. (2004). Bovine cumulus cell-oocyte gap junctional communication during *in vitro* maturation in response to manipulation of cell-specific cyclic adenosine 3′,5′-monophosphate levels. *Biology of Reproduction,* Vol.70, No.3, (March 2004), pp. 548-556, ISSN 0006-3363

Törnell, J., Billig, H. & Hillensjö, T. (1990). Resumption of rat oocyte meiosis is paralleled by a decrease in guanosine 3′, 5′-cyclic monophosphate (cGMP) and is inhibited by microinjection of cGMP. *Acta Physiologica Scandinavica,* Vol.139, No.3, (July 1990), pp.511-517, ISSN 0001-6772

Tosca, L., Uzbekova, S., Chabrolle, C. & Dupont, J. (2007). Possible role of 5′AMP-activated protein kinase in the metformin-mediated arrest of bovine oocytes at the germinal vesicle stage during *in vitro* maturation. *Biology of Reproduction,* Vol.77, No.3, (September 2007), pp. 452-465, ISSN 0006-3363

Tosti, E., Boni, R. & Cuomo, A. (2002). Fertilization and activation currents in bovine oocytes. *Reproduction,* Vol.124, No.6, (December 2002), pp. 835-846, ISSN 1470-1626

Tremoleda, J.L., Tharasanit, T., Van Tol, H.T.A., Stout, T.A.E., Colenbrander, B. & Bevers, M.M. (2003). Effects of follicular cells and FSH on the resumption of meiosis in equine oocytes matured *in vitro*. *Reproduction,* Vol.125, No.4, (April 2003), pp. 565-577, ISSN 1470-1626.

Tsafriri, A., Lindner, H.R., Zor, U. & Lamprecht, S.A. (1972). *In vitro* induction of meiotic division in follicle-enclosed rat oocytes by LH, cyclic AMP and prostaglandin $E_2$. *Journal of Reproduction and Fertility,* Vol.31, No.1, (October 1972), pp. 39-50, ISSN 0022-4251

Urner, F., Herrmann, W.L., Baulieu, E.E. & Schorderet-Slatkine, S. (1983). Inhibition of denuded mouse oocyte meiotic maturation by forskolin, an activator of adenylate cyclase. *Endocrinology,* Vol.113, No.3, (September 1983), pp. 1170-1172, ISSN 0013-7227

Vaccari, S., Weeks II, J.L., Hsieh, M., Menniti, F.S. & Conti, M. (2009). Cyclic GMP signalling is involved in the luteinizing hormone-dependent meiotic maturation of mouse oocytes. *Biology of Reproduction,* Vol.81, No.3, (September 2009), pp. 595-604, ISSN 0006-3363

Viana, K.S., Caldas-Bussière, M.C., Matta, S.G., Faes, M.R., de Carvalho, C.S. & Quirino, C.R. (2007). Effect of sodium nitroprusside, a nitric oxide donor, on the *in vitro* maturation of bovine oocytes. *Animal Reproduction Science,* Vol.102, No.3-4, (December 2007), pp. 217-227, ISSN 0378-4320

Vivarelli, E., Conti, M., De Felici, M. & Siracusa, G. (1983). Meiotic resumption and intracellular cAMP levels in mouse oocytes treated with compounds which act on cAMP metabolism. *Cell Differentiation,* Vol.12, No.5, (May 1983), pp. 271-276, ISSN 0045-6039

Ye, J., Flint, A.P., Luck, M.R. & Campbell, K.H. (2003). Independent activation of MAP kinase and MPF during the initiation of meiotic maturation in pig oocytes. *Reproduction*, Vol.125, No.5, (May 2003), pp. 645-656, ISSN 1470-1626

Zhou, G., Myers, R., Li, Y., Chen, Y., Shen, X., Fenyk-Melody, J., Wu, M., Ventre, J., Doebber, T., Furii, N., Musi, N., Hirshman, M.F., Goodyear, L.J. & Moller, D.E. (2001). Role of AMP-activated protein kinase in mechanism of metformin action. *Journal of Clinical Investigation*, Vol.8, No.8, (October 2001), pp. 1167-1174, ISSN 0021-9738

9

# Energy Metabolism Regulating Mammalian Oocyte Maturation

N. Songsasen
*Department of Reproductive Sciences, Center for Species Survival, Smithsonian Conservation Biology Institute, Front Royal, Virginia*

## 1. Introduction

Oocyte maturation is a final step of gamete development that follows a prolonged period of cell growth within a growing follicle. Unlike oocyte growth that takes several weeks or months, maturation process is a short (hours or days), dynamic process. The period of oocyte maturation varies among species, ranging from 10-13 hours in the mouse (Edwards & Gates, 1959) to 16-24 hours in the cow (Dominko & First, 1997) and 48 -72 hours in the dog (Reynaud et al., 2005, Songsasen & Wildt, 2007). For an oocyte to fully capable of fertilizing and developing into an embryo, the gamete needs to undergo nuclear and cytoplasmic maturation. Nuclear maturation encompasses events associated with the separation of homologous chromosomes during meiosis I and the segregation of sister chromatids during meiosis 2 (Albertini & Limback, 2009). Events occur during this process include nuclear envelope breakdown, rearrangement of the cortical cytoskeleton and meiotic spindle assembly. Cytoplasmic maturation includes events of post-transcriptional and post-translational processes, including mRNA synthesis, rearrangement of cytoplasmic organelles and glutathione production that are essential for successful fertilization and subsequent embryonic development (Albertini & Limback, 2009, Watson, 2007). For an oocyte to appropriately progress to these dynamic process of nuclear and cytoplasmic maturation, it requires enormous energy from various substrates, including glucose, amino acids and lipids (Sutton et al., 2003). In addition, tight regulation of reactive oxygen species (ROS) and calcium homeostasis are important during this process. This chapter will review current knowledge on mammalian oocyte development, the roles of mitochondria on cell functions and energy metabolism and its impact on gamete maturation.

## 2. Mammalian oocyte development

The oocyte arises from the primordial germ cells (PGCs) developed during the embryogenesis (Edson et al., 2009). Once formed, the PGCs proliferate and migrate to the undifferentiated gonad that later becomes the ovary. Within the gonad, PGCs enter mitosis with incomplete cytokinesis to form clusters of germ cell nest consisting of oogonia connected to each other by intercellular bridges (Tingen et al., 2009), and the syncytia units are surrounded by pre-granulosa and stromal mesenchymal cells of the ovary. Oogenesis occurs *in utero* in rodents, ruminants and primates, whereas that of the cat, dog and ferret takes place after birth (Peter & McNatty, 1980). During this process, oogonia within germ cell nests transform into the oocytes by, albeit asynchronously, entering the first meiotic prophase and being arrested at the late diplotene stage. The interval between the appearance of the first and the last oocytes within the ovary varies greatly among species, ranging from 2 days in the rat to 5 months in the human (Peter & McNatty, 1980).

Formation of the primordial follicle begins during the fetal life in the human, monkey, horse, cow and pig, but not until during neonatal period in the mouse and rat or later in the second or third weeks after birth in cats, dogs, ferrets, rabbits and minks (Peter & McNatty, 1980). Primordial follicle formation begins with the breakdown of germ cell nest involving the degeneration of vast numbers of oocytes and the invasion of pre-granulosa cells into the germ cell syncytia (Tingen et al., 2009). The loss of oocytes during germ cell nest breakdown is substantial and is believed to be part of quality control processes to ensure that only healthy oocytes are enclosed inside primordial follicles (Tingen et al., 2009). It has been suggested that genetic defects or the failure of germ cells to produce mitochondria are responsible for selective loss of oocytes during the nest breakdown process (Tingen et al., 2009). The surviving oocytes are individually surrounded by squamous pre-granulosa cells and the entire unit is referred to as the primordial follicle (Edson et al., 2009). To date, it has been suggested that several factors produced by the oocytes and somatic cells, including synaptonemal complex protein, Foxl2, NOBOX, members of Notch signaling pathway and transforming growth factor family play roles in germ cell nest breakdown and formation of primordial follicles (Tingen et al., 2009).

Most primordial follicles (90%) leave the resting pool via apoptosis, while the remainders are activated by poorly understood mechanisms to enter the growing follicle pool and develop into the primary, secondary and antral stage (Gougeon, 2010, Picton, 2001). During the early stage of follicle development, the oocyte rapidly increases in size; however, as folliculogenesis proceeds, the growth rate significantly decline and the gamete reaches the maximum size shortly after antral formation (Griffin et al., 2006, Reynaud et al., 2009, Songsasen et al., 2009). During oocyte growth, several organelles including, mitochondria, endoplasmic reticulum and golgi complexes become more abundant (Peter & McNatty, 1980), indicating that energy production and protein synthesis are essential during this process. In most mammalian species, the oocyte resumes meiosis in the preovulatory follicle shortly before ovulation. However, meiotic resumption occurs after the dog oocyte is released from the follicle (Songsasen & Wildt, 2007). At the initiation of meiotic resumption, the nucleus of the oocyte migrates from the central position to the periphery of the cell, and the nuclear membrane and nucleoli disappear as the chromosomes become condensed. This stage is referred to as germinal vesicle breakdown (GVBD). The GVBD oocyte progresses to the metaphase I (MI) stage as the chromosomes are firmly attached to the meiotic spindle. This stage is followed by the separation of homologous chromosomes; one set remain in the secondary oocyte and another set move into a small portion of cytoplasm that is extruded as the second polar body. The chromosomes within the secondary oocyte resume metaphase configuration (i.e., metaphase II [MII] stage) which remains until fertilization. Completion of meiosis occurs after a spermatozoon penetrating the oocyte. During this process, the gamete extrudes the secondary polar body. The remaining chromosomes are enclosed in the nuclear membrane and forming female pronucleus that later fuses with the male counterpart to become the zygote. During its developmental process, the oocyte is coupled to the surrounding granulosa cells through trans-zonal processes (Eppig et al., 1996). This intimate physical connection is crucial for follicle and oocyte development as it facilitates bi-directional communication between the gamete and the somatic cells via gap junction and paracrine signaling (Eppig et al., 1996).

## 3. Mitochondria are the key organelles regulating cell functions

The mitochondria are characterized by having double membranes and their own DNA (mtDNA) inherited from the maternal origin (Van Blerkom, 2004). These organelles play fundamental roles in cell functions, including, providing energy, regulating apoptotic pathway and $Ca^{2+}$ homeostasis (Van Blerkom, 2004, Ramalho-Santos et al., 2009). Dysfunction of mitochondria has been linked to several pathologies, such as heart diseases (Facecchia et al., 2011; Perrelli, et al. 2011), neurodegenerative (Facecchia et al., 2011) and infertility (Ramalho-Santos et al., 2009). The mitochondria provide ATP to cells via oxidative phosphorylation. During this process, high energy electrons derived from oxidation are carried by NADH + $H^+$ and $FADH_2$ to the inner mitochondrial membrane and transferred through cascades of electron transport chain that convert the electrons into ATP (Ramalho-Santos et al., 2009; Voet & Voet, 2004).

Mitochondria also participate in apoptotic pathways (Ramalho-Santos et al., 2009). Because mitochondria consume ~85% of cell's oxygen, these organelles are major producers of ROS (Ramalho-Santos et al., 2009). Excessive production of ROS can lead to DNA damage (especially mtDNA), oxidation of proteins and lipid, as well as release of cytochrome B into the extramitochondrial milieu (Ott et al., 2007). The release of cytochrome B into the cytosol triggers a series of events leading to proteolytic enzyme activation, including caspase 3, 6 and 7 that regulate cell death (Ott et al., 2007). Therefore, cells critically depend on the tight regulation of mitochondrial redox balance to maintain viability and proper functions. It has been shown that glutathione (GSH) and GSH-linked antioxidant enzymes, including Gpx1 and 4 play important roles in maintaining mitochondrial redox balance (Ott et al., 2007). Specifically, these enzymes catalyze the reduction of hydrogen peroxide and lipid peroxide (into $H_2O$) with GSH serves as the electron donor. Furthermore, mitochondrial thioredoxin has been shown to play roles in maintaining mitochondria protein in their reduce state, that in turn counter the reaction of ROS (Ott et al., 2007).

During folliculogenesis and oogenesis, mitochondria propagate simultaneously with the increase in cytoplasmic volume. Pre-migratory PGCs have < 10 mitochondria (Van Blerkom, 2004). However, the numbers of mitochondria within the germ cells increase 10-fold by the time PGCs reach the ovary and additional 2-fold after transformation into the oocyte. Primordial follicle oocytes contain 10,000 mitochondria which increase to 100,000 in mature gametes (Ramalho-Santos et al., 2009). The increase in number of mitochondria also coincides with changes in the distribution of the organelles (Rmalho-Santos et al., 2009). Specifically, mitochondria surround the nucleus in the primary follicle. As the follicle developing into secondary stage, mitochondria within the oocyte distribute throughout the cytoplasm (Peter & McNatty, 1980). In fully grown-germinal vesicle oocyte, the mitochondria homogenously distribute throughout the cell with some localization at the periphery (Sun et al., 2001). As the oocyte progresses through meiotic maturation, mitochondria relocate into the perinuclear region and aggregate into cluster (Yu et al., 2010; Van Blerkom et al., 2002; Sturmey et al., 2006); this event coincides with the rise in ATP levels (Yu et al., 2010). Therefore, the change in localization of mitochondria during oocyte growth is probably in response to energy demand during a given stage of development (Ramalho-Santos et al., 2009).

The oocyte contains two populations of mitochondria which differ in polarization (i.e., electrical and chemical gradient [$\Delta\Psi_M$]); one which is more abundant has low $\Delta\Psi_M$ and the smaller population is highly polarized (Ramalho-Santos et al., 2009; Acton et al., 2004, Van Blerkom et al., 2003). In mouse and human oocytes, highly polarized mitochondria are clustered in pericortical cytoplasm probably to (1) maintain sufficient ATP production in the sub-plasmalemma region in the preparation for fertilization and (2) play role in $Ca^{2+}$ regulation during oocyte activation (Ramalho-Santos et al., 2009; Van Blerkom et al., 2003; Van Blerkom & Davis, 2007). It also has been shown that mitochondrial polarity is associated with developmental capacity of the oocyte and embryo (Van Blerkom, 2004; Acton et al., 2004; Van Blerkom & Davis, 2007; Fujii & Funahashi, 2009). Specifically, mitochondrial membrane potential (MMP) increases as oocytes progress through meiotic maturation (Fujii & Funahashi, 2009), and inhibition of MMP rise decreases the ability of the gamete to form pronucleus and impairs embryonic development (Fujii & Funahashi, 2009).

## 4. Glucose is a key substrate for providing energy during oocyte maturation

Glucose metabolism is crucial for oocyte maturation and development post-fertilization in many mammalian species (Sutton-McDowall et al., 2010; Krisher et al., 2007). *In vitro* culture of oocytes in sub-optimal concentrations of glucose results in delayed meiotic maturation, fertilization and embryonic development (Sutton-McDowall et al., 2010; Sato et al., 2007; Zheng et al., 2001). Delayed resumption of meiosis in prepubertal cattle oocytes is associated with retarded glucose metabolism (Steeves & Gardner, 1999). Furthermore, pharmacological stimulation of glucose metabolism enhances the developmental competence of cow (Krisher & Bavister, 1999) and pig (Herrick et al., 2006) oocytes *in vitro*. Finally, it has been shown that diabetic mice experience abnormal cellular metabolism, mitochondrial dysfunction and meiotic defect (Wang et al., 2010; Colton, et al., 2002).

Glucose uptake into the oocyte occurs via facilitative glucose transporters (GLUT) in the mouse (Purcell & Moley, 2009), cow (Augustin et al., 2001), sheep (Pisani et al., 2008), human (Dan Goor et al., 1997) and rhesus monkey (Zheng et al., 2007). But mammalian oocytes also have low capacity to utilize this substrate (Sutton-McDowall et al., 2010; Steeves & Gardner, 1999; Purcell & Moley, 2009, Brinster, 1971), possibly due to having limited amount of a glycolytic enzyme phosphofructokinase (Cetica et al., 2002). Thus, most mammalian species appear to rely on cumulus cells that contain an additional GLUT with high affinity to this substrate and high phosphofructokinase activity to convert glucose into readily utilized substrates (i.e., pyruvate, NADPH; (Sutton-McDowall et al., 2010; Biggers, et al., 1967). However, we have recently found that dog oocytes utilize glucose at a much higher rate than that of other species (Songsasen et al., 2012). This finding indicates that dog gamete may contain additional GLUT or high levels of glycolytic enzyme compared to those in other species.

The cumulus-oocyte complexes (COCs) have been found to metabolize glucose through four pathways, including glycolysis, the pentose-phosphate- (PPP), hexoxamine (HBP)- and polyol pathways (Sutton-McDowall et al., 2010), with the first two known to affect nuclear and cytoplasmic maturation of mouse (Downs, 1995), pig (Herrick et al., 2006; Krisher et al.,

2007), cow (Krisher et al., 2007; Steeves & Gardner, 1999, Rieger & Loskutoff, 1994) and cat (Spindler et al., 2000) oocytes.

COCs utilize substantial amount of glucose via glycolytic pathway produces energy (ATP), pyruvate and lactate. Pyruvate and lactate then enter the oocyte and are metabolized via the tricarboxylic pathway (TCA) followed by oxidative phosphorylation within the mitochondria that produce substantial amount of ATP essential for oocyte development. Glycolytic metabolism has been shown to play key roles in developmental competence of cow (Steeves & Gardner, 1999, Rieger & Loskutoff, 1994), cat (Spindler et al., 2000) and pig oocytes (Herrick et al., 2006). Specifically, glucose metabolism increases as immature cat oocytes progress through meiotic maturation from the GV to MII stage (Spindler et al., 2000). These same investigators also demonstrated that developmental competence post-fertilization, including the ability to advance to the blastocyst embryos, directly depended on glycolytic rate.

Although PPP does not generate ATP, this pathway generates NADPH that is essential for cytoplasmic integrity and GSH production (Sutton-McDowall et al., 2010; Garcia, et al., 2010). Furthermore, PPP produces ribose-5-phosphate that is critical for DNA and RNA syntheses (Sutton-McDowall et al., 2010; Krisher et al., 2007; Newsholme, et al., 2003). It has been shown the mouse oocyte preferentially metabolize glucose via this pathway. Stimulation of the PPP in mouse oocytes significantly increases GVBD due to conversion of ribose-5 phosphate to phosphoribosyl pyrophosphate that is involved in the production of purine nucleotides, important precursors of DNA and RNA synthesis (Downs et al., 1998). PPP also plays roles in completion of meiosis after fertilization via production of NADPH followed by generation of ROS essential for signaling pathways (Urner & Sakkas, 2005). In the pig, PPP plays critical role in resumption of meiosis and transition of GVBD to MII stage oocytes (Sato et al., 2007; Herrick et al., 2006; Funahashi et al., 2008). Inhibiting PPP activity decreases glycolysis and production of GSH that, in turn compromise oocyte developmental potential in this species (Herrick et al.,2006).

Follicle stimulating hormone (FSH) is the primary regulator of ovarian folliculogenesis (Gougeon, 2010). FSH has been shown to support meiotic resumption by promoting glucose metabolism in mouse oocyte. Specifically, FSH increases glucose uptake (Roberts et al., 2004), as well as promotes glycolysis and PPP in the mouse (Downs & Utecht, 1999), and augment TCA in the cow (Zuelke & Brackett, 1992). Luteinizing hormone surge (LH) plays significant roles in meiotic maturation of mammalian oocytes (Gougeon, 2010; Son et al., 2011, Hsieh et al., 2011). LH surge causes a significant decline in gap junctions leading to dissociation of granulosa cells from the gamete and expansion of the cumulus cells. LH also activates its G-protein-coupled receptor on theca and granulosa cells, which in turn leads to elevation of intracellular cAMP that subsequently triggers multiple downstream pathways regulating meiotic maturation and ovulation (Hsieh et al., 2011, Sun et al., 2009). Finally, LH promotes cow oocytes maturation by modifying gamete's nutritional microenvironment via increasing glucose utilization through glycolysis and TCA cycle (Zuelke & Brackett, 1992).

## 5. Amino acids influence cell functions

Amino acids play important roles in cellular functions, as they serve as substrates for protein synthesis, energy production, organic osmolytes and intracellular buffer (Sutton et al., 2003; Bae & Foote, 1974). Furthermore, cysteine, proline and glutamine are precursors of GSH (Sutton et al., 2003). It has been shown that there are differences in amino acid composition within follicular fluid among species. Hystinine, phynylalanine, asparagines and glutamate are present in high concentrations in human follicular fluid (Jozwik et al., 2006; Jimena, et al., 1993). However, glycine, glutamine and alanine are most abundant in the cow (Orsi et al., 2005). Finally, glycine, alanine and serine, and glutamine, glycine and aspartate are found in high concentration in horses (Engle et al., 1984) and mice (Harris et al., 2005), respectively. These apparent differences in follicular amino acids composition among species suggest that there are variations in amino acid requirement during oocyte maturation among various taxa.

Amino acid concentrations fluctuate with ovarian follicle development. Specifically, in the pig, most amino acids are present in lower concentration in large follicles than in small counterparts (Hong & Lee, 2007). This may be attributed to the decrease in the amount of specific amino acids following preferred consumption by follicular cells or oocytes during follicular development. Culturing pig oocytes in the presence of glutamine, aspargine and valine enhances cytoplasmic maturation based on the improvement of monospermic fertilization and embryonic development (Hong & Lee, 2007). Furthermore, addition of essential amino acids to chemically defined maturation media enhances oocyte maternal mRNA synthesis, embryo developmental rates and cell numbers in blastocyst embryos in the cow (Watson et al., 2000).

Mammalian oocytes utilize amino acids via the cumulus cells. Cumulus cells contain high concentration of two essential enzymes for amino acid metabolism, alanine aminotransferase [ALT] and aspartate aminotransferase [AST] (Cetica, et al., 2003), suggesting that the somatic cells supplies the oocyte with amino acid or oxidative substrate. Because oocytes also possess ALT and AST activities, albeit lower than cumulus cells, they continue to utilize amino acids after being dissociated from the somatic cells during maturation (Cetica et al., 2003).

Glutamine is the most widely studied amino acid among those found in follicular fluid. This amino acid is recognized as a key substrate for GSH synthesis, protein translation and gluconeogenesis (Bae & Foote 1974; Newsholme et al. 2003). In cattle, glutamine metabolism through the TCA cycle increases steadily during oocyte maturation and reaches maximum at 18 to 24 of *in vitro* culture (Steeves & Gardner, 1999; Rieger & Loskutoff, 1994). This finding suggests that this amino acid is critical for promoting final nuclear maturation in this species (Rieger & Loskutoff, 1994). Addition of glutamine to maturation medium increases the number of cow oocytes completing nuclear maturation (Bilodeau-Goeseels, 2006). However, supplement culture medium with glutamine alone does not improve developmental competence of rhesus monkey oocytes (Zheng et al., 2002). Nevertheless, combination of glutamine and 20 amino acids enhances nuclear maturation in this species (Zheng et al., 2002). It has been shown that glutamine is an effective energy substrate to support rabbit oocyte maturation (Bae & Foote, 1974). Our earlier study demonstrates that glutamine uptake peaks at about 12 h after the onset of culturing dog oocytes (Songsasen et al., 2007), suggesting its role in meiotic resumption in this species. However, addition of glutamine to a culture medium does not improve nuclear maturation rate, suggesting that this amino acid plays role in cytoplasmic maturation in the dog (Songsasen et al., 2007). In the mouse, the use of glutamine as a sole energy source (i.e., without carbohydrate supplementation) is sufficient to initiate meiotic resumption, but not enough to support the transition of GVBD to MII oocytes (Downs & Hudson, 2000). Gonadotropins have been shown to promote glutamine metabolism. Specifically, in the presence of FSH, glutamine promotes nuclear maturation of hamster oocytes (Kito & Bavister, 1997). LH stimulates cumulus cells to convert glutamine to α-ketoglutarate, which is then oxidized through TCA cycle to generate ATP (Zuelke & Brackett, 1993).

## 6. Lipids are important endogenous energy source during oocyte maturation

Intracellular lipids play essential roles in oocyte development (Sturmey et al., 2009, 2006; Sturmey & Leese, 2003; Ferguson & Leese, 2006). Lipids serve as reservoir of endogenous energy source, substrates for water production during blastocoel development and precursors of second messengers modulating cell functions and purine synthesis (McEvoy et al., 2000). Furthermore, membrane bound phospholipids regulate various cell functions associated with calcium flux (e.g., cortical granule exocytosis and fertilization (McEvoy et al., 2000).

Mammalian oocytes contain an endogenous lipid reserve that varies in quantity among species (ranging from 4 ng total lipid per oocyte (Loewenstein & Cohen, 1964) in the mouse to 63 ng (McEvoy et al., 2000) in the cow to 161 ng the pig (Sturmey & Leese, 2003; McEvoy et al., 2000). Triglyceride is the main lipid found in mammalian oocytes (range for 30% in sheep to 60% of total lipid in pig) (Sturmey & Leese, 2003; Sturmey et al., 2009; Ferguson & Leese, 1999). It has been shown that triglyceride stores decrease as cows (Leese & Ferguson, 1999) and pigs (Sturmey & Leese, 2003) oocytes progress through meiotic maturation, and this process is coincides with increased lipolysis (Cetica et al., 2002). These findings indicate that triglyceride provides a rich energy supply for oocyte maturation (Cetica et al., 2002) and sustaining pre-implantation embryo growth (Sturmey et al., 2006, Ferguson & Leese, 2006). Sturmey et al. (2006) utilized the fluorescence resonance energy transfer technology to examine the relationship between mitochondria and cytoplasmic lipid droplets during pig oocyte maturation and reported that the two organelles co-localize in a molecular level and form 'metabolic units' at the periphery of the gamete. There are evidence indicating that free fatty acids cleaved from triglyceride molecules stored in lipid droplets can be directly transported across the mitochondrial membrane and oxidized via β-oxidation that results in the production of acetyl CoA, a substrate for the TCA cycle (Sturmey et al., 2006; Dunning et al., 2010). Culturing pig and cow oocytes (Ferguson & Leese, 2006) in the presence of an inhibitor of carnitine palmitoyl transferase, the enzyme responsible for the transport of free fatty acids into the mitochondrial matrix compromises embryo development post-fertilization (Sturmey et al., 2006). Enhancing lipid metabolism and mitochondrial activity by addition of L-carnitine to culture medium decreases ROS levels, as well as improves MII and cleavage rates (Somfai et al., 2011), although the treatment does not impact blastocyst formation. In the mouse, β-oxidation is significantly up-regulated during both *in vivo* and *in vitro* oocyte maturation (Dunning et al., 2010). Inhibition of β-oxidation compromises meiotic resumption (Downs et al., 2009) and impairs embryonic development formation following fertilization (Dunning et al., 2010), suggesting that lipid metabolism plays essential roles in both nuclear and cytoplasmic maturation in the mouse. Furthermore, enhancing β-oxidation by supplement L-carnitine to the culture medium during in vitro follicle culture and *in vitro* maturation significantly improves mouse oocyte developmental competence (Dunning et al., 2011, 2010).

## 7. Species specificity in preferentially differences in energy substrate

To date, studies have revealed that there are species-specific energy requirement for oocyte maturation. Mouse oocytes require exogenous energy substrate (especially pyruvate) to complete nuclear maturation (Downs & Hudson, 2000) probably due to the limited amount of intracellular lipid (Loewenstein & Cohen, 1964). Mouse oocytes cultured in the absence of glucose and pyruvate fail to progress to the MII stage (Downs & Hudson, 2000). In contrast, cow oocytes which contain 20 fold of total lipid mass compared to the mouse are able to complete nuclear maturation in the absence of exogenous energy substrates (Sturmey et al., 2009). Furthermore, inhibition of triglyceride metabolism compromises nuclear maturation in this species (Ferguson & Leese, 2006).

Mouse (Sturmey et al., 2009; Downs et al., 2002; Downs & Mastropolo, 1994; Biggers et al., 1967), cow (Steeves & Gardner, 1999) and cat oocytes (Spindler et al., 2000) appear to prefer pyruvate to glucose as an energy source. Pyruvate supports maturation, maintains viability and promotes cleavage of the fertilized oocyte in the absence of cumulus cells (Downs et al., 2002; Downs & Mastropolo, 1994; Biggers et al., 1967). The metabolism of pyruvate is related to the stage of meiosis, with arrested oocytes (GV or MII) metabolizing less pyruvate than oocytes progressing through meiosis (Downs et al., 2002). Cow oocytes utilize pyruvate produced by the cumulus cell via glycolysis (Cetica et al., 2002). Furthermore, cow oocytes have more G6PDH than phosphofructokinase, suggesting that the gamete preferentially metabolize glucose via PPP pathway rather than glycolysis (Cetica et al., 2002).

Pig and dog oocytes utilize glucose as their primary energy substrate (Krisher et al., 2007; Songsasen & Wildt, 2007). Recent study has shown that lipid metabolism plays significant roles in oocyte maturation in the pig (Sturmey & Leese, 2003). This is not surprising since pig oocytes contain a substantial amount of triglyceride compared to other species (Sturmey & Leese, 2003). To date, there is no information on roles of intracellular lipid in dog oocyte development.

## 8. Summary and future perspectives

Energy metabolism is critical for oocyte maturation. Development of appropriate systems for *in vitro* oocyte maturation requires a great understanding of factors, including energy metabolism involved in the acquisition of oocyte developmental competence during folliculogenesis and during the maturation period. To date, studies have been focused on the impact of exogenous substrates, especially glucose and pyruvate on meiotic and cytoplasmic maturation. Very little attention has been centered on roles of intracellular lipid in oocyte development. Fatty acids are several-fold more energy rich than glucose. For example, 130 mols of ATP result from the oxidation of one mol of palmitic acid (C16:0), as compared to 38 mols of ATP from one mol of glucose. Thus, energy-dense lipids have potential ability to support and promote oocyte maturation and embryo development. Indeed, there has been increasing evidence that enhancing mitochondrial activity and β-oxidation lipid plays important role improve oocyte developmental competence in the mouse, a species that have small amount of intracellular lipids (Dunning et al., 2010). Furthermore, increase β-oxidation during *in vitro* folliculogenesis has been shown to promote mouse oocyte developmental competence (Dunning et al., 2011). Therefore, further research is needed to understand how the oocyte and early embryo utilize lipid substrates for energy production and whether this form of metabolism is developmentally beneficial.

Certainly, there are species-specificities in oocyte metabolism. An *in vitro* condition developed for oocytes of a certain species cannot be directly applied to another. Thus, one of future research priorities should be advance our understanding about oocyte metabolic requirement for understudied species, especially carnivores. At last, current and future development of *in vitro* culture conditions for mammalian oocytes will certainly benefit from comparative studies conducted in different animal species.

## 9. References


Acton, B. M., Jurisicova, A. & Casper, R. F. (2004) Alterations in mitochondrial membrane potential during preimplantation stages of mouse and human embryo development. *Molecular Human Reproduction*, 10, 23-32.

Albertini, D. F. & Limback, S. D. (2009) The natural life cycle of the mammalian oocyte. In Borini, A. and Coticchio, G. (eds), *Preservation of Human Oocytes*. Informa Healthcare, London. pp. 83-94

Augustin, R., Pocar, P., Navarrete-Santos, A., Wrenzycki, C., Gandolfi, F., Niemann, H. & Fischer, B. (2001) Glucose transporter expression is developmentally regulated in *in vitro* derived bovine preimplantation embryos. *Molecular Reproduction and Development*, 60, 370-376.

Bae, I.-H. & Foote, R. H. (1974) Utilization of glutamine for energy and protein synthesis by cultured rabbit follicular oocytes. *Experimental Cell Research*, 90, 432-436.

Biggers, J. D., Whittingham, D. G. & Donahue, R. P. (1967) The pattern of energy metabolism in the mouse oocyte and zygote. *Proceedings of National Academy of Sciences USA*, 58, 560-567.

Bilodeau-Goeseels, S. (2006) Effects of culture media and energy sources on the inhibition of nuclear maturation in bovine oocytes. *Theriogenology*, 66, 297-306.

Brinster, R. L. (1971) Oxidation of pyruvate and glucose by oocytes of the mouse and rhesus monkey. *Journal of Reproduction and Fertility*, 24, 187-191.

Cetica, P., Pintos, L., Dalvit, G. & Beconi, M. (2002) Activity of key enzymes involved in glucose and triglyceride catabolism during bovine oocyte maturation *in vitro*. *Reproduction*, 124, 675-681.

Cetica, P., Pintos, L., Dalvit, G. & Beconi, M. (2003) Involvement of enzymes of amino acid metabolism and tricarboxylic acid cycle in bovine oocyte maturation *in vitro*. *Reproduction*, 126, 753-763.

Colton, S. A., Pieper, G. M. & Downs, S. M. (2002) Altered meiotic regulation in oocytes from diabetic mice. *Biology of Reproduction*, 67, 220-231.

Dan Goor, M., Sasson, S., Davarashvili A. & Almagor, M. (1997) Expression of glucose transporter and glucose uptake in human oocytes and preimplantation embryos. *Human Reproduction*, 12, 2508-2510.

Dominko, T. & First, N. L. (1997) Timing in meiotic progression in bovine oocytes and its effect on early embryo development. *Molecular Reproduction and Development*, 47, 456-467.

Downs, S. M. & Hudson, E. D. (2000) Energy substrates and the completion of spontaneous meiotic maturation. *Zygote*, 8, 339-351.

Downs, S. M. & Mastropolo, A. M. (1994) The participation of energy substrates in the control of meiotic maturation in murine oocytes. *Developmental Biology*, 162, 154-168.

Downs, S. M. & Utecht, A. M. (1999) Metabolism of radiolabeled glucose by mouse oocytes and oocyte-cumulus cell complexes. *Biology of Reproduction*, 60, 1146-1452.

Downs, S. M. (1995) The influences of glucose, cumulus cells, and metabolic coupling on ATP levels and meiotic control in the isolated mouse oocytes. *Developmental Biology*, 167, 502-512.

Downs, S. M., Humpherson, P. G. & Leese, H. J. (1998) Meiotic induction in cumulus cell-enclosed mouse oocytes: involvement of the pentose phosphate pathway. *Biology of Reproduction*, 58, 1084-1094.

Downs, S. M., Humpherson, P. G. & Leese, H. J. (2002) Pyruvate utilization by mouse oocytes is influenced by meiotic status and the cumulus oophorus. *Molecular Reproduction and Development*, 62, 113-123.

Downs, S. M., Mosey, J. L. & Klinger, J. (2009) Fatty acid oxidation and meiotic resumption mouse oocytes. *Molecular Reproduction and Development*, 76, 844-853.

Dunning, K. R., Akison, L. K., Russell, D. L., Norman, R. J. & Robker, R. L. (2011) Increased beta-oxidation and improved oocyte developmental competence in response to L-carnitine during ovarian *in vitro* follicle development in mice. *Biology of Reproduction*, 85, 548-555.

Dunning, K. R., Cashman, K., Russell, D. L., Thompson, J. G., Norman, R. J. & Robker, R. L. (2010) Beta oxidation is essential for mouse oocyte developmental competence. *Biology of Reproduction*, 83, 909-918.

Edson, M. A., Nagaraja, A. K. & Matzuk, M. M. (2009) The mammalian ovary from genesis to revelation. *Endocrine Review*, 30, 624-712.

Edwards, R. G. & Gates, A. H. (1959) Timing of the stages of the maturation divisions, ovulation, fertilization and the first cleavage of egg of adult mice treated with gonadotrophins. *Journal of Endocrinology*, 18, 292-304.

Engle, C. C., Foley, C. W., Plotka, E. D. & Witherspoon, D. M. (1984) Free amino acids and protein concentrations in reproductive tract fluids of the mare. *Theriogenology*, 21, 919-930.

Eppig, J. J., O'Brien, M. O. & Wigglesworth, K. (1996) Mammalian oocyte growth and development *in vitro*. *Molecular Reproduction and Development*, 44, 260-273.

Facecchia, K., Fochesato, L. A., Stohs, S. J. & Pandey, S. (2011) Oxidative toxicity in neurodegenerative dieseases: role of mitochondrial dysfunction and therapeutic strategies. *Journal of Toxicology*, 683728, 1-12.

Ferguson, E. M. & Leese, H. J. (1999) Triglyceride content of bovine oocytes and early embryos. *Reproduction*, 116, 373-378.

Ferguson, E. M. & Leese, H. J. (2006) A potential role for tryglyceride as an energy sources during bovine oocyte maturation and early embryo development. *Molecular Reproduction and Development*, 73, 1195-1201.

Fujii, W. & Funahashi, H. (2009) Exogenous adenosine reduces the mitochondrial membrane potential of murine oocytes during the latter half of *in vitro* maturation and pronuclear formation following chemical activation. *Journal of Reproduction and Development*, 55, 187-193.

Funahashi, H., Koike, T. & Sakai, R. (2008) Effect of glucose and pyruvate on nuclear and cytoplasmic maturation of porcine oocytes in a chemically defined medium. *Theriogenology*, 70, 1041-1047.

Garcia, J., Han, D., Sancheti, H., Yap, L. P., Kaplowitz, N. & Cadenas, E. (2010) Regulation of mitochondrial glutathione redox status and protein glutathionylation by respiratory substrates. *Journal of Biological Chemistry*, 285, 39646-39654.

Gougeon, A. (2010) Human ovarian follicular development: From activation of resting follicles to preovulatory maturation. *Annls d' Endocrinologie*, 71, 132-143.

Griffin, J., Emery, B. R., Huang, I., Peterson, C. M. & Carrell, D. T. (2006) Comparative analysis of follicle morphology and oocyte diameter in four mammalian species (mouse, hamster, pig and human). *Journal of Experimental Clinical and Assisted Reproduction*, 3, 2.

Harris, S. E., Gopichandran, N., Picton, H. M., Leese, H. J. & Orsi, N. M. (2005) Nutrient concentrations in murine follicular fluid and the female reproductive tract. *Theriogenology*, 64, 992-1006.

Herrick, J. R., Brad, A. M. & Krisher, R. L. (2006) Chemical manipulation of glucose metabolism in porcine oocytes: effects on nuclear and cytoplasmic maturation *in vitro*. *Reproduction*, 131, 289-298.

Hong, J. & Lee, E. (2007) Intrafollicular amino acid concentration and the effect of amino acids in a defined maturation medium on porcine oocyte maturation, fertilization and preimplantation development. *Theriogenology*, 68, 728-735.

Hsieh, M., Thao, K. & Conti, M. (2011) Genetic dissection of epidermal growth factor receptor signaling during luteinizing hormone-induced oocyte maturation. *PLoS One*, 6, e21574.

Jimena, P., Castilla, J., A., Peran, F., Ramirez, J. P., Gil, T. & Mozas, J. (1993) Distribution of free amino acids in human preovulatory follicles. *Hormone and Metabolism Research*, 25, 228-230.

Jozwik, M., Jozwik, M., Teng, C. & Battaglia, F. C. (2006) Amino acid, ammonia and urea concentration in human pre-ovulatory ovarian follicular fluid. *Human Reproduction*, 21, 2776-2782.

Kito, S. & Bavister, B. D. (1997) Gonadotropins, serum, and amino acids alter nuclear maturation, cumulus expansion, and oocyte morphology in hamster cumulus-oocyte complexes *in vitro*. *Biology of Reproduction*, 56, 1281-1289.

Krisher, R. L. & Bavister, B. D. (1999) Enhanced glycolysis after maturation of bovine oocytes *in vitro* is associated with increased developmental competence. *Molecular Reproduction and Development*, 53, 19-26.

Krisher, R. L., Brad, A. M., Herrick, J. R., Sparman, M. L. & Swain, J. E. (2007) A comparative analysis of metabolism and viability in porcine oocytes during *in vitro* maturation. *Animal Reproduction Science*, 98, 72-96.

Leese, H. J. & Ferguson, E. M. (1999) Triglyceride content of bovine oocytes and early embryos. *Journal of Reproduction and Fertility*, 116, 373-378.

Loewenstein, J. E. & Cohen, A. (1964) Dry mass, lipid content and protein content of the intact and zona--free mouse ovum. *Journal Embryology Experiment and Morphology*, 12, 113-121.

McEvoy, T. G., Coull, G. D., Broadbent, P. J., Hutchinson, J. S. & Speake, B. K. (2000) Fatty acid composition of lipids in immature cattle, pig and sheep oocytes with intact zona pellucida. *Journal of Reproduction and Fertility*, 118, 163-170.

Newsholme, P., Lima, M. M. R., Procopio, J., Pithon-Curi, T. C., Doi, S. Q., Bazotte, R. B. & Curi, R. (2003) Glutamine and glutamate as vital metabolites. *Brazilian Journal of Medical and Biological Research*, 36, 153-163.

Orsi, N. M., Gopichandran, N., Leese, H. J., Picton, H. M. & Harris, S. E. (2005) Fluctuations in bovine ovarian follicular fluid throughout the oestrous cycle: a comparison with plasma and a TCM-199-based maturation medium. *Reproduction*, 129, 229-334.

Ott, M., Gogvadze, V., Orrenious, S. & Zhivotovsky, B. (2007) Mitochondria, oxidative stress and cell death. *Apoptosis*, 12, 913-922.

Perrelli, M.-G., Pagliaro, P. & Penna, C. (2011) Ischemia/reperfusion injury and cardioprotective mechanisms: role of mitochondria and reactive oxygen species. *World Journal of Cardiology*, 3, 186-200.

Peter, H. & McNatty, K. P. (1980) *The Ovary*, University of California Press, Berkley and Los Angeles. 175 pp.

Picton, H. M. (2001) Activation of follicle development: the primordial follicle. *Theriogenology*, 55, 1193-1210.

Pisani, L., F., Antonini, S., Pocar, P., Ferrari, S., Brevini, T. A., Rhind, S. M. & Gandolfi, F. (2008) Effects of pre-mating nutrition on mRNA levels of developmentally relevant genes in sheep oocytes and granulosa cells. *Reproduction*, 136, 303-312.

Purcell, S. H. & Moley, K. H. (2009) Glucose transporters in gametes and preimplantation embryos. *Trends in Endocrinology and Metabolism*, 20, 483-489.

Ramalho-Santos, J., Varum, S., Amaral, S., Mota, P. C., Sousa, A. P. & Amaral, A. (2009) Mitochondrial functionality in reproduction: from gonads and gametes to embryos and embryonic stem cells. *Human Reproduction Update*, 15, 553-572.

Reynaud, K., Fontbonne, A., Marseloo, N., Thoumire, S., Chebrout, M., de Lesegno, C. V. & Chastant-Maillard, S. (2005) *In vivo* meiotic resumption, fertilization and early embryonic development in the bitch. *Reproduction*, 130, 193-201.

Reynaud, K., Gicquel, C., Thoumire, S., Chebrout, M., Ficheux, C., Bestandji, M. & Chastant-Maillard, S. (2009) Folliculogenesis and morphometry of oocyte and follicle growth in the feline ovary. *Repro Domes Anim*, 44, 174-179.

Rieger, D. & Loskutoff, N. M. (1994) Changes in the metabolism of glucose, pyruvate, glutamine and glycine during maturation of cattle oocytes *in vitro*. *Journal of Reproduction and Fertility*, 100, 257-262.

Roberts, R., Stark, J., Latropoulou, A., Becker, D. L., Franks, S. & Hardy, K. (2004) Energy substrate metabolism of mouse cumulus-oocyte complexes: response to follicle-stimulating hormone is mediated by the phosphatidylinositol 3-kinase pathway and is associated with oocyte maturation. *Biology of Reproduction*, 71, 199-209.

Sato, H., Iwata, H., Hayashi, T., Kimura, K., Kuwayama, T. & Monji, Y. (2007) The effect of glucose on the progression of the nuclear maturation of pig oocytes. *Animal Reproduction Science*, 99, 299-305.

Somfai, T., Kaneda, M., Akagi, S., Watanabe, S., Haraguchi, S., Mizutani, E., Dang-Nguyen, T. Q., Geshi, M., Kikuchi, K. & Nagai, T. (2011) Enhancement of lipid metabolism with L-carnitine during *in vitro* maturation improves nuclear maturation and cleavage ability of follicular porcine oocytes. *Reproduction Fertility and Development*, 23, 912-920.

Son, W. Y., Das, M., Shalom-Paz, E. & Holzer, H. (2011) Mechanisms of follicle selection and development. *Minerva Ginecologica*, 63, 89-102.

Songsasen, N. & Wildt, D. E. (2007) Oocyte biology and challenges in developing *in vitro* maturation systems in the domestic dog. *Animal Reproduction Science*, 98, 2-22.

Songsasen, N., Fickes, A., Pukazhenthi, B. S. & Wildt, D. E. (2009) Follicular morphology, oocyte diameter and localization of fibroblast growth factors in the domestic dog ovary. *Reproduction in Domestic Animals*, 44 (Suppl 2), 65-70.

Songsasen, N., Spindler, R. E. & Wildt, D. E. (2007) Requirement for, and patterns of, pyruvate and glutamine metabolism in the domestic dog oocyte *in vitro*. *Molecular Reproduction and Development*, 74, 870-877.

Songsasen, N., Wesselowski, S., Carpenter, J. W., Wildt, D. E. (2012) The ability to achieve meiotic maturation in the dog oocyte is linked to glycolysis and glutamine oxidation. *Molecular Reproduction and Development*, in press.

Spindler, R. E., Pukazhenthi, B. S. & Wildt, D. E. (2000) Oocyte metabolism predicts the development of cat embryos to blastocyst *in vitro*. *Molecular Reproduction and Development*, 56, 163-171.

Steeves, T. E. & Gardner, D. K. (1999) Metabolism of glucose, pyruvate and glutamine during the maturation of oocytes derived from pre-pubertal and adult cows. *Molecular Reproduction and Development*, 54, 92-101.

Sturmey, R. G. & Leese, H. J. (2003) Energy metabolism in pig oocytes and early embryos. *Reproduction*, 126, 197-204.

Sturmey, R. G., O'Toole, P. J. & Leese, H. J. (2006) Fluorescence resonance energy transfer analysis of mitochondrial lipid association in the porcine oocyte. *Reproduction*, 132, 829-837.

Sturmey, R. G., Reis, A., Leese, H. J. & McEvoy, T. G. (2009) Role of fatty acids in enery provision during oocyte maturation and early embryo development. *Reproduction of Domestic Animals*, 44, 50-58.

Sun, Q. Y., Miao, Y. L. & Schatten, H. (2009) Towards a new understanding on the regulation of mammalian oocyte meiotic resumption. *Cell Cycle*, 8, 2741-2747.

Sun, Q. Y., Wu, G. M., Lai, L., Park, K. W., Cabot, R., Cheong, H. T., Day, B. N., Prather, R. S. & Schatten, H. (2001) Translocation of active mitochondria during pig oocyte maturation, fertilization and early embryo development *in vitro*. *Reproduction*, 122, 155-163.

Sutton, M. L., Gilchrist, R. B. & Thompson, J. G. (2003) Effects of *in-vivo* and *in-vitro* environments on the metabolism of the cumulus-oocyte complex and its influence on oocyte developmental capacity. *Human Reproduction Update*, 9, 35-48.

Sutton-McDowall, M. L., Gilchrist, R. B. & Thompson, J. G. (2010) The pivotal role of glucose metabolism in determining oocyte developmental competence. *Reproduction*, 139, 685-695.

Tingen, C., Kim, A. & Woodruff, T. K. (2009) The primordial pool of follicles and nest breakdown in mammalian ovaries. *Molecular Human Reproduction*, 15, 795-803.

Urner, F. & Sakkas, D. (2005) Involvement of the pentose phosphate pathway and redox regulation in fertilization in the mouse. *Molecular Reproduction and Development*, 70, 494-503.

Van Blerkom, J. & Davis, P. (2007) Mitochondrial signaling and fertilization. *Molecular Human Reproduction*, 13, 759-779.

Van Blerkom, J. (2004) Mitochondria in human oogenesis and preimplantation embryogenesis: engines of metabolism, ionic regulation and developmental competence. *Reproduction*, 128, 269-280.

Van Blerkom, J., Davis, P. & Alexander, S. (2003) Inner mitochondrial membrane potential (DYm), cytoplasmic ATP content and free $Ca^{2+}$ levels in metaphase II mouse oocytes. *Human Reproduction*, 18, 2429-2440.

Van Blerkom, J., Davis, P., Mathwig, V. & Alexander, S. (2002) Domains of high-polarized and low-polarized mitochondria may occur in mouse and human oocytes and early embryos. *Human Reproduction*, 17, 393-406.

Voet, D. & Voet, J. G. (2004) *Biochemistry*. 3 edn, John, Wiley & Sons, Inc., Hoboken, NJ. 1591 pp.

Wang, Q., Frolova, A. I., Purcell, S., Adastra, K., Schoeller, E., Chi, M. M., Schedl, T. & Moley, K. H. (2010) Mitochondrial dysfunction and apoptosis in cumulus cells of type I diabetic mice. *PLoS One*, 5, e15901.

Watson, A. J. (2007) Oocyte cytoplasmic maturation: A key mediator of oocyte and embryo developmental competence. *Journal of Animal Sciences*, 85 (E. Suupl.), E1-E3.

Watson, A. J., de Sousa, P., Caveney, A., Barcroft, L., Natale, D., Urquhart, J. & Westhusin, M. E. (2000) Impact of bovine oocyte maturation media on oocyte transcript levels, blastocyst development, cell number, and apotosis. *Biology of Reproduction*, 62, 355-364.

Yu, Y., Dumollard, R., Rossbach, A., Lai, F. A. & Swann, K. (2010) Redistribution of mitochondria leads to bursts of ATP production during spontaneous mouse oocyte maturation. *Journal of Cellular Physiology*, 224, 672-680.

Zheng, P., Bavister, B. D. & Ji, W. (2001) Energy substrate requirement for *in vitro* maturation of oocytes from unstimulated adult rhesus monkeys. *Molecular Reproduction and Development*, 58, 348-355.

Zheng, P., Bavister, B. D. & Ji, W. Z. (2002) Amino acid requirements for maturation of rhesus monkey (*Macacca mulatta*) oocytes in culture. *Reproduction*, 124, 515-522.

Zheng, P., Vassena, R. & Latham, K. E. (2007) Effects of *in vitro* oocyte maturation and embryo culture on the expression of glucose transporters, glucose metabolism and insulin signaling genes in rhesus money oocytes and preimplantation embryos. *Molecular Human Reproduction*, 13, 361-371.

Zuelke, K. A. & Brackett, B. G. (1992) Effects of luteinizing hormone on glucose metabolism in cumulus-enclosed bovine oocytes matured *in vitro*. *Endocrinology*, 131, 2690-2696.

Zuelke, K. A. & Brackett, B. G. (1993) Increased glutamine metabolism in bovine cumulus cell-enclosed and denuded oocytes after *in vitro* maturation with lutenizing hormone. *Biology of Reproduction*, 48, 815-820.

# 10

# PKC Regulation of Gametogenesis and Early Development

James J. Faust, Madhavi Kalive, Anup Abraham and David G. Capco
*Arizona State University, USA*

## 1. Introduction

The protein kinase C (PKC) family is comprised of 11 isotypes and many can exist in a single cell simultaneously. There are three general categories of PKC based on their cofactor requirements for activation: The conventional, novel, and atypical PKCs. The first category, the conventional PKC isotypes, are PKCα, -βI, -βII, and -γ and are activated by diacylglycerol (DAG), and negatively charged phospholipids in a calcium-dependent manner. The second category, the novel PKCs, are composed of PKCδ, -ε, -θ, and -η and require negatively changed phospholipids and DAG, but act in a calcium-independent manner. Finally, the atypical PKCs are human ι/mouse λ and PKCζ and only require negatively charged phospholipids for activation. Each PKC isotype phosphorylates serine/threonine residues on protein substrates. There are several known substrates for PKC and they include MARCKS proteins, RACK proteins, Dynamin, EGFR, MEK5, the two subunits of MPF, $p34^{cdc2}$ and cyclin B, among others (Yu et al., 2004; Steinberg 2008; Meier et al., 2009).

Many PKC isotypes have overlapping substrate specificity. Since many isotypes function in different cellular locations and have different cofactor requirements for activation they provide for differential function during various cellular events. Germ cells (i.e. eggs and sperm) are highly specialized cells that eventually give rise to a new organism through several developmental transitions, these include: a) The oocyte must become mature as a fertilization-competent egg arrested in meiotic metaphase II of the cell cycle; b) Post fertilization events follow a series of time-dependent changes both at the structural and biochemical level that convert the egg to the zygote, and c) The zygote to the embryo through pivotal developmental transitions. Disruption of these time-dependent changes, likely results in spontaneous abortion or abnormal development. Equally important is the maturation process the sperm undergoes. Sperm cells require first that capacitation and later the acrosome reaction occur before becoming fertilization-competent. If these gametes interact without first undergoing these initial changes, the orchestration of fertilization will not take place. Indeed the egg should be thought of as a cell programmed for death, but rescued by the key developmental transition of fertilization. This chapter examines the involvement of PKC isotypes in oocytes and eggs. The involvement of PKC in sperm development is next considered - followed by examining the involvement of PKC in fertilization and development of the early embryo. The concluding section addresses methods for the study of PKC in eggs/embryos.

## 2. Oocytes and eggs

With the exception of M-phase at which point the spindle apparatus reorganizes from the nucleus, the cell can be thought of as partitioned into nuclear and cytoplasmic compartments. As such, the nuclear envelope provides a physical barrier permitting access of different signaling molecules to these two compartments. At the onset of M-phase the nuclear envelope is disassembled and, accompanied by the disassembly of the interphase array of microtubules and replacement with the meiotic spindle apparatus. Despite the absence of the nuclear envelope in partitioning the cell, differential enzyme substrate specificity can continue to afford unique enzyme action at different cellular locations. Thus, in a sense, it can be thought that the nuclear-cytoplasmic partition remains.

In mammals, oocytes are arrested in the diplotene state of the meiotic cell cycle within the ovary awaiting maturity. At this point in the cell's development the oocyte nucleus, also known as the germinal vesicle, is still present. Rupture of the follicles trigger resumption of meiosis and there is a release of oocytes each surrounded by a few layers of cumulus cells. During this time the oocyte is released from arrest at the diplotene state and progresses to the next cell cycle arrest point, meiotic metaphase II. Briefly, in mammals cumulus cells are responsible for physical support of the developing gamete and maintenance of a so-called microenvironment as reviewed elsewhere (Huang & Wells, 2010).

The presence of cumulus cells surrounding the oocyte can cause problems during experimental analysis, most notably when agonists or antagonists of signal transduction pathways are applied because they are applied externally. When applied in the short term these pharmacological agents necessarily act first on the cumulus cells surrounding the oocyte and then later on the cumulus-enclosed oocyte. Under these conditions the exact concentration of the pharmacological agent within the oocyte is unlikely to be consistent since the membrane-permeate, pharmacological agent must first interact with the "sponge-like" cumulus cells that surround the oocyte before diffusing into the oocyte. In addition, many pharmacological agents are foreign to cellular metabolism and thus any paracrine communication between not only cumulus cells, but also the cumulus cell and the oocyte may be altered. Thus, for investigations employing agents applied to oocytes, it is best to first remove the cumulus cells prior to application of a PKC agonist or antagonist. However, when the natural, unaltered distribution of PKC or some other endogenous component is to be studied, the experiment is benefited by the retention of the cumulus cells, since that is the natural state (Downs et al., 2006).

One such study (Avazeri et al., 2004) shows that all of the conventional PKC isotypes, except for PKCγ, undergo a change from a cytoplasmic to nuclear localization just prior to germinal vesicle breakdown. The investigators also injected antibodies directed against each of the previously mentioned PKC isotypes to block their biological activity. When injected into the nucleus, blocking PKCα and βII had the greatest effect on inhibition of germinal vesicle breakdown, followed by a lesser effect of antibodies to PKCβI and finally antibodies to PKCγ had no effect. Other studies examined a single PKC isotype and confirm the presence of PKCα (Quan et al., 2003), and PKCβI (Denys et al., 2007) in the nucleus prior to germinal vesicle breakdown. One study (Luria et al, 2000) examined PKCα, βI, βII and found all three isotypes present in the cytoplasm of the germinal vesicle stage oocyte which is in agreement with the above studies at the early germinal vesicle stage (Avazeri et al., 2004). The focus of the study by Luria and colleagues (2000) was to apply PMA as an agonist to activate PKCs. This treatment caused resumption of the meiotic cell cycle and consequent disruption of the germinal vesicle. Through biochemical techniques it was shown that PKCδ is localized in the germinal vesicle as well as the cytoplasm when PKC activity is elevated. Later, during meiosis I, PKCδ was shown to be associated with the spindle apparatus (Viveiros et al., 2001, 2003), and that its active form, p-PKCδ, was enriched at the spindle poles and colocalized with both pericentrin and γ-tubulin (Ma et al., 2008).

The fertilization-competent egg arrested at meiotic metaphase II features notable differences in PKC isotypes and their individual localization. Total antibody, that is, antibody that detects both the phosphorylated and unphosphorylated form of the kinase, directed against PKCα, -γ, -δ and –ζ were found not only in the cytoplasm, but also enriched on the spindle apparatus of the fertilization-competent egg (Baluch et al., 2004). The tightness of this PKC binding was assessed by detergent extraction, a process which removes the soluble components of the cell and retains the egg's cytoskeleton and associated proteins. Total PKCζ remained behind in the cytoskeleton after the detergent extraction process; the closeness of this binding was confirmed by FRET analysis between α-tubulin of the meiotic spindle and the PKC isotypes. FRET analysis demonstrated a close molecular proximity not only between α-tubulin and PKCζ, but also between α-tubulin and PKCδ (Baluch et al., 2004, Baluch & Capco, 2008). Other investigations have shown that PKCβ exists in the cytoplasm of the fertilization-competent egg (Raz et al., 1998). In mouse eggs, p-PKCζ is enriched at the ends of the acentrosomal spindle, whereas total PKCζ decorates the length of the spindle apparatus.

Upon fertilization PKCα, -β, and –γ localize to the plasma membrane (Raz et al., 1998; Baluch et al., 2004, Halet et al., 2004). Here these conventional PKCs are poised to become active, as they are in a prime location to interact with their co-factors (i.e. DAG and phospholipids) for activation. Intriguingly, total PKCζ and the phosphorylated form of PKCζ (p- PKCζ) remain associated with the spindle apparatus, from the arrest at meiotic metaphase II through the anaphase II transition. This result suggested that p-PKCζ may play a role in its association with the spindle. In fact, inhibition of p-PKCζ with a specific, membrane-permeate, peptide inhibitor caused inactivation of the isotype and appeared to result in a disruption of the spindle apparatus. Inhibitors that would block most other active isotypes of PKC, but not p-PKCζ, did not result in spindle disassembly.

Evidence exists that also suggests a role for p-PKCδ in spindle stability (Ma et al., 2008) as others have noted p-PKCδ is enriched in the same region of the spindle pole as p-PKCζ in the metaphase egg. A targeted knockdown of PKCδ expression with siRNA disrupts the spindle apparatus and also decreases the expression of pericentrin. However, these data leave open the possibility that the knockdown may have several effects on the egg's spindle apparatus (Ma et al., 2008), as the reduction of pericentrin would provide no sites for p-PKCζ to bind at the poles. This alternative interpretation could explain the disruption of the spindle since p-PKCζ activity is required for spindle stability as previously described (Baluch et al., 2004, 2008). Moreover, both immunopurification and FRET analysis at the spindle poles demonstrates that total and p-PKCζ are in close molecular proximity with γ-tubulin, Par6, and ser9-GSK3β (Baluch & Capco, 2008). The Par6/PKCζ/GSK3β pathway may have a role in microtubule stability (Baluch & Capco, 2008). When GSK3β is active, microtubule networks can be destabilized (Zhou & Snider, 2005). However, when GSK3β is rendered inactive by phosphorylation on serine 9, spindle microtubules are stabilized. Ser9 p-GSK3β and p-PKCζ are localized to the spindle poles and kinetochore regions of the mouse egg and FRET analysis demonstrates their close molecular proximity (Baluch & Capco, 2008). A knockdown of the PKCδ gene in mice using gene targeting strategy shows that mice are viable and fertile, and thus suggests no deleterious effects on the spindle apparatus (Leitges et al., 2001). This may suggest that cells have a "plan-B" to protect the spindle in the event of a complete gene knockout. However, the aim of that study was to investigate vein arteriosclerosis and therefore the spindle was not specifically examined, so it remains unclear if the PKCδ gene knockout triggered any other signaling events to occur regarding the spindle.

## 3. Sperm

Using a combination of biochemical and immunocytochemical methods, Rotem and coworkers (1990) demonstrated that cPKCs are present in sperm in the equatorial segment, the principal piece of the tail and occasionally visualized in the centriole region. Application of staurosporine, 2-amino-4-octadecene-1,3-diol (sphingosine), or 1-(5-isoquinoylinylsulfonyl)-2-methylpiperazine (H7) all older, concentration-dependent PKC inhibitors blocked sperm motility, while application of a phorbol ester, phorbol 12-myristate 13-acetate (PMA) which activates PKC, increased motility.

For sperm to become fertilization competent two separate events must first take place that is, capacitation and subsequently the acrosome reaction. Capacitation is a series of physiological changes in the sperm that typically occur as the sperm traverses the female reproductive tract to reach the egg. During capacitation, there is an efflux of cholesterol from the sperm plasma membrane followed by an increase in the level of intracellular-free calcium, and cAMP levels increase to activate PKA (Breitbart, 2003). Capacitation also induces a rise in free-calcium that itself could lower the requirement for PKC activation even in the absence of increased levels of DAG. However, the calcium-dependent isotype of PLC (PLCγ) is activated by calcium which could also generate DAG by hydrolysis of $PIP_2$, leading to the activation of many of the PKC isotypes (Breitbart, 2003) at the time of capacitation.

Capacitation is accompanied by assembly of an actin network between the outer acrosomal membrane and the overlying sperm plasma membrane. PKC itself or in concert with PLCγ and/or phospholipase D could mediate the formation of this network as both have been shown to be associated with the underlying actin network in this area (Breitbart 2002; Cohen et al., 2004). In order for the acrosome reaction to take place this cortical actin network must subsequently disassemble. Evidence that the disassembly of the actin network is necessary for completion of the acrosome comes from the application of an actin-stabilizing agent such as phalloidin which was shown to inhibit the acrosome reaction (Spungin et al., 1995). The opening of calcium channels is thought to be mediated by the binding of sperm to ligands in the zona pellucidaa and initiates the acrosome reaction (Breitbart 2002). This calcium influx induced by the zona pellucidaa could activate PLC which in turn can produce DAG, all of which are required for PKC activation. Studies on human sperm (Rotem et al., 1992) demonstrated that capacitated sperm could be induced to undergo the acrosome reaction in the absence of intracellular-free calcium via the non-specific PKC agonist, PMA. Both PKCα and -βII were found in a sharp band at the equatorial segment, whereas PKCβI and PKCε were found at the principal piece of the tail (Rotem et al., 1992).

The acrosome reaction is a secretory event in the sperm where the large secretory vesicle effectively a large lysosomal vesicle of the sperm head, the acrosome, vesiculates to release digestive enzymes. This permits the fertilization-competent sperm to burrow its way between cumulus cells to reach the egg zona pellucida. Here, through the use of digestive enzymes and other proteins released from the acrosome, the sperm is able to penetrate the zona pellucida to fuse with the egg plasma membrane. The zona pellucida is a glycoprotein-rich network exterior to the plasma membrane of the egg. The acrosome reaction is dependent on extracellular-free calcium (Yanagimachi & Usui, 1974; Florman et al., 1989); however, utilizing PMA to activate PKC induced the acrosome reaction independent of extracellular-free calcium (Rotem et al. 1992). PMA is not part of normal cellular metabolism and therefore the possibility exists that the calcium-independent acrosome reaction was an artifact. The notion, however, that PKC is involved in the acrosome reaction is supported by application of a diacylglycerol, a natural PKC agonist that also induced the acrosome reaction in the absence of extracellular-free calcium. Moreover, it was speculated that the increase in intracellular-free calcium required during the earlier capacitation event supplied sufficient calcium for the PKC-induced acrosome reaction while inhibitors to PKC blocked this response (O'Toole et al., 1996).

Although progesterone secreting cumulus cells surrounding the mammalian egg have been shown to trigger the acrosome reaction (Garcia & Meizel, 1999), PKC inhibitors block the acrosome in human sperm (O'Toole et al., 1996). In addition, some have shown that components of the egg zona pellucida are responsible for the acrosome reaction, but similarly the older drug inhibitor of PKC, Staurosporine, blocks the acrosome reaction (Liu and Baker, 1997).

It has also been reported that PKC is essential for the maintenance of sea urchin sperm motility, although other kinases such as PKA and tyrosine kinase are present, but not key for motility (White et al., 2007). Intriguingly, this article also reported the presence of PKM, the nonmembrane-bound catalytic subunit of PKC in the sea urchin sperm. PKC is cleaved to form PKM which has different substrate specificity than PKC. Since PKM is not membrane-bound it phosphorylates substrates in the sperm interior. PKM also has been reported in mammalian eggs and has been shown to phosphorylate cytoskeletal substrates in the egg interior as discussed in the fertilization section (Gallicano & Capco 1995). Although activation of PKC in sperm seems to result in similar developmental fates in a diversity of animals, it is not to be considered a universal activator since PKC activation in fowl sperm blocks the acrosome reaction (Ashizawa et al., 2006). Some level of PKC activity also has been implicated in retaining the proper volume in sperm as it traverses fluids of different osmolarity during its passage from the testis to the oviduct (Petrunkina et al., 2007).

## 4. Fertilization

The process of fertilization induces a number of structural and biochemical changes within the egg as the single sperm cell penetrates the egg to subsequently form the zygote. This pivotal developmental transition appears to be dependent on a series of signal transduction events initiated by sperm penetration (Figure 1). Increasing evidence suggest that phospholipase C (PLC) ζ, supplied by the sperm, initiates this developmental transition within the egg (Saunders et al., 2002; Knott et al., 2005; Lee et al., 2006; Swann et al., 2006; Yu et al., 2008). Once PLCζ is within the egg, it then hydrolyzes phosphatidylinositol 4,5-bisphosphate ($PIP_2$) to produce inositol triphosphate ($IP_3$) and DAG. $IP_3$ subsequently diffuses and binds to $IP_3$ receptors to initiate a rise in calcium from sequestered stores in the egg, which potentially initiates calcium oscillations through a calcium-induced activation of PLC or PKC.

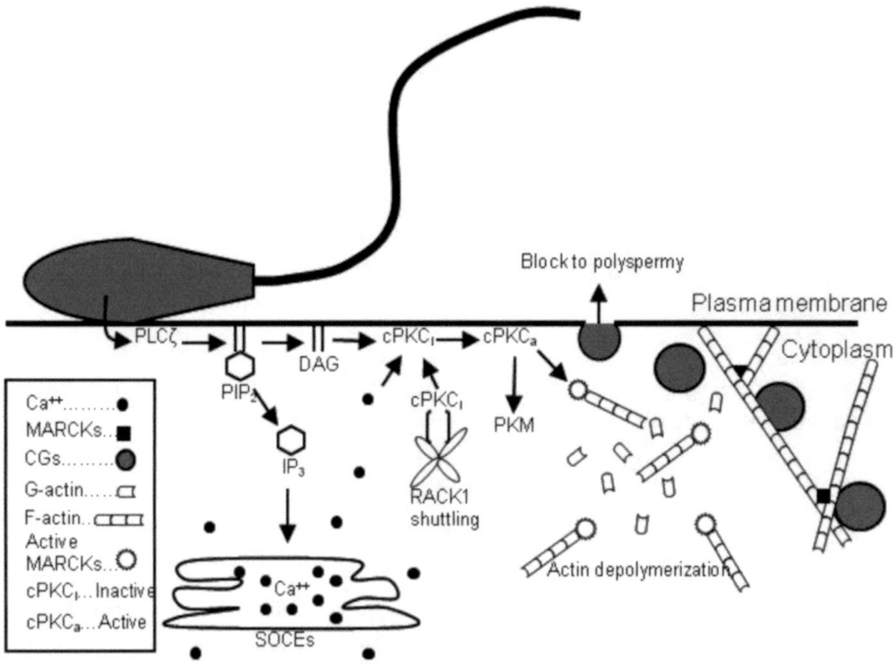


Fig. 1. Diagrammatic representation of PKC signaling events that may be involved in cortical granule exocytosis, the block to polyspermy, and subsequently fertilization.

Intracellular-free calcium along with DAG are essential cofactors for the activation of conventional PKCs. Translocation of the conventional PKC isotypes to the cell cortex indicates activation of the kinase and one study (Halet et al., 2004) has provided strong evidence that the cPKC, PKCα, is translocated to the egg plasma membrane after every calcium oscillation, and functions to induce calcium transients as part of a positive feedback loop that regulates store-operated calcium entry (SOCE). Others have shown the translocation of PKCs to the egg plasma membrane resulting from egg activation (Gallicano et al., 1995; Raz et al., 1998, Baluch et al., 2004; Carbone & Tatone, 2009) however, the investigation by Halet et al. (2004) clearly provided a link to calcium oscillations and shows that PKC has a role in the positive feedback loop that generates the calcium oscillations through SOCE.

After recruitment to the egg plasma membrane, perhaps in part by the proposed shuttling action of RACK1 (Haberman et al., 2010), activated PKCs are poised to phosphorylate MARCKS proteins. MARCKS proteins are substrates for PKC, and MARCKS have the ability to crosslink actin filaments into a network at the cell cortex (Eliyahu et al., 2005, 2006). However, once MARCKS are phosphorylated by PKC the actin network can then disassemble (Tsaadon et al., 2008). Disassembly of the actin network at the egg cortex could release cortical granules from the cortical actin network and allow them to reach the plasma membrane to exocytose (Tsaadon et al., 2008). Once cPKCs are activated, as part of their down regulation, the kinase is cleaved between its membrane-binding domain and catalytic subunit to form PKM (Jaken 1990; Hashimoto et al., 1991). PKM remains active in the cytosol and its altered folding provides for altered substrate specificities. Gallicano et al. (1995) demonstrated that PKM which forms as a consequence of fertilization acts to phosphorylate a specialized intermediate filament network known as cytoskeletal sheets (reviewed by Capco 2001). In addition, through a series of experiments it was also shown to remodel the cytoskeletal interior (Gallicano et al., 1995). The authors first determined that it was indeed PKC acting downstream of calcium responsible for the changes in the cytoskeletal interior by experimentally activating PKC while clamping calcium to low levels. Subsequently the distribution of PKC was mapped over time with the PKC reporter dye Rim-1 and PKC was found at the egg cortex indicating it was activated (Gallicano et al., 1995). Furthermore, it was noticed during a biochemical assay that utilized a monoclonal antibody to the catalytic subunit of PKCα that there was a change in the molecular weight of PKC from 80 to 50 kDa and that the kinase shifted compartments from the detergent-soluble fraction to the detergent-resistant, sheet-enriched fraction indicative of the formation of PKM. A further biochemical assay utilizing inhibitors to PKC, myosin light-chain kinase, and tyrosine kinase could not block the phosphorylation of exogenous substrate while an inhibitor to PKC/PKM blocked phosphorylation (Gallicano et al., 1995). Taken together these results suggest that the membrane-bound PKC downstream of calcium was cleaved forming PKM and that PKM bound to and phosphorylated the internal cytoskeletal elements. For these reasons the cPKCs were proposed to have a chronometer function that acts on the cell spatially and temporally. Through the action of PKC at the membrane the egg first blocks polyspermy by inducing cortical granule exocytosis and later, following each calcium oscillation, acts on substrates within the egg interior through the action of PKM as the egg remodels to form the cytoskeletal framework appropriate for the zygote.

There has been debate as to whether or not PKC acts alone to stimulate cortical granule exocytosis. Some reports suggest that another calcium-dependent kinase known as calcium/calmodulin-dependent protein kinase II (CaMKII) may be involved (Abbott & Ducibella, 2001; Abbott et al., 2001; Madgwick et al., 2005). In a series of experiments, Knott et al. (2006) injected constitutively active CaMKIIα into mouse eggs and it was reported that CaMKII was responsible for meiotic resumption and cortical granule exocytosis. Both PKC and CaMKII have several different isotypes, and the different isotypes have different substrate specifities. The δ subunit of CaMKII was shown to be effective in the resumption of mouse eggs (Johnson et al., 1998), while others have shown cell cycle resumption to be dependent on the γ subunit (Change et al., 2009; Backs et al., 2010). A plausible alternative explanation is upon injection the constitutively active CaMKIIα (Knott et al., 2006) could immediately phosphorylate substrates in the cytoplasm and alter the sequence of events leading to activation. As many others have noted, since the cortical granule block to polyspermy is key for continued development, redundant mechanisms regulating this important event are likely to be in place.

## 5. The early embryo

Various studies can demonstrate that the zygote and preimplantation embryo display a change in cellular localization of several PKC isotypes during postfertilization development. Both PKC ζ and -δ, which were enriched on the spindle apparatus prior to fertilization later appear enriched within the pronuclei at six hours postfertilization, while PKCα and -γ are absent from the pronuclei (Viveros et al. 2003; Baluch et al., 2004). By the two-cell stage PKCα, γ, δ, and ζ are enriched in the nuclei (Viveros et al. 2003; Baluch et al., 2004; Dehghani and Hahnel, 2005). Reports from Pauken and Capco (1999, 2000) have shown a marked reduction in the nuclear localization of these isotypes after the two-cell stage with the exception that PKCζ lines the nuclear periphery at the four-cell stage. However, these isotypes appear in unique locations poised to presumably interact during subsequent developmental transitions: At the time of compaction PKCα, γ, δ, and μ line the cell-cell boundaries to differing extents, and these isotypes are considerably absent from the nucleus (Pauken & Capco, 1999, 2000). During the late eight-cell stage just prior to compaction the ζ isotype is greatly enriched in the nuclei (Pauken & Capco, 2000). Moreover, when PKC was experimentally activated by the natural agonist (DiC8 a diacylglycerol and natural activator of PKC) it induces PKCα to localize at internal cell-cell boundaries. Then β-catenin becomes phosphorylated and accumulates at these internal cell-cell boundaries as the blastomeres begin to flatten out on each other during the process of embryonic compaction (Pauken & Capco, 1999). In addition, it was shown that immediately before compaction begins β-catenin becomes part of the detergent-resistant cytoskeleton at intercellular boundaries indicative of its association with the adherens junctions that are responsible for adhering and subsequently flattening of the blastomeres later during compaction (Pauken & Capco, 1999). Although PKCβI and -βII were not investigated in the aforementioned study, others (Dehghani and Hahnel, 2005) have shown that PKCβI accumulates in the nuclei of embryos at the four-cell stage and later during the postcompaction stage, while PKCβII appears to become uniformly distributed throughout the cytoplasm and nuclei from the four-cell stage until the blastocyst stage.

PKCδ and ε are reported to transiently enrich in nuclei of the four-cell embryo (Dehghani and Hahnel, 2005). In this study investigators blocked both PKCδ and ε with peptides that interfere with adapter sites to block movement of these isotypes, which subsequently altered transcription. This suggests that the location of the isotype may be involved in its activity and that both isotypes have a role in transcription at the four-cell stage.

## 6. Consideration of experimental procedures & methods

### 6.1 Pharmacological agents & PKC

To determine the role of a single type of kinase investigators often employ various pharmacological agents (Table 1).

| Common name | Also known as | Target kinase(s) | $IC_{50}$ |
|---|---|---|---|
| **Inhibitors** | | | |
| Staurosporine | N/A | PKA<br>CaMK<br>MLCK<br>PKC<br>PKG | 7 nM<br>20 nM<br>1.3 nM<br>700 pM<br>8.5 nM |
| Chelerythrine Chloride | N/A | PKC | 660 nM |
| Bisindolylmaleimide | BIM | PKC<br>GSK-3<br>GSK-3β<br>PKA | 10 nM<br>360 nM<br>170 nM<br>2 μM |
| Rottlerin | Mallotoxin | PKCδ/θ<br>PKCα/β/γ<br>PKCε/η/ζ<br>CaMKIII | 3-6 μM<br>30-40 μM<br>80-100 μM<br>5 μM |
| H-7 | 1-(5-Isoquinolinylsulfonyl)-2-methylpiperazine dihydrochloride, Isoquinoline-5-sulfonic 2-methyl-1-piperazide dihydrochloride | PKA<br>PKC | Determine empirically |
| Myristoylated PKCζ Pseudosubstrate | N/A | PKCζ | Determine empirically |
| Myristoylated PKCθ Pseudosubstrate | N/A | PKCθ | Determine empirically |
| Myristoylated PKCη Pseudosubstrate | N/A | PKCη | Determine empirically |
| **Activators** | | | |
| PMA | TPA, phorbol 12-myristate 13-acetate | PKC | Determine empirically |
| OAG | 1-(cis-9-Octadecenoyl)-2-acetyl-sn-glycerol, 2-Acetyl-1-oleoyl-sn-glycerol | PKC | Determine empirically |
| DiC8 | 1,2-Dioctanoyl-*sn*-glycerol | PKC<br>PKC | Determine empirically |

Table 1. A large variety of agonists/antagonists exist for the experimental study of PKC. Some PKC inhibitors have the ability to interact with multiple kinases since the concentration of the drug increases as it accumulates within the cell over time.

While their use is essential, it is important to understand their limitations and design experiments containing the proper controls when conclusions are drawn from their uses. Ideally, a log-fold dose response curve should be conducted prior to experimentation to determine the lowest working concentration to activate/inhibit a single type of kinase of interest. The lowest working concentration should be used in subsequent experiments as many agonists/antagonists have the ability to interact with multiple kinases as the cell continues to absorb the membrane-permeate pharmacological agent over time. Examples include the PKC inhibitors *3-[1-[3-(dimethylamino)propyl]-1H-indol-3-yl]-4-(1H-indol-3-yl)-1H-pyrrole-2,5-dione* (BIM, also referred to as Gö 6850, or GF 10923X), Staurosporin, and Rottlerin, among others. An alternative to pharmacological inhibitors of PKC are membrane–permeant peptide inhibitors, which exist for some of the PKC isotypes and other kinases and have a greater degree of specificity since their peptide sequence is designed to block the active site of the specific kinase. In addition to membrane-permeant peptide inhibitors, it would be wise to employ two structurally and chemically distinct inhibitors to reduce the possibility of misinterpretation of experimental data (Stricker et al., 2010).

It also is wise to adopt natural agonists such as a diacylglycerol (DAG); for instance OAG or DiC8 can be routinely used in parallel when pharmacological agents are employed (Gallicano et al., 1995; Pauken & Capco, 1999; Eliyahu & Shalgi, 2002; Halet et al., 2004). In addition, it is useful to confirm the activity of the PKC isotype. A rapid method to determine whether a kinase is active is to employ an antibody specific to the phosphorylated/active form of the isotype during immunocytochemical or western blot analysis.

Some molecular strategies at the DNA or RNA level have been developed to remove or knockdown a specific PKC isotype. Knockout mice have been developed for PKCα, PKCβ, PKCγ, PKCδ, PKCε, PKCθ, and PKCζ and the effects of gene knockout have been studied (Abeliovich et al., 1993; Leitges et al., 1996, 2001a, 2001b, 2002; Sun et al., 2000; Meier et al., 2007). Care should be taken when interpreting experimental data from these models as PKC operates within many other signaling pathways.

### 6.2 Introduction to the handling and procurement of mouse eggs

There exist several technical challenges concerning the procurement and manipulation of mammalian eggs/embryos. For starters, the mouse egg is about 80 μm in diameter. This small size requires the use of a finely pulled, flame-polished Pasteur pipette attached to a pipetting apparatus; a 1 mL syringe attached to a 24" piece of flexible tubing through which suction can be created for aspiration or expulsion. Under optimal conditions, only 20-40 eggs can be obtained from a single female, and consequently any loss of sample during handling can significantly decrease the amount of material for study. In order to obtain 20-40 eggs/embryos female mice are superovulated by an injection regimen of gonadotropins. An outbred mouse strain CD-1 (Charles River Laboratories) is routinely used in this laboratory and maintained under a 14-hour light/ 10-hour dark schedule and given *ad libitum* access to food and water.

#### 6.2.1 Procedure for the procurement of cumulus-free eggs

1. Pregnant mare serum gonadotropin (PMSG) administration is accomplished by intraperitoneally (i.p.) injection of 5.0 IU PMSG in a 0.1 mL sterile volume of 100 mM Phosphate-buffered saline (PBS) at approximated 3:00 p.m.
2. Approximately 48 hours later, inject sterile human chorionic gonadotropin (5 IU).
3. Approximately 15 hours post-hCG injection, females are euthanized according to the established IUCUC protocol for the given institution.
4. Oviducts are removed by gently cutting away the mesometrium while holding the uterine horn near the oviduct. Remove the fat that allows the ovary to adhere to the

abdominal viscera. Cut between the oviduct and ovary followed by a cut at the top of the uterine horn to remove the oviduct. Place the oviduct in a Petri dish with pre-equilibrated FHM-BSA. All subsequent steps are conducted under a dissection microscope equipped with a stage warmer set to 37°C and fiber-optic lighting. Locate the cumulus mass. Removal of the cumulus mass is accomplished by carefully immobilizing one side of the oviduct with Dumont no. 5 forceps while gently slicing the oviduct on the opposite side with a clean hypodermic needle. If the cumulus mass does not immediately "pop" out of the oviduct, gently tease it out with the blunt side of the needle. Alternatively, a 26 or 30G needle coupled to a syringe filled with medium can be inserted in the ostium and flushed with excess medium to release the cumulus mass from the opposite end of the oviduct.

5. Collect cumulus masses with aid from a fire polished unpulled, 5" glass Pasteur pipette and place in the pre-equilibrated medium FHM-BSA (Millipore, product number MR-024-D) containing 300 μg/mL hyaluronidase and observe to determine when cumulus cells are released.
6. Once denuded, immediately transfer eggs through several drops (approximately 1 mL) of FHM-BSA to wash away any remaining hyaluronidase. Proceed immediately to the next step in the experiment (e.g. treatment with peptide inhibitors or pharmacological agents, immobilization for cytological fixation, or production of a lysate for a biochemical kinase assay, etc.) as spontaneous activation will begin at approximately 9 A.M.

The above procedure details the procurement of cumulus-free mouse eggs for experimental purposes. However, this protocol can be modified to collect fertilized eggs and embryos. To produce fertilized eggs and embryos a male is placed with a female for copulation after hCG injection. The following morning the female is checked for a white copulation (vaginal) plug to indicate that copulation occurred. The day at which the plug is detected is 0.5 days post coitum (dpc), since fertilization is assumed to occur at midnight. Two-cell embryos can be collected at noon 1.5 dpc and four-cell embryos approximately 8-12 hours later. Eight-cell embryos are collected on the morning of 2.5 dpc, while morulas are collected in the evening.

It is most efficient to flush the oviducts with approximately 0.1 mL of FHM-BSA since, beginning at the two-cell stage and beyond, the cumulus cells sloughed off which makes them difficult to locate.

### 6.3 Detergent extraction

The cytoskeleton is the cellular framework composed of actin filaments, intermediate filaments, microtubules and associated protein that regularly reorganize in response to stimuli. Each filament has a subset of signaling proteins responsible for cytoskeletal reorganization. During meiosis, the egg undergoes a remodeling of the cytoskeleton in preparation of the developmental transition of fertilization. If one is interested in studying the cytoskeleton and its associated proteins at a morphological and biochemical level a technique known as detergent extraction can be employed.

Detergent extraction removes the soluble components of the cell through the use of a non-ionic detergent in an intracellular buffer (ICB) that mimics the intracellular milieu. As a result of this process approximately one-third of the egg's total protein is extracted into a cell fraction referred to as the soluble fraction. Two-thirds remains insoluble and constitutes the detergent-resistant, cytoskeletal fraction. This latter fraction (i.e. the cytoskeletal fraction) contains all three filament systems and those proteins that are tightly bound to each cytoskeletal framework. For eggs and embryos the detergent extraction medium is ICB (Aggeler et al., 1983; Webster and McGaughey, 1990) made 1% with Tween-20 and 200 μg/mL with the protease inhibitor 4-(2-Aminoethyl) benzenesulfonyl fluoride hydrochloride (AEBSF). ICB is composed of 100 mM KCl, 5 mM $MgCl_2$, 3 mM EGTA, 20 mM HEPES, (pH 6.8). Tween-20 is the non-ionic detergent used for eggs and embryos as Triton X-100 was shown to remove selective peptides from and destabilize the cytoskeletal network in mammalian eggs and embryos (Gallicano et al., 1991, 1994).

How long does it take to completely detergent extract cells? The answer to this question is dependent on the cell type the investigator employs and should be determined empirically. To determine the proper extraction time the investigator should detergent extract the cells and take aliquots of the medium at increasing time intervals. The protein containing medium can then be analyzed to determine protein concentration and the plateau at which the proteins are no longer rapidly released from cells. The time that corresponds to the establishment of a plateau should then be used in replicate experiments as the extraction end-point and clearly indicated in the methods section of the manuscript.

### 6.3.1 Detergent extraction procedure for eggs/embryos

1. Eggs/embryos are washed through 3 drops of PBS and placed in detergent extraction medium (ICB made 1% with Tween-20 and 200 μg/mL AEBSF).
2. Prepare the soluble-fraction and detergent-resistant cytoskeleton as in the detergent extraction section. For biochemical analysis (i.e. gel electrophoresis), eggs/embryos can be transferred into SDS-sample buffer executing caution not to transfer excess fluid with the cytoskeleton. The detergent-soluble fraction is isolated in a large volume and needs to be concentrated; this is done by precipitating the soluble-fraction in ice-cold 95% ethanol and subsequently incubating it at -20°C overnight. Centrifuge the precipitated soluble fraction into a pellet and decant the supernatant. The pellet containing the soluble-fraction can then be solubilized by the addition of SDS-sample buffer.
3. The fixative is largely dependent on the type of microscopic analysis being conducted. The detergent-resistant cytoskeleton of eggs/embryos is processed for observation by light or electron microscopy. For instance, if immunocytochemistry is the form of analysis, the detergent-extracted specimen is cytologically fixed by the addition of 0.05% glutaraldehyde 2% formaldehyde made in ICB for 5 minutes at room temperature and then transferred to 2% formaldehyde made in ICB for 25 minutes at room temperature. Any remaining free aldehyde groups are inactivated, and sticky sites are mitigated by transferring eggs/embryos through the blocking solution ICB-BSA (ICB made 1% with bovine serum albumin). This treatment allows the specimen to be transferred through antibody-containing solutions to view specific proteins.

## 6.4 Conventional and embedment-free electron microscopy

Conventional, resin-embedded transmission electron microscopy has been utilized by investigators as a powerful tool to interrogate the ultrastructural changes that accompany fertilization (Bement and Capco, 1989; 1991; Gallicano et al., 1991, 1994, 1995). However, mammalian eggs and embryos do not afford high contrast images in resin-embedded, ultrathin sections (silver to gold interference patterns corresponding to 60-70 nm). To mitigate the inherent low-contrast of eggs and embryos the authors routinely employ 0.1% tannic acid during glutaraldehyde fixation. Tannic acid acts as a mordant allowing $OsO_4$ to more effectively bind. Alternatively, *en block* staining in aqueous 2% uranyl acetate prior to dehydration can be used to further improve contrast of the biological material. The aforementioned steps produce marked electron density for resin-embedded ultrathin sections and provide detail unattainable at the level of the light microscope.

Further detail and three-dimensional information is afforded by removing the embedding medium entirely. This requires employing embedding medium that can be removed without damaging the specimen. By implementing the embedment medium, diethylene glycol disterate (DGD, also referred to as Pentament), Capco and coworkers (1984) refined a procedure for the complete removal of the DGD in HeLa and Madin-Darby Canine Kidney cultured cells for its use in transmission and scanning electron microscopy. Removing embedment not only provides high resolution images, but significantly increased electron density in biological material due to the absence of a resin, and also allowed for the use of thick sections (200 nm sections and greater corresponding to purple interference) at the level of the electron microscope. Gallicano and coworkers exploited the use of DGD in detergent extracted mammalian eggs and for the first time novel cytoskeletal elements known as "sheets" were characterized in mammalian eggs (Gallicano et al., 1991).

### 6.4.1 Procedure for embedment-free electron microscopy for use with eggs/embryos

1. Before obtaining eggs/embryos coverslips are prepared by cleaning no. 1 coverglass in a beaker containing acetone by sonication for 3x for 5 minutes each followed by sonication in distilled water for 3x for 5 minutes each. Allow coverslips to dry by placing them on Whatman no. 1 filter paper in a Petri dish protected from dust. Poly-L-lysine (10% w/v) is spread evenly over the surface of the coverslips and placed on a 37°C slide warmer until dry.
2. Obtain eggs/embryos (see Procurement section) and wash through 3 drops of PBS at 37°C.
3. In a glass Petri dish, eggs/embryos are added to prepared coverslips immersed in an excess volume of PBS. The specimens should adhere immediately. If specimens fail to adhere, they are reaspirated washed again and added to a different prepared coverslip. Care should be exercised during manipulation as poly-L-lysine will clog the tip of the micropipette in the event that the tip touches the poly-L-lysine and this is typically followed by a significant loss of sample. Using a disposable, fire polished, 5" glass Pasteur pipette, remove three-fourths total volume of PBS and slowly add copious amounts of extraction buffer. The density of the extraction buffer will displace the PBS. Repeat the controlled addition of extraction buffer 1x. Allow specimens to extract.
4. Remove three-fourths total volume of the extraction buffer and add fresh extraction buffer containing 2% (v/v) glutaraldehye and 1% formaldehyde for 30 minutes at room temperature.
5. Remove three-fourths total volume of the fixation medium for 3x 15 minutes with 100 mM sodium cacodylate.

6. Post fixation occurs by removal of three-fourths total volume of sodium cacodylate wash buffer and the addition of fresh 1% (v/v) $OsO_4$ in sodium cacodylate at 4°C in the dark for 1 hour. Upon completion of secondary fixation specimens are washed 3x for 15 minutes in sodium cacodylate containing no $OsO_4$.
7. Specimens are then dehydrated through a series of increasing ethanol concentrations starting with 10% ethanol. Remove three-fourths volume of sodium cacodylate wash buffer and add 10% ethanol. Repeat 1x and allow 10-15 minutes time for the specimen to equilibrate. This procedure should be repeated for 30, 50, 70, 90, and 100% ethanol. Exchange 100% ethanol 3x for 20 minutes each with 1:1 100% ethanol: 100% *n*-butyl alcohol. After the third change allow the specimens to equilibrate for 30 minutes. Remove three-fourths volume 1:1 100% ethanol: 100% *n*-butyl alcohol, and replace with 100% *n*-butyl alcohol 3x for 20 minutes each change. After the third change allow the specimens to equilibrate for 30 minutes. Place the Petri dish in a 70°C oven for 15 minutes. Pour off the *n*-butyl alcohol and immediately add prewarmed 1:1 100% *n*-butyl alcohol: 100% DGD. Repeat this 3x for 30 minutes each. Pour off 1:1 100% *n*-butyl alcohol: 100% DGD and add fresh DGD 3x for 30 minutes each.
8. Preheat the flat embedding mold (Ted Pella, Inc., Redding CA; product 10505) in an oven. Add molten DGD to each block of a Teflon-coated flat-embedding mold under a heat lamp. Carefully remove eggs/embryos from the poly-L-lysine with the blunt end of a prewarmed needle. Using a prewarmed, fire-polished pulled pipette, immediately transfer eggs/embryos to the embedding mold and allow the wax to solidify at room temperature. It is necessary to add additional DGD as the block begins to cool and contract. Remove blocks carefully once solidified, as they tend to stick if left for extended periods of time.
9. Trim the block face to produce a square. Blocks are sectioned on an ultramicrotome with a knife angle adjusted to10° (Capco et al., 1993). 200 nm sections are collected on formvar-coated, carbon-stabilized grids precoated with poly-L-lysine and subsequently dried overnight in a vacuum desiccator.
10. Removal of the wax is accomplished by placing the formvar-coated, carbon-stabilized grids containing thick sections into excess 100% *n*-butyl alcohol for 1 hour at room temperature in a glass Petri dish. After 1 hour gently swirl the dish containing 100% *n*-butyl alcohol and let sit for an additional 15 minutes. Remove the grids and place into a fresh Petri dish containing the transition fluid 1:1 100% ethanol: 100% *n*-butyl alcohol for 15 minutes. Remove the grdis and place into 100% ethanol for 1 hour. After 1 hour, carefully swirl the 100% ethanol and let sit for an additional 15 minutes.
11. Dry the specimens through the $CO_2$ critical point and immediately view the sample with a conventional transmission electron microscope with an accelerating voltage of 60 kV.

## 7. Conclusion

The 11 isotype family of PKC has been identified within both the sperm and egg during key developmental transitions such as gametogenesis, fertilization, and early development, and this suggests that the PKC family may take on multiple, essential tasks. Differential regulation of individual isotypes can occur in a number of ways, most notably through different cofactor requirements for activation of individual isotypes, differential substrate specificity of individual isotypes, and localization or enrichment of individual iostypes.

These mechanisms likely serve to impart distinction among isotypes regarding the function of the kinase.

Elucidation of the possible involvement of PKC during each developmental transition will be expedited by the use of antibodies and inhibitors specific to individual isotypes. For instance, the use of a pan- (i.e. total) antibody directed against all of the PKC isotypes has been previously studied in great detail in this area, and is therefore counterproductive for use in a manuscript. In addition, care should be employed with the use of older, concentration-dependent PKC inhibitors as the interpretation of the results obtained by the use of these inhibitors can be difficult as these inhibitors can interact with multiple kinases. Furthermore, investigations focusing on localization or enrichment of specific PKC isotypes will likely reveal signaling-mediated changes during developmental transitions. These studies may expose the possible redundancy of specific isotypes, i.e. are there backup mechanisms in place in the event of a complete dysfunction of an individual isotype? Lastly, few have studied the potential role of PKM, the catalytic subunit of cPKCs that was shown to interact in the egg cytoskeletal interior. Studies directed towards PKM may reveal time-dependent changes in the egg interior that have long been ignored.

## 8. References

Abbott, A.L. & Ducibella, T. (2001). Calcium and the control of mammalian cortical granule exocytosis. *Froniers in Bioscencesi*, Vol. 6, No. D, July 2001, pp. 792-806.

Abbott, A.L., Fissore, R.A. & Ducibella, T. (2001). Identification of a translocation deficiency in cortical granule secretion in preovulatory mouse oocytes. *Biology of Reproduction*, Vol. 65, No. 6, December 2001, pp. 1640-1647.

Abeliovich, A., Paylor, R., Chen, C., Kim, J.J., Wehner, J.M. & Tonegawa, S. (1993). PKC$\gamma$ mutant micr exhibit mild deficits in spatial and contextual learning. *Cell*, Vol. 75, No. 7, December 1993, pp. 1263-1271.

Aggeler, J., Takemura, R. & Werb, Z. (1983). High-resolution three-dimensional views of membrane-associated clatherin and cytoskeleton critical-point-dried macrophages. *Journal of Cell Biology*, Vol. 97, No. 5, November 1983, pp. 1452-1458.

Ashizawa, K., Wishart, G.J., Katayama, S., Takano, D., Ranasinghe, A.R., Narumi, K. & Tsuzuki, Y. (2006). Regulation of acrosome reaction of fowl spermatozoa: evidence for the involvement of protein kinase C and protein phosphatase-type 1 and/or -type 2A. *Reproduction*, Vol. 131, No. 6, June 2006, pp. 1017-1024.

Avazeri, N; Courtot, A.M. & Lefevre, B. (2004). Regulation of spontaneous meiosis resumption in mouse oocytes by various conventional PKC isozymes depends on cellular compartmentalization. *Journal of Cell Science*, Vol. 117, No. 21, October 2004, pp. 4969-4978.

Backs, J., Stein, P., Backs, T., Duncan, F.E., Grueter, C.E., McAnally, J., Qi, X., Schultz, R.M. & Olson, E.N. (2010). The $\gamma$ isoform of CaM Kinase II controls mouse egg activation by regulating cell cycle resumption. *Proceedings from the National Academy of Science*, Vol. 107, No. 1, January 2010, pp. 81-86.

Baluch, D.P., Koeneman, B.A., Hatch, K.R., McGaughey, R.W. & Capco, D.G. (2004). PKC isotypes in post-activated and fertilized mouse eggs: association with the meiotic spindle. *Developmental Biology*, Vol. 274, No. 1, October 2004, pp. 45-55.

Baluch, D.P. & Capco, D.G. (2008). GSK3 beta mediates acentromeric spindle stabilization by activated PKC zeta. *Developmental Biology*, Vol. 317 No. 1, May 2008, pp. 46-58.

Bement, W.M. & Capco, D.G. (1989). Activators of protein kinase C triggers cortical granule exocytosis, cortical contraction, and cleavage furrow formation in Xenopus laevis oocytes and eggs. *Journal of Cell Biology*, Vol. 108, No. 3, March 1989, pp. 885-892.

Bement, W.M. & Capco, D.G. (1991). Parallel pathways of cell cycle control during Xenopus egg activation. *Proceedings from the National Academy of Science*, Vol. 88, No. 12, June 1991, pp. 5172-5176.

Breitbart, H. (2002). Intracellular calcium regulation in sperm capacitation and acrosomal reaction. *Mol Cell Endocrinol*, Vol. 187, No. 1-2, February 2002, pp. 139-144.

Breitbart, H. (2003). Signaling pathways in sperm capacitation and acrosome reaction. *Cell Mol Biol*, Vol. 49, No. 3, May 2003, pp. 321-327.

Capco, D.G. (2001). Molecular and biochemical regulation of early mammalian development. *International Review of Cytology*, Vol. 207, 2001, pp. 195-235.

Capco, D.G., Gallicano, G.I., McGaughey, R.W., Downing K.H. & Larabell, C.A. (1993). Cytoskeletal sheets of mammalian eggs and embryos: a lattice-like network of intermediate filaments. *Cell Motility and the Cytoskeleton*, Vol. 24, No. 2, 1993, pp. 85-99.

Capco, D.G., Krochmalnic, G. & Penman, S. (1984). A new method of preparing embedment-free sections for transmission electron microscopy: applications to the cytoskeletal framework and other three-dimensional networks. *Journal of Cell Biology*, Vol. 98, No. 5, May 1984, pp. 1978-1985.

Carbone, M.C. & Tatone, C. (2009). Alterations in protein kinase c signaling activated by a parthenogentic agent in oocytes from reproductively old mice. *Molecular Reproduction and Development*, Vol. 76, No. 2, February 2009, pp. 122-131.

Chang, H-Y., Minahan, K., Merriman, J.A. & Jones, K.T. (2009). Calmodulin-dependent protein kinase gamma 3 (CamKIIγ3) mediates the cell cycle resumption of metaphase II eggs in mouse. *Development*, Vol. 136, No. 24, September 2009, pp. 4077-4081.

Cohen, G., Rubinstein, S., Gur, Y. & Breitbart, H. (2004). Crosstalk between protein kinase A and C regulates phospholipase D and F-actin formation during sperm capacitation. *Developmental Biology*, Vol. 267, No. 1, pp. 230-241.

Dehghani, H. & Hahnel, A.C. (2005). Expression profile of protein kinase C isozymes in preimplantation mouse development. *Reproduction*, Vol. 130, No. 4, October 2005, pp. 441-451.

Dehghani, H., Reith, C. & Hahnel, A.C. (2005). Subcellular localization of protein kinase C delta and epsilon affects transcriptional and post-transcriptional processes in four-cell mouse embryos. *Reproduction*, 130, No. 4, October 2005, pp. 453-465.

Denys, A., Avazeri, N. & Lefevre, B. (2007). The PKC pathway and in particular its beta1 isoform is clearly involved in meiotic arrest maintenance but poorly in FSH-induced meiosis resumption of the mouse cumulus cell enclosed oocyte. *Molecular Reproduction and Development*, Vol. 74, No. 12, December 2007, pp. 1575-1580.

Downs, S.M., Gilles, R., Canderhoef, C., Humpherson, P.G. & Leese, H.J. (2006). Differential response of cumulus cell-enclosed and denuded mouse oocytes in a meiotic induction model system. *Molecular Reporduction and Development*, Vol. 73, No. 3, March 2006, pp. 379-389.

Eliyahu, E. & Shalgi, R. (2002). A role for protein kinase c during rat egg activation. *Biology of Reproduction*, Vol. 67, No. 1, July 2002, pp. 189-195.

Eliyahu, E., Shtraizent, N., Tsaadon, A. & Shalgi, R. (2006). Association between myristoylated alanin-rich C kinase substrate (MARCKS) translocation and cortical granule exocytosis in rat eggs. *Reproduction*, Vol. 131, No. 2, February 2006, pp. 221-231.

Eliyahu, E., Tsaadon, A., Shtraizent, N. & Shalgi, R. (2005). The involvement of protein kinase C and actin filaments in cortical granule exocytosis in the rat. *Reproduction*, Vol. 129, No. 2, February 2005, pp. 161-170.

Florman, H.M., Tombes, R.M., First, N.L. & Babcock, D.F. (1989). An adhesion-associated agonist from the zona pellucida activates G protein-promoted elevations of internal Ca2+ and pH that mediate mammalian sperm acrosomal exocytosis. *Developmental Biology*, Vol. 135, No. 1, September 1989, pp. 133-146.

Gallicano, G.I. & Capco, D.G. (1995). Remodeling of the specialized intermediate filament network in mammalian eggs and embryos during development: regulation by protein kinase C and protein kinase M. *Current Topics in Developmental Biology*, Vol. 31, 1995, pp. 277-320.

Gallicano, G.I., Larabell, C.A., McGaughey, R.W. & Capco, D.G. (1994). Novel cytoskeletal elements in mammalian eggs are composed of a unique arrangement of intermediate filaments. *Mechanisms of Development*. Vol. 45, No. 3, March 1994, pp. 211-226.

Gallicano, G.I., McGaughey, R.W. & Capco, D.G. (1995). Protein kinase M, the cytosolic counterpart of protein kinase C, remodels the internal cytoskeleton of the mammalian egg during activation. *Developmental Biology*, Vol. 167, No. 2, February 1995, pp. 482-501.

Gallicano, G.I., McGaughey, R.W. & Capco, D.G. (1991). The cytoskeleton of the mouse egg and embryo: Reorganization of planar elements. *Cell Motility and Cytoskeleton*, Vol. 18, No. 2, 1991, pp. 143-154.

Garcia, M.A. & Meizel, S. (1999). Progesterone-mediated calcium influx and acrosome reaction of human spermatozoa: pharmacological investigation of T-type calcium channels. *Biology of Reproduction*, Vol. 60, No. 1, January 1999, pp. 102-109.

Haberman, Y., Tsaadon, L., Eliyahu, E. & Shalgi, R., (2010). Receptor for activated c kinase (RACK) and protein kinase c (PKC) in egg activation. *Theriogenology*, Vol. 75, No. 1, January 2011, pp. 80-89.

Hashimoto, E., Takeuch,i F. & Yamamura, H. (1991). Studies on protein kinase C tightly-bound to rat liver plasma membrane and its protease-activated form. *The International Journal of Biochemistry*, Vol. 23, No. 4, 1991, pp. 395-403.

Halet, G., Tunwell, R., Parkinson, S.J. & Carroll, J. (2004). Conventional PKCs regulate the temporal pattern of Ca2+ oscillations at fertilization in mouse eggs. *The Journal of Cell Biology*, Vol. 164, No. 7, March 2004, pp. 1033-1044.

Huang, Z. & Wells, D. (2010). The human oocyte and cumuls cells relationship: new insights from the cumulus cell transcriptome. *Molecular human reproduction*, Vol. 16, No. 10, April 2010, pp. 715-725.

Jaken, S. (1990). Protein kinase C and tumor promoters. *Current opinion in Cell Biology*, Vol. 2, No. 2, April 1990, pp. 192-197.

Johnson, J., Bierle, B.M., Gallicano, G.I. & Capco, DG. (1998). Calcium/calmodulin-dependent protein kinase II and calmodulin: regulators of the meiotic spindle in mouse eggs. *Developmental Biology*, Vol. 204, No. 2, December 1998, pp. 464-477.

Knott, J.G., Gardner, A.J., Madgwick, S., Jones, K.T., Williams, C.J. & Schultz, R.M. (2006). Calmodulin-dependent protein kinase II triggers mouse egg activation and embryo development in the absence of Ca2+ oscillations. *Developmental Biology*, Vol. 296, No. 2, August 2006, pp. 388-395.

Knott, J.G., Kurokawa, M., Fissore, R.A., Schultz, R.M. & Williams, C.J. (2005). Transgenic RNA interference reveals role for mouse sperm phospholipase Czeta in triggering Ca2+ oscillations during fertilization. *Biology of Reproduction*, Vol. 72, No. 4, April 2005, pp. 992-996.

Lee, B., Yoon, S.Y. & Fissore, R.A. (2006). Regulation of fertilization-initiated [Ca2+]i oscillations in mammalian eggs: a multi-pronged approach. *Seminars in Cell & Developmental Biology*, Vol. 17, No. 2, April 2006, pp. 274-284.

Leitges, M., Mayr, M., Braun, U., Mayr, U., Li, C., Pfister, G., Ghaffari-Tabrizi, N., Baier, G., Hu, Y. & Xu, Q. (2001a). Exacerbated vein graft arteriosclerosis in protein kinase Cδ-null mice. *J Clin. Invest.*, Vol. 108, No. 10, November 2001, pp. 1505-1512.

Leitges, M., Plomann, M., Standaert, M.L., Bandyopadhyay, G., Sajan, M.P., Kanoh, Y. & Farese, R.V. (2002). Knockout of PKCα enhances insulin signaling through PI3K. *Molecular Endocrinology*. Vol. 16, No. 4, April 2002, pp. 847-858.

Leitges, M., Sanz, L., Martin, P., Duran, A., Braun, U., Garcia, J.F., Camacho, F., Diaz-Meco, M., Rennert, P.D. & Moscat, J. (2001b). Targeted disruption of the ζPKC gene results in the impairment of the NF-κB pathway. *Molecular Cell*, Vol. 8, No. 4, October 2001, pp. 771-780.

Leitges, M., Schmedt, C., Guinamard, R., Davoust, J., Schaal, S., Stabel, S. & Tarahovsky, A. Immunodeficiency in protein kinase cbeta-deficient mice. *Science*, Vol. 273, No. 5276, August 1996, pp. 788-791.

Liu, D.Y. & Baker, H.W. (1997). Protein kinase C plays an important role in the human zona pellucida-induced acrosome reaction. *Molecular Human Reproduction*, Vol. 3, No. 12, December 1997, pp. 1037-1043.

Luria, A., Tennenbaum, T., Sun, Q.Y., Rubinstein, S. & Breitbart, H. (2000). Differential localization of conventional protein kinase C isoforms during mouse oocyte development. *Biology of Reproduction*, Vol. 62, No. 6, June 2000, pp. 1564-1570.

Madgwick, S., Levasseur, M. & Jones, K.T. (2005). Calmodulin-dependent protein kinase II, and not protein kinase C, is sufficient for triggering cell-cycle resumption in mammalian eggs. *Journal of Cell Science*, Vol. 118, No. 17, August 2005, pp. 3849-3859.

Ma, W., Koch, J.A. & Viveiros, M.M. (2008). Protein kinase C delta (PKCdelta) interacts with microtubule organizing center (MTOC)-associated proteins and participates in meiotic spindle organization. *Developmental Biology*, Vol. 320, No. 2, August 2008, pp. 414-425.

Meier, M., Menne, J. & Haller, H. (2009). Targeting the protein kinase c family in diabetic kidney: lessons from analysis of mutant mice. *Diabetologia*, Vol. 52, No. 5, May 2009, pp. 765-775.

Meier, M., Menne, J., Holtz, M., Gueler, F., Kirsch, T., Schiffer, M., Mengel, M., Lindschau, C., Leitges, M. & Haller, H. (2007). Deletion of protein kinase c-epsilon signaling pathway induces glomerulosclerosis and tubelointerstitial fibrosis in vivo. *Journal of the American Society of Nephrology*, Vol. 18, No. 4, April 2007, pp. 1190-1198.

Odeon, M.M., Salatino, A.E., Rodriguez, C.B., Scolari, M.J. & Acosta, G.B. (2010). The response to postnatal stress: amino acids transporters and PKC activity. *Neurochem. Research*, Vol. 35, No. 7, July 2010, pp. 967-975.

O'Toole, C.M., Roldan, E.R. & Fraser, L.R. (1996). Protein kinase C activation during progesterone-stimulated acrosomal exocytosis in human spermatozoa. *Molecular Human Reproduction*, Vol. 2, No. 12, December 1996, pp. 921-927.

Pauken, C.M. & Capco, D.G. (1999). Regulation of cell adhesion during embryonic compaction of mammalian embryos: roles for PKC and beta-catenin. *Molecular Reproduction and Development*, Vol. 54, No. 2, October 1999, pp. 135-144.

Pauken, C.M. & Capco, D.G. (2000). The expression and stage-specific localization of protein kinase C isotypes during mouse preimplantation development. *Developmental Biology*, Vol. 223, No. 2, July 2000, pp. 411-421.

Petrunkina, A.M., Harrison, R.A., Tsolova, M., Jebe, E. & Topfer-Petersen, E. (2007). Signalling pathways involved in the control of sperm cell volume. *Reproduction*, Vol. 133, No. 1, January 2007, pp. 61-73.

Quan, H.M., Fan, H.Y., Meng, X.Q., Huo, L.J., Chen, D.Y., Schatten, H., Yang ,P.M. & Sun, Q.Y. (2003). Effects of PKC activation on the meiotic maturation, fertilization and early embryonic development of mouse oocytes. *Zygote*, Vol. 11, No. 4, November 2003, pp. 329-337.

Raz, T., Ben-Yose,f D. & Shalgi, R. (1998). Segregation of the pathways leading to cortical reaction and cell cycle activation in the rat egg. *Biology of Reproduction*, Vol. 58, No. 1, January 1998, pp. 94-102.

Rotem, R., Paz, G.F., Homonnai, Z.T., Kalina, M., Lax, J., Breitbart, H. & Naor, Z. (1992). Ca(2+)-independent induction of acrosome reaction by protein kinase C in human sperm. *Endocrinology*, Vol. 131, No. 5, November 1992, pp. 2235-2243.

Rotem, R., Paz, G.F., Homonnai, Z.T., Kalina, M. & Noar, Z. (1990). Protein kinase c is present in human sperm: possible role in flagellar motility. *Proceedings from the National Academy of Science*, Vol. 87, No. 18, September 1990, pp. 7305-7308.

Saunders, C.M., Larman, M.G., Parrington, J., Cox, L.J., Royse, J., Blayney, L.M., Swann, K. & Lai, F.A. (2002). PLC zeta: a sperm-specific trigger of Ca(2+) oscillations in eggs and embryo development. *Development*, Vol. 129, No. 15, August 2002, pp. 3533-3544.

Sun, Z., A, C.W., Ellmeier, W., Schaeffer, E.M., Sunshine, M.J., Gandhi, L., Annes, J., Petrzilka, D., Kupfer, A., Schwartzberg, P.L. & Littman, D.R. (2000). PKC-θ is required for TCR-induced NF-κB activation in mature but not immature T lymphocytes. *Nature*, Vol. 404, No. 6776, March 2000, pp. 402-407.

Spungin, B., Margalit, I. & Breitbart, H. (1995). Sperm exocytosis reconstructed in a cell-free system: evidence for the involvement of phospholipase C and actin filaments in membrane fusion. *Journal of Cell Science*, Vol. 108, No. 6, pp. 2525-2535.

Stricker, S., Escalona, J., Abernathy, S. & Marquardt, A. (2010) Pharmacological analysis of protein kinases regulating egg maturation in marine nemertean worms: A review and comparison with mammalian eggs. *Marine Drugs*, Vol. 2010, No. 8, August 2010, pp. 2417-2434, 1660-3397

Steinberg, S.F. (2008). Structural basis of protein kinase c isoform function. *Physiological Reviews*, Vol. 88, No. 4, October 2008, pp. 1341-1378.

Swann, K., Saunders, C.M., Rogers, N.T. & Lai, F.A. (2006). PLCzeta(zeta): a sperm protein that triggers Ca2+ oscillations and egg activation in mammals. *Seminars in Cell & Developmental Biology*, Vol. 17, No. 2, April 2006, pp. 264-273.

Tsaadon, L., Kaplan-Kraicer, R. & Shalgi, R. (2008). Myristoylated alanine-rich C kinase substrate, but not Ca2+/calmodulin-dependent protein kinase II, is the mediator in cortical granules exocytosis. *Reproduction*, Vol. 135, No. 5, May 2008, pp. 613-624.

Viveiros, M.M., Hirao, Y. & Eppig, J.J. (2001). Evidence that protein kinase C (PKC) participates in the meiosis I to meiosis II transition in mouse oocytes. *Developmental Biology*, Vol. 235, No. 2, July 2001, pp. 330-342.

Viveiros, M.M., O'Brien, M., Wigglesworth, K. & Eppig, J.J. (2003). Characterization of protein kinase C-delta in mouse oocytes throughout meiotic maturation and following egg activation. *Biology of Reproduction*, Vol. 69, No. 5, November 2003, pp. 1494-1499.

Webster, S.D. & McGaughey, R.W. (1990). The cortical cytoskeleton and its role in sperm penetration of the mammalian egg. *Developmental Biology*, Vol. 142, No. 1, November 1990, pp. 61-67.

White D., de Lamirande, E. & Gagnon, C. (2007). Protein kinase C is an important signaling mediator associated with motility of intact sea urchin spermatozoa. *J Exp Biol*, Vol. 210, No. 22, November 2007, pp. 4053-4064.

Xiao, J., Lui, C., Hou, J., Cui, C., Wu, C., Fan, H., Sun, X., Meng, J., Yang, F., Wang, E. & Yu, B. (2011). $Ser^{149}$ is another potential PKA phosphorylation target of Cdc25B in $G_2$/M transition of fertilized mouse eggs. *The Journal of Biological Chemistry*, Vol. 286, No. 12, January 2011, pp. 10356-10366.

Yanagimachi, R. & Usui, N. (1974). Calcium dependence of the acrosome reaction and activation of guinea pig spermatozoa. *Experimental Cell Research*, Vol. 89, No. 1, November 1974, pp. 161-174.

Yu, Y., Halet, G, Lai, F.A. & Swann, K. (2008). Regulation of diacylglycerol production and protein kinase C stimulation during sperm- and PLCzeta-mediated mouse egg activation. *Biol Cell*, Vol. 100, No. 11, November 2008, pp. 633-643.

Yu, B.Z., Zheng, J., Yu, A.M., Shi, W.Y., Liu, Y., Wu, D.D., Fu, W. & Yang, J. (2004). Effects of protin kinase c on M-phase promoting factor in early development of fertilized mouse eggs. *Cell Biochem. Funct*, Vol. 22, No. 5, September 2004, pp. 291-298.

Zhou, F.Q. & Snider, W.D. (2005). GSK-3beta and microtubule assembly in axons. *Science*, Vol. 308, No. 5719, April 2005, pp. 211-214.

# 11

# Role of Bcl2l10 in Regulation of Meiotic Cell Cycle in the Mouse Oocyte

Kyung-Ah Lee[1], Se-Jin Yoon[2], Eun-Young Kim[1], Jeehyeon Bae[3], Hyun-Seo Lee[1], Su-Yeon Lee[1] and Eun-Ah Kim[1]
[1]*Department of Biomedical Science, College of Life Science, CHA University,*
[2]*Department of Genetics, Stanford University,*
[3]*Department of Pharmacy, College of Pharmacy, CHA University,*
[1,3]*Korea*
[2]*USA*

## 1. Introduction

Bcl2l10, also known as Diva or Boo, is a member of the Bcl2 family. This factor is known to have opposing apoptotic functions in various tissues. That is, it can act as either a pro-apoptotic or an anti-apoptotic factor depending on the cellular milieu (Ke et al., 2001; Lee et al., 2001).

The pro-apoptotic factor Bad is expressed in various tissues including rat ovaries and testes (Kaipia et al., 1997). Bok, anti-apoptotic factor, has been detected in granulosa cells as well as in several reproductive tissues such as the ovaries, testes, and uterus (Hsu et al., 1997). Several anti-apoptotic Bcl2 homologs are expressed in the ovary. Mcl1, Bcl2, Bcl2l1 (Bcl-x), and other Bcl2 family members have also been detected in ovarian tissues (Hsu et al., 1997; Hsu and Hsueh, 2000; Kim and Tilly, 2004; Tilly et al., 1995). However, the expression patterns of these Bcl2 family members are quite different from those of Bcl2l10, which exhibits ovary- and oocyte-specific expression. Murine Bcl2l10 was first identified in expressed sequence tag clones from unfertilized, fertilized, and two-cell-stage mouse eggs (Inohara et al., 1998). Expression of this factor is restricted to the ovary and testis in adult mice (Inohara et al., 1998).

## 2. Expression of Bcl2l10 in the ovary

In a previous study, we used the annealing control primer-PCR method to investigate differentially expressed genes in the mouse oocytes. Using this approach, we found that Bcl2l10 was highly expressed in oocytes (Yoon et al., 2005). We confirmed that Bcl2l10 is constantly expressed in oocytes during oocyte maturation and found that its expression disappeared after the four-cell stage (Figure 1).

Since Bcl2l10 is a member of Bcl2 family, we first evaluated the relationship between Bcl2l10 expression and apoptosis in the ovary. Surprisingly, Bcl2l10 expression did not appear to be related to granulosa cell apoptosis in ovarian follicles (Figure 2). Analysis of serial ovarian sections using immunohistochemical labeling for Bcl2l10 and TUNEL assay revealed that BCL2L10 expression is oocyte-specific but that this expression is mismatched with the apoptotic death of follicular granulosa cells. Therefore, Bcl2l10 may have a function that is not related to the regulation of apoptosis in oocytes.

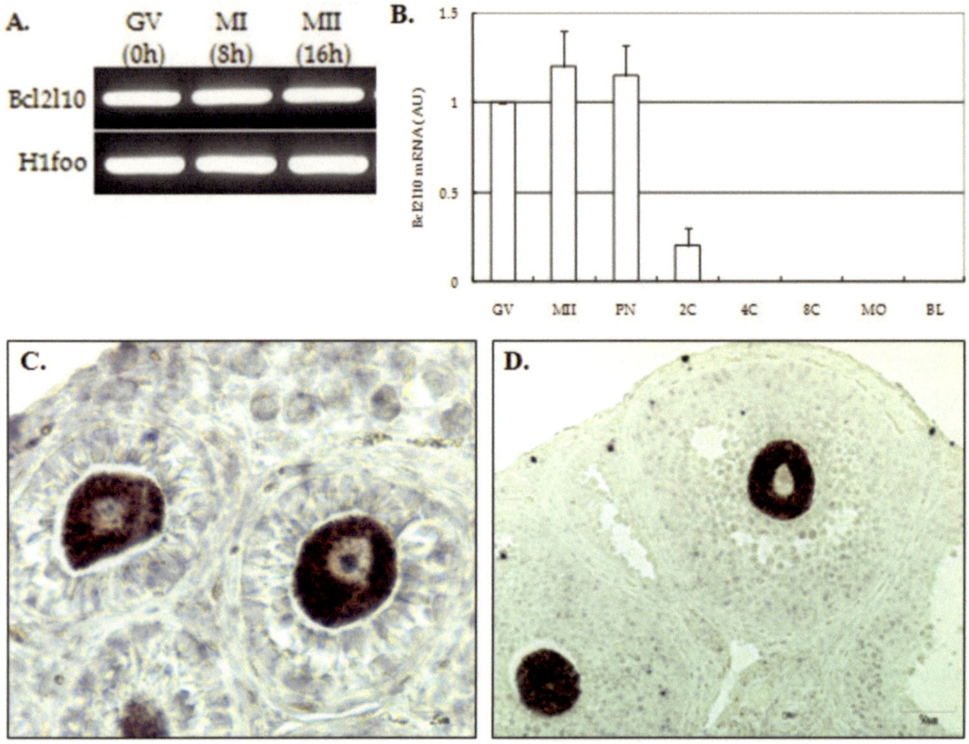


Fig. 1. Expression of Bcl2l10 mRNA in oocytes and preimplantational embryos. A) Semiquantitative RT-PCR analysis of Bcl2l10 expression during spontaneous oocyte maturation *in vitro*. GV, germinal vesicle-stage oocytes; MI, meiosis I oocytes collected after 8 h of culture; MII, meiosis II-stage oocytes collected after 16 h of in culture. B) Quantitative real-time RT-PCR of Bcl2l10 mRNA in oocytes and embryos. Messenger RNA isolated from oocytes and at various embryonic stages was reverse transcribed. For PCR, the cDNA from a single oocyte or an embryo equivalent served as a template for amplification. The expression level was calculated from the cycle threshold values (CT) based on the fluorescence detected within the geometric region of the semi-log plot, and the mRNA ratio (arbitrary units) was calculated with respect to that of GV oocytes. Experiments were repeated at least three times, and data are expressed as the mean ± SEM. PN, pronucleus one-cell zygote; 2C, two-cell; 4C, four-cell; 8C, eight-cell; MO, morula; BL, blastocyst-stage embryo. C, D) *In situ* hybridization of Bcl2l10 mRNA. Mouse ovaries of 2-week-old (C) and 4-week-old (D) were used, and we observed the oocyte-specific Bcl2l10 mRNA expression. Scale bars represent 25 □m and 50□m for C and D, respectively (C, D cited in Yoon et al., 2006, *Korean J Fertil Steril*).

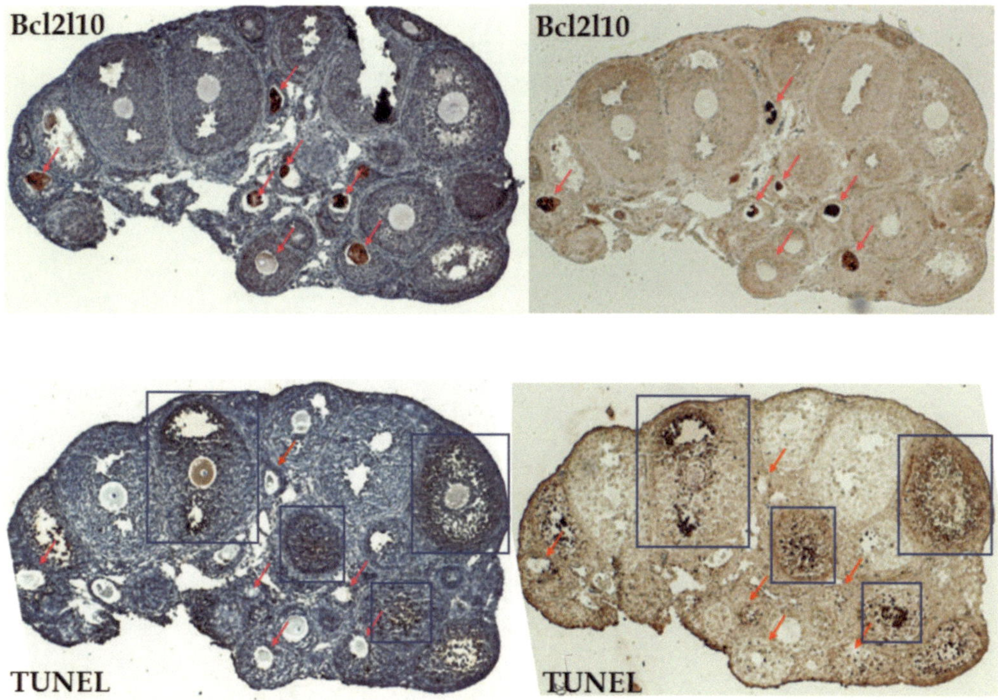


Fig. 2. BCL2L10 immunohistochemical labeling and TUNEL assay in serial sections. Tissue sections were obtained from 4-week mouse ovaries. Arrows indicate peculiar BCL2L10 expression in oocytes of preantral follicles, while boxes indicate apoptotic follicles with TUNEL-positive granulosa cells.

## 3. Bcl2l10 binding proteins

Next, we tried to identify the working partner(s) of Bcl2l10 using immunoprecipitation followed by mass spectrometry (Yoon et al., 2006). We transiently expressed FLAG-Bcl2l10 in NIH/3T3 cells and purified Bcl2l10-associated proteins (Figure 3). Specifically detected 14 bands were excised in the Coomassie Blue-stained 12% SDS-PAGE gels and identified using LC/MS/MS analysis. The protein band specific for Diva was identified as Bcl2-like 10 in the size of 21 kDa (Fig. 3, gel slice number 2) suggesting a successful IP analysis using monoclonal anti-FLAG antibody. List of potential Bcl2l10-binding partners is summarized in Table 1. Interestingly, many of the identified Bcl2l10-associated proteins are known to be associated with the cytoskeletal system. The identification of actin-related proteins such as actin, α-actinin, gelsolin, myosin, tropomyosin, and tropomodulin 3 as Diva-binding proteins suggests that Diva protein associates with the components of actin filaments. Actin was the most abundant Diva-associated protein as shown in Figure 3 (gel slice number 6). All these proteins, with the exception of actin, are known to bind actin to form, stabilize, and cross-linking the microfilaments.

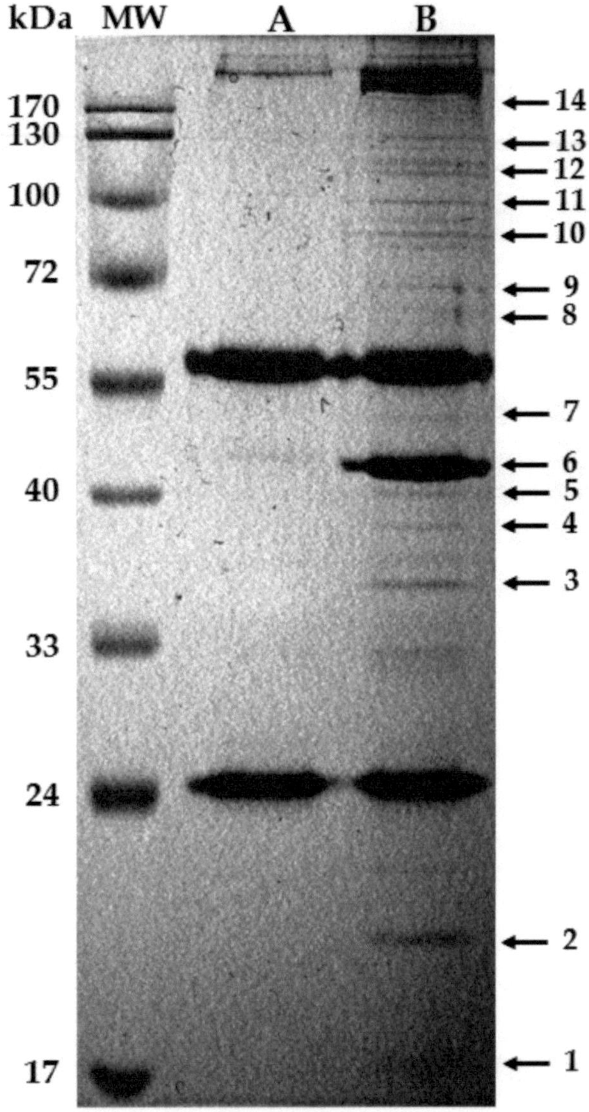


Fig. 3. Identification of BCL2L10-associated proteins. NIH/3T3 cells were transiently transfected for 24 h with empty vector or FLAG-BCL2L10-expressing vector. Total protein extracts were incubated with anti-FLAG-agarose beads. Anti-FLAG-agarose elutes from an equivalent amount of transfected cells (500 µg) were analyzed by 12% SDS polyacrylamide gel electrophoresis, and proteins were visualized by Coomassie Blue staining. The positions and relative molecular masses in kilodaltons (kDa) of protein size markers are indicated on the left. Protein-containing bands, as indicated by numbers on the right, were excised, and proteins present in gel slices were identified by mass spectrometry. MW, protein size markers; A) NIH/3T3, anti-FLAG-agarose elutes from NIH/3T3 cells transfected with pCMV-FLAG empty vector; B) FLAG-BCL2L10, NIH/3T3 cells transfected with pCMV-FLAG-BCL2L10 vector (Yoon et al., 2006).

| Gel slice number | Accession No. | Score | Description | Unigene |
|---|---|---|---|---|
| 1 | gi_16307437 | 95 | RIKEN cDNA 2900073G15 | 2900073G15Rik |
| 2 | gi_30851239 | 69 | Bcl2l10 | Bcl2l10 |
| 3 | gi_1351289 | 69 | Tropomyosin 1 alpha chain (alpha-tropomyosin) | Tpm1 |
| 4 | gi_19353393 | 79 | Tpm2 protein; Tropomyosin 2, beta | Tpm2 |
| 5 | gi_52139168 | 90 | Tropomodulin 3 | Tmod3 |
| 6 | gi_49868 | 109 | Beta-actin (aa 27-375); Actin, beta, cytoplasmic | Actb |
| 7 | gi_80478706 | 45 | ARP3 actin-related protein 3 homolog (yeast) | Actr3 |
| 8 | gi_194362 | 123 | Igh-4 protein | Igh-4 |
| 9 | gi_27369615 | 29 | PIF1 homolo: Expressed sequence AI449441 | AI449441 |
| 10 | gi_34871482 | 34 | PREDICTED: similar to Transcription initiation factor | Taf6 |
| 11 | gi_90508 | 39 | Gelsolin, cytosolic | Gsn |
| 12 | gi_61097906 | 35 | Actinin, alpha 1 | Actn1 |
| 13 | gi_47847434 | 42 | mFLJ00150 protein: Centrosomal protein 110 | Cep110 |
| 14 | gi_17978023 | 80 | Myosin, heavy polypeptide 9, non-muscle | Myh9 |

Table 1. Bcl2l10-associated proteins identified by immunoprecipitation and mass spectrometry.

Immunoprecipitation/Western blot analysis of ovarian tissue homogenates confirmed the association of actin and tropomyosin with Bcl2110 (Figure 4). These findings suggest that, in the ovary, Bcl2l10 plays roles unrelated to apoptosis and instead participates in the regulation of cytoskeletal systems. During meiosis, actin filaments have roles in migration of chromosomes, segregation of homologous chromosomes, development and maintenance of the cortex, formation of polarity, movement of peripheral cortical granules, and extrusion of the first polar body (Sun and Schatten, 2006).

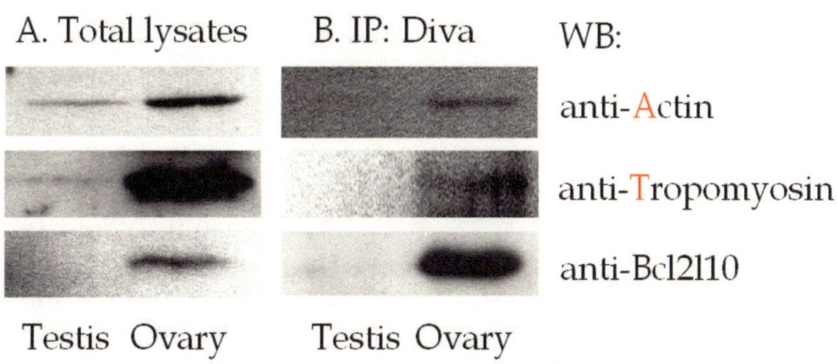


Fig. 4. Identification of BCL2L10-associated proteins using immunoprecipitation (IP)/Western blot analysis (WB). A) WB analysis. Total protein lysates (20 µg) from mouse testes and ovaries were electrophoresed and probed with anti-actin, anti-tropomyosin, or anti-BCL2L10 antibody. Testes lysates served as a negative control for BCL2L10 protein expression. B) IP/WB analysis. Total protein lysates from testes and ovaries (500 µg) were subjected to IP using anti-Bcl2l10 antibody. Anti-BCL2L10-agarose elutes were then electrophoresed and probed with anti-actin, anti-tropomyosin, or anti-BCL2L10 antibody to confirm of the association of actin and tropomyosin with BCL2L10 (as cited in Yoon et al., 2006, *Korean J Fertil Steril*).

A non-apoptotic function of Bcl2l10 has also been demonstrated. Specifically, Bcl2l10 plays a role in Huntington-interacting protein 1-related (HIP1R) protein-mediated endocytosis as well as in the regulation of actin machinery in 293T cells. HIP1R regulates clathrin-mediated endocytotic apparatus and actin assembly. An interaction between endogenous BCL2L10 and HIP1R has been shown by immunoprecipitation and Far-Western analysis (Kim et al., 2009).

## 4. Function of Bcl2l10 in oocytes

We have investigated the role of Bcl2l10 not only in the ovary, but also in oocytes. RNA interference (RNAi) was used for this purpose. To determine the role of Bcl2l10 during oocyte maturation, we microinjected *in vitro* transcribed dsRNA for Bcl2l10 into the cytoplasm of germinal vesicle-stage (GV) oocytes and monitored *in vitro* oocyte maturation. Bcl2l10 RNAi selectively reduced levels of endogenous Bcl2l10 and resulted in incomplete meiosis that was arrested in meiosis I (MI) (Yoon et al., 2009). MI-arrested oocytes had abnormalities in the spindles and chromosomes. The most prominent changes were the disappearance of spindles and aggregation of chromosomes (Figure 5).

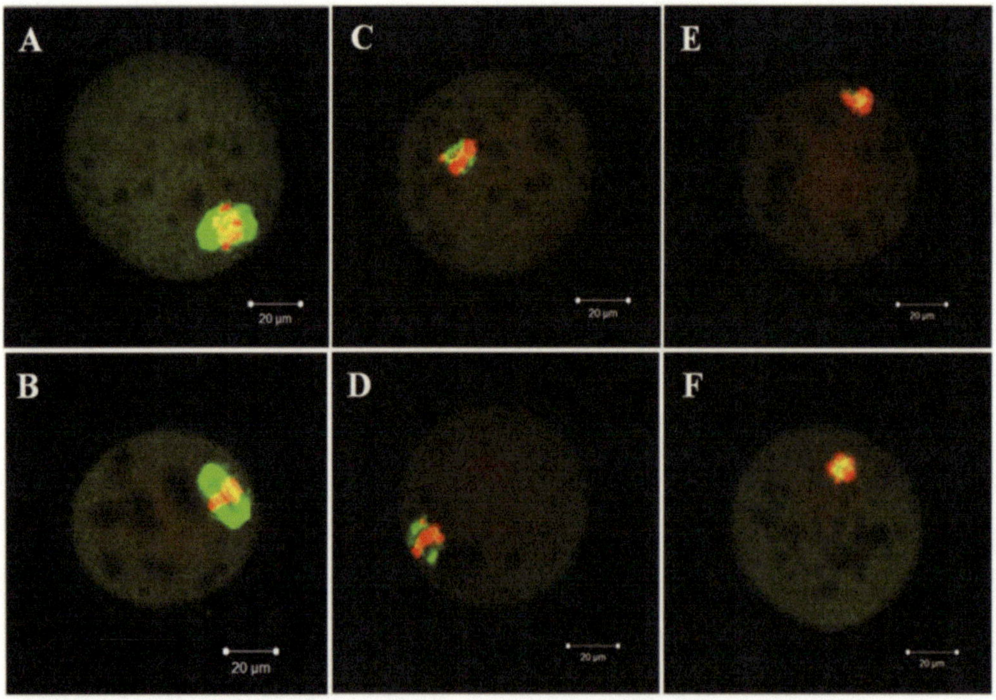


Fig. 5. Bcl2l10 RNAi-induced abnormalities in oocytes, as seen by α-tubulin immunofluorescent staining and chromosomal staining. Germinal vesicle oocytes were injected with Bcl2l10 dsRNA and cultured for 16 h. Oocytes were then fixed in 4% paraformaldehyde and stained with an α-tubulin antibody (green). Chromosome material was counterstained with propidium iodide (red). A) Control, uninjected oocyte. B) Buffer-injected control oocyte. C-F) Bcl2l10 dsRNA-injected oocytes arrested in meiosis I (as cited in Yoon et al., 2010, From Biol Reprod). Bars represent 20 μm.

## 5. Genes downstream of Bcl2l10

After discovering that Bcl2l10 RNAi induced changes in spindles and chromosomes, we set out to identify the network of factors acting downstream of Bcl2l10 in oocytes so that we could better understand the regulatory mechanisms underlying meiosis in oocytes. To identify downstream genes, we conducted microarray analysis of Bcl2l10 RNAi-induced changes in gene expression in mouse oocytes (Kim et al., 2011).

Due to the small amounts of initial total RNA obtained from the 350 oocytes, we performed an amplifying two-cycle target labeling assay so that we could obtain sufficient amounts of labeled cRNA target for microarray analysis. The labeled cRNA was hybridized to the Affymetrix GeneChip Mouse Genome 430 2.0 Array, which covers transcripts and variants from 34,000 well-characterized mouse genes.

Bcl2l10 RNAi induced a more than 2-fold up-regulation of 644 genes and down-regulation of 1,166 genes. Notably, the top 20 up-regulated genes included five enzymes (*i.e.*, pyrophosphate synthase, N-methyltransferase, and three kinases). The top 20 down-regulated genes were related to cytoskeletal organization (Table 2). These genes encoded proteins such as Tpx2, Cep192, Kir20b, Myo6, and Cd2ap. Tpx2 functions in spindle assembly, Cep192 in microtubule nucleation, Kir20b in microtubule-based movement, Myo6 in physical interactions, and Cd2ap in actin polymerization.

| Genes | Gene title | Fold change |
|---|---|---|
| Tpx2 | TPX2, microtubule-associated protein homolog (*Xenopus laevis*) | - 16.1 |
| Rbm12b | RNA binding motif protein 12B | - 15.3 |
| Ptp4a1 | protein tyrosine phosphatase 4a1-like | - 14.6 |
| Ranbp2 | RAN binding protein 2 | - 10.1 |
| Eea1 | early endosome antigen 1 | - 9.3 |
| Arid4a | AT rich interactive domain 4A (RBP1-like) | - 9.1 |
| Cep192 | centrosomal protein 192 | - 8.2 |
| Kif20b | kinesin family member 20B | - 7.9 |
| Psip1 | PC4 and SFRS1 interacting protein 1 | - 7.8 |
| Atad2b | ATPase family, AAA domain containing 2B | - 7.5 |
| Mki67 | antigen identified by monoclonal antibody Ki 67 | - 7.4 |
| Nexn | nexilin | - 7.2 |
| Eif4g3 | eukaryotic translation initiation factor 4 gamma, 3 | - 6.9 |
| Ccnb3 | cyclin B3 | - 6.9 |
| C430048L16Rik | RIKEN cDNA C430048L16 gene | - 6.8 |
| Cenpm | centromere protein M | - 6.8 |
| Leo1 | Leo1, Paf1/RNA polymerase II complex component | - 6.7 |
| Myo6 | myosin VI | - 6.6 |
| Tnfaip8 | tumor necrosis factor, alpha-induced protein 8 | - 6.6 |
| Cd2ap | CD2-associated protein | - 6.5 |

Table 2. Top 20 genes down-regulated more than 2-fold by Bcl2l10 RNAi.

Tpx2 was found to be down-regulated by 16.1-fold and Cep192 by 8.2-fold. The functions of these proteins are intimately related. Interfering with TPX2 function in HeLa cells causes defects in microtubule organization during mitosis, and Tpx2 RNAi produces abnormalities in spindle formation (Gruss et al., 2002). Tpx2, a microtubule-binding protein, and Cep192, a centromere protein, are well-known cofactors of Aurora A kinase. Both proteins act to control the activity and localization of this kinase (Joukov et al., 2011). Eukaryotes have one to three members of the Aurora family of serine-threonine kinases. Aurora A is an important oncogenic kinase that has well-established roles in spindle assembly (Xu et al., 2011). During mitosis, a fraction of Aurora A binds Tpx2, activates the kinase, and targets it to spindle microtubules (Eyers et al., 2003, Kufer et al., 2002, Ozlu et al., 2005, Tsai et al., 2003). Tpx2 controls localization of Aurora A at centrosomes, whereas Cep192 controls its activity in microtubules (Joukov et al., 2010).

Our finding that Bcl2l10 RNAi induced concurrent down-regulation of Tpx2 and Cep192 leads us to conclude that Bcl2l10 may have important roles in regulating oocyte meiosis through its ability to act as an upstream regulator of Tpx2 and Cep192. Association between Bcl2l10 and Aurora kinase A is an interesting new area that warrants further investigation.

## 6. Conclusion

We have identified Bcl2l10 expression in oocytes and uncovered a role for this factor in regulating meiosis. Our findings point to new non-apoptotic function for this Bcl2 family member and open a challenging new area of research on Bcl2l10 regulation of meiosis through Bcl2l10 involvement in spindle assembly. We propose that Bcl2l10 is an important regulator of meiotic spindle formation and works closely with Tpx2, Cep192, and Aurora A kinase. The molecular mechanisms underlying meiotic regulation by Bcl2l10 and its downstream genes (Tpx2 and Cep192) as well as the relationship between Bcl2l10 and Aurora A kinase are currently under careful investigation.

## 7. Acknowledgment

This research was supported by the Basic Science Research Program through the National Research Foundation of Korea (NRF) funded by the Ministry of Education, Science, and Technology (20100022600 and 2009-0068363), by the Priority Research Centers Program through the NRF of Korea funded by the Ministry of Education, Science and Technology (2009-0093821), and by a Korea Research Foundation Grant funded by the Korean Government (KRF-2008-314-E00120).

## 8. References

Eyers PA, Erikson E, Chen LG & Maller JL. (2003). A novel mechanism for activation of the protein kinase Aurora A. *Current Biology*, 13, 8, pp.691-697, ISSN 0960-9822

Gruss OJ, Wittmann M, Yokoyama H, Pepperkok R, Kufer T, Sillje H, Karsenti E, Mattaj IW & Vernos I. (2002). Chromosome-induced microtubule assembly mediated by TPX2 is required for spindle formation in HeLa cells. *Nature Cell Biology*, 4, 11, pp.871-879, ISSN 1465-7392

Hsu SY & Hsueh AJ. (2000). Tissue-specific Bcl-2 protein partners in apoptosis: an ovarian paradigm. *Physiological Reviews*, 80, 2, pp.593–614, ISSN 0031-9333

Hsu SY, Kaipia A, McGee E, Lomeli M & Hsueh AJ. (1997). Bok is a pro-apoptotic Bcl-2 protein with restricted expression in reproductive tissues and heterodimerizes with selective anti-apoptotic Bcl-2 family members. *Proceedings of the National Academy of Sciences of the United States of America*, 94, 23, pp.12401-12406, ISSN 0027-8424

Inohara N, Gourley TS, Carrio R, Muniz M, Merino J, Garcia I, Koseki T, Hu Y, Chen S & Nunez G. (1998). Diva, a Bcl-2 homologue that binds directly to Apaf-1 and induces BH3-independent cell death. *Journal of Biological Chemistry*, 273, 49, pp.32479-32486, ISSN 0021-9258

Joukov V, De Nicolo A, Rodriguez A & Walter JC. Livingston DM. (2010). Centrosomal protein of 192 kDa (Cep192) promotes centrosome-driven spindle assembly by engaging in organelle-specific Aurora A activation. *Proceedings of the National Academy of Sciences of the United States of America*, 107, 49, pp.21022-21027, ISSN 0027-8424

Joukov, V. (2011). Aurora kinases and spindle assembly: Variations on a common theme? *Cell Cycle*, 10, 6, pp.895-903, ISSN 1538-4101

Kaipia A, Hsu SY & Hsueh AJ. (1997). Expression and function of a proapoptotic Bcl-2 family member Bcl-XL/Bcl-2-associated death promoter (BAD) in rat ovary. *Endocrinology*, 138, 12, pp.5497-5504, ISSN 0013-7227

Ke N, Godzik A & Reed JC. (2001). Bcl-B, a novel bcl-2 family member that differentially binds and regulates bax and bak. *Journal of Biological Chemistry*, 276, 16, pp.12481-12484, 0021-9258

Kim EA, Kim KH, Lee HS, Lee SY, Kim EY, Seo YM, Bae J, Lee KA. (2011). Downstream genes regulated by Bcl2l10 RNAi in the mouse oocytes. *Development and Reproduction*, 15, 1, pp.61-69, ISSN 1226-6752

Kim JD, Won M, Yoon S, Ko JJ, Lee KA, Lee K & Bae J. (2009). HIP1R interacts with a member of Bcl-2 family, BCL2L10, and induces moderate apoptosis. *Cellular Physiology and Biochemistry*, 23, 1-3, pp.43-52, ISSN 1015-8987

Kim MR & Tilly JL. (2004). Current concepts in Bcl-2 family member regulation of female germ cell development and survival. *Biochimica and Biophysica Acta*, 1644, 2-3, pp.205–210, ISSN 1672-9145

Kufer TA, Sillje HH, Korner R, Gruss OJ, Meraldi P, Nigg EA. (2002). Human TPX2 is required for targeting Aurora-A kinase to the spindle. *Journal of Cell Biology*, 158, 4, pp.617-623, ISSN 0021-9525

Lee R, Chen J, Matthews CP, McDougall JK & Neiman PE. (2001). Characterization of nr13-related human cell death regulator, boo/diva, in normal and cancer tissues. *Biochimica and Biophysica Acta*, 1520, 3, pp.187-194, ISSN 1672-9145

Ozlu N, Srayko M, Kinoshita K, Habermann B, O'toole ET, Müller-Reichert T, Schmalz N, Desai A & Hyman AA. (2005). An essential function of the C. elegans ortholog of TPX2 is to localize activated aurora A kinase to mitotic spindles. *Developmental Cell*, 9, 2, pp.237-248, ISSN 1534-5807

Sun QY, & Schatten H. (2006). Regulation of dynamic events by microfilaments during oocyte maturation and fertilization. *Reproduction*, 131, 2, pp.193-205, ISSN 1470-1626

Tilly JL, Tilly KI, Kenton ML & Johnson AL. (1995). Expression of members of the Bcl-2 gene family in the immature rat ovary: equine chorionic gonadotropin-mediated inhibition of granulosa cell apoptosis is associated with decreased Bax and constitutive Bcl-2 and Bcl-xlong messenger ribonucleic acid levels. *Endocrinology*, 136, 1, pp.232–241, ISSN 0013-7227

Tsai MY, Wiese C & Cao K. (2003). A Ran signaling pathway mediated by the mitotic kinase Aurora A in spindle assembly. *Nature Cell Biology*, 5, 3, pp.242-248, ISSN 1465-7392

Xu X, Wang X, Xiao Z, Li Y & Wang Y. (2011). Two TPX2-dependent switches control the activity of Aurora A. *PLoS ONE*, 6, 2, e16757, ISSN 1932-6203

Yoon SJ, Chung HM, Cha KY, Kim NH & Lee KA. (2005). Identification of differential gene expression in GV vs. MII mouse oocytes by using annealing control primers. *Fertility and Sterility*, 83, S4, pp.1293-1296, ISSN 0015-0282

Yoon SJ, Kim EY, Kim YS, Lee HS, Kim KH, Bae J, & Lee KA. (2009). Role of Bcl2-like 10 (Bcl2l10) in regulating mouse oocyte maturation. *Biology of Reproduction*, 81, 3, pp.497-506, ISSN 0006-3363

Yoon SJ, Kim JW, Choi KH, Lee SH & Lee KA. (2006). Identification of oocyte-specific Diva-associated proteins using mass spectrometry. *Korean Journal of Fertility and Sterility*, 33, 3, pp.189-198, ISSN 1226-2951

# 12

# Nuage Components and Their Contents in Mammalian Spermatogenic Cells, as Revealed by Immunoelectron Microscopy

Yuko Onohara and Sadaki Yokota
*Nagasaki International University,*
*Japan*

## 1. Introduction

The nuage is a germ cell-specific organelle that has been studied for more than a hundred years. It was first discovered in spermatogenic cells as a perinuclear granule stained by basic dyes and visualized using a light microscope. Morphological studies using electron microscopes demonstrated that "chromatoid body (CB)" is a nuage component in spermatids, and that "inter-mitochondrial cement (IMC)" is another nuage component found in spermatocytes. During meiosis, the IMC disappears, but the CB soon reforms in post-meiotic spermatids. Recent morphological and molecular biological studies have identified many components of nuage, and suggest that they play roles in the silencing, decay, and storage of RNA, and in the aggresome system. In this report, we summarize recent findings related to nuage and discuss their functions in spermatogenic cells.

## 2. Historical aspect of nuage components in germ line cells

By the 19th century, the basic techniques for histology, including preparation of tissue sections and staining of sections with various dyes, had largely been established, and light microscopic studies of tissues and cells from various animals and plants had begun to increase in terms of both number and detail. The subcellular structures in spermatogenic cells strongly attracting histologists' interest were strongly stained by basic dyes such as safranin, crystal violet, and Heidenhain's iron-hematoxylin. Two types of structures that today correspond to the chromatoid body (CB) were first described by von Brunn, who termed them "Protoplasmaanhäufungen" (protoplasmic depositions) and followed their fate, concluding that one formed the acrosome cap and the other moved to the caudal portion of spermatids to create the flagellum of spermatozoa (von Brunn, 1876). Afterwards, many histologists described similar structures using various names, such as "Nebenkörper" in spermatogenic cells from salamander and mouse (Herman 1889); "chromatoide Nebenkörper," derived from "intranuclearkörper" (the intranuclear body), which is different from the nucleolus (von Ebner, 1888; Benda, 1891); "corps chromatoides," which were stained black by iron-hematoxylin and deep red by safranin and finally degraded to "corps résiduel" (Regaud, 1901); and "chromatoide Körpers," which appeared as "chromatoiden Nuckeolens" in the nucleus and were dispersed in the cytoplasm (Schreiner & Schreiner, 1905). In the first half of the 20th century, CBs from various animals including insects (Wilson, 1913; Pollister, 1930), crustaceans (Fasten, 1914), arachnids (von Korff, 1902), fish (Schreiner & Schreiner, 1905), fowl (Zlotnik, 1947), and mammals (Duesberg, 1908; Wodsedalek, 1914; Gatenby & Beams, 1935) were studied extensively by light microscopy. In these classic studies, the potential origins of CBs were discussed. The arguments can be summarized into two ideas: 1) that the CB appears from the beginning in the cytoplasm of spermatocytes or spermatids, and 2) that the CB arises within the nucleoplasm and then moves to the cytoplasm. The fate of CBs can be summarized as follows: the CB exists in a perinuclear area and forms a part of the acrosome or the axis of the flagellum, or enters the bag-like structure that is formed in the cytoplasm at the base of the flagellum, and is degraded there. The studies cited above only involved observing stained tissue sections by light microscopy. Although most of these ideas have been shown to be incorrect, some of them have been accepted.

## 3. Ultrastructural characteristics of nuage components in mammalian spermatogenic cells

### 3.1 The CB as a representative nuage structure in mammalian spermatogenic cells

Electron microscopic studies of mammalian spermatogenic cells commenced in the 1950s (Watson, 1952; Challice, 1953). Burgos and Fawcett (1955) were the first to observe the CB by electron microscopy (Figure 1).

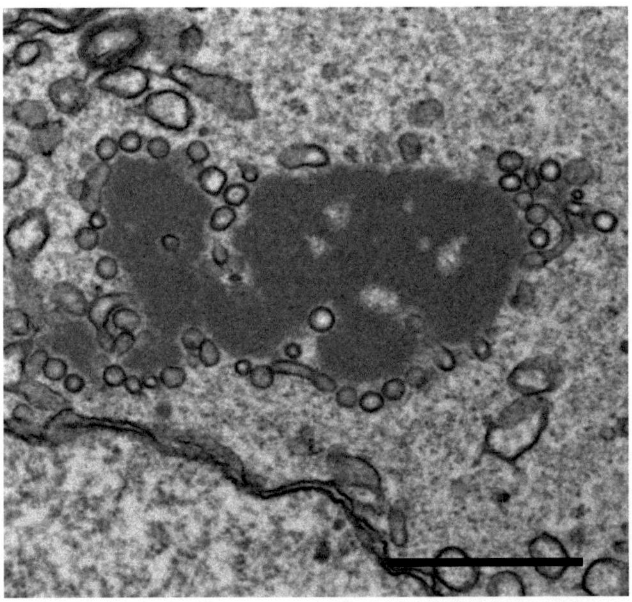

Fig. 1. Electron micrograph of a typical CB of a step 4 spermatid. The CB consists of an electron-dense matrix and is surrounded by small clear vesicles and tubules. The CB has no limiting membrane. Bar = 1 μm.

Burgos and Fawcett described an irregular and osmiophilic component corresponding to the "chromatic body" or "accessory body" detected by light microscopy. This structure was initially found near the Golgi complex, subsequently moving towards the caudal region in late spermatids. In 1955, Minamino described the material as an "idiosome remnant." In 1959, Sasa reported the ultrastructure of the rat testis, and referred to "Chromatoider

Nebenkörper." He suggested that osmiophilic components derived from the cluster of cytoplasmic vesicles might fuse to each other to form the big honeycomb structure.

In 1970, Fawcett et al. studied the origin and fate of CBs and satellite bodies during spermatogenesis in several mammals at the ultrastructural level. They presented evidence that the CB was not derived from the nucleus, as had been reported previously. CBs were not present in spermatocytes. Instead, they were found between clusters of mitochondria, in the dense interstitial material that is today known as inter-mitochondrial cement (IMC) (Figure 2). Because its texture and density were similar to those of CB, the researchers assumed that IMC might be the origin of the CB, and that two CBs might be assembled from IMC and possibly distributed to two daughter cells during meiosis I. In late spermatids, the CB became associated with the base of the flagellum, so they assumed that it might contribute to formation of the "annulus," a ring associated with the plasma membrane in spermatids and subsequently located at the junction of the middle and principal pieces in spermatozoa.

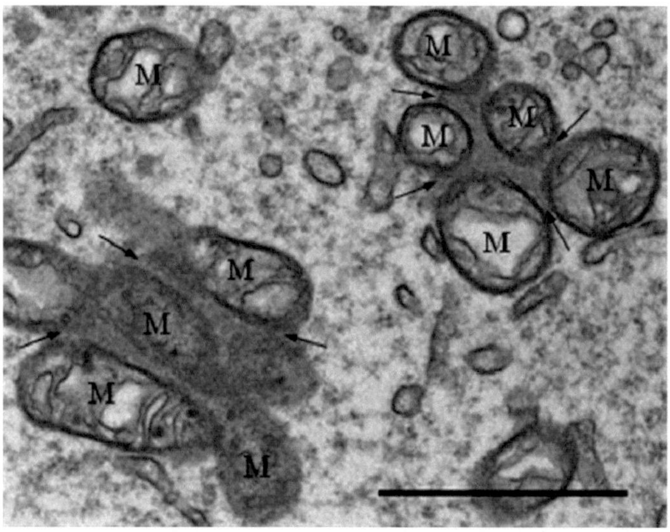


Fig. 2. Electron micrograph of typical IMC in a stage X pachytene spermatocyte. IMC appears as a dense interstitial material (arrows) between the clustered mitochondria (M). Bar = 1 μm.

Susi and Clermont (1970) studied the morphology and fate of CBs by routine electron microscopy. In spermatocytes, the CB was composed of two elements: 1) an electron-dense material with a sponge-like texture; and 2) numerous small vesicles with a diameter of 40–80 nm, located in the cytoplasm near the nuclear envelope. In step 1–7 spermatids, the CB was observed as a single irregular granule with a diameter of 1–2 μm, whose material was more condensed compared with CBs in spermatocytes. It was located proximal to the nuclear envelope, or sometimes near the Golgi apparatus, and was occasionally associated with the "multivesicular body (MB)." The CB and MB were found in the caudal region of the nucleus in step 8 spermatids. In step 9–10 spermatids, the CB was spherical, had a diameter of 1.5 μm, and was surrounded by vesicles positive for glycoproteins (stained by the periodic acid-chromic acid-silver methenamine method). In later spermatids, the CB was fragmented into smaller masses. Susi and Clermont suggested that the CB might be highly active in dramatically changing its form.

Based on the results of indium trichloride staining, Eddy (1970) concluded that no RNA existed in the CB. Similarly, the results of radioautography with isotope-labeled bases suggested that the dense granules observed in oocytes from *Rana* spp. contained neither RNA nor any other nucleic acid (Eddy & Ito, 1971). These results conflicted with previous reports (Daoust & Clermont, 1955).

In 1974, Eddy studied "nuage" (clouds in French) structures in primordial germ cells from rats of both sexes. He identified nuage in both male and female cells, and proposed that the nuage is the characteristic component of mammalian germ cells. He further compared the nuage with the "polar granule" found in insects (Dhainaut, 1970; Mahowald, 1962) and with "germinal plasm" found in amphibians (Nieuwkoop & Faber, 1956). These structures were previously speculated to play a role in germ cell determination. Eddy noted the common morphological profile and distribution of nuage with these components, which led him to suggest that nuage might be involved in the determination of mammalian germ cells, as had been reported for insects and amphibians. In terms of mammals, nuage was identified in guinea pig (Adams & Hertig, 1964), hamster (Weakley, 1969; Fawcett et al., 1970), rabbit (Nicander & Plöen, 1969), mouse (Fawcett et al., 1970), rat (Brökelmann, 1963), and human (Burgos et al., 1970). In germ cells of both sexes, nuage appeared either as a discrete mass or in association with mitochondrial clusters during the different stages of oogenesis and spermatogenesis. Eddy (1974) suggested that that the CB was a component of the nuage in spermatogenic cells.

In the same year, Kerr and Dixon (1974) studied germ plasm, which they regarded as a nuage found in spermatogenic cells, based on its appearance, expression stage, and association with mitochondria. They assumed that germ plasm might be a precursor of the CB. Russell and Frank (1978) classified nuage into six different types based on its form, distribution, and interrelationships with other organelles: 1) 70–90 nm spherical particles: fine fibrous and partly high-dense material found in spermatogonia, secondary spermatocytes, and intermediate forms; 2) sponge bodies: loosely organized masses, not only perinuclear but found throughout the cytoplasm in spermatocytes of all stages, and occasionally in spermatogonia and early spermatids; 3) IMC: 0.1 µm or narrower loosely organized strands, whose density and appearance resemble those of the sponge body, observed mainly in early spermatocytes and occasionally in spermatogonia; 4) 30 nm particles: clusters of dense particles different from ribosomes in the cytoplasm of meiosis I cells and secondary spermatocytes; 5) CBs: located in the cytoplasm proximal to the nucleus in pachytene spermatocytes; and 6) definitive CBs. Temporary CBs had been described previously as large spherical bodies with a diameter of approximately 0.5 µm that were closely associated with the few mitochondria observed in secondary spermatocytes and spermatids. Russell and Frank (1978) first classified the CB into two types that were present during different stages of spermatogenesis, although it was unclear whether the two types were the same in terms of their composition. They further reported that the CBs were not found in diplotene spermatocytes or during meiosis I. During meiosis II, they found numerous CBs in the cytoplasm. These CBs were separated into two components, one of which had a large, round honeycomb structure, and the other of which was a loose network of irregularly shaped dense strands.

The ultrastructural studies of CBs described above can be summarized as follows: 1) the CB is a component of nuage that was specifically detected in spermatogenic cells; 2) CBs displayed irregular shapes, comprising dense fibrous material surrounded by small vesicles, and had no limiting membrane; 3) CBs appeared first in spermatocytes, disappeared during meiosis, and reappeared in spermatids.

### 3.2 Relationship between the CB and the nuclear envelope

In classical studies, CBs were assumed to be derived from the intranuclear structure, based on the similarity in safranin staining in both structures (Benda, 1891; Regaud, 1901). Sud (1961) first suggested the presence of highly polymerized RNA and arginine-rich basic proteins in CBs based on the results of histochemical studies.

In 1970, Fawcett et al. proposed a new idea: that CB originated not from nucleus, but from the dense materials between clustered mitochondrial, i.e., IMC, which appeared during early spermatocytes. IMC was gradually deposited there as spermatocytes differentiated. Their hypothesis that CB is derived from IMC was supported by the facts that 1) no dense substance was observed on the intranuclear side of nuclear pores when the CB was in contact with the cytoplasmic side, and 2) that CBs already existed in spermatocytes before the CB made contact with nuclear pores. Although the CB is not derived from the nucleus, Fawcett et al. (1970) assumed that some kind of exchange might take place between the nucleus and the CB. On the other hand, in 1972, Comings and Okada observed that a nuclear granule exited to the cytoplasm of primary spermatocytes via the nuclear pore, and therefore concluded that the CB originated from the nucleus. This idea was discussed by Eddy in 1974.

The movement of CBs in the rat testis was studied using time-lapse cinemicrography, the results of which revealed that the CB rapidly moved around the nuclear envelope and Golgi complex, and occasionally seemed to be detected as an intranuclear particle (Parvinen & Jokelainen, 1974; Parvinen & Parvinen, 1979). Based on these observations, they assumed that the CB played a role in the transport of haploid gene products in early spermatids.

Ventelä et al. (2003) reported that the CB moved from one spermatid to another through the cytoplasmic bridge, and that this movement was inhibited by the microtubule-depolymerizing agents, nocodazole and vincristine. These results demonstrated that the microtubular network is involved in CB mobility.

Communication between the CB and nucleus, suggested by the results of classic light microscopic studies, was confirmed by electron microscopic studies. Cinemicrography studies showing real-time movement of CBs provided clear evidence of CB-nucleus communication (Parvinen & Jokelainen, 1974). Consequently, it was concluded that the CB may not be derived from the nucleus, but communicates with the nucleus via the nuclear pore complex during spermatogenesis.

### 3.3 Clusters of 30–40 nm particles

Russell and Frank (1978) observed clusters of small, 30–40 nm particles in dividing meiosis I cells and pachytene spermatocytes, which were morphologically different from ribosomes and glycogen particles. These clusters were composed of hundreds of aggregated 30–40 nm particles, and contained a filamentous material. Russell and Frank suggested that these particles might stabilize RNAs encoding proteins required for the subsequent development of spermatids.

### 3.4 IMC as an origin of the CB

Some concluded that IMC was a precursor of mitochondria because its density was similar to that of the mitochondrial matrix (Odor, 1965; André, 1962). However, this hypothesis was disproved by confirmation of the striking difference in the density of the two components after improved fixation (Fawcett, et al., 1970). As mentioned above, Fawcett et al. proposed that the CB was derived from IMC (Fawcett, et al. 1970). According to them, IMC gradually increased in size by coalescence as spermatids developed, subsequently dissociated from the mitochondria, and assembled to form the CB.

Russell and Frank (1978) reported that IMC appeared when mitochondria were noticeably clustered in pachytene spermatocytes, and that there was no evidence of IMC during or after the first meiotic metaphase, when the mitochondria dispersed.

### 3.5 Satellite body (SB, sponge body) and its origin

Sud (1961) first named the structure the "satellite," and described its localization near to, and sometimes in contact with, the CB. The chemical composition of the satellite differed from that of the CB. Sud proposed that the satellite might form the basal body of the axial filament.

Fawcett et al. (1970) described the characteristics, origin, and fate of the satellite body (SB), which they referred it "chromatoid body satellite", and first described the distinction between the SB and the CB at the ultrastructural level. He reported that the SB was present in zygotene and pachytene spermatocytes prior to the appearance of the CB, and had a more regular shape and contained less filamentous material than the CB. In the report of Fawcett et al. (1970), they hypothesized that clusters of small particles of 40–60 nm in diameter, which had previously been suggested to be precursors of centrioles (Stockinger & Cirelli, 1965; Sorokin, 1968), were in fact the source of the SB, because they were the only conceivable precursor of the SB and had a strikingly resemblance to the SB. The fate of the SB was unknown, but it was found to move from the Golgi region to the caudal region of the nucleus in spermatids. In late spermatids, a spherical mass was found near the developing connecting piece, and was assumed to be derived from the SB on the basis of its size.

Russell and Frank (1978) described the SB as a "sponge body" found in the cytoplasm of secondary spermatocytes and young spermatids, and very occasionally spermatogonia. They indicated that the density and appearance of the SB resembled those of IMC.

### 3.6 Nuage components in meiotic cells

Nuage was found to dissociate from mitochondrial clusters during the pachytene phase of meiosis, forming the CBs in spermatids (Eddy, 1974). Eddy also observed that after meiosis II, the CB was dispersed in the cytoplasm as small dark masses. However, in step 1 spermatids the CB was reconstructed. Russell and Frank (1978) reported that while the CB was rarely seen in dividing meiosis I cells, there was loose, dense material that was irregularly shaped and contained granular materials on its inner surface. As mentioned above, the clusters of 30 nm particles were found in dividing meiosis I cells and were thought to possibly contain mRNAs. Russell and Frank assumed that these clusters might contain RNAs that had been transferred from the nucleus to cytoplasm, and that these RNAs might encode proteins involved in the later stages of spermatogenesis. They also reported that the definitive CB was observed in secondary spermatocytes proximal to meiosis II cells. CB was suggested to be a storage organelle for haploid gene products during meiosis, and to possibly participate in the transport of these products from the nucleus to the cytoplasm (Söderström & Parvinen, 1976; Parvinen & Parvinen, 1979). Söderström (1978) reported that the condensed CB was present during meiotic prophase, and that new materials were formed in the nucleus in cells of meiotic prophase and spermatids, and proposed that the materials might be transported to the cytoplasm and be added to the CB. We ourselves have shown that the small particles partly associated with mitochondria during meiosis stain positive for the nuage marker protein DDX4. This suggests that nuage components might dissociate into small particles during meiosis, allowing them to be apportioned to the daughter cells evenly (Figure 3).

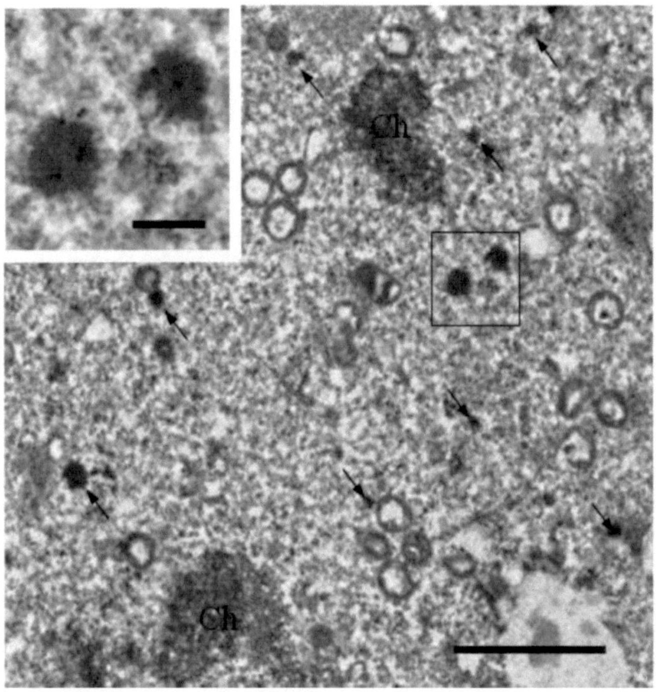


Fig. 3. Rat spermatocyte during meiosis. A dividing chromosome (Ch) is present. No aggregates of particles are seen, but small particles are present (arrows). These particles are positive for DDX4 (inset). Bar = 2 µm (main image) and 0.5 µm (inset).

## 4. Immunoelectron microscopic localization of nuage proteins in spermatogenic cells

### 4.1 Argonaute/Piwi and Tudor families in nuage components

The Argonaute/Piwi family of proteins can be split into CB and nuage components. Members of the Argonaute/Piwi family commonly have PAZ and PIWI domains, and are classified into the Ago1 and PIWI subfamilies based on their sequences. Ago 1–4 belong to the Ago1 subfamily, are highly expressed in various tissues, and function in the RNA-induced silencing complex (RISC) pathway (Meister et al., 2004). In contrast, members of the PIWI subfamily are specifically expressed in germ cells, with MIWI and MILI performing particularly important roles in spermatogenesis (Sasaki et al., 2003; Deng & Lin, 2002). MIWI was localized to the CB in spermatids. In a MIWI-null mouse model, the fully compacted CB was not found, with a non-compacted and diffuse CB instead being observed (Kotaja et al., 2006b), which suggests the importance of MIWI for the construction of the compacted CB. The Tudor family proteins Tudor repeat domain containing protein (TDRD)-1, -4, -5, -6, -7, and -9 were reported to be expressed in germ cells, and were shown to co-localize with Piwi family proteins in nuage. TDRD-1 has been detected in nuage in spermatogonia, in IMC in spermatocytes, and in CBs in round spermatids (Chuma et al., 2003). The analysis of a TDRD-1-null mouse model revealed that TDRD-1 was essential for piRNA biogenesis, formation of IMC, and the correct localization of DDX4 in the CB (Hosokawa et al., 2007). In pachytene spermatocytes, TDRD-5 co-localized in IMC and the CB with TDRD-1, MIWI, MILI, and DDX4. In mid-pachytene spermatocytes, TDRD-5 was partly co-localized with TDRD-6 and -7; in diplotene spermatocytes, it was mainly co-localized with TDRD-6. In round spermatids, TDRD-5 co-localized in the CB with DDX4, MIWI, TDRD-1, -6, and -9, and interestingly, at the same time, TDRD-7 localized to another perinuclear structure distal from the CB (Yabuta et al., 2011), which seemed to be the second nuage component. In a TDRD-6-null mouse model, CB was not condensed, but rather was dispersed (Vasileva et al., 2009).

### 4.2 RNF17/TDRD-4 in nuage components

*RNF17/TDRD-4* was first described as a germ cell-specific gene that contains repeated Tudor domains and a RING finger motif, which is present in ubiquitin E3 ligase. Yin et al. (1999, 2001) reported that RNF17 interacted with Mad family proteins and repressed transcription of the gene encoding the oncoprotein Myc. RNF17 contributes to activation of the transcription of Myc-responsive genes by supplying Mad proteins. In RNF17-null mice, which are sterile, spermatogenesis completely stops at the round spermatid stage (Pan et al., 2005), which indicates the importance of RNF17 in the development of spermatids. Pan et al. (2005) described a new dense granule that is positive for RNF17 and located in the perinuclear region near to the CB throughout spermatogenesis, and named it the "RNF17 granule." The morphological appearance of the RNF17 granule closely resembles that of the SB. If the SB contains RNF17, it would be one of the first SB components to be identified. Our preliminary data show that MAELSTRÖM (MAEL) is also localized to the SB, as well as other nuage components (Fig. 4).

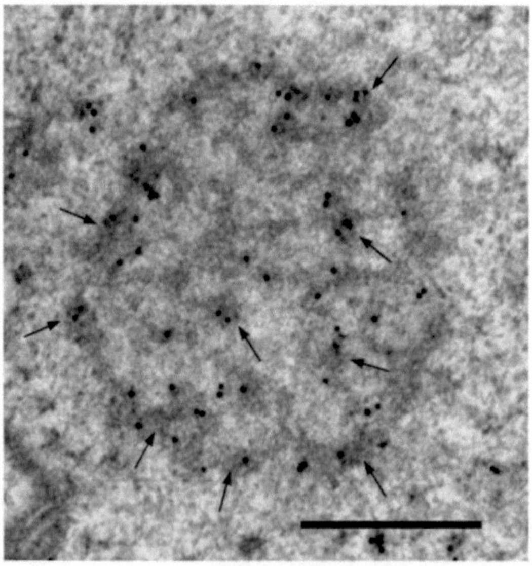

Fig. 4. Typical SB of a stage X pachytene spermatocyte stained for MAEL by immunoelectron microscopy (IEM). Gold particles showing MAEL antigenic sites are present on denser patches (arrows). The SB is 0.5–1.5 μm in diameter, and consists of a network of fibrils overlaid by denser patches of amorphous material. Bar = 0.5 μm.

### 4.3 DDX4 in nuage components

DDX4, the mouse homolog of the *Drosophila* vasa gene MVH, is an ATP-dependent RNA helicase belonging to the DEAD box family. DDX4 has been studied as a CB marker protein (Noce et al., 2001; Kotaja et al., 2006a; Kotaja & Sassone-Corsi, 2007; Onohara et al., 2010). In DDX4-null mice, spermatogenesis arrests at the prophase of meiosis, and most spermatocytes undergo degeneration. Furthermore, the amount of IMC in the spermatocytes is greatly reduced (Tanaka et al., 2000; Chuma et al., 2006). DDX4 was reported to interact with MIWI and MILI. Moreover, MILI$^{-/-}$ and DDX4$^{-/-}$ mice have similar phenotypes, which suggest that these proteins work cooperatively (Kuramachi-Miyagawa et al., 2004). In MILI-null mice, DDX4 was not detected in the nuage components (Kuramachi-Miyagawa et al., 2004), which suggests that DDX4 requires MILI to localize to the nuage components.

We previously reported the ultrastructual localization of DDX4 in nuage components during rat spermatogenesis (Onohara et al., 2010). Our report showed the wide expression of DDX4 in nuage components and other structures. In pachytene spermatocytes, DDX4 mainly localized to the surface of IMC, while loose aggregates were observed in the juxtanuclear area (Figure 5). The loose aggregate consisted of 70–90 nm particles and the material was dissociated from the IMC. In meiosis, structures positive for DDX4 disappeared, but small particles were identified in the cytoplasm (Figure 3). In spermatids, DDX4 mainly localized to the CB until step 6, after which the signal became gradually weaker, which suggests that the expression of CB proteins was dependent on spermatid step. No DDX4 signal was observed in the SB.

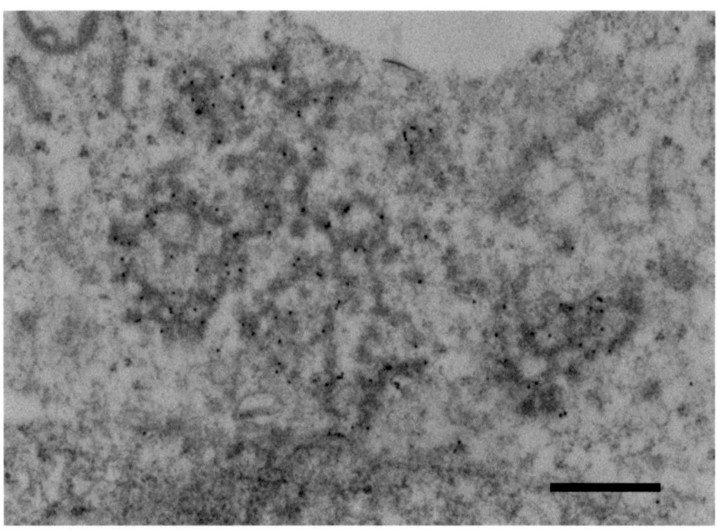

Fig. 5. IEM image of the loose aggregate consisting of 70–90 nm particles. Note that the particles contain gold particles used to label DDX4. Bar = 0.5 μm.

### 4.4 DDX25/GRTH in nuage components

DDX25 belongs to the DEAD-box family, and is essential for the completion of spermatogenesis. DDX25 acts as a hormone-dependent RNA helicase in Leydig cells and germ cells, and is referred to as a gonadotropin-regulated testicular helicase (GRTH) (Tang et al., 1999). DDX25-null mice, which are sterile, showed arrest of spermatogenesis at the round spermatid stage (Sheng et al., 2006). Sato et al. (2010) treated spermatogenic cells with inhibitors of RNA polymerase and nuclear protein export. As a result, the amount of DDX25 in the nucleus increased, while the amount in the cytoplasm decreased. Furthermore, after treatment, the CB became smaller and condensed, as observed in DDX25-deficient mice. The results of co-immunoprecipitation studies using an anti-DDX25 antibody revealed that DDX25 bound to mRNAs, including DDX25 mRNA, in both the nucleus and cytoplasm. This suggested that the main function of DDX25 is to transport mRNA from the nucleus to cytoplasm, and to transport DDX25-ribonucleoprotein (RNP) complexes essential for controlling CB construction.

We ourselves found that DDX25 was abundant in small particles and loose aggregates of 70–90 nm particles in spermatocytes, but was less abundant in IMC (in press). The loose aggregate is closely associated with the nuclear envelope (Onohara et al., 2010). In spermatids, DDX25 is also localized to CB, but rarely or not at all to the SB.

### 4.5 Other proteins in nuage components

Haraguchi et al. (2005) reported the localization of the ubiquitin-conjugating enzyme cytochrome oxidase subunit I (COXI), Hsp70, and phospholipid hydroperoxide glutathione peroxidase (PHGPx) to the CB, and the localization of vimentin, the 20S proteasome subunit, and Lamp1 in the region around the CB. The protein composition of the CB overlapped with that of the aggresome, which indicates that the CB has a role not only in protein synthesis, but also in degradation, as an aggresome system.

Dicer, a key protein in the biogenesis of mature microRNAs and small-interfering RNAs (siRNAs), has a highly dynamic expression pattern in the CBs of meiotic spermatocytes and round spermatids, and interacts with DDX4 at its C-terminus, as revealed by immunoprecipitation (Kotaja et al., 2006a). The localization of Ago2, -3, Dcp1a, and GW182 to the CB has been reported. Because these proteins are known to be markers of the processing body (P-body), a dense granule present in the cytoplasm in somatic cells (Kedersha et al., 2005), the CB may have functions in common with the P-body.

The Kinesin motor protein KIF17b is involved in the nucleus-to-cytoplasm transport of RNA, and was reported to co-localize with MIWI in the CB of round spermatids (Kotaja et al., 2006b). It may therefore be involved in the microtubule-mediated transport of CBs.

Brunol2/CUG-BP1/CELF1 is a homolog of the *Drosophila melanogaster* protein Bruno, and is a member of the CELF family that controls the splicing of pre-mRNAs. Bruno was found in nuage in ovaries and embryos (Snee & Macdonald, 2004). Spermatogenesis was arrested in step 7 spermatids in Brunol2-deficient mice (Kress et al., 2007). Recently we showed that Brunol2 localizes to the CB and other nuage components during rat spermatogenesis (in press).

HuR, an RNA-binding protein in somatic cells that controls the stability or translation of AU-rich mRNAs, was found in the CB and co-localized with DDX4 (Nguyen et al., 2009). HuR is involved in the shuttling of mRNAs from the nucleus to the CB for storage and protection against degradation.

MAEL, which is an ortholog of the *Drosophila* protein, MAELSTROM, is localized to the CB and unsynapsed chromosomes in spermatocytes, and has been implicated in the silencing of unsynapsed chromatin in spermatocytes during meiosis (Costa et al., 2006). MAEL co-localizes with DDX4, MIWI2, TDRD-9, and the P-body components Dcp1a, DDX6, GW182, and Xrn1 in the CB, but does not localize to the IMC. In MAEL-knockout mice, Piwi-interacting RNA (piRNA) production and post-transcriptional transposon silencing are perturbed in fetal gonocytes, suggesting that MAEL may be involved in these processes (Aravin et al., 2009).

GASZ, a germ cell protein with ankyrin repeats, a sterile alpha motif, and a leucine zipper, is localized to the CB. In GASZ-null mice, levels of MILI/piRNAs in the CB were dramatically reduced, and spermatogenesis was arrested before meiosis (Ma et al., 2009).

In 2010, MOV10L1, a member of the DEAD-box RNA helicase family essential for retrotransposon silencing in mouse germ cells, was reported to be expressed in spermatogonia, pachytene spermatocytes, and all intermediate forms in the mouse testis, and to interact with MILI, MIWI, and heat shock 70 kDa protein 2 (Frost et al., 2010). MOV10L1 appeared in a complex termed "MIWI-MILI block," which may be identical to IMC.

MitoPLD, a member of the phospholipase D superfamily, is abundant in the outer membrane of mitochondria, and degrades cardiolipin, yielding the lipid signaling molecule phosphatidic acid (PA). In MitoPLD-knockout mice, the nuage was arranged like a donut in the perinuclear region, and γ-tubulin was detected in the center of the aberrant nuage in spermatogonia, suggesting that MitoPLD may be involved in microtubule-dependent nuage transport. Furthermore, in MitoPLD-null mice, spermatogenesis arrests in late or post-meiotic spermatocytes, and the IMC is absent from spermatocytes. In addition, TDRD-1 and mitochondria aggregate to the pericentriolar region instead of the perinuclear region in gonocytes. In mice lacking Lipin1, which metabolizes PA, nuage increases in size and density, and the localization of TDRD-1 is altered. These results suggest that MitoPLD and/or PA may be involved in the generation of IMC and the correct localization of nuage and maintenance of its components (Huang et al., 2011; Watanabe et al., 2011).

NANOS, which is essential for primordial germ cell (PGC) in *Drosophila*, plays a critical role in spermatogenesis, particularly during meiosis. NANOS2 blocks meiosis by suppressing Stra8, an inducer of meiosis (Saga, 2008). NANOS1, which is known to regulate the translation of specific mRNAs, is found in the CB and co-localizes with PUMILIO protein, as well as the microRNA biogenesis factor GEMIN3 (Ginter-Matuszewska et al., 2011).

During the last decade, many nuage constituent proteins have been identified. Above all, it is noteworthy that RNA-binding proteins and RNA-regulating proteins are abundant in nuage, indicating that nuage may contribute to RNA silencing and RNA decay during spermatogenesis. Many nuage proteins co-localize simultaneously with other proteins in the same compartment, suggesting that most nuage components may function cooperatively during germ cell development. Functional nuage proteins are listed in Table 1.

| Component | Domain/Function | Where found | References |
|---|---|---|---|
| TDRD-1 | Tudor proteins; contain Tudor domains; essential for piRNA biosynthesis | Spermatogonia, spermatocytes, round spermatids | Chuma et al., 2003 |
| TDRD-5 | | Spermatocytes, spermatids | Yabuta et al., 2011 |
| TDRD-6 | | Spermatocytes, spermatids | Vasileva et al., 2009; Yabuta et al., 2011 |
| TDRD-7 | | Spermatids | Tanaka et al., 2000; Yabuta et al., 2011 |
| TDRD-9 | Tudor protein; ATPase/DExH-type helicase; essential for piRNA biosynthesis | Spermatocytes | Shoji et al., 2009 |
| TDRD-4/RNF17 | Tudor protein; contains a RING finger motif | Spermatogonia, spermatocytes, round spermatids | Pan et al., 2005 |
| Ago2/Ago3 | Argonaute family protein; component of the RISC | Spermatids | Kotaja et al., 2006a |
| MILI | Piwi family proteins; associate with piRNA | Spermatocytes | Sasaki et al., 2003; Kotaja et al., 2006b |
| MIWI2 | | Spermatids | Sasaki et al., 2003; Kotaja et al., 2006b |
| DDX4/MVH | DEAD box RNA helicases | Spermatocytes, spermatids | Noce et al., 2001; Kotaja et al., 2006a |
| DDX6 | | Spermatocytes | Aravin et al., 2009 |
| DDX25 | | Spermatocytes, spermatids | Sheng et al., 2006; Sato et al., 2010 |
| MOV10L1 | DEAD box RNA helicase family; silencing retrotransposons in germ cells | Spermatogonia to pachytene spermatocytes | Frost et al., 2010 |
| Dicer | RNase III; major protein in the biogenesis of small RNAs | Spermatocytes, round spermatids | Kotaja et al., 2006a |
| Dcp1a | P-body markers | Pachytene spermatocytes, spermatids | Kotaja et al., 2006a |
| GW182 | | Spermatids | Kotaja et al., 2006a; Aravin et al., 2009 |
| Xnt1 | | Spermatids | Aravin et al., 2009 |
| Brunol2/CUG-BP1 | CELF family protein; controls the splicing of pre-mRNAs | Spermatocytes, spermatids | Kress et al., 2007 |
| GASZ | Essential for fertility in females and spermatogenesis | PGCs, gonocytes, spermatogonia, spermatocytes | Ma et al., 2009 |
| HuR | RNA-binding protein in somatic cells; controls the stability or translation of AU-rich mRNAs | Spermatids | Nguyen et al., 2009 |
| KIF17b | Kinesin motor protein | Round spermatids | Kotaja et al., 2006b; Aravin et al., 2011 |
| MAEL | HMG box protein | Gonocytes, meiosis, spermatocytes, round spermatids | Costa et al., 2006; Aravin et al., 2009 |
| NANOS1 | Suppression of meiosis; regulates the translation of specific mRNA | PGCs, gonocytes, meiosis, spermatids | Ginter-Matuszewska et al., 2011 |
| PUMILIO2 | RNA-binding protein; translational regulation | Round spermatids | Ginter-Matuszewska et al., 2011 |
| GEMIN3 | MicroRNA biogenesis factor | Round spermatids | Ginter-Matuszewska et al., 2011 |

Table 1. Functional nuage-related proteins that play roles in RNA silencing, RNA decay, and nuage morphogenesis.

## 5. Functions of nuage proteins and their relationships to morphological features

### 5.1 A transcription context specific for spermatogenic cells

Proteins such as Dicer and PIWI family proteins that are involved in the posttranscriptional regulation of microRNAs during spermatogenesis are highly concentrated in nuage. Dicer processes the precursors of both siRNAs and microRNAs (miRNAs) into small mature RNAs in the cytoplasm in somatic cells. These small mature RNAs are assembled into an RISC, which contains Argonaute family proteins and causes translational repression or mRNA cleavage in the cytoplasm in somatic cells (Stefani & Slack, 2008). Ago family proteins, Dicer, miRNAs, and miRNA-repressed mRNA are localized to the P-bodies of somatic cells, suggesting that RNA silencing and RNA disruption may occur there (Sen & Blau, 2005). Some P-body markers are also expressed in the CB, suggesting that the CBs of germ cells may be involved in RNA silencing and RNA disruption, as in the P-bodies of somatic cells (Kotaja et al., 2006a). The function of the P-body in somatic cells has been studied extensively (Sen & Blau, 2005). The CB has many features in common with the P-body, strongly suggesting that the CB may play similar roles to the P-body.

### 5.2 Function of the CB in mRNA storage and transport

Söderström and Parvinen (1976) studied RNA synthesis during spermatogenesis by autoradiography using tritiated uridine. In step 1–8 spermatids, the rate of RNA synthesis was low in the cell as a whole, but very high in the CB, and was arrest in step 8 spermatids in both places. Therefore, it is likely that CBs in spermatids contain RNAs, which may encode proteins involved in the regulation of spermiogenesis in late spermatids.

Kotaja et al. (2006a) performed *in situ* hybridization to determine whether or not the CB contains miRNA, and demonstrated the localization of miRNAs in the CB. HuR is involved in the transport of mRNAs from the nucleus to the CB so that they can be stored and protected against degradation (Nguyen et al., 2009). Kotaja et al. (2006b) detected KIF17b, known to bind to mRNAs, in the CB, and suggested that the CB might be involved in the transport of mRNAs in early spermatids.

These studies strongly suggest that the CB is also a site for the storage and transport of mRNAs that encode proteins with roles in late spermatids.

### 5.3 The function of nuage components other than the CB

During the differentiation of spermatogonia and spermatocytes, several nuage structures with specific shapes appear, persist for a period of time, and then disappear, as described above. The other organelles, including mitochondria, the Golgi complex, and lysosomes, do not undergo marked changes in morphology. However, the differentiation of spermatids to spermatozoa is dynamic and dramatic. Spermatids transform into spermatozoa, whose role is to enable transport of DNA to the target cell, the oocyte, through an extraordinarily intricate process of cell differentiation termed spermiogenesis, which lasts approximately 20 days in rats (Clermont et al., 1959) and 24 days in humans (Heller & Clermont, 1964). Major events that occur during spermiogenesis include formation of the acrosome, nuclear condensation, formation of the tail, trimming of the cytoplasm, and organelle reorganization (de Kretser & Kerr, 1988; Clermont et al., 1993). Ultrastructural studies have described various specialized structures, including the radial body-annulate lamellae complex; small puffs of a fine, filamentous, fuzzy material; a granulated body composed of fine, dense granular materials; a reticulated body consisting of several dense anastomosed cords; and a large, dense granule surrounded by crescentic mitochondria (Clermont et al., 1993), which we termed the mitochondria-associated granule (MAG).

Our own IEM studies provide evidence that some of these structures contain nuage proteins.

1. The radial body-annulate lamellae complex, a membrane-bound structure that is continuous with the endoplasmic reticulum (ER), is observed in the cytoplasmic lobe of late spermatids, and is believed to be the site at which resorption of the ER membrane occurs (Clermont & Rambourg, 1978). No nuage proteins have yet been detected in this structure. Therefore, it seems that it is not a structural site for the function of nuage proteins.
2. Small puffs have no limiting membrane, are attached to the cytoplasmic surface of the ER, and are observed in step 8–10 spermatids. The only nuage protein to have been detected in the puffs so far is Brunol2 (in press).
3. Granulated bodies appear in the cytoplasmic lobes of step 14 spermatids, are most abundant in step 17 spermatids, and decrease in number during subsequent stages of spermatogenesis. It was reported by Clermont et al. (1990) that they contain outer dense fiber (ODF) proteins. It is assumed that ODF polypeptides are temporarily stored in these bodies (Clermont et al., 1993). However, their function remains unclear. Our preliminary IEM studies detected BRUNOL2, DDX25, NANOS1, and MAEL in these bodies, but not DDX4 (unpublished data). Gold particles that were used to label these nuage proteins were confined to the fine granular matrix.
4. The reticulated body first appears in the cytoplasm of step 14 spermatids and completely disappears in step 18 spermatids (Clermont et al. 1990). The body is characterized by several dense, anastomosed cords with a width of 80–100 nm. We detected BRUNOL2, DDX25, NANOS1, and MAEL in this structure by IEM, but not DDX4. Other than the nuage proteins, only cathepsin H has so far been detected in the structure (Haraguchi et al., 2003). The nature and function of this structure remains unclear.
5. The MAG is 1–2 μm in diameter, is composed of a fine granular material, and appears in the elongated cytoplasmic lobes of step 9–17 spermatids (Figure 6). Its strongest characteristic is its close association with mitochondria (Clermont et al., 1990). We detected the nuage proteins BRUNOL2, DDX4, DDX25, NANOS1, and MAEL in this structure in our preliminary studies (unpublished data). Although dense materials in the MAG were assumed to be a source of ODF proteins, the results of IEM experiments that detected no ODF protein signals in the MAG indicates that this is not the case (Clermont et al., 1990). No proteins other than the above five nuage proteins have so far been detected in this structure. Although the nature and function of the MAG are unknown, the existence of nuage proteins may provide important clues about the function of the MAG.

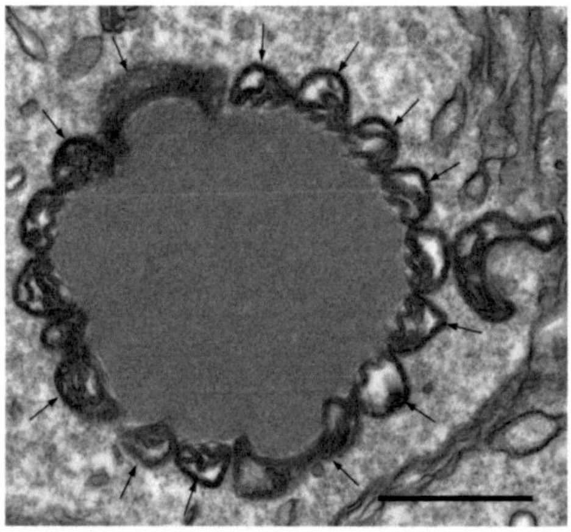

Fig. 6. Electron micrograph of an MAG in a step 16 spermatid. The MAG is a large spherical mass with a diameter of 1–2 µm, composed of granular material and surrounded by mitochondria. Bar = 1 µm.

In the neck cytoplasm of step 11 spermatids, small, discrete, dense masses are frequently observed (Fawcett & Phillips, 1969), closely associated with other structures or free in the cytoplasm. One, which is associated with the plasma membrane and subsequently moves to a position at the junction of the middle and principal regions of the tail, is known as the annulus. It was assumed that the annulus was derived from the CB (Fawcett et al., 1970). However, our study (Onohara et al., 2010) and preliminary results (unpublished data) indicate a lack of signals in the annulus for the nuage proteins listed above, indicating that the CB and the nuage proteins are not involved in the formation of the annulus. Spherical masses are frequently observed at the base of the flagellum of late spermatids (Fawcett & Phillips, 1969). Our IEM studies show that these masses are positive for Dicer1 and MAEL (unpublished data). Interestingly, these Dicer1-positive particles are maintained in epididymal sperm, suggesting that they are carried into the cytoplasm of the ovum. Furthermore, a less electron-dense mass composed of fine filamentous materials surrounds the connecting piece in late spermatids (Clermont et al., 1993). This structure is positive for BRUNOL2 (unpublished data). In the neck region, small dense particles are present. These particles contain small amounts of the nuage proteins BRUNOL2, DDX25, NANOS1, and MAEL. In addition, BRUNOL2 and MAEL have been detected in large aggregates of free ribosomes and other unknown materials in the residual bodies of step 19 spermatids (unpublished data). Thus, nuage proteins are associated with various structures that are unrelated to the nuage. Although it is not clear whether the nuage proteins function there, it is likely that they are active in some of the structures mentioned above.

## 6. Conclusion - Future nuage research

In classic reports, the CB was detected in either the nucleus or the cytoplasm, but there was no obvious evidence to confirm either location. More recent studies have suggested that the IMC is a source of the CB. However, in TDRD-1-null mice, CBs were present in spite of the fact that the IMC disappeared (Chuma et al., 2006). It therefore appears that IMC is not essential for the formation of the CB. Recently, Meikar et al. (2010) purified the CB by immunoprecipitation and found that it contained more than 100 proteins. MitoPLD is essential for the formation of IMC, while PA, which is produced by MitoPLD, affects the architecture of the CB (Huang et al., 2011; Watanabe et al., 2011), suggesting that various proteins and factors are involved in the construction of nuage. Nuage has various forms and is associated with other subcellular organelles such as the nucleus, mitochondria, and the Golgi apparatus (Parvinen, 2005), suggesting that communication between nuage and the other organelles is important for the completion of spermatogenesis. More detailed studies of the properties of nuage will elucidate its function and origin.

One big question remains to be answered: during meiosis, after chromosome recombination has occurred, where do the nuage components go, how are they divided between the daughter cells equally, and how is the nuage reformed? It is also unclear how nuage or nuage components contribute to meiosis. MAEL suppresses transcription via the small RNA pathway during meiosis (Costa et al., 2006). Defects in several nuage components cause the arrest of spermatogenesis before meiosis, suggesting that the correct function of these components is essential for spermatogenesis. Microtubule-dependent movement of the CB is critical to enable communication with other organelles (Kotaja et al., 2006b; Huang et al., 2011; Watanabe et al., 2011).

Frost et al. (2010) suggested that the piRNA silencing complex may be constructed hierarchically. In other reports, nuage protein immunofluorescence staining patterns in some cases overlap completely, but in others only partially, even in the same stage of spermatogenesis (Figure 7). These observations suggest that nuage is formed hierarchically by the coalescence of small complexes assembled from a few proteins. To confirm whether this is indeed the case, we need to clarify the precise relationships among nuage components.

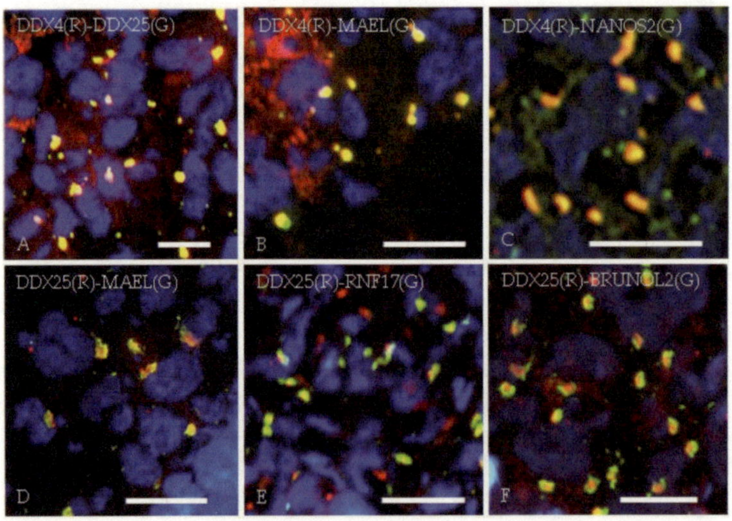


Fig. 7. Immunofluorescence staining of rat seminiferous epithelium with a combination of two different antibodies. Different antigens were stained using Alexa Fluor® 488 and Alexa Fluor® 568. The images were merged using Adobe Photoshop®. Staining for (A) DDX4 and DDX25, (B) DDX4 and MAEL, (C) DDX4 and NANOS2, (D) DDX25 and MAEL, (E) DDX25 and RNF17, and (F) DDX25 and BRUNOL2. All proteins examined were localized to CBs and two staining patterns were seen: 1) the patterns for both proteins completely overlapped within the CBs (A–C); and 2) the patterns for both proteins partially overlapped within the CBs (D–F). This clearly indicates that some nuage proteins distribute homogeneously, while others are segregated within CBs. Bar = 50 μm.

Figure 8 summarizes the possible functions of nuage in molecular biology and morphology. While the function and significance of nuage in spermatogenic cells have begun to be elucidated, they still remain largely unclear. Collecting information on nuage components and clarifying the function of other nuage-like structures may reveal insights into the significance of nuage in the development and maintenance of germ cells.

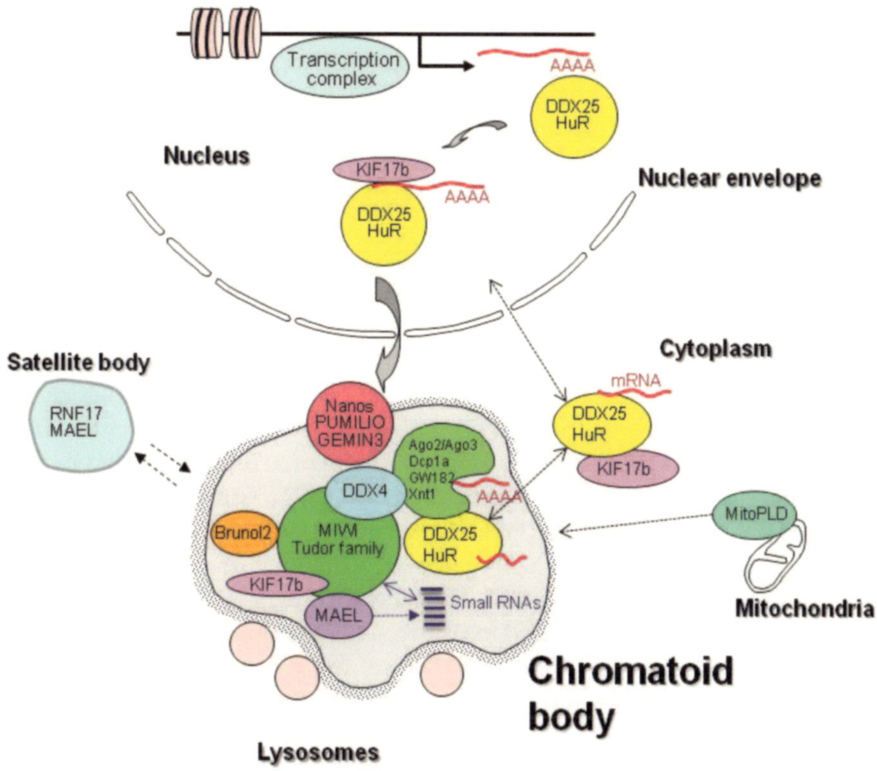


Fig. 8. Possible functions of nuage. Haploid gene products, including RNA binding proteins such as DDX25 and HuR, and microtubule-associated proteins such as KIF17b, bind to RNP. The mRNA-RNP complex is transported from the nucleus to the cytoplasm via the nuclear pore complex, or directly, to the CB. The movement of this complex is known to be supported by the microtubule network. In the cytoplasm, the CB frequently associates with the nuclear pores to interact with mRNAs. The CB contains RNA-binding and RNA-processing proteins such as DDX4, DDX6, and DDX25, and components of the RNA silencing and RNA decay pathways, such as small RNAs, Dicer, MAEL, Piwi family proteins, and Tudor family proteins. Furthermore, the CB contains P-body components such as Ago2, Dcp1a, GW182, and Xnt1, and thus, like the P-body, functions as a post-transcriptional regulator. The CB also contains an RNA-protecting protein, HuR. mRNAs stored in the CB are released into the cytoplasm in response to appropriate stimuli and are translated. Dicer produces small RNAs from their precursors in the CB. The mitochondrial membrane protein MitoPLD is involved in the movement and construction of the CB. The CB also contains the ubiquitin-conjugating enzyme E2. Some CB proteins are polyubiquitinated and degraded by proteasomes located on the surface of the CB (dots). Other components are degraded by lysosomes in close contact with the CB.

## 7. References

Adams, E.C. & Hertig, A.T. (1964) Studies on guinea pig oocytes. I. Electron microscopic observation on the development of cytoplasmic organelles in oocytes of primordial and primary follicles. *J. Cell Biol.* Vol. 21, pp. 397–427, ISSN 0021-9525

André J. (1962) Contribution of à la conaissance du chondriome. *J. Ultrastruct. Res.* Vol. 6, No. 3, pp. 1-185, ISSN 0022-5320

Aravin, A.A., van der Heijden, G.W., Castañeda, J., Vagin, V.V., Hannon, G.J. & Bortvin, A. (2009) Cytoplasmic compartmentalization of the fetal piRNA pathway in mice. *PLoS Genet.* Vol. 5, No. 12, pp e1000764. ISSN 1553-7404

Benda, C. (1891) Neue Mittheilungen über die Entwickelung der Genitadrüsen und über die Metamorphose der Samenzellen (Histogenese der Spermatozoen) *Arch. Anat. Physiol. Physiol.* Vol. 30, pp. 549–552

Brökelmann, J. (1963) Fine structure of germ cells and Sertoli cells during the cycle of the seminiferous epithelium in the rat. *Z. Zellforsch.* Vol. 59, pp. 820-850, ISSN 0340-0336

Burgos, M.H. & Fawcett, D.W. (1955) Studies on the structure of the mammalian testis. I. Differentiation of the spermatids in the cat (Felis domestica) *J. Biophys. Biochem. Cytol.* Vol. 1, pp. 287–315, ISSN 0095-9901

Burgos, M.H., Vitale-Calpe, R. & Aoki, A. (1970) Fine structure of the testis and its functional significance Vol. 1. In: "The Testis", Johnson, A.D., Gomes, W.R. & Vandemark, N.L. (Ed.) pp. 552–649, Acad. Press, New York.

Challice, C.E. (1953) Electron microscopic studies of spermiogenesis in some rodents. *J. Roy. Micros. Soc.* Vol. 73, No. 3, pp. 115–127, ISSN 0368-3974

Chuma, S., Hiyoshi, M., Yamamoto, A., Hosokawa, M., Takamune, K. & Nakatsuji, N. (2003) Mouse Tudor Repeat-1 (MTR-1) is a novel component of chromatoid bodies/nuages in male germ cells and forms a complex with snRNPs. *Mech Dev.* Vol. 120, No. 9, pp. 979-990, ISSN 1872-6356

Chuma, S., Hosokawa, M., Kitamura, K., Kasai, S., Fujioka, M., Hiyoshi, M., Takamune, K., Noce, T. & Nakatsuji, N. (2006) Tdrd1/Mtr-1, a tudor-related gene, is essential for male germ-cell differentiation and nuage/germinal granule formation in mice. *Proc Natl Acad Sci U S A.* Vol. 103, No. 43, pp. 15894-15899, ISSN 1091-6490

Clermont, Y., Leblond, C.P. & Meissier, B. (1959) Durée du cycle de l'épithélium séminal du rat. *Arch. Anat. Micrscop. Morphol. Exptl.* Vol. 48, pp. 37-56.

Clermont, Y., Oko, R. & Hermo, L. (1990) Immunocytochemical localization of proteins utilized in the formation of outer dense fibers and fibrous sheath in rat spermatids: An electron microscope study. Vol. 227, No.4, pp. 447-457, ISSN 1097-0185

Clermont, Y., Oko, R. & Hermo, L. (1993) Cell Biology of Mammalian Spermiogenesis, In: *Cell and Molecular Biology of the Testis,* Desjardins, C. & Ewing, L.L. (eds.) pp. 332-376

Clermont, Y. & Rambourg, A. (1978) Evolution of the endoplasmic reticulum during rat spermiogenesis. *Am. J. Anat.* Vol. 151, No. 2, pp. 191-212, ISSN 0002-9106

Comings, D.E. & Okada, T A. (1972) The chromatoid body in mouse spermatogenesis: evidence that it may be formed by the extrusion of nucleolar components. J. Ultrastruct. Res. Vol. 39, No.,1 pp. 15-23, ISSN 0022-5320

Costa, Y., Speed, R.M., Gautier, P., Semple, C.A., Maratou, K., Turner, J.M. & Cooke, H.J. (2006) Mouse MAELSTROM: the link between meiotic silencing of unsynapsed chromatin and microRNA pathway? *Hum Mol Genet,* Vol. 15, No.15, pp. 2324-2334, ISSN 0964-6906

Daoust, R. & Clermont, Y. (1955) Distribution of nucleic acids in germ cells during the cycle of the seminiferous epithelium in the rat. *Am J Anat.* Vol. 96, No. 2, pp. 255-83, ISSN 0002-9106

De Kretser, D.M. & Kerr, J.B. (1988) The cytology of the testis, In: *The Physiology of Reproduction,* Knobil, E. Neill, J. D. et al. (eds.) pp. 837-932, Raven Press, New York.

Deng, W. & Lin, H. (2002) miwi, a murine homolog of piwi, encodes a cytoplasmic protein essential for spermatogenesis. *Dev Cell.* Vol. 2, No. 6, pp. 819-830, ISSN 1878-1551

Dhainaut, A. (1970) Etude en microscopie électronique et par autoradiographie á haute résolution des extrusions nucléaires au cours de l'ovogenèse de Nereis pelagica (Annélide polychète) *J. Microscopie.* Vol. 9, pp. 99–118

Duesberg, J. (1908) Les division des spermatocytes chez le rat (Mus decumanus Pall., variété albinos) *Arch. Zellforsch.* Vol.1, pp. 399–449

Eddy, E.M. (1970) Cytochemical observations on the chromatoid body of the male germ cells. *Biol. Reprod.* Vol. 2, No. 1, pp. 114–128, ISSN 1529-7268

Eddy, E.M. (1974) Fine structural observations on the form and distribution of nuage in germ cells of the rat. *Anat Rec.* Vol. 178, No. 4, pp. 731-757, ISSN 1097-0185

Eddy, E.M. & Ito, S. (1971) Fine structural and radioautographic observations on dense perinuclear cytoplasmic material in tadpole oocytes. *J Cell Biol.,* Vol. 49, No.1, pp. 90-108, ISSN 1540-8140

Fasten, N. (1914) Spermatogenesis of the American grayfish, *Cambarus virilis* and *Cambrarus immunis* (?), with special reference to synapsis and the chromatoid bodies. *J. Morph.* Vol. 25, pp. 587–649, ISSN 1097-4687

Fawcett, D.W., Eddy, E.M. & Phillips, DM. (1970) Observations on the fine structure and relationships of the chromatoid body in mammalian spermatogenesis. *Biol Reprod.* Vol. 2, No. 1, pp. 129-153, ISSN 1529-7268

Fawcett, D.W. & Phillips, D.M. (1969) The fine structure and development of the neck region of the mammalian spermatozoon. *Anat. Rec.* Vol. 165, pp. 153-184, ISSN 1097-0185

Frost, R.J., Hamra, F.K., Richardson, J.A., Qi X., Bassel-Duby, R. & Olson, E.N. (2010) MOV10L1 is necessary for protection of spermatocytes against retrotransposons by Piwi-interacting RNAs *Proc Natl Acad Sci U S A.* Vol. 107, No. 26, pp. 11847-11852, ISSN 1091-6490

Gatenby, J.E. & Beams, H.W. (1935) The cytoplasmic inclusions in the spermatogenesis of man. *Q. J. Microsc. Sci.* Vol. 18, pp. 1-33, ISSN 0370-2952

Ginter-Matuszewska, B., Kusz, K., Spik, A., Grzeszkowiak, D., Rembiszewska, A., Kupryjanczyk, J. & Jaruzelska, J. (2011) NANOS1 and PUMILIO2 bind microRNA biogenesis factor GEMIN3, within chromatoid body in human germ cells. *Histochem Cell Biol.* Vol.136, No. 3, pp.279-287

Haraguchi, C.M., Ishido, K., Kominami, E. & Yokota, S. (2003) Expression of cathepsin H in differentiating rat spermatids: Immnuoelectron microscopic study. *Histochem. Cell Biol.* Vol. 120, No. 1, pp. 63-71, ISSN 0948-6143

Haraguchi, C. M., Mabuchi, T., Hirata, S., Shoda, T., Hoshi, K., Akasaki, K. & Yokota, S. (2005) Chromatoid bodies: Aggresome-like characteristics and degradation sites for organelles of spermiogenic cells. *J. Histochem. Cytochem.* Vol. 53, No. 4, pp. 455–465, ISSN 0022-1554

Heller, C.G. & Clermont, Y. (1964) Kinetics of the germinal epithelium in man. *Rec. Prog. Hormone Res.* Vol. 20, pp. 545-575

Hermann, F. (1889) Beiträge zur Histologie des Hodens. *Arch. f. mikr. Anat.* Vol. 34, pp. 58-105

Hosokawa, M., Shoji, M., Kitamura, K., Tanaka, T., Noce, T., Chuma, S. & Nakatsuji, N. (2007) Tudor-related proteins TDRD1/MTR-1, TDRD6 and TDRD7/TRAP: domain composition, intracellular localization, and function in male germ cells in mice. *Dev Biol.* Vol. 301, No. 1, pp. 38-52, ISSN 0012-1606

Huang, H., Gao, Q., Peng, X., Choi, S.Y., Sarma, K., Ren, H., Morris, A.J. & Frohman, MA. (2011) piRNA-associated germline nuage formation and spermatogenesis require MitoPLD profusogenic mitochondrial-surface lipid signaling. *Dev Cell.* Vol. 20, No. 3, pp. 376-387, ISSN 1878-1551

Kedersha, N., Stoecklin, G., Ayodele, M., Yacono, P., Lykke-Andersen, J., Fritzler, M.J., Scheuner, D., Kaufman, R.J., Golan, D.E. & Anderson, P. (2005) Stress granules and processing bodies are dynamically linked sites of mRNP remodeling. *J Cell Biol.* Vol. 169, No. 6, pp. 871-884, ISSN 1540-8140

Kerr, J.B. & Dixon, K.E. (1974) An ultrastructural study of germ plasm in spermatogenesis of *Xenopus laevis. J Embryol Exp Morphol.* Vol. 32, No. 3, pp. 573-592, ISSN 0022-0752

Kirino, Y., Vourekas, A., Kim, N., de Lima Alves F., Rappsilber J., Klein P.S., Jongens T.A. & Mourelatos Z. (2010) Arginine methylation of vasa protein is conserved across phyla. *J Biol Chem.* Vol. 285, No. 11,pp. 8148-8154, ISSN 0021-9258

Kotaja, N., Bhattacharyya, S.N., Jaskiewicz, L., Kimmins, S., Parvinen, M., Filipowicz, W. & Sassone-Corsi P. (2006a) The chromatoid body of male germ cells: similarity with processing bodies and presence of Dicer and microRNA pathway components. *Proc Natl Acad Sci U S A.* Vol. 103, No. 8, pp. 2647-52, ISSN 1091-6490.

Kotaja, N., Lin, H., Parvinen, M. & Sassone-Corsi, P. (2006b) Interplay of PIWI/argonaute protein MIWI and kinesin KIF17b in chromatoid bodies of male germ cells. *J. Cell Sci.* Vol. 119, No. 13, pp. 2819-2825, ISSN 0021-9533

Kotaja, N. & Sassone-Corsi, P. (2007) The chromatoid body: a germ-cell-specific RNA-processing centre. *Nat Rev Mol Cell Biol.* Vol. 8, pp. 85-90, ISSN 1471-0072

Kress, C., Gautier-Courteille, C., Osborne, H.B., Babinet, C. & Paillard, L. (2007) Inactivation of CUG-BP1/CELF1 causes growth, viability, and spermatogenesis defects in mice. *Mol Cell Biol.* Vol. 27, No. 3, pp. 1146-1157, ISSN 0270-7360

Kuramochi-Miyagawa, S., Kimura, T., Ijiri, T.W., Isobe, T., Asada, N., Fujita, Y., Ikawa, M., Iwai, N., Okabe, M., Deng, W., Lin, H., Matsuda, Y. & Nakano, T. (2004) Mili, a mammalian member of piwi family gene, is essential for spermatogenesis. *Development.* Vol. 131, No. 4, pp. 839-849, ISSN 0959-1991

Ma, L., Buchold, G.M., Greenbaum, M.P., Roy, A., Burns, K.H., Zhu, H., Han, D.Y., Harris, R.A., Coarfa, C., Gunaratne, P.H., Yan, W. & Matzuk, M.M. (2009) GASZ is essential for male meiosis and suppression of retrotransposon expression in the male germline. *PLoS Genet.* Vol. 5, No. 9, pp. e1000635, ISSN 1553-7390

Mahowald, A.P. (1962) Fine structure of pole cells and polar granules in *Drosophila melanogaster. J. Exp. Zool.* Vol. 151, No. 3, pp. 201-215, ISSN 0022-104X

Meikar, O., Da Ros, M., Liljenbäck, H., Toppari, J. & Kotaja, N. (2010) Accumulation of piRNAs in the chromatoid bodies purified by a novel isolation protocol. *Exp Cell Res.* Vol. 316, No. 9, pp. 1567-1575, ISSN 0014-4827

Meister, G., Landthaler, M., Patkaniowska, A., Dorsett, Y., Teng, G. & Tuschl, T. (2004) Human Argonaute2 mediates RNA cleavage targeted by miRNAs and siRNAs. *Mol Cell.* Vol. 15, No. 2, pp. 185-197, ISSN 1097-2765

Minamino, T. (1955) Spermiogenesis in the albino rat as revealed by electron microscopy. *Electron Microsc.* Vol. 4, pp. 249-253

Nguyen, C.M., Chalmel, .F, Agius, E., Vanz,o N., Khabar, K.S., Jégou, B. & Morello, D.. (2009) Temporally regulated traffic of HuR and its associated ARE-containing mRNAs from the chromatoid body to polysomes during mouse spermatogenesis. PLoS One. Vol. 4, No. 3, pp. e4900 (1-13), ISSN 1932-6203

Nicander, L. & Plöen, L. (1969) Fine structure of spermatogonia and primary spermatocytes in rabbits. *Z. Zellforsch.* Vol. 99, pp. 221-234

Nieuwkoop, P.D. & Faber, J. (1956) *Normal table of Xenopus laevis (Daudin).* North Holland Publ. Co., Amsterdam.

Noce, T., Okamoto-Ito, S. & Tsunekawa, N. (2001) Vasa homolog genes in mammalian germ cell development. *Cell Struct Funct.* Vol. 26, No. 3, pp. 131-136, ISSN 0386-7196

Odor, D.L. (1965) The ultrastructure of unilaminar follicles of the hamster ovary. *Am. J. Anat.* Vol. 116, pp. 493–522, 0002-9106

Onohara, Y., Fujiwara, T., Yasukochi, T., Himeno, M. & Yokota, S. (2010) Localization of mouse vasa homolog protein in chromatoid body and related nuage structures of mammalian spermatogenic cells during spermatogenesis. *Histochem Cell Biol.* Vol. 133, No. 6, pp. 627-639, ISSN 0948-6143

Pan, J., Goodheart, M., Chuma, S., Nakatsuji, N., Page, D.C. & Wang, P.J. (2005) RNF17, a component of the mammalian germ cell nuage, is essential for spermatogenesis. *Development.* 132:4029–4039.

Parvinen, M. (2005) The chromatoid body in spermatogenesis. *Int. J. Androl.* Vol. 28, No. 4, pp. 189-201

Parvinen, M. & Jokelainen, PT. (1974) Rapid movements of the chromatoid body in living early spermatids of the rat. *Biol Reprod.* Vol. 11, No. 1, pp. 85-92, ISSN 1529-7268

Parvinen, M. & Parvinen, L.M. (1979) Active movements of the chromatoid body. A possible transport mechanism for haploid gene products. *J. Cell Biol.* Vol. 80, No. 3, pp. 621-628, ISSN 1540-8140

Pollister, A.W. (1930) Cytoplasmic phenomena in the Gerris. *J. Morph.* Vol. 49, pp. 455-507, ISSN 1097-4687

Regaud, C.L. (1901) Études sur la structure des tubes séminifères et sur la spermatogénèse chez les Mammifères. *Arch. Anat. Micr. Morphol. Exp.* Vol. 4, pp. 231–380

Russell, L. & Frank, B. (1978) Ultrastructural characterization of nuage in spermatocytes of the rat testis. *Anat Rec.* Vol. 190, No. 1, pp. 79-97, ISSN 1097-0185

Saga, Y. (2008) Sexual development of mouse germ cells; Nanos2 promotes the male germ cell fate by suppressing the female pathway. *Develop. Growth Differ.* Vol. 50, Supple. 1, pp. S141-S147, ISSN 0012-1592

Sasa, S. (1959) On the ultrastructure of the spermatogenic cells of the albino rat. *J. Chiba Med. Soc.* Vol. 34, pp. 1698-1721, ISSN 0009-3459

Sasaki, T., Shiohama, A., Minoshima, .S. & Shimizu, N. (2003) Identification of eight members of the Argonaute family in the human genome small star, filled. *Genomics.* Vol. 82, No. 3, pp. 323-330, ISSN 0888-7543

Sato, H., Tsai-Morris, C.H. & Dufau, M.L. (2010) Relevance of gonadotropin-regulated testicular RNA helicase (GRTH/DDX25) in the structural integrity of the chromatoid body during spermatogenesis. *Biochim Biophys Acta.* Vol. 1803, No. 5, pp. 534-543, ISSN 0006-3002

Schreiner, A. & Schreiner, K.E. (1905) Über die Entwickelung der männlichen Geschlechtszellen von Myxine glutinosa. *Arch. Biol.* Vol. 21, pp. 183-355

Sen, G.L. & Blau, H.M. (2005) Argonaute 2/RISC resides in sites of mammalian mRNA decay known as cytoplasmic bodies. *Nat Cell Biol.* Vol. 7, No.6, pp. 633-636, ISSN 1465-7392

Sheng, Y., Tsai-Morris, C.H., Gutti, R., Maeda, Y. & Dufau, M.L. (2006) Gonadotropin-regulated testicular RNA helicase (GRTH/Ddx25) is a transport protein involved in gene-specific mRNA export and protein translation during spermatogenesis. *J Biol Chem.* Vol. 281, No. 46, pp. 35048-35056, ISSN 0021-9258

Shoji, M., Tanaka, T., Hosokawa, M., Reuter, M., Stark, A., Kato, Y., Kondoh, G., Okawa, K., Chujo, T., Suzuki, T., Hata, K., Martin, S.L., Noce, T., Kuramochi-Miyagawa, S., Nakano, T., Sasaki, H., Pillai, R.S., Nakatsuji, N. & Chuma, S. (2009) The TDRD9-MIWI2 complex is essential for piRNA-mediated retrotransposon silencing in the mouse male germline. *Dev Cell.* Vol. 17, No. 6, pp. 775-787, ISSN 1878-1551

Snee, M.J. & Macdonald, P.M. (2004) Live imaging of nuage and polar granules: evidence against a precursor-product relationship and a novel role for Oskar in stabilization of polar granule components. *J Cell Sci.* Vol. 117, Pt. 10, pp. 2109-2020, ISSN 0021-9533

Söderström, K.O. (1978) Formation of chromatoid body during rat spermatogenesis. *Z Mikrosk Anat Forsch.* Vol. 92, No. 3, pp. 417-430, ISSN 0044-3107

Söderström, K.O. & Parvinen, M. (1976) In corporation of [3H]uridine by the chromatoid body during rat spermatogenesis. *J. Cell. Biol.* Vol. 70, No. 1, pp. 239-246, ISSN1540-8140

Sorokin, S.P. (1968) Reconstruction of centriole formation and ciliogenesis in mammalian lungs. *J. Cell Sci.* Vol. 3, No. 2, pp. 207-230, ISSN 0021-9533

Stefani, G. & Slack, G. (2008) Small non-coding RNAs in animal development. *Nature review,* Vol. 9, No. 3, pp. 219-230, ISSN9;219-230

Stockinger, .L. & Cirelli, E. (1965) Eine bisher unbekannte Art der Zentiolenvermehrung. *Z. Zellforsh. Mikroscop. Anat. Abt. Histochem.* Vol. 68, pp. 233-740

Sud, B.N. (1961). Morphological and cytochemical studies of the chromatoid body and related elements in the spermatogenesis of the rat. *Q J Microsc Sci* Vol. 102, pp. 495-505, ISSN 0370-2952

Susi, F.R. & Clermont, Y. (1970) Fine structural modifications of the rat chromatoid body during spermiogenesis. *Am J Anat.* Vol. 129, No. 2, pp. 177-191, ISSN 0002-9106

Tanaka, S.S., Toyooka, Y., Akasu, R., Katoh-Fukui, Y., Nakahara, Y., Suzuki, R., Yokoyama, M. & Noce, T. (2000) The mouse homolog of Drosophila Vasa is required for the development of male germ cells. Genes Dev. Vol. 14, No. 7, pp. 841-853, ISSN 0890-9369

Tang, P.Z., Tsai-Morris, C.H. & Dufau, M.L. (1999) A novel gonadotropin-regulated testicular RNA helicase. A new member of the dead-box family. *J Biol Chem.* Vol. 274, No. 53, pp. 37932-37940, ISSN 0021-9258

Vasileva, A., Tiedau, D., Firooznia, A., Müller-Reichert, T. & Jessberger, R. (2009) Tdrd6 is required for spermiogenesis, chromatoid body architecture, and regulation of miRNA expression. *Curr Biol.* Vol. 19, No. 8, pp. 630-639, ISSN 0960-9822

Ventelä, S., Toppari, J. & Parvinen, M. (2003) Intracellular organelle traffic through cytoplasmic bridges in early spermatids of the rat; mechanism of haploid gene product sharing. *Mol. Biol. Cell* Vol. 14, No. 7, pp. 2768-2780, ISSN 1059-1524

von Brunn, A.V. Beiträge zur Entwicklungsgeschiche der Samenkörper. (1876) Arch. f. Mikr. Anat. Vol. 12, pp. 528-536

von Ebner, V. (1888) Zur Spermatogenese bei den Säugethieren. *Arch. f. Mikr. Anat.* Vol. 31, pp. 236-292

von Korff, K. (1902) Zur histogenese der spermien von Phalangista vulpine. *Arch. f. Mikr. Anat.* Vol. 60, pp. 232-260

Watanabe, T., Chuma, S., Yamamoto, Y., Kuramochi-Miyagawa, S., Totoki, Y., Toyoda, A., Hoki, Y., Fujiyama, A., Shibata, T., Sado, T., Noce, T., Nakano, T., Nakatsuji, N., Lin, H. & Sasaki, H. (2011) MITOPLD is a mitochondrial protein essential for nuage formation and piRNA biogenesis in the mouse germline. *Dev Cell.* Vol. 20, No. 3, pp. 364-375, ISSN 1878-1551

Watson, M.L. (1952) Spermatogenesis in the albino rat as revealed by electron microscopy. *Biochim. Biophys. Acta.* Vol. 8, No. 4, pp. 369-374, ISSN 0006-3002

Weakley B.S. (1969) Granular cytoplasmic bodies in oocytes of the golden hamster during the post-natal period. *Z. Zellforsch. Mikrosk. Anat.* Vol. 101, No. 3, pp. 394-400, ISSN 0340-0336

Wilson, E.B. (1913) A chromatoid body simulating an accessory chromosome in pentatoma. *Biol. Bull.* Vol. 24, No. 6, pp. 392-411, ISSN 0006-3185

Wodesdalek, J.E. (1914) Spermatogenesis of the horse with special reference to the accessory chromosome and the chromatoid body. *Biol. Bull.* Vol. 27, No. 6, pp. 295-325, ISSN 0006-3185

Yabuta, Y., Ohta, H., Abe, T., Kurimoto, K., Chuma, S. & Saitou, M. (2011) TDRD5 is required for retrotransposon silencing, chromatoid body assembly, and spermiogenesis in mice. *J Cell Biol.* Vol. 192, No. 5, pp. 781-795, ISSN 1540-8140

Yin, X.Y., Gupta, K., Han, W.P., Levitan, E.S. & Prochownik, E.V. (1999) Mmip-2, a novel RING finger protein that interacts with mad members of the Myc oncoprotein network. *Oncogene.* Vol. 18, No. 48, pp. 6621-6634, ISSN 0950-9232

Yin, X.Y, Grove, L.E. & Prochownik, E.V. (2001) Mmip-2/Rnf-17 enhances c-Myc function and regulates some target genes in common with glucocorticoid hormones. *Oncogene*. Vol. 20, No. 23, pp. 2908-2917, ISSN 0950-9232

Zlotnik, I. (1947) The cytplasmic components of germ-cells during spermatogenesis in the domestic fowl. *Q. J. Microsc. Sci.* Vol. 88, No. 3, pp. 353-365, ISSN 0370-2952

13

# Meiotic Behaviour of Chromosomes Involved in Structural Chromosomal Abnormalities Determined by Preimplantation Genetic Diagnosis

L. Xanthopoulou and H. Ghevaria
*University College London, UK*

## 1. Introduction

### 1.1 The origin of structural chromosomal abnormalities

Structural rearrangements can arise premeiotically, during meiosis or during postzygotic mitotic divisions. The main causes leading to chromosomal aberrations are illegitimate recombination due to chromosome misalignment and asymmetric pairing in meiosis and mitosis, defective DNA repair mechanisms and aberrant behaviour at the replication fork (Gardner and Sutherland, 2004).

Chromosome rearrangement breakpoints are not uniformly found throughout the genome (Lupski, 2004) and certain genomic regions, especially subtelomeric and pericentromeric regions (Shaw and Lupski, 2004) are more likely to be involved in a chromosomal rearrangement. This clustering of chromosomal rearrangements around hotspots creates considerable genomic instability (Shaw and Lupski, 2004). Such regions of genomic instability involve low copy repeats (LCRs).

LCRs act as substrates for non-allelic homologous recombination (NAHR), by erroneously facilitating different chromosome regions of the same or of different chromosomes to come together. Chromatin structure can also be involved in the generation of chromosomal aberrations, with areas which are less compacted being more accessible to double strand breaks and DNA damage (Shaw and Lupski, 2004).

There are also non-recurrent rearrangements, whose breakpoints are scattered around the genome and which often occur at unique sequences (Shaw and Lupski, 2004) but even in those cases the breakpoints often involve intronic motifs of smaller repetitive sequences which are usually involved in inducing susceptibility to double strand breaks (Toffolatti et al., 2002). Such rearrangements with unique breakpoints are created by non-homologous DNA end-joining (NHEJ), which is an error prone mechanism (Lieber et al., 2003) of repairing double strand breaks in multicellular organisms (Shaw and Lupski, 2005). NHEJ can result in genomic alterations by generating deletions or duplications through erroneously joining together the ends of double strand breaks from different chromosomes (Pfeiffer et al., 2004).

## 2. Structural chromosomal abnormalities and meiosis: Focussing on translocations

Structural chromosomal abnormalities involve chromosome breakage followed by the rejoining of chromosome parts into a different configuration. These structural rearrangements can be mainly categorised into translocations (reciprocal or robertsonian), insertions, inversions (pericentric or pericentric), deletions, duplications, ring chromosomes and isochromosomes. In the case of a structural rearrangement, each chromosome pair consists of a normal and a derivative chromosome.

Many structural abnormalities are associated with clinical charactteristics, such as mental retardation, characteristic dysmophic features and often other malformations and developmental delay. For example the cri-du-chat syndrome caused by a terminal deletion on chromosome 5, or the DiGeorge syndrome caused by a microdeletion on the long arm of chromosome 22. Duplication syndromes are also known to be associated with abnormal phenotypes, such as Charcot Marie Tooth disease Type I caused by a duplication in 17p12. Other structural aberrations such as inversions, translocations and ring chromosomes do not cause any abnormalities in balanced carriers when there is no gain or loss of genetic material, however these individuals are faced with reproductive problems.

The most common type of structural chromosomal abnormality in humans is translocation, most specifically reciprocal translocations that are seen in about 1 in 500 live births (Jacobs et al., 1992) and involve the exchange of genetic material between different chromosomes. In carriers of reciprocal translcoations, each chromosome pair consists of a normal and a derivative chromosome, as shown in figure 1i. Carriers are phenotypically normal since there is no loss of genetic material unless the breakpoints disrupt important genes (Gardner and Sutherland, 2004). However they are faced with unfavourable meiotic segregation patterns when the chromosomes involved in the translocation pair up at prophase forming a quadrivalent (also known as pachytene) as shown in figure 1ii. The chromosomal status of the gametes produced by a carrier of a reciprocal translocation depends on the segregation pattern that took place in meiosis. As shown in figure 1iii, the chromosomes in the quadrivalent can segregate in a 2:2 mode, whereby each daughter cell will receive 2 chromosomes, in a 3:1 segregation mode, whereby one daughter cell receives 3 chromosomes and the other daughter call receives just one or there might be complete non disjunction in a 4:0 mode of segregation.

Robertsonian translocations have a prevalence of 1 in 1000 and involve the centric fusion of two acrocentric chromosomes (in 75% of the cases chromosomes 13 and 14 are involved) and the loss of the short arms (Garner and Sutherland, 2004). As a result a derivative chromosome is formed as shown in figure 2i, which comprises of the two long arms of the chromosomes involved in the translocation and at meiosis the chromosomes pair up as shown in figure 2ii. The total chromosome number of carriers of Robertsonian translocations is 45. Although all acrocentric chromosomes have been found to be involved in Robertsonian translocations, rob(13q14q) and rob(14q21q) constitute around 85% of all Robertsonian translocations (Therman et al., 1989).

Balanced carriers of a structural chromosomal rearrangement are usually phenotypically normal since there is no loss of genetic material, unless the breakpoints are within important genes. They are however faced with unfavourable meiotic segregation patterns when the normal and derivative chromosome(s) involved in the abnormality pair up at meiosis I. Carriers therefore are at a high risk of producing unbalanced gametes and hence genetically abnormal embryos that are associated with recurrent miscarriage, infertility as well as unbalanced offspring (Gardner and Surtherland, 2004).

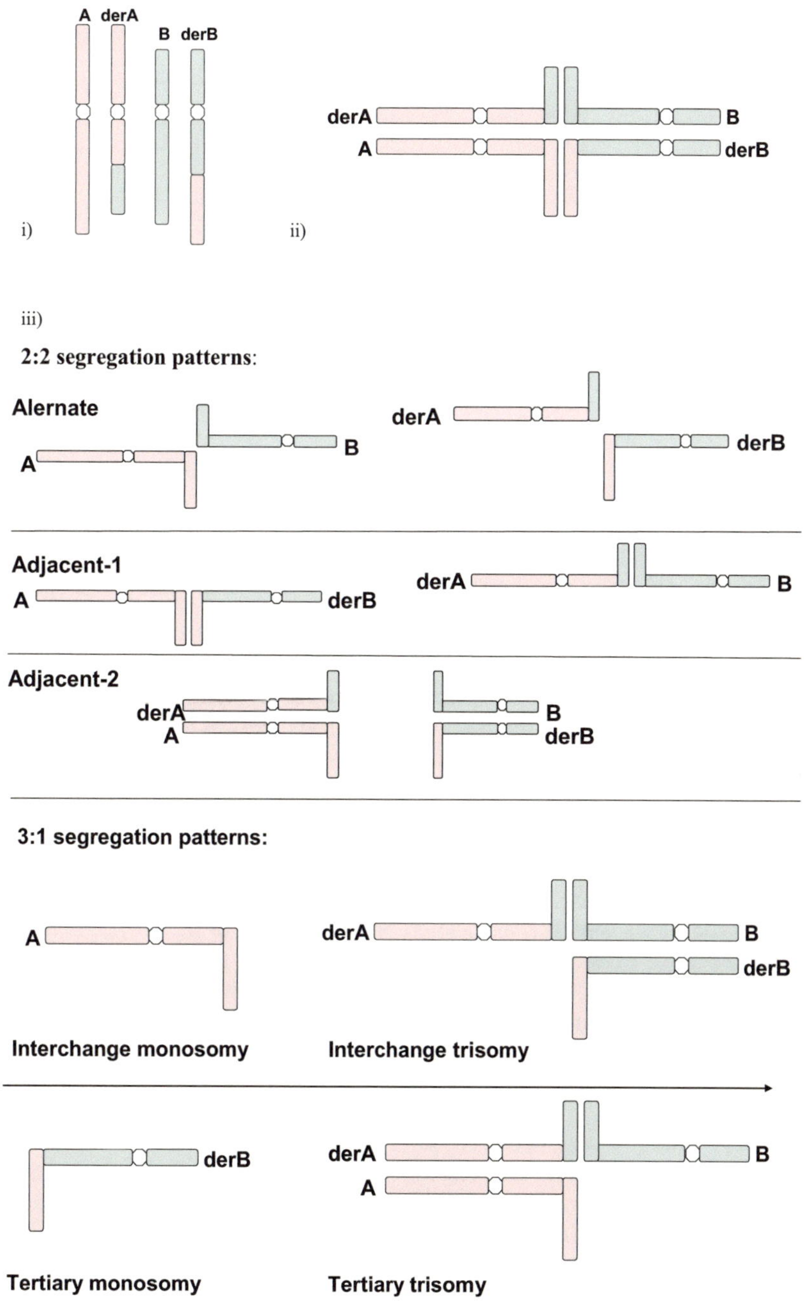


Fig. 1. i) Chromosomes in a cell of a carrier of a reciprocal translocation, ii) Pachytene configuration of the quadrivalent cross during meiosis in a carrier of a reciprocal translocation, iii) possible segregation modes seen at meiosis (4:0 segregants not shown here).

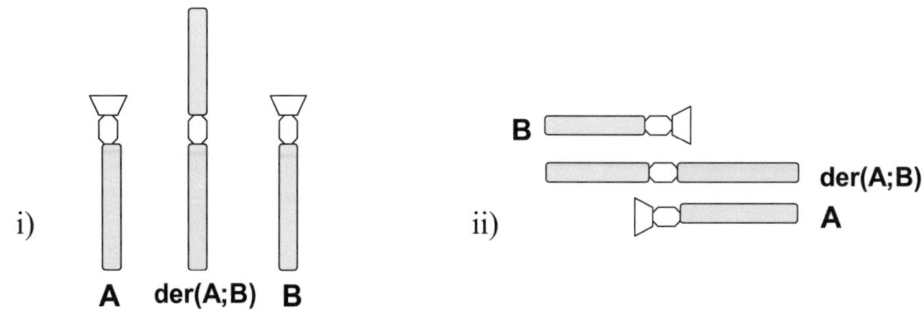


Fig. 2. i) Carrier of a Robertsonian translocation, ii) Pairing up of chromosomes, forming a trivalent during meiosis in a carrier of a Robertsonian translocation.

## 3. Preimplantation genetic diagnosis (PGD)

Preimplantation genetic diagnosis provides an alternative to prenatal diagnosis for couples at risk of having a child with a specific genetic or chromosomal abnormality. It involves the removal and testing of material from the oocyte or the developing embryo. First and second polar bodies for instance can be analysed in order to determine the genetic status of the oocyte (Verlinsky et al., 1990) or material can be biopsied from embryos generated through *in vitro* fertilization (IVF). In the case of embryo biopsy, one or two single blastomeres can be removed during the cleavage stage or material can be biopsied from the trophectoderm at the blastocyst stage (Dokras et al., 1990).

The biopsied material is then analysed by the polymerase chain reaction (PCR) for single gene disorders (Findlay et al., 1996) or fluorescent in situ hybridisation (FISH) for structural or numerical chromosomal abnormalities (Griffin et al., 1991, Coonen et al., 1998, Conn et al., 1998) whereas recently array comparative genomic hybridization (aCGH) has also been introduced (Alfarawati *et al.*, 2011). In this way unaffected embryos are selected and transferred to the uterus, aiming to establish an unaffected pregnancy.

Couples that are at risk of having a child with a specific single gene or chromosomal abnormality may opt to have PGD in order to avoid an affected pregnancy and to avoid having prenatal diagnosis which is associated with a 1% risk of miscarriage; moreover their decision to have PGD is often linked to the couple's view on pregnancy termination. At the same time other couples that seek PGD have difficulty achieving a pregnancy due to reasons of infertility or subfertility or are victims of repeated pregnancy loss.

## 4. PGD for structural chromosomal abnormalities: strategies and outcome

PGD provides a unique opportunity to investigate the meiotic behaviour of the chromosomes involved in a structural rearrangement. Until recently structural chromosomal abnormalities were tested for at PGD with FISH, using probes for the chromosomes involved in the translocation.

The main FISH probe strategies used in PGD for recirocal translocations, involve the use of probes flanking the breakpoint in one of the chromosomes, in conjunction with another probe on the other chromosome. In this way on one chromosome one probe distal to the breakpoint (i.e. a subtelomeric probe specific to the segment that is translocated) and one probe proximal to the breakpoint (i.e. a centromeric probe of any other probe that will be used for the enumeration of that chromosome) are used, together with another probe on the other chromosome, which can either be distal or proximal to the breakpoint on the second chromosome (Scriven et al.1998). So the main two strategies involve using two centromeric and one subtelomeric probe or one centromeric and two subtelomeric probes, where the subtelomeric probes will always be on the segments that are translocated. The aim of these probe strategies is to be able to detect all possible segregation patterns, so they need to be informative for both normal and boh derivative chromosomes.

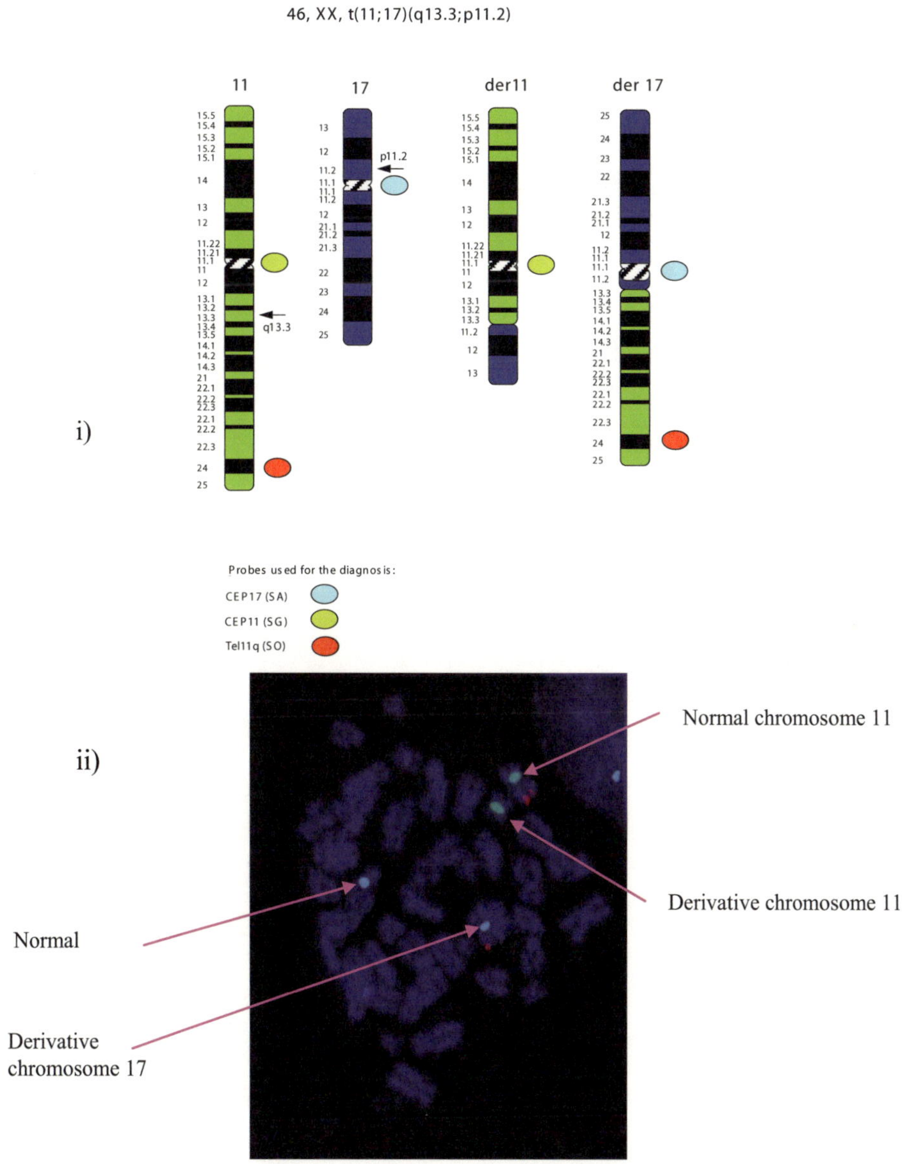


Fig. 3. i) Probe strategy for PGD for translocation 46, XX, t(11;17)(q13.3;p11.2), ii) Metaphase nucleus of the carrier of 46, XX, t(11;17)(q13.3;p11.2) after FISH with the probes for centromere of 11 and 17 and the telomere of 11q.

The probe strategy chosen for PGD for each srtuctural abnormality case is tested prior to clinical application on control lymphocyte slides from the parents of the couple seeking PGD. For example figure 3 below shows an example of a translocation between chromosomes 11 and 17, carried by the female partner: 46, XX, t(11;17)(q13.3;p11.2).

The centromeric probe for chromosome 11 in spectrum green and the centromeric probe for chromosome 17 in spectrum aqua were used together with the subtelomeric probe for 11q in psectrum orange. The probes were tested on parental lymphocytes and in figure 3ii it is clear that the probes chosen pick up the abnormality and allow us to distinuish between the normal and derivative chromosomes on the metaphase spread.

| Segregation mode in the gamete | | Chromosomes present in the gamete of the carrier parent | FISH signals seen in the embryo | Outcome |
|---|---|---|---|---|
| 2:2 segregation modes | Alternate | 11 and 17 | 2xCEP11, 2xTel11p, 2xCEP17 | Balanced |
| | | Der11 and der17 | 2xCEP11, 2xTel11p, 2xCEP17 | Balanced |
| | Adjacent-1 | 11 and der17 | 2xCEP11, 3xTel11p, 2xCEP17 | Partial trisomy 11, partial monosomy 17 |
| | | Der11 and 17 | 2xCEP11, 1xTel11p, 2xCEP17 | Partial monosomy 11, partial trisomy 17 |
| | Adjacent-2 | 11 and der11 | 3xCEP11, 2xTel11p, 1xCEP17 | Partial trisomy 11, partial monosomy 17 |
| | | 17 and der17 | 1xCEP11, 2xTel11p, 3xCEP17 | Partial monosomy 11, partial trisomy 17 |
| 3:1 segregation modes | 3 → | 11, der11 and 17 | 3xCEP11, 2xTel11p, 2xCEP17 | Partial trisomy 11 and 17 |
| | 1 → | Der17 | 1xCEP11, 2xTel11p, 2xCEP17 | Partial monosomy 11 partial monosomy 17 |
| | 3 → | 11, der11, der17 | 3xCEP11, 3xTel11p, 2xCEP17 | Trisomy 11 |
| | 1 → | 17 | 1xCEP11, 1xTel11p, 2xCEP17 | Monosomy 11 |
| | 3 → | Der11, 17, der17 | 2xCEP11, 2xTel11p, 3xCEP17 | Trisomy 17 |
| | 1 → | 11 | 2xCEP11, 2xTel11p, 1xCEP17 | Monosomy 17 |
| | 3 → | 11, 17, der17 | 2xCEP11, 3xTel11p, 3xCEP17 | Partial trisomy 11, partial trisomy 17 |
| | 1 → | Der11 | 2xCEP11, 1xTel11p, 1xCEP17 | Partial monosomy 11, partial monosomy 17 |

Table 1. Possible segregation patterns for the carrier of 46, XX, t(11;17)(q13.3;p11.2).

Once it has been established that a particular probe strategy is informative for the translocation chromosomes, the conditions of the FISH protocols are optimised and the couple can commence their stimulation to undergo their IVF cycle. The biopsied samples are then tested at PGD using the optimised protocol and embryos are diagnosed as balanced or unbalanced. Due to the fact that in the majority of cases of the nuclei of the biopsied cells during cleavage stage biopsy are in the interphase stage, it is not possuble to distinguish between balanced embryos that will be balanced carriers of the structural aberration and normal embryos (Munne, 2005). By considering the FISH signals for each embryo it is then possible to determine the segregation pattern that took place in the gamete of the carreir parent, as shown in table 1, although crossing over events between the centromere and the breakpoint can complicate the situation further and affect the interpretation of the results (Hulten, 2011). Only biopsied samples with two signals for each probe used will be balanced as two signals indicate diploid status for the loci tested. Any other combination of signals is unbalanced for the translocation chromosomes bue to chromosome malsegregation at meiosis.

Figure 4 shows another example of a reciprocal translocation between chromosomes 10 and 11, 46,XY,t(11;19)(q12.3;q13.1), the probe strategy used at PGD (figure 4ii) and images from single blastomeres that were biopsied on day 3 from cleavage stage embryos (figure 4ii).

i)

ii)

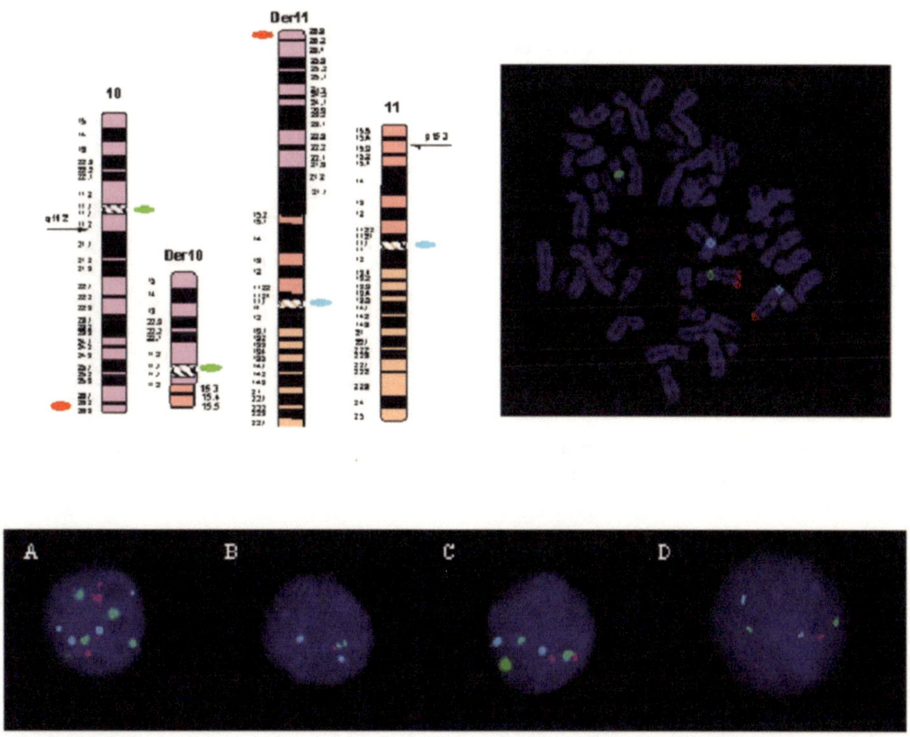


Fig. 4. Probe strategy for translocation 46,XY,t(11;19)(q12.3;q13.1) and FISH on the lymphocytes of the carrier parent and ii) images from the biopsied single cells from cleavage stage embryos at PGD. Only nucleus D is balanced for the translocation, whereas nucleus A is unbalanced and polyploid, nucleus B shows partial monosomy 10q and nucleus C shows partial trisomy 10.

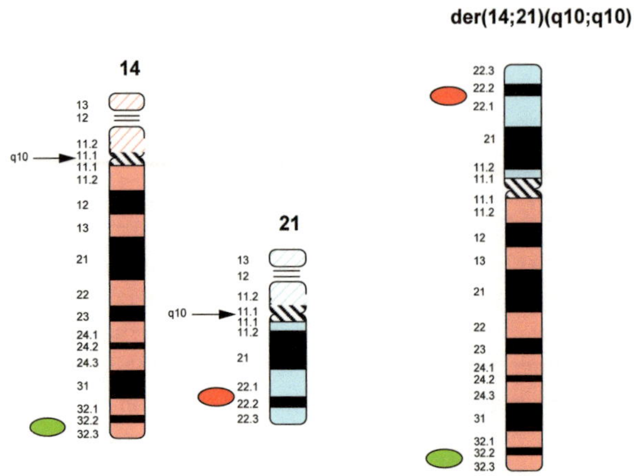


Fig. 5. Probe strategy for PGD for the Robertsonian translocation between chromosomes 14 and 21.

For Robertsonian translocations, the expected segregation patterns can also be worked out as shown in table 2. The resulting gametes are either nullisomic or disomic for either of the chromosomes involved in the translocation, resulting in monosomic or trisomic embryos (Scriven et al., 2001).

| **Segregation of the translocation chromosomes present in the gamete of the carrier parent** | **FISH signals seen in the embryo** | **Outcome** |
|---|---|---|
| 14, 21 | 2xTel14q, 2xLSI21 | Normal |
| Der14/21 | 2xTel14q, 2xLSI21 | Balanced |
| 14, der14/21 | 3xTel14q, 2xLSI21 | Trisomy 14 |
| 21 | 1xTel14q, 2xLSI21 | Monosomy 14 |
| 14 | 2xTel14q,1xLSI21 | Monosomy 21 |
| 21, der14/21 | 3xTel14q, 2xLSI21 | Trisomy 21 |

Table 2. Different possible segregation patterns at meiosis for the carrier of the Robertsonian translocation between chromosomes 14 and 21.

Since the first clinical PGD cases for carriers of translocations and structural abnormalities FISH was the method of choice for embryo testing in order to select those embryos that were balanced. A disadvantage of FISH however is that it only gives information for the chromosomes for which probes were used. Additional probes can be included in a subsequent round of hybridization for other chromosomes in order to test for the main chromosomes at risk of being aneuploid. Recently the application of aCGH has been reported in PGD for carriers of reciprocal or Robertsonian translocations as well as inversions (Alfarawati et al., 2011.) which allows the complete enumeration of all chromosome sets in a sample.

Results from PGD cycles for structural abnormalities using array CGH, have revealed aneuploidies for chromosomes other than those involved in the translocation, which could account for the poorer PGD outcome for women of advanced maternal age. Array CGH can also be used for the detection of other structural abnormalities, provided that the smallest translocated segment is detectable by the resolution of the array platform used. Alternatively when the segments are small FISH can be used. In the case of other structural aberrations, such as inversions, insertions, duplications and deletions, FISH involves the use probes that are included in the segment that is inverted, inserted, duplicated or deleted and one or two other probes on either side (proximally and distally) of that segment in order to be able to detect all different meiotic outcome combinations. Figure 6 below shows examples of strategies used in PGD for an inversion and an intrachromosomal insertion.

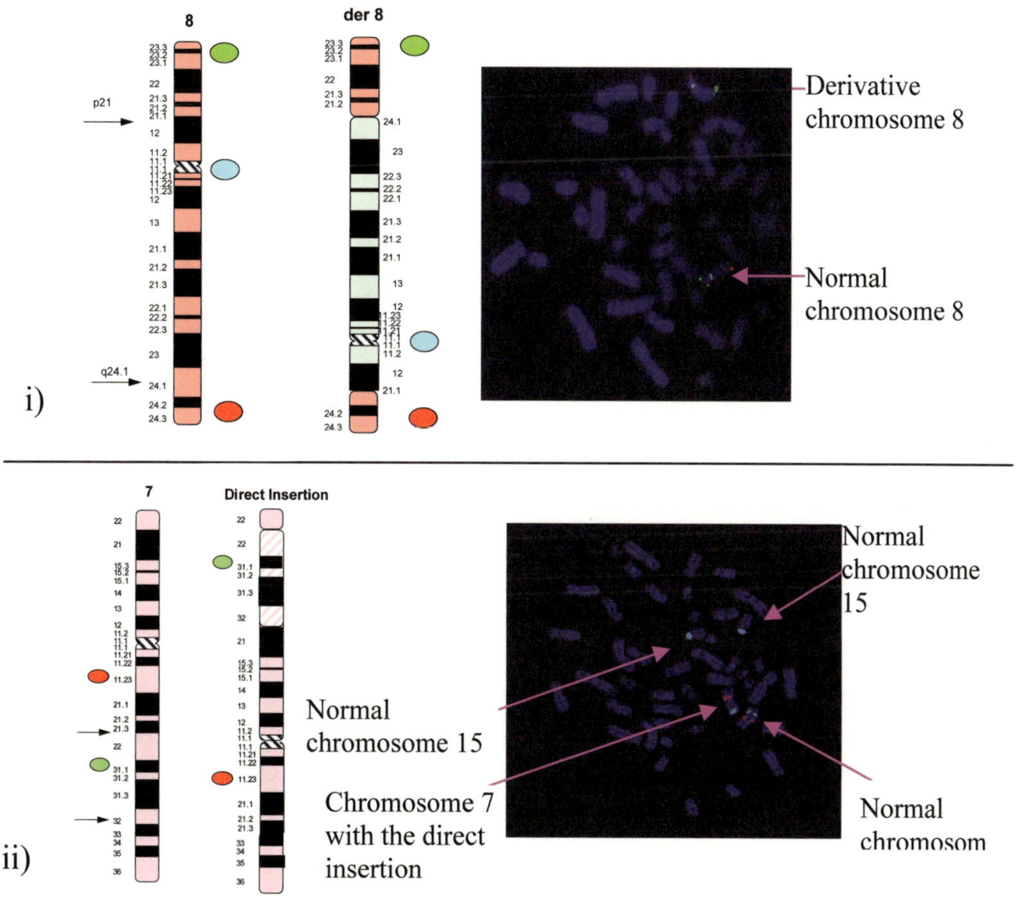


Fig. 6. i) Probe strategy for PGD for an intrachromosomal inversion, 46, XX, inv(8)(p21;q24.1) and FISH on the lymphocytes of the carrier parent, ii) probe stratege for PGD for an intrachromosomal insertion, 46, XY, dir ins (7)(p22q32q31.1) FISH on the lymphocytes of the carrier parent. An extra probe was used in this protocol for chromosome 15 to check for ploidy.

## 5. Evidence obtained from PGD treatment cycles relevant to the meiotic segregation of chromosomes involved in structural abnormalities

What is unique about studying preimplantation embryos is that all the products from all different modes of segregation from a structural aberration can be seen, which are not viable at later stages of development. Moreover in cases where the structural aberration involves a small segment, unbalanced forms are more likely to be tolerated until later stages of development.

For carriers of reciprocal translocations overall alternate segregation is reported as being the most common segregation pattern (Scriven et al., 2000), followed by adjacent-1 (25%), 3:1 (15%), adjacent-2 (10%) and 4:0 (2%), where most 3:1 segregations came from female carriers (Ogilvie and Scriven, 2002).

However each translocation is unique in terms of the position of the breakpoints and in terms of the length of the translocated segments. As a result different translocations will form different quadrivalents at meiosis I and in each case the configuration of the quadrivalent cross will be different. The quadrivalent configuration partly influences which spindle fibre gets attached to which centromere thus determining the way in which the translocation chromosomes will segregate (Gardner and Sutherland, 2004). The number and the position of chiasmata is also important (Scriven et al., 1998). Each translocation therefore behaves differently at meiosis (Conn et al., 1999) and hence for each translocation the frequency of each mode of segregation will be different and a particular segregation mode might occur at a higher frequency that others (Jalbert et al., 1980). In this way particular translocations will have a prediscposition towards a specific mode of segregation. In order to confirm the meiotic segregation patterns seen on PGD, full follow up analysis is required on the untransferred embryos, which allows us to study the chromosomal ploidy status of those embryos.

For Robertsonian translocations sperm studies have shown that the most common segregation pattern in carriers of Robertsonian translocations is alternate segregation that results in normal or balanced gametes (Ogur et al., 2006), whereas an interchromosomal effect was also seen, as aneuploidy for other chromosomes that were not involved in the translocation were seen. This interchromosomal effect, referring to the translocation chromosomes affecting the recombination and segregation of other chromosomes was also suggested for reciprocal translocations by Estop et al. (2000), but it was not detected in later studies (Oliver-Bonet et al., 2004).

Follow up analysis on untransferred embryos has revealed that cleavage stage embryos show a high level of mosaicism, a situation whereby more than one different cell lines is present in the embryo (Munne et al., 1993, Harper et al., 1995, Delhanty and Handyside, 1995). An extreme form of mosaicism is chaoticism, whereby almost every nucleus present in the embryo will have a different chromosome constitution. Mosaicism has been reported not only in arrested or fragmented embryos but also in embryos of good quality (Delhanty et al., 1997) and has been observed in the embryos of both young and older women (Munne et al., 1995). Different factors are thought to be involved in the formation of mosaic embryos, such as the ovarian stimulation protocol used or the embryo culture conditions, as well as the fact that cell-cycle checkpoints are not fully functional at those early stages of preimplantation embryo development (Delhanty and Handyside, 1995).

A high level of mosaicism has been reported in embryos from reciprocal translocation carriers (Simopoulou et al., 2003), Robertsonian translocation carriers (Conn et al., 1998) as well as other forms of structural abnormalities such as intrachromosomal insertions (Xanthopoulou et al., 2010). As far as the embryos from translocation carriers are concerned, Iwarsson et al. (2000) reported that the chromosomes involved in the translocation show an even higher degree of mosaicism when compared to control chromosomes. This suggests that the translocation chromosomes not only have a high risk of meiotic malsegregation leading to embryos with unbalanced genomes, but also have a predisposition to segregate unfavourably during the following postzygotic divisions and produce highly mosaic, chaotic embryos (Simopoulou et al., 2003). As a result errors in chromosome segregation during subsequent mitotic divisions can complicate the situation further (Conn et al., 1999). The chaotic nature of the chromosomes in the biopsied samples therefore might therefore produce signals that are not characteristic of a particular segregation pattern. Furthermore Delhanty et al. (1997) observed that there is a patient-related predisposition towards the production of chaotic embryos.

In addition to meiotic malsegregation and postzygotic errors resulting in mosaicism, recently testing embryos at PGD using aCGH has revealed a high level of abnormalities affecting other chromosomes apart from those involved in the structural aberration. More specifically Alfarawati et al. (2011) report that 28.9% of the embryos that were balanced for the aberration chromosomes had an aneuploidy for other chromosomes. Follow up analysis on the untransferred embryos can reveal whether there aneuploidies for other chromosomes are meiotic in origin. Figure 7 below shows results from aCGH PGD cases for reciprocal and Robertsonian translocations. In each case the karyotype of the carrier parent is shown together with the abnormalities detected at PGD. Figure 7i shows a normal, euploid profile, whereas the rest of the images show different abnormalities present, which are highlighted.

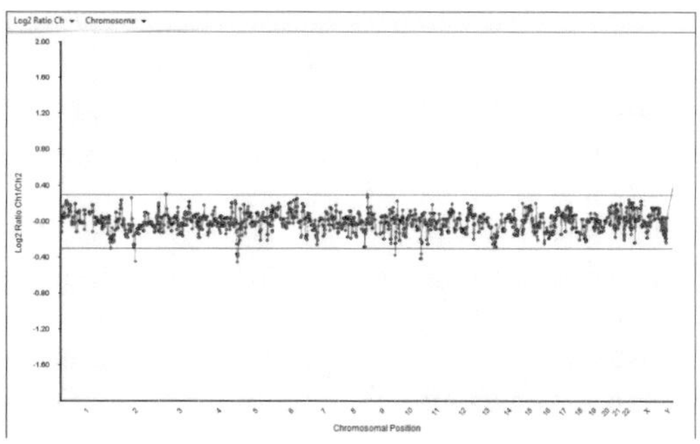

Fig. 7i. Normal euploid aCGH profile of a male embryo

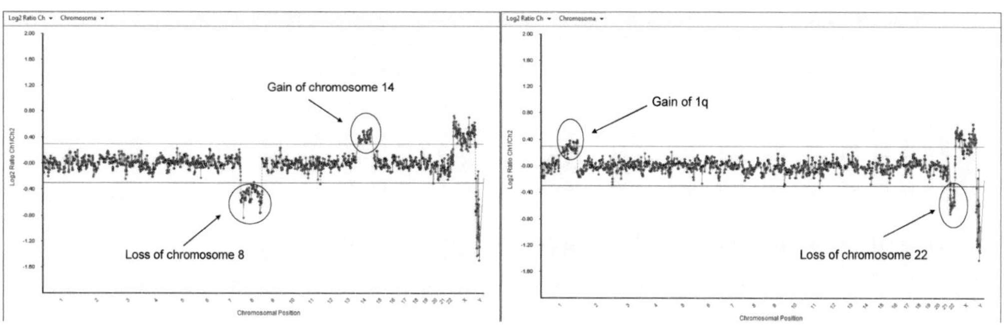


Fig. 7ii. aCGH profiles from cleavage stage embryos from 45, XX, der(13;14)(q10;q10)

The image on the left shows a female embryo with a gain of chromosome 14 as a result of the translocation, but also a loss of chromosome 8. The image on the right shows a female embryo that is balanced for the translocation chromosomes but has a gain of 1q and a loss of chromosome 22.

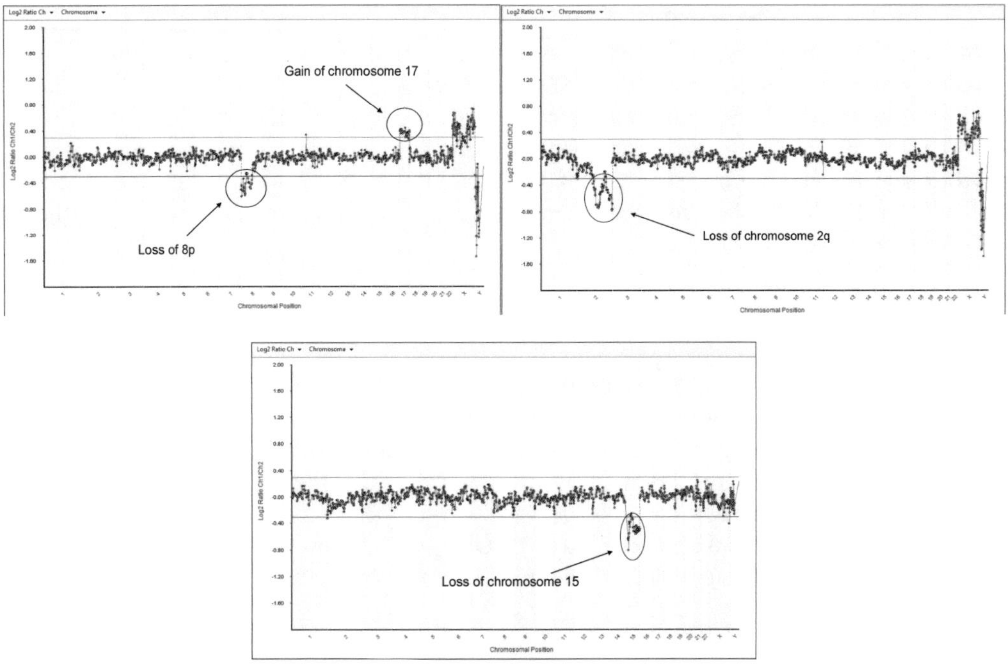


Fig. 7iii. aCGH profiles from trophectoderm after blastocyst stage biopsy for the reciprocal translocation 46, XX, t(8;17) (q21.1;p11.2).

The image on the top left shows a female embryo with a loss of 8p and a gain of chromosome 17 as a result of the translocation, whereas the image on the top right shows a female embryo that was balanced for the translocation chromosomes but had a loss of 2q. The image in the middle shows a male embryo that was balanced for the translocation chromosomes but had loss of chromosome 15.

As a result, apart from unfavourable meiotic segregation, mosaicism and postzygotic errors contribute to the reproductive challenges faces by couples carrying structural abnormalities. Array CGH therefore might be a more appropriate method for PGD for those patients as it allows screening of all chromosomes and therefore aids in choosing those embryos that are viable.

## 6. Other factors affecting chromosome segregation at meiosis in carriers of reciprocal translocations

### 6.1 Sex of the carrier parent and segregation mode at meiosis

For couples treated with PGD for reciprocal translocations the overall number of balanced embryos does not seem to be different between male and female carriers (Xanthopoulou et al., 2011). Munne et al. (2000) reported that the meiotic segregation patterns found at female carriers of Robertsonian translocations were different from those described in male carriers, with females showing a higher level of unbalanced gametes, however this observation was not confirmed by later studies (Munne, 2005). However for one family with an intrachromosomal insertion there seemed to be an effect of the sex of the carrier parent on the mode of segregation (Xanthopoulou et al., 2010).

Chromosomal insertions are rare forms of structural chromosomal abnormalities, that involve breakpoints on the same chromosome and they can be interchromosomal or intrachromosomal depending on whether the material that is broken off from one chromosome is inserted at another site within the same chromosome or is inserted on another chromosome. Moreover insertions can be direct or inverted depending on whether the orientation of the inserted segment is the same or changes with relation to the centromere. An example of an intrachromosomal insertion and the way that chromosomes can segregate at meiosis is shown in figure 8.

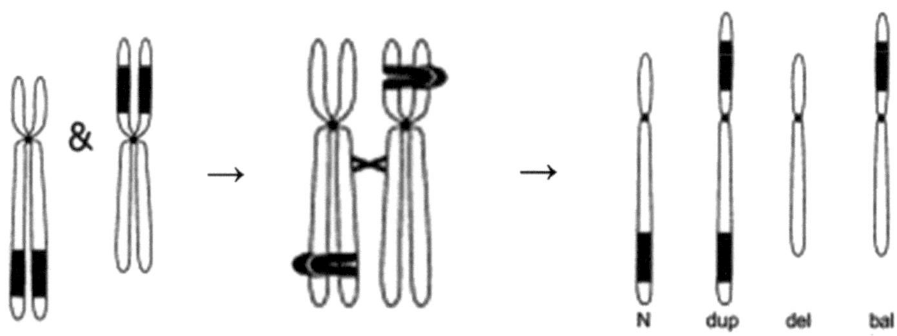


Fig. 8. Chromosome segregation in a carrier of an intrachromosomal insertion at meiosis. Key: N: normal, dupl: duplication of the inserted segment, del: deletion of the inserted segment, bal ins: balanced chromosome that carries the insertion

Balanced carriers of direct intrachromosomal insertions are phenotypically normal but are at risk of unbalanced meiotic segregation due to crossing over. At PGD it is possible to study all possible segregation modes, which might not be viable in later stages of development.

Full follow up analysis on 22 untransferred embryos from a female carrier and 19 embryos from a male carrier of the same intrachromosomal insertion, indicated that the female carrier produced far more balanced embryos (45% versus 16%, Xanthopoulou et al., 2010).

### 6.2 Maternal age

Advanced maternal age has long been associated with an increase in the rate of aneuploidy, for example trisomy 21, whereas preimplantation embryos from women of advanced maternal age referred for Preimplantation Genetic Screening (PGS) also seem to have an increased level of meiotic errors (Mantzouratou et al., 2007).

Ogilvie and Scriven (2002) reported a higher percentage of 3:1 segregation modes in female carriers of reciprocal translocations, resembrling aneuploidy non-disjunction, but no maternal age associations were made. Advanced maternal age is not considered to increase levels of aneuploidy for the chromosomes involved in a structural abnormality in embryos.

However women of advanced maternal age referred for PGD for reciprocal translocations have reduced chances of achieving a pregnancy (Xanthopoulou et al., 2010) due to the high level of meiotic aneuploidy for chromosomes other than the ones involved in the aberration as well as due to malsegregation of the aberration chromosomes.

## 7. Conclusion

PGD provides a unique opportunity to study the behaviour of chromosomes involved in structural abnormalities during meiosis. At those early stages of human preimplantation development all the different modes of meiotic segregation which might not be viable at later stages of development can be seen. As described above carriers of structural chromosomal abnormalities face a high risk of malsegregation at meiosis.

## 8. References

Alfarawati S, Fragouli E, Colls P, Wells D, 2011, First births after preimplantation genetic diagnosis of structural chromosome abnormalities using comparative genomic hybridization and microarray analysis, *Hum Reprod.*;26(6):1560-74.

Cohen O, Cans C, Mermet MA, Demongeot J, Jalbert P, 1994, Viability thresholds for partial trisomies and monosomies. A study of 1,159 viable unbalanced reciprocal translocations, *Hum Genet.*; 93(2):188-94.

Conn CM, Harper JC, Winston RM, Delhanty JD, 1998, Infertile couples with Robertsonian translocations: preimplantation genetic analysis of embryos reveals chaotic cleavage divisions, *Hum Genet.*; 102(1):117-23.

Conn CM, Cozzi J, Harper JC, Winston RM, Delhanty JD, 1999, Preimplantation genetic diagnosis for couples at high risk of Down syndrome pregnancy owing to parental translocation or mosaicism, *J Med Genet.*; 36(1):45-50.

Coonen E, Hopman AH, Geraedts JP, Ramaekers FC, 1998, Application of in-situ hybridization techniques to study human preimplantation embryos: a review, *Hum Reprod Update.;4(2):135-52.*

Delhanty JD, Handyside AH, 1995, The origin of genetic defects in the human and their detection in the preimplantation embryo, *Hum Reprod Update.; 1(3):201-15.*

Delhanty JD, Harper JC, Ao A, Handyside AH, Winston RM, 1997, Multicolour FISH detects frequent chromosomal mosaicism and chaotic division in normal preimplantation embryos from fertile patients, *Hum Genet.*; 99(6):755-60.

Dokras A, Sargent IL, Ross C, Gardner RL, Barlow DH, 1990, Trophectoderm biopsy in human blastocysts, *Hum Reprod.;5(7):821-5.*

Estop AM, Cieply K, Munne S, Surti U, Wakim A, Feingold E, 2000, Is there an interchromosomal effect in reciprocal translocation carriers? Sperm FISH studies, *Hum Genet.*; 106(5):517-24.

Findlay I, Quirke P, Hall J, Rutherford A, 1996, Fluorescent PCR: a new technique for PGD of sex and single-gene defects, *J Assist Reprod Genet.;13(2):96-103.*

Gardner RJM, Sutherland GR, 2004, Chromosome abnormalities and gentic counceling, 3rd Edition, Oxford University Press, New York.

Griffin DK, Handyside AH, Penketh RJ, Winston RM, Delhanty JD, 1991, Fluorescent in-situ hybridization to interphase nuclei of human preimplantation embryos with X and Y chromosome specific probes, *Hum Reprod.;6(1):101-5.*

Harper JC, Coonen E, Handyside AH, Winston RM, Hopman AH, Delhanty JD, 1995, Mosaicism of autosomes and sex chromosomes in morphologically normal, monospermic preimplantation human embryos, Prenat Diagn.; 15(1):41-9.

Hultén MA, 2011, On the origin of crossover interference: A chromosome oscillatory movement (COM) model, Mol Cytogenet.; 8;4:10.

Iwarsson E, Malmgren H, Inzunza J, Ahrlund-Richter L, Sjöblom P, Rosenlund B, Fridström M, Hovatta O, Nordenskjöld M, Blennow E, 2000, Highly abnormal cleavage divisions in preimplantation embryos from translocation carriers, *Prenat Diagn.;20(13):1038-47.*

Jacobs PA, Browne C, Gregson N, Joyce C, White H, 1992, Estimates of the frequency of chromosome abnormalities detectable in unselected newborns using moderate levels of banding, *J Med Genet.;29(2):103-8.*

Jalbert P, Sele B, Jalbert H, 1980, Reciprocal translocations: a way to predict the mode of imbalanced segregation by pachytene-diagram drawing, *Hum Genet.;* 55(2):209-22.

Lieber MR, Ma Y, Pannicke U, Schwarz K, 2003, Mechanism and regulation of human non-homologous DNA end-joining, *Nat Rev Mol Cell Bio*, 4(9):712-20.

Lupski JR, 2004, Hotspots of homologous recombination in the human genome: not all homologous sequences are equal, *Genome Biol.*;5(10):242.

Mantzouratou A, Mania A, Fragouli E, Xanthopoulou L, Tashkandi S, Fordham K, Ranieri DM, Doshi A, Nuttall S, Harper JC, Serhal P, Delhanty JD, 2007, Variable aneuploidy mechanisms in embryos from couples with poor reproductive histories undergoing preimplantation genetic screening, *Hum Reprod.*; 22(7):1844-53.

Munné S, Lee A, Rosenwaks Z, Grifo J, Cohen J, 1993, Diagnosis of major chromosome aneuploidies in human preimplantation embryos, *Hum Reprod.*; 8(12):2185-91.

Munné S, Alikani M, Tomkin G, Grifo J, Cohen J, 1995, Embryo morphology, developmental rates, and maternal age are correlated with chromosome abnormalities, *Fertil Steril.;64(2):382-91.*

Munné S, Escudero T, Sandalinas M, Sable D, Cohen J, 2000, Gamete segregation in female carriers of Robertsonian translocations, *Cytogenet Cell Genet.*; 90(3-4):303-8.

Munne S, 2005, Analysis of chromosome segregation during preimplantation genetic diagnosis in both male and female translocation heterozygotes, *Cytogenet Genome Res*; 111:305-309.

Mackie Ogilvie C, Scriven PN, 2002, Meiotic outcomes in reciprocal translocation carriers ascertained in 3-day human embryos, *Eur J Hum Genet.*; 10(12):801-6.

Ogur G, Van Assche E, Vegetti W, Verheyen G, Tournaye H, Bonduelle M, Van Steirteghem A, Liebaers I, 2006, Chromosomal segregation in spermatozoa of 14 Robertsonian translocation carriers, *Mol Hum Reprod.*;12(3):209-15.

Oliver-Bonet M, Navarro J, Codina-Pascual M, Abad C, Guitart M, Egozcue J, Benet J, 2004, From spermatocytes to sperm: meiotic behaviour of human male reciprocal translocations, *Hum Reprod.*; 19(11):2515-22.

Pfeiffer P, Goedecke W, Kuhfittig-Kulle S, Obe G, 2004, Pathways of DNA double-strand break repair and their impact on the prevention and formation of chromosomal aberrations, *Cytogenet Genome Res.*, 104(1-4):7-13.

Scriven PN, Handyside AH, Ogilvie C, 1998, Chromosome translocations: segregation modes and strategies for preimplantation genetic diagnosis, *Prenat Diagn*; 18:1437-1449.

Scriven PN, O'Mahony F, Bickerstaff H, Yeong CT, Braude P, Mackie Ogilvie C, 2000, Clinical pregnancy following blastomere biopsy and PGD for a reciprocal translocation carrier: analysis of meiotic outcomes and embryo quality in two IVF cycles, *Prenat Diagn.;20(7):587-92.*

Scriven PN, Flinter FA, Braude PR, Ogilvie CM, 2001, Robertsonian translocations--reproductive risks and indications for preimplantation genetic diagnosis, *Hum Reprod.*; 16(11):2267-73.

Shaw CJ, Lupski JR, 2004, Implications of human genome architecture for rearrangement-based disorders: the genomic basis of disease, *Hum Molec Genet*, 13(1):R57-R64.

Shaw CJ, Lupski JR, 2005, Non-recurrent 17q11.2 deletions are generated by homologous and non-homologous mechanisms, *Hum Genet*, 116:1-7.

Simopoulou M, Harper JC, Fragouli E, Mantzouratou A, Speyer BE, Serhal P, Ranieri DM, Doshi A, Henderson J, Rodeck CH, Delhanty JD, 2003, Preimplantation genetic diagnosis of chromosome abnormalities: implications from the outcome for couples with chromosomal rearrangements, *Prenat Diagn; 23(8):652-62.*

Therman E, Susman B, Denniston C, 1989, The nonrandom participation of human acrocentric chromosomes in Robertsonian translocations, *Ann Hum Genet.*; 53(Pt 1):49-65.

Toffolatti L, Cardazzo B, Nobile C, Danieli GA, Gualandi F, Muntoni F, Abbs S, Zanetti P, Angelini C, Ferlini A, Fanin M, Patarnello T, 2002, Investigating the mechanism of chromosomal deletion: characterization of 39 deletion breakpoints in introns 47 and 48 of the human dystrophin gene, *Genomics*; 80(5):523-30.

Verlinsky Y, Pergament E, Strom C, 1990, The preimplantation genetic diagnosis of genetic diseases, *J In Vitro Fert Embryo Transf.;7(1):1-5.*

Xanthopoulou L, Mantzouratou A, Mania A, Cawood S, Doshi A, Ranieri DM, Delhanty JD, 2010, Male and female meiotic behaviour of an intrachromosomal insertion determined by preimplantation genetic diagnosis, *Mol Cytogenet.*; 3(1):2.

Xanthopoulou L, Mantzouratou A, Mania A, Ghevaria H, Ghebo C, Serhal P, Delhanty JD, 2011, When is old too old for preimplantation genetic diagnosis for reciprocal translocations? *Prenat Diagn.* Jun 28. doi: 10.1002/pd.2813. [Epub ahead of print]

14

# OMICS for the Identification of Biomarkers for Oocyte Competence, with Special Reference to the Mare as a Prospective Model for Human Reproductive Medicine

Maria Elena Dell'Aquila[1], Yoon Sung Cho[2], Nicola Antonio Martino[1], Manuel Filioli Uranio[1], Lucia Rutigliano[1] and Katrin Hinrichs[3]
[1]*Dept. Animal Production, University of Bari "Aldo Moro", Bari,*
[2]*Assisted Procreation Unit - Ospedale Accreditato Clinica Santa Maria, Bari,*
[3]*Dept. Physiology and Pharmacology, Texas A&M University, College Station,*
[1,2]*Italy,*
[3]*USA*

## 1. Introduction

A crucial component of Assisted Reproductive Technologies (ART) is the assessment of oocyte developmental potential, to allow selection of those oocytes most likely to result in fertilization and pregnancy. Currently, oocyte quality assessment is largely based on the morphological appearance of the cumulus-oocyte complex, however the accuracy of morphological methods, as predictive of oocyte competence, is still suboptimal. Therefore, the development of objective, accurate, fast and reliable tests for assessing oocyte developmental potential remains an important aim of human and veterinary reproductive medicine. The process of oocyte meiotic maturation, which is central to the developmental competence of the oocyte, is regulated by numerous genes (Matzuk & Lamb, 2008; Fauser et al., 2011) and protein pathways (Kubiak, 2011) and is accompanied by significant changes within the oocyte at many levels. Better understanding of oocyte meiotic maturation would allow better support of this process to increase the success of reproductive biotechnologies, and thus overcome some forms of infertility. Recently, global assessment strategies, namely OMICS, investigating genomic, transcriptomic, proteomic, lipidomic, and glycomic profiles of oocytes, cumulus or granulosa cells have become increasingly applied to the study of oocyte physiology and pathology. Also being investigated is the oocyte-cumulus metabolome, via measurements of metabolites in biological fluids, such as follicular or tubal fluid, or in culture media. The establishment of these technologies, which are in their initial stages of application to reproductive biology, can require large sample numbers; only animal models can meet this requirement. Because of their wide availability and the body of existing knowledge regarding their biology, oocytes of large animals provide useful models for investigating the relationship between oocyte developmental competence and OMICS biomarkers. This review summarizes recent literature on the application of OMICS strategies to evaluating developmental competence of human oocytes and oocytes of large animals. Among the available animal models, the mare is uniquely applicable to investigation of oocyte developmental competence. Horses represent the most economically valuable domestic animal, with progeny from specific mares worth hundreds of thousands of euros. Thus, there is obvious practical interest in the use of assisted reproduction in this species. In addition, similarities between equine and human follicle growth and oocyte maturation make the mare a particularly valuable model for topics at the interface between animal breeding and biomedical research, such as age-related and obesity-related oocyte dysfunction and the effects of exposure to environmental toxicants, as well as for fundamental research on factors involved in meiotic maturation. For these reasons, particular attention will be dedicated in this review to recent OMICS results obtained in the equine species and to discussion of the potential application of this animal model in future investigations.

## 2. OMICS as innovative strategies for evaluating oocyte quality

Systems biology is a new and rapidly developing research area in which, by quantitatively describing the interactions among the components of a cell, a systems-level understanding of a biological response can be achieved. Therefore, it requires high-throughput measurement technologies, that is, technologies that can investigate a large number of biological molecules at once. OMICS technologies -- in which aspects of cellular structure or function, such as proteins or RNA transcripts, are studied in their totality (global assessment strategies) -- are opening wider and wider doors into the understanding of all branches of the biology, physiology, and pathology of living organisms. It is likely that information obtained using OMICS will change our concept of "normal" and "pathological," and will enable the efficient evaluation of the effects of extrinsic factors on the status of living systems. Initial studies on the application of OMICS strategies to the oocyte have appeared in the past decade, starting with genomics and transcriptomics, and progressing to the newer fields of glycomics and metabolomics. As noted above, a major concern in the production of viable and competent embryos in vitro is the evaluation of initial oocyte quality and the support of optimal nuclear and cytoplasmic maturation. OMICS approaches to the oocyte will significantly contribute not only to accurate assessment of oocyte quality, but also to the clarification of the mechanisms involved in cell cycle regulation and cell differentiation, thus contributing to the effective utilization of recovered oocytes. Because meiotic maturation and early embryo development involve regulation of the cell cycle and evolution from differentiated, to pluripotent, back to differentiated cells, data generated from study of these processes may also relate to the establishment of innovative targeted cancer treatments and stem cell-based therapies. To introduce the sequential phases of the meiotic process, changes occurring within the oocyte and some of their fundamental regulating factors are briefly described. Upon the luteinizing hormone (LH) surge, M-phase promoting factor (MPF) and the mitogen-activated protein (MAP) kinase ERK 2 (extracellularly-regulated kinase 2) are activated within the oocyte. The oocyte, which at this time is in prophase of meiosis, has replicated chomosomes contained within a nucleus (termed the germinal vesicle, GV). Activation of MPF and ERK 2 trigger nuclear envelope breakdown and chromatin condensation. The condensed chromosomes are subsequently aligned on the spindle of the first meiotic division, forming the metaphase I plate. At this time MPF levels decrease, while ERK 2 levels remain high. The homologous chromosomes separate: one set of sister chromatids is discarded as the polar body; the other set, in response to a recrudescence of MPF, lines up on a spindle, forming the second metaphase plate (MII). Fertilization causes inactivation of MPF and ERK 2, and the second meiotic division occurs, separating the sister chromatids. One set of chromatids is discarded, as the second polar body; the other set becomes the female pronucleus. For a comprehensive description of major pathways involved in oocyte M-phase entry, see Kubiak et al., 2011 and Tosti & Boni, 2011. Detailed descriptions of OMICS techniques go beyond the intent of this article; corresponding references are provided in the text. We instead focus on the most significant results obtained using these techniques, the role of large animal models in experimental designs that cannot be performed in humans, and on actual and potential contributions of different animal models to understanding of oocyte biology, with particular interest in the equine species.

### 2.1 The mare as a model for human oocyte biology

Large animal models allow the establishment of a wide variety of experimental designs that can not be applied in humans for obvious ethical reasons, or due to the limited and highly regulated availability of human biological samples. Among large animals, the mare has many attributes that make her a good model for reproduction in women (Carnevale, 2008). These include a long follicular phase, a long interovulatory interval (22 days), presence of a single dominant follicle, formation a large diameter follicle (~40 mm) with a large volume of follicular fluid -- the same volume:body weight ratio as in women; a relatively long time from LH stimulation to ovulation (36 h for both human and horse) and, like the human oocyte, formation of a markedly dense chromatin mass within the germinal vesicle as the oocyte gains meiotic competence or undergoes atresia (Parfenov et al, 1989; Hinrichs et al., 1993). Although seasonality does not occur in women, the equine characteristic of seasonal reproductive activity provides the potential to examine the influence of applied factors when cyclic hormonal patterns are not occurring (Carnevale, 2008). Horses are the best animal model for studies on age-related infertility. Because mares can be of great value, many mares continue to be bred until they experience subfertility, thus animals with naturally-occuring age-related subfertility are available for study. Horses have a long lifespan, thus age-related subfertility occurs at an age (~20-25 years) much closer to that observed in women than is seen in other animal models. In addition, horses, unlike other large domestic species, are selected for attributes other than fertility, such as conformation, athletic prowess, or behavior. Individuals showing subfertility may be worked with intensively to try to obtain foals, thus, they provide an excellent naturally-occurring model for many intrinsic causes of subfertility. Horses have similar metabolic responses to nutrient intake to that in humans, and are used for a wide variety of athletic purposes, thus they can serve to model important physiological or pathological situations affecting reproduction in humans (such as stress, life-style, sports activity, obesity or metabolic syndrome) as well as to examine the effects of external factors such as acute or long-term exposure to drugs or environmental toxicants. In addition to mimicking the situation in humans, the development of particularly large follicles allows the possibility of collecting large amounts of mural granulosa cells (GC) issuing from the follicular wall as well as large amounts of follicular fluid (30 to 50 ml/follicle) that may be used for OMICS studies in a 1:1 comparison with the developmental status of the enclosed oocyte. The cumulus-oocyte complex (COC) of the mare is particularly large, thus allowing a 1:1 evaluation of biological parameters of cumulus cells (CCs) predictive of oocyte meiotic and developmental competence. Moreover, follicular COCs in the mare can be recovered from immature follicles, with initial COC morphological features indicating viability (compact cumulus) or atresia (apoptosis, expanded cumulus) of their surrounding follicle, thus supporting study of the effects of follicle immaturity and early or late atresia on oocyte competence (Hinrichs and Williams, 1997; Dell'Aquila et al., 2003). The equine oocyte is approximately 200 microns in diameter, with good visibility of the perivitelline space and the first polar body (PB), so that mature oocytes are easily identified on morphological examination. The horse oocyte possesses a unique distribution of cytoplasmic lipid droplets, which assume polar aggregation in metaphase II (MII) oocytes, and whose biological meaning is under investigation (Ambruosi et al., 2009). Horses make a valuable model for oocyte assessments associated with penetration of the zona pellucida (e.g. PB biopsy) because, in contrast to species such as cattle and sheep, methods for fertilization via intracytoplasmic sperm injection (ICSI) are well established in the horse (Hinrichs et al., 2005; Choi et al., 2006). Sperm injection is necessary to achieve fertilization after penetration of the zona pellucida for investigative purposes, as the defect in the zona would lead to polyspermy if standard in vitro fertilization (IVF) were to be performed. These features make the equine oocyte a particularly useful model for the establishment of OMICS strategies that could be not only applied to better understanding of human assisted reproductive medicine, but also directly applicable to the horse industry.

### 2.2 Oocyte genomics – The polar body biopsy and genomic analysis for predicting half of the DNA constitution of an embryo: from FISH to CGH/CNV/SNP-based arrays

The genomic DNA constitution of the oocyte determines the sequence of produced transcripts and proteins, and constitutes half of the early embryo phenotype. The most widely used diagnostic tool for oocyte and embryo genomic investigation to date has been Fluorescent In Situ Hybridization (FISH), a cytogenetic technique which identifies specific DNA sequences on chromosomes by means of fluorescent probes that bind to those parts of the chromosome with which they show a high degree of sequence similarity.

Since the first report in humans (Griffin et al., 1992), several studies have been published reporting the evaluation of human day 3 embryos (4-8 cell stage) for up to 8 pairs of chromosomes (chromosomes 13, 15, 16, 17, 18, 21, 22, and X/Y; review by Seli et al., 2010). However, in recent meta-analysis studies, reported from 2008 to 2010, it has become clear that preimplantation genetic screening by using FISH is not justified. This is because it causes damage to the embryo, it requires embryo cryopreservation and transfer in a subsequent cycle, and it does not significantly contribute to the identification and exclusion of aneuploid embryos. Use of FISH has been reported to be associated with lower implantation rates and it shows errors such as false positives due to mosaicism or false negatives due to the limited number of chromosomes analyzed and the limited targeted regions. Therefore, authoritative scientific committees, including the European Society of Human Reproduction and Embryology (ESHRE) and the American Society of Reproductive Medicine (ASRM), decided to conduct a study to determine whether biopsy of the first and second polar bodies (PBs) of the oocyte would enable the timely identification of the chromosomal status of an oocyte. This aim could be reached by analyzing the complete chromosome complement of the two PBs by Comparative Genomic Hybridization (CGH; reviews by Seli et al., 2010; Geraedts et al., 2010).

Conventional CGH, initially developed by cancer biologists, was applied to human early embryos around 10 years ago (Voullaire et al., 2000 reviewed by Geraedts et al., 2010). These authors performed CGH in association with whole genome amplification by degenerate oligonucleotide-primed polymerase chain reaction. CGH is a competitive hybridization of two fragmented genomes (test and reference genomes) to the chromosomes of a metaphase plate of a normal subject. The tested and subject genomes are labeled with different (red and green) fluorescent dyes so that an increase of red staining will indicate the presence of duplicated regions, an increase of green staining will indicate the presence of deleted regions, whereas the lack of predominance of one of the two colors will indicate normal chromosome structure. This technique allows examination of the whole chromosomal complement, but requires extensive time to get the results. In recent years, CGH-microarray tools have been developed in which the labeled DNAs are affixed to DNA on a microscope slide rather than to metaphase chromosomes. A variety of microarray-CGH platforms are available. As an example, the Cambridge-based company BlueGnome offers an array-based CGH protocol which allows analysis of biopsied PBs within 11 hrs (SurePlex amplification protocol; 24sure analysis, BlueGnome; "http://www.bluegnome.co.uk/"; Geraedts et al., 2010). As regard, Geraedts et al., (2011) and Magli et al., (2011) reported clinical results and technical aspects of a proof-of-principle study performed in associated ART centers in which all mature metaphase II oocytes from patients who consented to the study, fertilized by ICSI, were analyzed. The first and second PBs were biopsied and analysed separately for chromosome copy number by array CGH. If either or both of the PBs were found to be aneuploid, the corresponding zygote was then also processed by array CGH for concordance analysis. It was concluded that the ploidy of a zygote can be predicted with acceptable accuracy by array CGH analysis on both PBs. Interestingly, on the male side, the application of CGH arrays to single human sperm cells has been recently reported (Antonello et al., 2011).

In the aim to move from chromosomal structure to single mutation analysis, SNP (Single Nucleotide Polymorphism) arrays have been developed. A single-nucleotide polymorphism (SNP, pronounced snip) is a DNA sequence variation occurring when a single nucleotide – Adenine (A), Thymine (T), Cytosine (C), or Guanine (G) – differs in a sequence between members of a species or paired chromosomes in an individual. Many common SNPs have only two alleles. Within a population, SNPs can be assigned a minor allele frequency – the lesser of the two allele frequencies for a population. There are variations among human populations, so a SNP allele that is common in one geographical or ethnic group may be rare in another. Unlike the CGH-microarray platforms which involve simultaneous hybridization of differentially labeled DNAs to the same microarray, SNP-microarrays assess test and reference samples, separately, in parallel. From 10.000 to 500.000 SNPs may be evaluated simultaneously. For example, using the Affymetrix platform, analysis of 250.000 SNPs in first PB biopsies (Treff et al., 2010a) and in Day-3 embryos (Treff et al., 2010b) have been reported (review by Seli et al., 2010). The Illumina platform allows the analysis of 370.000 human SNPs.

Because of their utility in recognizing variations associated with disease, recent genetic epidemiology studies have been dominated by genome-wide association studies using

SNPs. However, another form of structural genomic variation, termed copy number variation (CNV), is also widespread throughout the genome. These genomic structural variations range from 1 to 5 Mb and can be highly polymorphic between individuals, and thus can be used for epidemiological study. CNVs in the form of large-scale insertions and deletions, as well as inversions and translocations, may have important roles in meiotic recombination, human genome evolution and gene expression. Many genetic diseases are based on CNVs. However, because they consist of quantitative rather than qualitative changes, show variability in copy numbers and are confounded by the diploidy of the human genome, the detailed genetic structure of CNVs cannot be readily studied by available techniques. Thus, the establishment CNV-microarrays is currently under investigation. New microarray-based technologies will enable more accurate mapping of CNVs, and CNV maps of the human genome are being refined with increasing resolution. The study of CNVs and their effects on human health and disease therefore present a dynamic and exciting challenge for researchers in the field of genetic epidemiology (Wain and Tobin, 2011). The importance of CNVs in human preimplantation genetic screening, or to animal oocyte and embryo testing, has not been reported to date.

Although there is potential economic interest for the application of PB biopsy and subsequent analysis of the chromosomal complement or genome by CGH-, CNV- or SNP arrays in animal husbandry and breeding, to the best of our knowledge no studies have been published to date in large animals. The field is therefore open to future investigations, pending the establishment of the different genomic arrays in these species. A recent report (Le Bourhis et al., 2011) presented for the first time bovine embryo biopsy and genotyping using a 50K SNP Illumina chip. In this study, biopsies of 5 to 10 cells were obtained from *in vitro*-cultured morulae and blastocysts and kept frozen or at room temperature. The genomic DNA of each biopsy was amplified by using a whole-genome amplification kit and was genotyped using a custom CRV 50K Illumina chip. Call rates were calculated from 50.905 SNPs. Percentage of allele drop-out was estimated from the number of heterozygous markers present [% allele drop-out = (calculated heterozygous–observed heterozygous) /calculated heterozygous]. Parentage error was estimated by using the genotypes of the parents of the embryos. A greater quantity of DNA was obtained after amplification of biopsies that were sent frozen to the laboratory than from those at room temperature ($P<0.05$). However, the SNP call rate, % allele drop-out, and parentage error did not differ between groups. These results indicate that genotyping from embryo biopsies following whole genome amplification can be achieved with good efficiency when using high-density marker chips. To the best of our knowledge no studies have been reported to date on genomic analysis in the equine oocyte. A recent paper in the horse by Choi et al., (2010) reports the identification of disease-causing mutations in trophoblastic biopsies from equine in vivo-recovered pre-implantation embryos. These authors demonstrated for the first time the correct identification, by embryo biopsy and whole genome amplification, of sex and genotype at the causative mutation sites for two disease-linked genes (SCN4A and PPIB). The biopsies were performed on Day-6 and Day-7 equine embryos, and after biopsy these embryos were able to produce pregnancies leading to term delivered, normal foals. These two recent studies demonstrate that OMICS technologies have the potential in animal breeding for both marker-assisted selection and for preimplantation diagnosis of genetic diseases.

Another promising genomic investigation area is Epigenetics, the study of changes in gene expression and thus cellular phenotype caused by mechanisms other than changes in the underlying DNA sequence - hence the name *epi-* (Greek: *επι-* over, above, outer) *genetics*. Examples of such changes are DNA methylation and deacetylation of the histones, the proteins around which DNA are wrapped. Both of these changes serve to suppress gene expression without altering the sequence of the silenced genes. These changes may remain through cell divisions for the remainder of the cell's life, and some epigenetic changes in germ cells may potentially last for multiple generations. Epigenetic changes in eukaryotic biology are the basis of the process of cell differentiation. During embryonic morphogenesis, the totipotent cells of the zygote become the various pluripotent cell lines of the embryo, which in turn become fully differentiated cells. This is accomplished by activating some genes while inhibiting others. Current epigenetic research focuses on chromatin modifications occurring during sequential phases of fertilization (sperm chromatin decondensation, pronuclear formation with DNA duplication and syngamy) and early development (chromosome condensation and assembly in the first metaphase plate of the first mitotic division and the subsequent series of mitotic divisions to the blastocyst stage; Burton & Torres Padilla, 2011). These events may be studied by comparing embryos produced in vivo with those obtained using different technologies, such as IVF, ICSI, parthenogenesis or somatic cell nuclear transfer (Cremer & Zakhartchenko, 2011). Soon, the emergence of quantitative high-throughput microarray technology should allow the development of epigenomic arrays for the evaluation of embryo whole-genome epigenetic status, thus opening the new field of epigenomics (Callinan & Feinberg, 2006) to the study of oocyte and embryo competence.

The methylation pattern of DNA in oocytes may be a key factor for the improvement of efficiency of in vitro embryo production, because it is related to oocyte competence. A recent study (Simarro Fagundes et al., 2011) reported on a differentially-methylated region located in exon 10 of the imprinted gene *IGF2* This study evaluated immature vs *in vitro*-matured bovine oocytes from small (1–3 mm in diameter) and large follicles (≥ 8.1 mm in diameter). It was observed that after IVM, oocytes from ≥ 8.1 mm follicles were less methylated (18.51%) than were those from 1- to 3-mm follicles (49.62%). As oocytes from the larger follicles are more developmentally competent, the less methylated pattern appears to be associated with higher oocyte quality. It was concluded that the methylation pattern of specific genes could be used as a molecular marker for epigenetic reprogramming status in oocytes, helping the development of new in vitro embryo production protocols. A broader study on this wave (Smallwood et al., 2011) reported the first integrated epigenomic analysis of mammalian oocytes (GV vs MII oocytes) and preimplantation embryos (blastocyst stage) identifying over a thousand CG islands methylated in matured oocytes. The authors observed that CG islands were preferentially located within active transcription units, supporting a general transcription-dependent mechanism of methylation, and that very few CG islands were protected from post-fertilization reprogramming, the majority showing incomplete demethylation in Day-3 blastocysts. This study revealed the extent and dynamics of CG island methylation in oocytes, which is a prerequisite for defining the full repertoire of imprinted genes and the mechanistic basis of parent-of-origin expression effects in somatic tissues.

Epigenomic studies have not been reported to date in equine oocytes; however, in the promising field of genomic investigations, the equine oocyte would serve as an excellent model for the comparison of oocyte (metaphase plate) and polar body genomes and epigenomic modifications, due to the ability to investigate the developmental competence of biopsied equine oocytes after fertilization via ICSI.

### 2.3 Oocyte transcriptomics – The global analysis of oocyte mRNA transcripts

In addition to the genomic constitution of the embryo, it is necessary to know its phenotype: which genes are being utilized at this particular stage of development? Initially, embryonic phenotype is determined by those mRNAs already transcribed and present in the oocyte cytoplasm at the time of fertilization (maternal mRNAs). Evaluation of maternal mRNA content is particularly attractive in the study of developmental biology and for diagnostic and applied purposes in ART (e.g. nuclear reprogramming in cloning, and stem cell research). However, transcriptome analysis of mammalian oocytes and embryos faces three main challenges: 1) the small amount of material available; 2) differing total RNA content in the subsequently-occurring developmental stages, making comparison among stages difficult; 3) existence of oocyte-specific genes often absent from commercially available microarrays (Dalbies-Tran and Mermillod, 2003; Thelie et al., 2009).

Via transcriptomics, it is possible to thoroughly investigate the functional status of a cell line or tissue. Rapidly developing methods consist of RNA extraction, reverse transcription (RT), amplification and labeling, array hybridization, chip scanning, and data interpretation by bioinformatic analysis with subsequent validation by Real Time RT-PCR. Detailed reviews of microarray analysis strategies and interpretation of transcriptomic profiles have been presented by White and Salamonsen, 2005 and Rodriguez-Zas et al., 2008. Some of the public or commercially available software commonly used for trascriptome analysis are:

Public:

- GENE ONTOLOGY: http://www.geneontology.org;
- NCBI Entrez Gene: http://www.ncbi.nlm.nih.gov.sites/entrez?db=gene);
- NCBI Gene Expression Omnibus GEO: http://www.ncbi.nlm.nih.gov/geo;
- KEGG pathway database: http://www.genome.jp/kegg/pathway.html;

Commercially available:

- INGENUITY pathway analysis http://www.ingenuity.com;
- PANTHER Applied Biosystem http://www.pantherdb.org);
- AFFYMETRIX (http://www.affymetrix.com/products/arrays/specific/bovine.affx).

A major aim in oocyte transcriptomics is the analysis of differences among maturation stages, especially between the germinal vesicle (GV) and the metaphase II (MII) stage, as well as differential expression between in vivo- (in vivo-MII) and in vitro- (IVM-MII) matured oocytes. The correct molecular control of meiotic maturation is a fundamental prerequisite for successful development of an early embryo (Tosti & Boni, 2011). Transcriptome microarray technologies have been developed, first in the mouse and more recently in large animals (review by Thelie et al., 2009). At the moment, cattle take center stage in the cast of large animals used as models for human reproductive medicine.

### 2.3.1 Studies in bovine oocytes

**GV vs MII oocyte** A pioneering study on oocyte gene expression was conducted at INRA (France) by Dalbies-Tran and Mermillod, in 2003. These authors analyzed gene expression in bovine oocytes before and after IVM, using heterologous hybridization onto a cDNA array. Total RNA was purified from pools of over 200 oocytes either immediately after aspiration from follicles of slaughterhouse cow ovaries, or following IVM. Radiolabeled cDNA probes were generated by RT followed by linear PCR amplification and were hybridized to Atlas human cDNA arrays. To the best of our knowledge, this was the first report of gene expression profiling by this technology in the bovine oocyte. The results demonstrated that cDNA array screening is a suitable method for analyzing the transcription pattern in oocytes, as about 300 identified genes were reproducibly shown to be expressed in the bovine oocyte. The relative abundance of most messenger RNAs appeared stable during IVM; however, it was observed that 70 transcripts underwent a significant differential regulation between meiotic stages (by a factor of at least two). Information obtained in this study constituted the first molecular signature of oocyte cytoplasmic maturation.

**GV oocyte vs embryo** In a subsequent study at INRA (Thelie et al., 2009) results of an RNA-amplification protocol for bovine oocytes and blastocysts was reported. Using RT-PCR, these authors confirmed that the profiles of both abundant and scarce polyadenylated transcripts were conserved after RNA amplification. Next, amplified probes generated from immature oocytes, in vitro-matured oocytes, and in vitro-produced hatched blastocysts were hybridized onto an in-house cDNA macroarray that included oocyte-specific genes (934 expressed sequence tags of interest including markers of oocyte maturation; Thelie et al., 2009). Following an original approach, two normalization procedures, based on either the median signal or an exogenous standard, were compared and the expected difference in sets of differential genes, depending on the normalization procedure, were calculated. Using a 1.5-fold threshold, no transcript was found to be up-regulated when data were normalized to an exogenous standard, which reflects the absence of transcription during oocyte IVM. In blastocysts, the majority of genes found to be preferentially expressed in oocytes (after normalization) were not activated. This study shed new light on and complemented previous transcriptomic analyses of the bovine oocyte-to-embryo transition using commercial platforms (i.e.: Misirlioglu et al., 2006; Fair et al., 2007; reviewed by Thelie et al., 2009).

**In vivo-MII vs IVM-MII oocyte** The differences in the MII oocyte transcriptome between oocytes matured in vivo and in vitro were investigated in cattle by Katz-Jaffe et al., (2009). In this study, the Affymetrix Gene Chip Bovine Genome Array, a platform containing over 23.000 bovine transcripts, was used. Transcripts identified as being differentially expressed between the two groups were classified according to gene ontology. Statistical analysis of microarray data identified several processes affected by IVM, including metabolism, energy pathways, cell biogenesis and organization, and cell growth and maintenance. In particular, it was found that 4 genes of the tricarboxylic acid cycle and 14 genes of oxidative phosphorylation were down-regulated in IVM-MII compared with in vivo-MII.

**GV vs MII oocyte** Mamo et al., (2011) used the Affymetrix GeneChip Bovine Genome Array to perform global mRNA expression analysis of immature (GV) and in-vitro matured (IVM) bovine oocytes. They then used a variety of approaches, including the analysis of transcript abundance in oocytes matured in the presence of alpha-amanitin (a transcription inhibitor), to determine whether the transcriptional changes observed during IVM were real or were artifacts of the techniques used during analysis. It was found that 8489 transcripts were detected across the two oocyte groups, of which ~25.0% (2117 transcripts) were differentially expressed ($p<0.001$); corresponding to 589 over-expressed and 1528 under-expressed transcripts in the IVM oocytes compared to their immature counterparts. Subsets of the differentially expressed genes were validated by quantitative RT-PCR and the gene expression data was classified according to gene ontology and pathway enrichment. Numerous cell-cycle linked (CDC2, CDK5, CDK8, HSPA2, MAPK14, TXNL4B), molecular transport (STX5, STX17, SEC22A, SEC22B), and differentiation (NACA) related genes were found to be among the over-expressed transcripts in GV oocytes compared to their mature counterparts, while other genes (ANXA1, PLAU, STC1and LUM) were among the over-expressed genes after maturation. This data set provided a unique reference resource for studies of the molecular mechanisms controlling oocyte meiotic maturation in cattle, and by extension to other species, and through use of the alpha-amanitin, addressed the existing conflicting issue of transcription during meiotic maturation.

**Adult vs prepubertal oocyte** (Romar et al., 2011) This study, rather than applying global OMICS strategies, analyzed the differential expression profile of adult vs prepubertal bovine oocytes by using a specialized panel for genes involved in the maturation process, such as genes known to specifically affect early development after fertilization (maternal-effect genes, shown via mouse knock-outs), biomarkers of oocyte competence or redox metabolism, or genes involved in the regulation of meiotic progression. It was found that some genes (particularly redox genes) are significantly underexpressed in oocytes from prepubertal subjects. This kind of comparison would benefit greatly by using OMICS technologies and underscores the value of animal models, as it would be difficult to perform in humans due to low availability of oocytes from young girls and women.

### 2.3.2 Studies in human oocytes

Transcriptomic studies have been reported in human oocytes. Kocabas et al., 2006 reported the use of a comprehensive human microarray platform (Affymetrix Human Genome U133 Plus 2.0 GeneChips) to identify the gene transcripts present in **early MII oocytes**, tested within minutes after isolation from the ovary.

In the study by Wells and Patrizio (2008), unfertilized **GV, in vivo-MII** and **IVM-MII** oocytes were analyzed. The study used the Applied Biosystem Human Genome Survey Microarray with 32.878 60mer oligonucleotide probes for the interrogation of 29.098 genes, including 8000 genes not previously included in any commercial array. By bioinformatic analysis, a Venn diagram can be obtained in which each circle represents the transcriptome of a specific cell type, and overlapping areas indicate commonly-expressed genes. The three oocyte categories expressed 12.219, 9.735 and 8.510 genes, respectively. There were extensive overlaps among the three groups, but also some significant differences. In particular, in vivo-MII and IVM-MII oocytes shared similar patterns of gene expression. However, some immature patterns of expression, reminiscent of GVs, persisted in IVM-MIIs. In humans, in-vitro maturation is an attractive strategy for IVF treatment; however, currently IVM oocytes perform poorly after IVF. Data from the this study indicates that although IVM-MII oocytes closely resemble in vivo-MII oocytes in cellular pathways related to nuclear maturity, several pathways associated with cytoplasmic functions continue to be expressed in an immature manner. Additionally, it was shown that IVM-MII oocytes differ in the expression of genes related to cellular storage and homeostasis. Such differentially expressed genes and their pathways provide clues for the optimization of IVM techniques, and, importantly, a method to assess the effects of those techniques on oocyte competence without having to evaluate development after fertilization, which could raise ethical issues in humans.

**In vivo-MII vs IVM-MII** In the study by Jones et al., (2008), more than 2000 genes were identified as expressed at more than 2-fold higher levels in oocytes recovered from gonadotropin-stimulated cycles and matured in vitro than those matured in vivo, and 162 of these were expressed at 10-fold or greater levels (this study used Codelink Whole Human Genome Bioarrays, GE Healthcare Biosciences). It was concluded that the overabundance of transcripts in immature oocytes recovered from gonadotropin stimulated cycles, then matured in vitro could be due to dysregulation of either gene transcription or post-transcriptional modifications, resulting in incorrect temporal utilization of genes, culminating in developmental oocyte incompetence.

**GV vs IVM-MII vs embryo** Zhang et al., 2009a followed the transcriptome changes occurring in human preimplantation development by applying microarray analysis (Affymetrix two-cycle GeneChip Eukaryotic small sample target labeling assay version II; HG-U133 Plus 2.0 array) to human oocytes and embryos at six developmental stages. They observed a dramatic reprogramming of transcription and translation during preimplantation development in a stage-specific manner, with two main transitions (MII to Day 2 and Day 3 to Day 5). Over 47.000 transcripts expressed in oocytes and early embryos were reported, thus providing a fundamental resource for understanding the genetic control of human early development. There was a significant underrepresentation of transcripts responsible for cell signaling and communication (genes associated with the G protein coupled receptor - GPCR - protein signaling pathway, cell communication, immune response, response to external stimuli, cell adhesion, sensory perception and cell-surface receptor-linked signal transduction pathways) in both oocytes and embryos, when compared to adult tissue; the authors concluded that human preimplantation development is almost self-directed -- i.e., oocytes and embryos apparently do not need to communicate with the "external world" to the same degree as adult tissues do. This paper also performed evolutionary comparisons between humans and mice, dogs and chimpanzees. Genes that were highly expressed in human oocytes and embryos varied less from those of other species than did genes of adult tissues: the conclusion was that these "pre-implantation genes" are highly conserved.

Microarray analysis of human oocytes has been subsequently applied to a variety of reproductive issues. Wood et al., (2007) found differences in gene expression between **normal** and **PCOS** (polycystic ovarian syndrome) oocytes for 8123 transcripts, 374 of which were genes related to meiotic spindle dynamics. Grondahl et al., (2010), evaulated 15 independent replicates of single **in vivo-MII** oocytes using the Affymetrix HG-U133 Plus 2.0 gene chip array, which tests around 48.000 well identified genes by using around 56.000 probe sets, and the Affymetrix gene array 2500 scanner. These authors identified 7.470 genes (10.428 transcripts) as present in human in vivo-MII oocytes. Of these, 342 genes showed a significantly different expression level between **young** and **aged** women; notably, genes annotated to be involved in cell cycle regulation, chromosome alignment (e.g. MAD2L1 binding protein), sister chromatid separation (e.g. separase), oxidative stress and ubiquitination. The top signaling network affected by age was 'cell cycle and organism development' (e.g. SMAD2 and activin B1 receptor). Thus, this study provided information on processes that may be associated with lowered oocyte developmental competence due to ageing.

### 2.3.3 The common gene expression signatures of oocytes and embryonic stem cells

Another interesting research area for transcriptomic investigations is the comparison of the transcriptomic profile between MII oocytes and stem cells. Data have been published on the comparison between human **MII oocytes** and human **embryonic stem cells (ESC)**. Both of these cells types are able to reprogram differentiated nuclei towards pluripotency, either by somatic cell nuclear transfer or by cell fusion, respectively. Comparison of the transcriptome of these two cell types may highlight genes that are involved in induction of pluripotency. Based on a microarray compendium of 205 samples, Assou et al., 2009 compared the gene expression profile of MII oocytes and human ESC to that of somatic tissues. A common oocyte/hESC gene expression profile was identified, which included a strong cell cycle signature, genes associated with pluripotency such as *LIN28* and *TDGF1*, a large chromatin remodelling network (*TOP2A, DNMT3B, JARID2, SMARCA5, CBX1, CBX5*), 18 different zinc finger transcription factors, including *ZNF84*, and several still-poorly annotated genes such as *KLHL7, MRS2,* and Selenophosphate synthetase 1 (*SEPHS1*). Interestingly, a large set of genes in both cell types was found to code for proteins involved in the ubiquitination-proteasome pathway. Upon ESC differentiation into embryoid bodies, the transcription of genes in this pathway declined. In vitro, a selective sensitivity of human ESC to inhibition of proteasome activity was observed. These results shed light on the gene networks that are concurrently overexpressed by the two cell types with somatic cell reprogramming properties.

### 2.3.4 Prediction of oocyte competence based on analysis of accessory cells (polar bodies, cumulus cells or granulosa cells)

A major problem of reproductive biotechnologies is predicting which oocytes are destined to develop into viable embryos. Analysis of accessory cells, such as PBs, CCs and GCs, allows oocyte quality assessment without interfering with use of the oocyte in ART.

**Polar Body** Klatsky et al., (2010) reported detection and quantification of mRNA from single human polar bodies, a minimally invasive test of the oocyte gene-expression profile. Gene expression of 12 candidate genes was investigated in PB biopsies and the oocytes from which they originated, and polar-body mRNA was detected for 11 out of 12 genes. This method would allow detection and comparison of individual differences in oocyte gene expression without harming the oocyte.

**Granulosa cells** The comparative evaluation of the effects of FSH vs human menopausal gonadotrophin on GCs has been reported (Grondahl et al., 2009). These authors found that the drugs used for controlled ovarian hyperstimulation have a significant impact on the gene expression profile of human granulosa cells. Interesting differences were observed for genes involved in the regulation of preovulatory events. For GC in the mare, see the work by Fahiminiya et al., 2010 in section 2.3.5

**Cumulus cells** The bi-directional communication between the oocyte and its companion CCs is crucial for the development and function of both cell types. Regassa et al. (2001) investigated the transcripts that are exclusively expressed either in oocytes or in CCs, and the molecular mechanisms affected when communication between the two cell types is removed. The transcriptomic profile of different oocyte and CC samples was analyzed by using Affymetrix GeneChip Bovine Genome array containing 23000 transcripts. Out of 13162 genes detected in GV oocytes and their companion CCs, 1516 and 2727 were exclusively expressed in oocytes and in CCs, respectively, while 8919 were expressed in both. Similarly, of 13602 genes detected in MII oocytes and CCs, 1423 and 3100 were exclusively expressed in oocytes and in CCs, respectively, while 9079 were expressed in both. A total of 265 transcripts were differentially expressed between oocytes cultured with (OO+CCs) and without (OO-CCs) CCs, of which 217 and 48 were over-expressed in the former and the latter groups, respectively. Similarly, 566 transcripts were differentially expressed when CCs were cultured with (CCs+OO) or without (CCs-OO) their enclosed oocytes. Of these, 320 and 246 were over-expressed in CCs+OO and CCs-OO, respectively. While oocyte-specific transcripts include those involved in transcription (IRF6, POU5F1, MYF5, MED18) and translation (EIF2AK1, EIF4ENIF1), CC-specific transcripts include those involved in carbohydrate metabolism (HYAL1, PFKL, PYGL, MPI), protein metabolic processes (IHH, APOA1, PLOD1) and steroid biosynthetic process (APOA1, CYP11A1, HSD3B1, HSD3B7). Similarly, while transcripts over expressed in OO+CCs were involved in carbohydrate metabolism (ACO1, 2), molecular transport (GAPDH, GFPT1) and nucleic acid metabolism (CBS, NOS2), those over expressed in CCs+OO were involved in cellular growth and proliferation (FOS, GADD45A), cell cycle (HAS2, VEGFA), cellular development (AMD1, AURKA, DPP4) and gene expression (FOSB, TGFB2). This study generated large-scale gene expression data that provide insights into gene function and interactions within and across different pathways that are involved in the maturation of bovine oocytes. Moreover, the presence or absence of oocyte and CC factors during bovine oocyte maturation has a profound effect on transcript abundance in the different cell types, showing the important molecular cross-talk between oocytes and their CCs. This kind of study has not yet been performed in humans.

A more recent study reported the transcriptomic analysis, by using the Affymetrix Bovine Expression Array, of granulosa cells and oocytes from newborn sheep ovaries (primordial, primary, secondary and small antral follicles) isolated by Laser Capture Microdissection (Bonnet et al., 2011). This study will significantly support clinical programs for rescue of fertility (oocyte production potential) in young women affected by ovarian pathologies or undergoing cancer therapy.

### 2.3.5 Preliminary data and prospective use of equine oocytes

The equine oocyte would make a valid animal model for transcriptomic studies of predictive markers of oocyte quality via analysis of PBs, CCs and GCs. Its peculiarly large PB size and the unique opportunity, due to large follicle size, to perform 1:1 oocyte:somatic cell ratios could allow reliable identification of predictive parameters of oocyte competence by analyzing the PB, CC or GC transcriptome.

Recently, molecular studies preliminary to OMICS applications have been performed in equine embryos. Paris et al., (2011) identified and validated a set of **reference genes** suitable for studying gene expression during equine embryo development. The expression of four carefully-selected reference genes and one developmentally-regulated gene was examined by quantitative PCR in equine in vivo-produced embryos, from the morula to the expanded blastocyst stage. SRP14, RPL4 and PGK1 were identified by geNorm analysis as stably-expressed reference genes suitable for data normalisation. RPL13A expression was less stable and changed significantly during the period of development examined, rendering it unsuitable as a reference gene. As anticipated, CDX2 expression increased significantly during embryo development, supporting its possible role in trophoectoderm specification in the horse. In summary, it was demonstrated that evidence-based selection of potential reference genes aids in validation of stable gene expression in an experimental system, which is particularly useful when dealing with tissues that yield small amounts of mRNA.

Smits et al., (2011) evaluated the difference between **in vivo-** and **in vitro-produced** (IVP) **equine blastocysts** at the genetic level. Suppression subtractive hybridization (SSH) was used to construct a cDNA library enriched for transcripts preferentially expressed in in vivo-derived equine blastocysts compared with IVP blastocysts. Of the 62 different genes identified in this way, six genes involved in embryonic development (BEX2, FABP3, HSP90AA1, MOBKL3, MCM7 and ODC) were selected to confirm this differential expression by RT-quantitative PCR. Five genes were confirmed to be significantly upregulated in in vivo-derived blastocysts (FABP3, HSP90AA1, ODC, MOBKL3 and BEX2), confirming the results of the SSH, however, there was no significant difference in MCM7 expression. Because of their possible importance in embryonic development, the expression of these genes can be used as a marker to evaluate in vitro embryo production systems in the horse, and can be used to compare their roles in embryo development of other species.

Previous studies of functional transcriptomics of individual or associated gene sequences in the **equine oocyte** have been reported by our laboratory (Dell'Aquila et al., 2004 for connexin 43, cyclooxygenase-2 and FSH receptor; Caillaud et al., 2009 for interleukin 1β and its receptors; Dell'Aquila et al., 2008 for the mu opioid receptor; De Santis et al., 2009 for the extracellular calcium-sensing receptor; Lange Consiglio/Cremonesi et al., 2009 for leptin and its ObR receptor) and other groups (Lindbloom et al., 2008 for EGF-like growth factors; Lupole et al., 2010 for ZP genes). To the best of our knowledge, few studies have been performed to date with OMICS technologies in equine reproductive cells or tissues. Fahiminiya et al., (2010) investigated the transcriptome of **granulosa** and **theca cells** from equine follicles at different developmental stages. An equine gene-expression microarray (Agilent technologies Inc., CA, USA) with 44.000 probes was used. Cells were examined from early dominant vs late dominant follicles, and from preovulatory follicles 34 h after injection of crude equine gonadotrophin. It was found that 8349 transcripts were differentially expressed in GC and 2338 in theca cells between preovulatory and late dominant follicles, and that 1602 transcripts were differentially expressed in GC and 8 in theca cells in late dominant vs. early dominant follicles. Thus, it appears that the GC have a highly dynamic nature during the development of dominant follicles. In additional work, Das et al. (2010) analyzed **sperm** and **testis** transcriptomes using the Texas A&M equine whole genome 21351-element oligoarray. Bruemmer et al. (2010) analyzed the **endometrium** transcriptome using the Horse gene expression Agilent microrray for 43000 transcripts. Slough et al., (2011) studied the gene expression (StAR, 3β-HSD, cox, and caspase-3) profile of equine corpus luteum tissue recovered by in vivo biopsy.

### 2.4 Oocyte proteome: The direct representation of the oocyte phenotype

Oocyte mRNA is not a direct representation of the factors that drive oocyte phenotype. The identified mRNA represent potential proteins, but the degree to which the mRNA are being translated is unknown. Thus, an OMICs goal is the identification and measurement of all proteins expressed in the oocyte or embryo. There are two main protein-containing oocyte compartments, the cytoplasm and the zona pellucida. The protein makeup of the oocyte is important for more than simply evaluating oocyte viability; as noted above, the mammalian oocyte cytoplasm possesses factors which can reprogram terminally-differentiated germ cells (sperm) or somatic cells within a few cell cycles. Moreover, it has been suggested that use of oocyte-derived transcripts may enhance the generation of induced pluripotent stem cells. The zona pellucida is composed of glycoproteins involved in the sperm-oocyte interactions which modulate sperm penetration and the fertilization process. Thus, improving our knowledge of oocyte global protein composition is of great interest.

The main phases of proteomic analysis consist of protein extraction, digestion, separation of proteins by gel- or non gel-based methods, mass spectrometry evaluation of digested and separated or electrosprayed peptides, and bioinformatic data analysis (for detailed proteomic methods, see Seli et al., 2010; Wang et al., 2010 and Arnold & Frohlich, 2011). A major problem in oocyte proteome analysis is the requirement of large numbers (thousands) of oocytes. This problem has limited the possibility of performing studies in the human; studies performed to date have been conducted in the mouse and in large animals.

#### 2.4.1 Proteomic studies in the mouse oocyte

Studies in the mouse have incorporated qualitative proteomic approaches, with the intention of generating a protein database to be used for the molecular characterization of the oocyte and developing embryo.

In a pioneering study by Meng et al. (2007), proteomic profiling of mouse mature **COCs** was performed, using two-dimensional electrophoresis and mass spectrometry. A total of 259 protein spots were identified, corresponding to 156 individual proteins. Functional classification of the identified proteins, performed manually according to the biological function of their coding genes, indicated that 12% were involved in cell signaling/communication, 7% in cell division, 31% in gene/protein expression, 24% in cell metabolism, 10% in cell structure and motility, 12% in cell/organism defense, and 4% were unknown.

In a subsequent study by Ma et al., (2008), two-dimensional electrophoresis of mouse **metaphase-II (MII) ooplasmic** proteins (the ZP was removed by digestion before protein extraction) was performed to describe the proteome and phosphoproteome of oocytes derived from ICR mice. A total of 869 selected protein spots, corresponding to 380 unique proteins, were identified successfully by mass spectrometry. Of these, 90 protein spots, representing 53 unique proteins, were stained by Pro-Q Diamond dye, indicating that, within the MII oocyte cytoplasm, they are in phosphorylated forms. All identified proteins were bioinformatically annotated and compared to the embryonic stem-cell proteome. A proteome reference database for the mouse oocyte was established from the protein data generated in this study (http://reprod.njmu.edu.cn/2d).

A subsequent study (Zhang et al., 2009b) applied one-dimensional sodium dodecyl sulfate polyacrylamide gel electrophoresis and reverse-phase liquid chromatography tandem mass spectrometry to analyze the **mature oocyte proteome** of the mouse in depth. Using this high-performance proteomic approach, the authors successfully identified 625 different proteins from 2700 mature mouse oocytes denuded of their zonae pellucidae. They identified 76 maternal proteins having high levels of mRNA expression both in oocytes and fertilized eggs. Many well-known maternal-effect proteins were included in this subset, including MATER and NPM2. In addition, the observed mouse oocyte proteome was compared with a recently published mouse **embryonic stem cell (ESC) proteome** (Van Hoof et al., 2006, see ref. in Zhang et al., 2009), and 371 overlapping proteins were identified.

In a more recent study by Wang et al. (2010), 7,000 mouse oocytes at different developmental stages, including the **GV stage**, the **MII stage**, and **fertilized oocytes (zygotes)**, were evaluated. The authors successfully identified 2,781 proteins present in GV-stage oocytes, 2,973 proteins in MII oocytes, and 2,082 proteins in zygotes, through semiquantitative mass spectrometry. The results of the bioinformatics analysis indicated that different protein compositions were correlated with oocyte characteristics at different developmental stages. For example, specific transcription factors and chromatin remodeling factors were more abundant in MII oocytes, which may be crucial for the epigenetic reprogramming of sperm or somatic nuclei. These results provided important knowledge for better understanding of the molecular mechanisms associated with early development, and may improve the generation of induced pluripotent stem cells.

A more recent study (Pfeiffer et al., 2011) reported the proteome of MII mouse oocytes to a depth of 3699 proteins, which extends the number of proteins identified to date in mouse oocytes to a comparable size to that of the proteome of undifferentiated mouse ES cells. Twenty-eight oocyte proteins, also detected in ES cells, matched the criteria of the multilevel approach reported in this study to screen for reprogramming factors, namely nuclear localization, chromatin modification, and catalytic activity, thus advancing the definition of "reprogrammome", the set of molecules (proteins, RNAs, lipids, and small molecules) that enable nuclear reprogramming.

### 2.4.2 Proteomic studies in farm animal oocytes

Studies in farm animals, such as cattle and pigs, have been performed for both qualitative database generation and for quantification of proteome changes during oocyte IVM (bovine: Coenen et al., 2004; Bhojwani et al., 2006; Massicotte et al., 2006; Memili et al., 2007; Berendt et al., 2009; pig: Ellederova et al., 2004; Susor et al., 2007, reviewed by Ma et al., 2008; Zhang et al., 2009; Arnold & Frohlich, 2011).

Berendt et al. (2009) performed two-dimensional gel electrophoresis saturation labeling to detect quantitative differences in the proteomes of immature versus IVM-MII **bovine oocytes**. From 250 ng of sample analyzed per gel, quantitative analysis revealed an average of 2244 spots in pH 4–7 images and 1291 spots in pH 6–9 images. Focusing on the pH 4-7 images, 38 spots with different intensities between oocyte stages were detected. Spots on a gel from 2200 immature oocytes were identified by nano-LC-MS/MS analysis. The ten spots which could be unambiguously identified include the translationally controlled tumor protein, enzymes of the Krebs and pentose phosphate cycles, clusterin, 14-3-3 ε protein and redox enzymes. In addition, the cellular distribution of two differentially-expressed proteins (14-3-3 ε protein, a mediator of Cdc25 phosphatase inhibition, and TCTP, translationally controlled tumor protein) was determined by confocal laser-scanning microscopy. The quantitative and cellular distribution differences of proteins identified in this study may help to identify attractive candidate proteins for oocyte quality evaluation.

To the best of our knowledge, no proteomics studies have been performed to date in the **equine oocyte**. In our group, the functional role of individual proteins involved in the regulation of meiotic maturation has been investigated by means of western blot or immunostaining and confocal microscopy (Dell'Aquila et al., 2008, De Santis et al., 2009; Lange Consiglio et al., 2009). Equine oocytes could be excellent models for oocyte proteomic studies due to the high abundance of maternal proteins accumulated in their large cytoplasm (160 to 180 microns in diameter) during oogenesis. The relatively large cytoplasmic volume is an important feature as it reduces the number of oocytes needed for effective protein extraction, thus increasing the specificity of the proteome analysis. A recent study performed in Xenopus laevis oocytes, chosen due to their abundant ooplasm, identified a number of proteins involved in the regulation of M-phase entry (Kubiak et al., 2011). The equilibrium among activites of these proteins is responsible for the quality of oocytes and the extent of embryo development, via their participation in decision whether to resume meiosis. Identification of cell-cycle control protein activities in mammalian oocytes may have a great impact on the study not only of oocyte quality but also of cancer growth regulation, and thus establishment of targeted therapies.

On the male side, the global proteome of **sperm** and **seminal plasma of fertile stallions** has been investigated (Novak et al., 2010) to determine whether associations exist between the observed proteome and in vivo fertility. Semen was collected throughout the breeding season from 7 stallions at stud in a commercial breeding station. The stallions were bred to a total of 164 mares to determine conception rates. On three occasions during the breeding season, raw semen was obtained from a regular collection and subjected to proteomic analysis using two-dimensional electrophoresis. The semen sample was also assessed for routine semen-quality end points. The first cycle conception rate was negatively related to ejaculate volume ($r = -0.43$, $P = 0.05$) and total IGF1 content (ng) per ejaculate ($r = -0.58$, $P=0.006$), whereas the overall pregnancy rate was positively related to sperm concentration ($r = 0.56$, $P = 0.01$). The abundance of three proteins known to be involved in carbohydrate metabolism in sperm was positively related to fertility. Abundance of cysteine-rich secretory protein 3 (CRISP3) was positively related to first cycle conception rate ($r = 0.495$, $P = 0.027$) and may provide a good marker of fertility. The abundance of four seminal plasma proteins was negatively related to fertility; these were identified as kallikrein-1E2 (KLK2), clusterin, and seminal plasma proteins 1 (SP1) and 2 (SP2). Based on stepwise regression analysis, low levels of clusterin and SP1 in seminal plasma together with abundance of sperm citrate synthase were predictive of fertility ($r=0.77$, $P< 0.0001$). This study identified proteins within sperm and seminal plasma that could serve as biomarkers of semen quality and fertility in stallions, and may present valid models for sperm fertility biomarkers in humans.

### 2.5 Oocyte lipid fingerprint – Investigating the biological role of structural and reserve lipids

Recently, a new OMIC strategy, namely lipidomics, which utilizes mass spectrometry (MS), chromatography and computer-assisted data analysis, has been proposed. In this approach, lipid molecules are extracted from cells and analyzed by matrix-assisted laser desorption ionization-time of flight (MALDI-TOF) MS (Huang et al., 2005). Like other OMICS, lipidomics is a subject which is both technology-driven and technology-driving, allowing changes in lipid metabolism, including the appearance of new species and the disappearance of others, and compartimentalization of specific lipid species, to be investigated. The underlying fundamentals of different lipidomic experimental approaches and the application of these approaches to the identification of inborn errors of metabolism were reported by Griffiths et al. (2011). Maturing mammalian oocytes, particularly those of farm animals, contain large numbers of cytoplasmic lipid droplets (LDs) whose functional role is still under investigation (Ambruosi et al., 2009). Lipid droplets are discrete organelles present in most cell types and in organisms including bacteria, yeast, plants, insects and animals. Long considered as passive storage deposits, recent proteomic and lipidomic analyses show that LDs are dynamic organelles involved in multiple cellular functions. They serve not only as main reservoirs of neutral lipids such as triglycerides and cholesterol but also contain structural proteins, proteins involved in lipid synthesis and transmembrane proteins (review by Kalantari et al., 2010). A recent study (Ferreira et al., 2010) reported the direct lipid analysis by MALDI-MS of single and intact human, bovine, sheep and fish oocytes. Characteristic lipid profiles, mainly represented by phosphatidylcholines, sphingomyelins and triacylglycerols, were obtained. This study demonstrated that MALDI-MS is capable of providing a reproducible lipid fingerprint from a single oocyte and can be used to investigate developmental modifications or the effects of culture conditions. To our knowledge, no lipidomic studies have been reported to date in the equine oocyte. The equine oocyte, being characterized by polar aggregation of cytoplasmic LDs during maturation, could help to significantly clarify the role of LDs in the maturation and fertilization processes, and in early embryonic development.

### 2.6 Oocyte glycomic analysis – Post-translational protein-carbohydrate modifications

Glycomics deals with the structure and function of glycans or carbohydrates. Lectin-based diagnostics are the main tool aimed at the detection of diseases associated with alterations of the glycosylation profiles of cells. Lectins are proteins that specifically bind to carbohydrates, of either mono- or oligosaccaridic structure. Certain lectins even recognize cell determinants which are not detected by available antibodies. The increasing use of lectins in biomedical diagnostics is leading rapidly to the development of **lectin/glycan microarrays** which could provide efficient, rapid screening tools to detect normal or altered glycosylation patterns in biological samples. Information on glycomics, concerning methods for use of recombinant and artificial lectins and a recently-launched detection platform using lectin microarrays, as well as their application, were reported by Mislovicova et al., 2009 and Gemeiner et al., 2009. A Glycomics DataBase - a data integration platform for glycans and their structures has been recently created (http://www.glycomics.bcf.ku.edu). To our knowledge no studies have been performed to date using large lectin arrays to evaluate oocyte quality. A recent paper by our research unit (Desantis et al., 2009) reported the use of a 13-lectin panel to evaluate differences of the glycoconjugate pattern between equine oocytes surrounded by compact (viable) or expanded (early atretic) cumulus oophorus. It was found that: 1) equine COCs have a species-specific carbohydrate composition; 2) biosynthesis of glycosylated ZP proteins occurs in both CCs and oocytes; 3) viable (compact) and atretic (expanded) COCs express different lectin-binding patterns in their CCs, ZP and ooplasm. This paper also reviewed numerous studies published on the glycoconjugate pattern of cumulus cells, ZP and ooplasm in several species, including humans. These data confirm that the mare is a good model for evaluation the glycome of oocytes of different quality, developmental stage or functional status, and that the application of lectin arrays could be of great value in evaluating oocyte pathology or the effects of culture conditions.

### 2.7 Oocyte metabolic profiling – The instantaneous snapshot of oocyte physiology

Following in the wake of OMICS revolutions, new fields of research are emerging. Among them is metabolomics, a field that holds great promise for the study of oocyte and embryo physiology. The metabolome, that is, the compounds produced by the oocyte, provides the natural complement to the genome and proteome. The physicochemical diversity of the metabolome leads to a subdivision of metabolites into compounds soluble in aqueous solutions or those soluble in organic solvents. A complete molecular and quantitative investigation of the latter when isolated from tissue, fluid or cells is a subset of lipidomics (see Section 2.5). A high-priority aim in evaluating oocyte quality is to establish a non-invasive quantification method. Analysis of oocyte metabolism, by evaluating the follicular fluid (FF) or culture media metabolome could be a useful predictor of pregnancy outcome (Sing & Sinclair, 2007; Nel-Themaat & Nagy, 2011). An important aspect limiting this kind of study in humans is the availability of FF aspirated from individual follicles or availability of culture media of individual oocytes. To correlate FF substances with oocyte quality, it is imperative that each follicle is aspirated individually. The procedure of single follicle aspiration is problematic, both for the patient and for the physician, because it requires multiple vaginal punctures (Revelli et al., 2009). Moreover, needle flushing with culture medium after every puncture must be performed, with a standard volume of flushing medium, in order to avoid cross-contamination and to control the dilution of FF substances. In this context, the availability of animal models from which large numbers of individual specimens may be obtained is of great help. A recent review by Revelli et al. (2009) provides an overview on the current knowledge of biochemical predictors of oocyte quality in FF, starting from studies on single biochemical markers and concluding with the most recent studies on metabolomics. Another study (Nagy et al., 2009) evaluated whether near-infrared spectroscopy-generated metabolomic data, obtained from individual oocyte culture media samples, would correlate with nuclear maturity status and subsequent embryo development. Drops (15-20 µl) of in vitro culture media from 3 h culture of individual oocytes recovered from patients undergoing controlled ovarian hyperstimulation were used to obtain a "viability index" of near-infrared spectroscopy metabolomic profiles. Oocytes at different meiotic stages showed significantly different indices, with a higher viability index related to nuclear maturity (MII stage), embryo grade at Day 3 and Day 5 (grade A) and pregnancy rate (human chorionic gonadotropin-positive).

## 3. Conclusions

OMICS are promising strategies for oocyte quality evaluation in the field of ART, and will lead to a greater understanding of the mechanisms involved in normal oocyte maturation, fertilization and embryo development. It is increasingly clear that large animal models, particularly those species such as horses, whose reproductive management is aimed not only to productivity but also to overcoming infertility, can provide a clinical and biological model for human reproductive phenomena. In addition to their value related to the understanding of human and animal reproduction, "oocyte OMICS" will undoubtedly reveal unexpected and invaluable information that will significantly contribute to the study of stem cell and cancer biology.

## 4. Acknowledgments

M.E. Dell'Aquila would like to thank all students, technicians, clinicians, breeders and local slaughterhouse staff for their invaluable contributions, given in last 25 years, to research activities on oocyte physiology performed at the Department of Animal Production in Bari. A special thought to Professor Paolo Minoia, our mentor in initiating the exciting adventure of the study of farm animal oocytes. This study was supported by COFIN PRIN MIUR 2008 University of Bari, Italy cod. 2008YTYNKE_001 (Resp. Sci. M.E. Dell'Aquila) and Fondi d'Ateneo 2010 University of Bari, Italy cod. ORBA10YTAK (Resp. Sci. M.E. Dell'Aquila).

## 5. References

Ambruosi, B.; Lacalandra, G.M.; Iorga, A.I.; De Santis, T.; Mugnier, S.; Matarrese, R.; Goudet, G. & Dell'Aquila M.E. (2009). Cytoplasmic lipid droplets and mitochondrial distribution in equine oocytes: implications on oocyte maturation, fertilization and developmental competence after ICSI. *Theriogenology*, Vol. 71, No. 7, (April 2009), pp. 1093–1104, ISSN 0093-691X.

Antonello, J.; Patassini, C.; Bottacin, A.; Ferlin, A. & Foresta, C. (2011) Ottimizzazione di un protocollo CGH-array su singolo spermatozoo. Proc. I Congress of Federazione Italiana Società Scientifiche della Riproduzione (FISSR, Riccione 26-28 Maggio 2011) pp. 13-14.

Arnold, G.J. & Frohlich, T. (2010). Dynamic proteome signatures in gametes, embryos and their maternal environment. *Reproduction, Fertility and Development,* Vol. 23, No. 1 (December 2010), pp 81-93, ISSN 1031-3613.

Assou, S.; Cerecedo, D.; Tondeur, S.; Pantesco, V.; Hovatta, O.; Klein, B.; Hamamah, S. & De Vos, J. (2009). A gene expression signature by human mature oocytes and embryonic stem cells. *BMC Genomics,* Vol. 8, N. 10 (January 2009), pag. 10, ISSN 1471-2164.

Berendt, F.J.; Frohlich, T.; Bolbrinker, P.; Boelhauve, M.; Gungor, T.; Habermann, F.A.; Wolf, E. & Arnold G.J. (2009) Highly sensitive saturation labeling reveals changes in abundance of cell cycle-associated proteins and redox enzyme variants during oocyte maturation in vitro. *Proteomics* Vol. 9 (February 2009) pp. 550-564, ISSN 1615-9861.

Bonnet, A.; Bevilacqua, C.; Benne, F.; Bodin, L.; Cotinot, C.; Liaubet, L.; Sancristobal, M.; Sarry, J.; Terenina, E.; Martin, P.; Tosser-Klopp, G. & Mandon-Pepin, B. (2011). Trascriptome profiling of sheep granulosa cells and oocytes during early follicular development obtained by Laser Capture Microdissection. *BMC genomics*, Vol 12. (August 2011), pp. 417, ISSN 1471-2164.

Bruemmer, J.E.; Bouma, J.G.; Hess, A.; Hansen, T.R. & Squires, E.L. Gene expression in the equine endometrium during maternal recognition of pregnancy. *Animal Reproduction Science* Vol. 121 (Suppl. 1-2) (2010) S286-S287, ISSN 0378-4320.

Burton, A. & Torres-Padilla, M.E. (2011) Epigenetic reprogramming and development: a unique heterochromatin organization in the preimplantation mouse embryo. *Briefings in Functional Genomics,* Vol. 9, No. 5-6 (December 2010), pp. 444-454, ISSN 2041-2649.

Caillaud, M.; Dell'Aquila, M.E.; De Santis, T.; Nicassio, M.; Lacalandra, G.M.; Goudet, G.; & Gérard, N. (2008). In vitro equine oocyte maturation in pure follicular fluid plus interleukin-1 and fertilization following ICSI. *Animal Reproduction Sciences*, Vol. 106, No. 3-4 (July 2008), pp. 431-439, ISSN 0378-4320.

Callinan, P.A. & Feinberg, A.P. (2006) The emerging science of epigenomics. *Human Molecular Genetics,* Vol. 15, n°1 (April 2006), pp. R95-R101, ISSN 0964-6906.

Carnevale, E.M. (2008). The mare model for follicular maturation and reproductive aging in the woman. *Theriogenology*, Vol. 69, No. 1, (January 2008) pp. 23-30, ISSN 0093-691X.

Choi, Y.H.; Love, L.B.; Varner, D.D. & Hinrichs, K. (2006). Holding immature equine oocytes in the absence of meiotic inhibitors: Effect on germinal vesicle chromatin and blastocyst development after intracytoplasmic sperm injection. *Theriogenology,* Vol. 66, No. 4 (September 2006), pp. 955-63, ISSN 0093-691X.

Choi, Y.H.; Gustafson-Seabury, A.; Velez, J.C.; Hartman, D.L.; Bliss, S.; Riera, F.L.; Roldan, J.E.; Chowdhary, B.; Hinrichs, K. (2010). Viability of equine embryos after puncture of the capsule and biopsy for preimplantation genetic diagnosis. *Reproduction* Vol 140 No. 6 (December 2010), pp. 893-902, ISSN 1470-1626.

Cremer, T. & Zakhartchenko V (2011) Nuclear architecture in developmental biology and cell specialization. *Reproduction, Fertility and Development* Vol. 23, No. 1 (2011), pp. 94-106, ISSN 1031-3613

Dalbiès-Tran, R. & Mermillod, P. (2003) Use of heterologous complementary DNA array screening to analyze bovine oocyte transcriptome and its evolution during in vitro maturation. *Biology of Reproduction,* Vol. 68, No. 1 (January 2003), pp. 252-261, ISSN 0006-3363.

Das P.J.; Vishnoi, M.; Kachroo, P.; Wang, J.; Love, C.C.; Varner, D.D.; Chowdary B.P.; Raudsepp, T. Expression microarray profiling of sperm and testis mRNA of reproductively normal stallions. *Animal Reproduction Science* Vol. 121 (Suppl. 1-2) (2010) S175, ISSN 0378-4320.

Dell'Aquila, M.E.; Albrizio, M.; Maritato, F.; Minoia, P.; Hinrichs, K. (2003). Meiotic competence of equine oocytes and pronucleus formation after intracytoplasmic sperm injection (ICSI) as related to granulosa cell apoptosis. *Biology of Reproduction,* Vol, 68, No. 6 (June 2003) pp. 2065-72, ISSN 0006-3363.

Dell'Aquila, M.E.; Caillaud, M.; Maritato, F.; Martoriati, A.; Gérard, N.; Aiudi, G.; Minoia, P. & Goudet G. (2004). Cumulus expansion, nuclear maturation and connexin 43, cyclooxygenase-2 and FSH receptor mRNA expression in equine cumulus-oocyte complexes cultured in vitro in the presence of FSH and precursors for hyaluronic acid synthesis. *Reproductive Biology and Endocrinology*. Vol. 2 (June 2004), p. 44, ISSN 1477-7827.

Dell'Aquila, M.E.; Albrizio, M.; Guaricci, A.C.; De Santis, T.; Maritato, F.; Tremoleda, J.L.; Colenbrander, B.; Guerra, L.; Casavola, V. & Minoia P. (2008). Expression and localization of the mu-opioid receptor (MOR) in the equine cumulus-oocyte complex and its involvement in the seasonal regulation of oocyte meiotic competence. *Molecular Reproduction and Development*, Vol. 75, No. 8 (August 2008), pp. 1229-46, ISSN 1040-452X.

De Santis, T.; Casavola, V.; Reshkin, S.J.; Guerra, L.; Ambruosi, B.; Fiandanese, N.; Dalbies-Tran, R.; Goudet, G. & Dell'Aquila, M.E. (2009). The extracellular calcium-sensing receptor is expressed in the cumulus-oocyte complex in mammals and modulates oocyte meiotic maturation. *Reproduction*, Vol. 138, No. 3 (September 2009), pp. 439-452, ISSN 1470-1626.

Desantis, S.; Ventriglia, G.; Zizza, S.; De Santis, T.; Di Summa, A.; De Metrio, G. & Dell'Aquila M.E. (2009). Lectin-binding sites in isolated equine cumulus-oocyte complexes: differential expression of glycosidic residues in complexes recovered with compact or expanded cumulus. *Theriogenology*, Vol. 72, No. 3 (August 2009), pp. 300-309, ISSN 0093-691X.

Fahiminiya, S.; Waddington, D.; Donadeu, X. & Gerard, N. (2010) Transcriptomic analysis of dominant follicle development in mares. *Animal Reproduction Science* Vol. 121 (Suppl. 1-2) (2010) S41, ISSN 0378-4320.

Fauser, B.C.; Diedrich, K.; Bouchard, P.; Domínguez, F.; Matzuk, M.; Franks, S.; Hamamah, S.; Simón, C.; Devroey, P.; Ezcurra, D. & Howles, C.M. (2011). Contemporary genetic technologies and female reproduction. *Human Reproduction Update*, doi: 10.1093/humupd/dmr033 (September 2011), ISSN 1355-4786.

Ferreira, C.R.; Saraiva, S.A.; Catharino, R.R.; Garcia, J.S.; Gozzo, F.C.; Sanvido, G.B.; Santos, L.F.A, Lo Turco, E.G.; Pontes, J.H.F.; Basso, A.C.; Bertolla, R.P.; Sartori, R.; Guardieiro, M.M.; Perecin, F.; Meirelles, F.V.; Sangalli, J.R. & Eberlin M.N. (2010). Single embryo and oocyte lipid fingersprinting by mass spectrometry. *Journal of Lipid Research*, Vol. 51, No. 5 (May 2010), pp. 1218-1227, ISSN 0022-2275.

Geraedts, J.; Collins, J.; Gianaroli, L.; Goossens, V.; Handyside, A.; Harper, J.; Montag, M.; Repping, S. & Schmutzler, A. (2010). What next for preimplantation genetic screening? A polar body approach! *Human Reproduction*, Vol. 25, No. 3 (March 2010), pp. 575-577, ISSN 0268-1161.

Geraedts, J.; Montag, M.; Magli, M.C.; Repping, S.; Handyside, A.H.; Staessen, C.; Harper, J.; Schmutzler, A.; Collins, J.; Goossens, V.; Van der Ven, H.; Vesela, K. & Gianaroli, L. (2011). Polar body array CGH for prediction of the status of the corresponding oocyte. Part I: clinical results. *Human Reproduction*, doi: 10.1093/humrep/der294 (September 2011), ISSN 0268-1161.

Gemeiner, P.; Mislovicova, D.; Tkac, J.; Svitel, J.; Patoprsty, V.; Hrabarova, E.; Kogan, G.; Kozar, T. Lectinomics II. (2009). A highway to biomedical/clinical diagnostics. *Biotecnology Advances* Vol. 27, No. 1 (January-February 2009), pp. 1-15, ISSN 0734-9750.

Griffin, D.K.; Wilton, L.J.; Handyside, A.H.; Winston, R.M.K. & Dehanty, J.D.A. (1992). Dual fluorescent in situ hybridisation for simultaneous detection of X and Y chromosome-specific probes for the sexing of human preimplantation embryonic nuclei. *Human Genetics*. Vol. 89, No. 1 (April 1992), pp. 18-22, ISSN 0340-6717.

Griffiths W.J.; Ogundare M.; Williams C.M. & Wang Y. (2011) On the future of "omics": lipidomics. *Journal of Inherited Metabolic Diseases*, Vol. 34, No. 3 (June 2011), pp. 583-592, ISSN 0141-8955.

Grøndahl, M.L.; Borup R.; Lee Y.B.; Myrhoj, V.; Meinertz, H. & Soresen S. (2009). Differences in gene expression of granulosa cells from women undergoing controlled ovarian hyperstimulation with either recombinant FSH or highly purified hMG. *Fertility and Sterility*, Vol. 91, No. 5 (May 2009), pp. 1820-1830, ISSN 0015-0282.

Grøndahl, M.L.; Yding Andersen, C.; Bogstad, J.; Nielsen, F.C.; Meinertz, H. & Borup, R. (2010). Gene expression profiles of single human mature oocytes in relation to age. *Human Reproduction*, Vol. 25, No. 4 (April 2010), pp. 957-968, ISSN 0268-1161.

Hinrichs, K.; Schmidt, A.L.; Friedman, P.P.; Selgrath, J.P. & Martin, M.G. (1993). In vitro maturation of horse oocytes: characterization of chromatin configuration using fluorescence microscopy. *Biology of Reproduction*, Vol. 48, No. 2 (February 1993), pp. 363-370, ISSN 0006-3363.

Hinrichs, K. & Williams, K.A. (1997). Relationships among oocyte-cumulus morphology, folicular atresia, initial chromatin configuration, and oocyte meiotic competence in the horse. *Biology of Reproduction*, Vol. 57, No. 2 (August 1997), pp. 377-384, ISSN 0006-3363.

Hinrichs, K.; Choi, Y.H.; Love, L.B.; Varner, D.D., Love C.C. & Walckenaer, B.E. (2005) Chromatin configuration within the germinal vesicle of horse oocytes: changes post mortem and relationship to meiotic and developmental competence. *Biology of Reproduction*. Vol. 72, n. 5 (May 2005), pp. 1142-1150, ISSN 0006-3363.

Huang, Y.; Shen, J.; Wang, T.; Yu, Y.K.; Chen, F.F.; Yang, J. (2005). A lipidomic study of the effects of N-methyl-N'-nitro-N-nitrosoguanidine on sphingomyelin metabolism. *Acta Biochim Biophys Sin (Shanghai)*, Vol. 37, No. 8 (August 2005), pp. 515-524, ISSN 1672-9145.

Jones, G.M.; Cram, D.S.; Song, B.; Magli, M.C.; Gianaroli, L.; Lacham-Kaplan, O.; Findlay, J.K.; Jenkin, G. & Trounson A.O. (2008) Gene expression profiling of human oocytes following in vivo or in vitro maturation. *Human Reproduction*, Vol. 23, No. 5 (May 2008), pp. 1138-1144, ISSN 0268-1161.

Kalantari, F.; Bergeron, J.J. & Nilsson T. (2010). Biogenesis of lipid droplets-how cells get fatter. *Molecular Membrane Biology* Vol. 27, No. 8 (November 2010), pp. 462-468, ISSN 0968-7688.

Katz-Jaffe, M.G.; McCallie, B.R.; Preis, K.A.; Filipovits, J. & Gardner, D.K. (2009) Transcriptome analysis of in vivo vs in vitro matured bovine MII oocytes. *Theriogenology*, Vol. 71, No. 6 (April 2009), pp. 939-946, ISSN 0093-691X.

Klatsky PC, Wessel GM, Carson SA. (2010). Detection and quantification of mRNA in single human polar bodies: a minimally invasive test of gene expression during oogenesis. *Molecular Human Reproductin*, Vol. 16, No. 12 (December 2010), pp. 938-943, ISSN1360-9947.

Kocabas, A.M.; Crosby, J.; Ross, P.J.; Otu, H.H.; Beyhan, Z.; Can, H.; Tam, W.L.; Rosa, G.J.M.; Halgren, R.G.; Lim, B.; Fernandez, E. & Cibelli, J.B. (2006). The trascriptome of human oocytes. *PNAS*, Vol. 103, No. 38 (September 2006), pp. 14027-14032, ISSN 1091-6490.

Kubiak, J.Z. (2011). Proteomics of M-phase entry: "Omnen" vs. "More" the battle for oocyte quality and beyond. *Folia Histochemica et Cytobiologica*, Vol. 49, No. 1 (2011), pp. 1-7, ISSN 0239-8508.

Lange Consiglio, A.; Dell'Aquila, M.E.; Fiandanese, N.; Ambruosi, B.; Cho, Y.S.; Bosi, G.; Arrighi, S.; Lacalandra, G.M. & Cremonesi, F. (2009). Effects of leptin on in vitro maturation, fertilization and embryonic cleavage after ICSI and early developmental expression of leptin (Ob) and leptin receptor (ObR) proteins in the horse. *Reproductive Biology and Endocrinology*, Vol 7. (October 2009), p. 113, ISSN 1477-7827.

Le Bourhis, A.D.; Mullaart, E.; Humblot, P.; Coppieters, W.; Ponsart, C. (2011). Bovine embryo genotyping using a 50k single nucleotide polymorphism chip. *Reproduction, Fertility and Development* Vol.23 (2011), p. 197, ISSN 1031-3613.

Lindbloom, S.M.; Farmerie, T.A.; Clay, C.M.; Seidel, G.E. Jr & Carnevale, E.M. (2008). Potential involvement of EGF-like growth factors and phosphodiesterases in initiation of equine oocyte maturation. *Animal Reproduction Sciences,* Vol. 103, No. 1-2 (January 2008), pp. 187-192, ISSN 0378-4320.

Lupole, R.E.; Bouma, G.J.; Clay, C.M.; Seidel, G.E.Jr & Carnevale E.M. (2010) Effect of mare age on gene expression of equine zona pellucida proteins and sperm binding. *Animal Reproduction Science* Vol. 121 (Suppl. 1-2) (2010) S252-253, ISSN 0378-4320.

Ma, M.; Guo, X.; Wang, F.; Zhao, C.; Liu, Z.; Shi, Z.; Wang, Y.; Zhang, P.; Zhang, K.; Wang, N.; Lin, M.; Zhou, Z.; Liu, J.; Li, Q.; Wang, L.; Huo, R.; Sha, J. & Zhou, Q. (2008). Protein expression profile of the Mouse Metaphase II oocyte. *Journal of Proteome Research* Vol. 7, No. 11 (November 2008), pp. 4821-4830, ISSN 1535-3893.

Magli, M.C.; Montag, M.; Koster, M.; Muzi, L.; Geraedts, J.; Collins, J.; Goossens, V.; Handyside, A.H.; Harper, J.; Repping, S.; Schmutzler, A.; Vesela, K. & Gianaroli, L. (2011). Polar body array CGH for prediction of the status of the corresponding oocyte. Part II: technical aspects. *Human Reproduction,* doi: 10.1093/humrep/der295 (September 2011), ISSN 0268-1161.

Mamo, S.; Carter, F.; Lonergan, P.; Leal, C.V.L.; Al Naib, A.; McGettigan, P.; Mehta, J.P.; Evans, A.C.O. & Fair, T. (2011). Sequential analysis of global gene expression profiles in immature and in vitro matured bovine oocytes: potential molecular markers of oocyte maturation. *BMC Genomics,* Vol 12 (March 2011), pp. 151, ISSN 1471-2164.

Matzuk, M.M. & Lamb, D.J. (2008). The biology of infertility: research advances and clinical challenges. *Nature Medicine* Vol. 14, No. 11(November 2008), ISSN 1078-8956.

Mislovicova, D.; Gemeiner, P.; Kozarova, A. & Kozar, T. (2009). Lectinomics I. Relevance of exogenus plant lectins in biomedical diagnostics. *Biologia*. Vol. 64, No. 1 (2009), pp. 1-19, ISSN 0006-3088.

Meng, Y.; Xiao-hui, L.; Shen, Y.; Fan, L.; Leng, J.; Liu, J. & Sha, J. (2007). The protein profile of mouse mature cumulus-oocyte complex. *Biochimica et Biophysica Acta,* Vol. 1774, No. 11 (November 2007), pp. 1477-1490, ISSN 0304-4165.

Nagy, Z.P.; Jones-Colon, S.; Roos, P.; Botros, L.; Greco, E.; Dasig, J. & Behr, B. (2009). Metabolomic assessment of oocyte viability. *Reproductive BioMedicine Online*. Vol 18, No. 2 (February 2009), pp 219-225, ISSN 1472-6483.

Nel-Themaat, L. & Nagy, Z.P. (2011). A review of the promises and pitfalls of oocyte and embryo metabolomics. *Placenta,* Vol 32, No. Suppl 3 (September 2011), pp. 5257-5263, ISSN 0143-4004.

Novak, S.; Smith, T.A.; Paradis, F.; Burwash, L.; Dyck, M.K.; Foxcroft, G.R. & Dixon, W.T. (2010). Biomarkers of in vivo fertility in sperm and seminal plasma of fertile stallions. *Theriogenology* Vol. 74, No. 6 (October 2010), pp. 956-67, ISSN 0093-691X.

Parfenov, V.; Potchukalina, G.; Dudina, L.; Kostyuchek, K. & Gruzova, M. (1989). Human antral follicles: oocyte nucleus and the karyosphere formation (electron microscopic and autoradiographic data). *Gamete Research,* Vol. 22, No. 2 (February 1989), pp. 219-231, ISSN 0148-7280.

Paris, D.B.; Kuijk, E.W.; Roelen, B.A. & Stout, T.A. (2011). Establishing reference genes for use in real time quantitative PCR analysis of early equine embryo. *Reproduction Fertility and Development,* Vol. 23, No. 2 (January 2011), pp. 353-363, ISSN 1031-3613.

Pfeiffer, M.J.; Siatkowski, M.; Paudel, Y.; Balbach, S.T.; Baeumer, N.; Crosetto, N.; Drexler, H.C.A.; Fuellen, G. & Boiani, M. (2011). Proteomic analysis of mouse oocytes reveals 28 candidate factors for the "Reprogammome". *Journal of Proteomic Research,* Vol. 10 , No. 5 (May 2011), pp. 2140-2153, ISSN 1535-3893.

Regassa, A.; Rings, F.; Hoelker,,M.; Tholen, E.; Looft, C.; Schellander, K. & Tesfaye, D. (2001) Transcriptome dynamics and molecular cross-talk between bovine oocyte and its companion cumulus cells. *BMC Genomics,* Vol 12 (January 2011), pp. 57, ISSN 1471-2164.

Revelli, A.; Delle Piane, L.; Casano, S.; Molinari, E.; Massobrio, M. & Rinaudo, P. (2009). Follicular fluid content and oocyte quality: from single biochemical markers to metabolics. *Reprodutive Biology and Endocrinology* Vol. 7 (May 2009), p. 40, ISSN 1477-7827.

Rodrigues-Zas, S.L.; Schellander, K. & Lewin H.A. (2008). Biological interpretation of transcriptomic profiles in mammalian oocytes and embryos. *Reproduction,* Vol. 135, No. 2 (February 2008), pp. 129-139, ISSN 1470-1626.

Romar, R.; De Santis, T.; Papillier, P.; Perreau, C.; Thelie, A.; Dell'Aquila, M.E.; Mermillod, P. & Dalbies-Tran, R. (2011). Expression of maternal transcripts during bovine oocyte In vitro maturation is affected by donor age. *Rerpoduction in domestic animals.* Vol. 46, No. 1 (February 2011), pp. e23-e30, ISSN 0936-6768.

Seli, E.; Robert, C. & Sirard, M.A. (2010). OMICS in assisted reproduction: possibilities and pitfalls. *Molecular Human Reproduction,* Vol. 16, No. 8 (August 2010), pp. 513-530, ISSN 1360-9947.

Simarro Fagundes, N.; Michalczechen Lacerda, V.A.; Siqueira Caixeta, E.; Marinheiro Machado, G.; de Oliveira Melo, E.; Rumpf, R.; Alves Nunes Dode, M. & Machaim Franco, M. (2010) Methylation pattern of a differentially methylated region located in the last exon of the *igf2* gene in oocytes from nellore cows *Reproduction Fertility and Development* Vol.22, (January 2010) p. 283 ISSN 1031-3613.

Singh, R. & Sinclair, K.D. (2007). Metabolomics: approaches to assessing oocyte and embryo quality. *Theriogenology,* 2007, 68 (Suppl I): S56-S62.

Slough, T.L.; Rispoli, L.A.; Carnevale, E.M.; Niswender G.D. & Bruemmer J.E. (2011) Temporal gene expression in equine corpora lutea based on serial biopsies in vivo. *Journal of Animal Sciences,* Vol 89, No. 2 (February 2011) pp. 389-396, ISNN 0021-8812.

Smallwood, S.A.; Tomizawa, S.; Krueger, F.; Ruf, N.; Carli, N.; Segonds-Pichon, A.; Sato, S.; Hata, K.; Andrews, S.R. & Kelsey, G. (2011). Dynamic CpG island methylation landscape in oocytes and preimplantation embryos. *Nature genetics,* Vol. 43, n. 8 (August 2011), pp. 811-815, ISSN 1061-4036.

Smits, K.; Goossens, K.; Van Soom, A.; Govaere, J.; Hoogewijs, M. & Peelman, L.J. (2011). In vivo derived horse blastocysts show transcriptional up-regulation of developmentally important genes compared with in vitro produced horse blastocysts. *Reproduction, Fertility and Development,* Vol. 23, No. 2 (2011), pp. 364-375, ISSN 1031-3613.

Thelie, A.; Papillier, P.; Perreau, C.; Uzbekova, S.; Hennequet-Antier, C. & Dalbies-Tran, R. (2009). Regulation of bovine oocyte-specific transcripts during in vitro oocyte maturation and after maternal-embryonic transition analyzed using a transcriptomic approach. *Molecular Reproduction and Development,* Vol. 76, No. 8 (August 2009), pp. 773–782, ISSN 1040-452X.

Treff, N.R.; Su, J.; Kasabwala, N.; Tao, X.; Miller, K.A. & Scott, R.T.J. (2010). Robust embryo identification using first polar body single nucleotide polymorphism microarray-based DNA fingerprinting. *Fertility and Sterility.* Vol. 93, No. 7 (May 2010), pp. 2453-2455, ISSN 0015-0282. (a)

Treff, N.R.; Su, J.; Tao, X.; Levy, B. & Scott, R.T.Jr. (2010). Accurate single cell 24 chromosome aneuploidy screening using whole genome amplification and single nucleotide polymorphism microarrays. *Fertility and Sterility.* Vol. 94, No. 6 (November 2010), pp. 2017-2021, ISSN 0015-0282. (b)

Tosti, E. & Boni, R. (2011). *Oocyte maturation and fertilization: a long history for a short event.* Bentham Books. ISBN 978-1-60805-182-3.

Wain, L.V. & Tobin, M.D. (2011) Copy number variation, In: *Genetic Epidemiology,* M. Dawn Dawn Teare (Ed.), Humana Press, New York, NY - USA Vol. 713 Methods in Molecular Biology pp.167-183, ISSN 1064-3745.

Wang, S.; Kou, Z.; Jing, Z.; Zhang, Y.; Guo, X.; Dong, M.; Wilmut, I. & Gao, S. (2010). Proteome of mouse oocytes at different developmental stages. *Proceedings of the National Academy of Sciences (PNAS) U S A,* Vol. 107, No. 41, (October 2010), pp. 17639-44, ISSN 0027-8424.

White, C.A. & Salamonsen, L.A. (2005). A guide to issues in microarray analysis: application to endometrial biology. *Reproduction,* Vol. 130, No. 1 (July 2005), pp. 1-13, ISSN 1470-1626.

Wells, D. & Patrizio, P. (2008). Gene expression profiling of human oocytes at different maturational stages and after in vitro maturation. *American Journal of Obstetrics and Gynecology* Vol. 198, No. 4 (April 2008), pp. 455.e1-455.e11, ISSN 00029378.

Wood, J.R.; Dumesic, D.A.; Abbot, D.H. & Strauss, J.F. (2007). Molecular abnormalities in oocytes from women with polycystic ovary syndrome revealed by microarray analysis. *The Journal of Clinical Endocrinology and Metabolism,* Vol. 92, No. 2 (February 2007), pp. 705-713, ISSN 0021-972X.

Zhang, P.; Zucchelli, M.; Bruce, S.; Hambiliki, F.; Stavreus-Evers, A.; Levkov, L.; Skottman, H.; Kerkelä, E.; Kere, J. & Hovatta, O. (2009). Transcriptome profiling of human pre-implantation development. *PLoS One,* Vol. 4, No. 11 (November 2009), pp. e7844, ISSN 1932-6203 (a).

Zhang, P.; Ni, X.; Guo, Y.; Guo, X.; Wang, Y.; Zhou, Z.; Huo, R. & Sha, J. (2009). Proteomic-based identification of maternal proteins in mature mouse oocytes. *BMC Genomics,* Vol 10 (August 2009), ISSN 1471-2164 (b).

15

# Insight Into the Molecular Program of Meiosis

Hiba Waldman Ben-Asher and Jeremy Don*
*The Mina & Everard Goodman Faculty of Life Sciences, Bar-Ilan University, Israel*

## 1. Introduction

"We estimate that >2,300 genes (~4% of the mouse genome) are dedicated to male germ cell-specific transcripts, 99% of which are first expressed during or after meiosis". This quotation from a paper published by Schultz et al. (2003), reflects the tremendous complexity of gamete production, the essence of which is meiosis. Meiosis is a differantiative process in which seemingly contradicting molecular pathways are activated simultaneously. On one hand the regular components and checkpoints of the cell division machinery, which is complex enough by itself, are utilized, but on the other hand a whole array of genes are activated to enable the unique characteristics of the meiotic division, such as partition of homologous chromosomes, and not the sister chromatides, in meiosis I, or executing cell division without a prior DNA duplication in meiosis II. On one hand double strand breaks are deliberately formed to ensure pairing of homologous chromosomes and recombination, but on the other hand a whole array of genes involved in DNA repair and safeguarding genome integrity are alerted. The meiotic complexity is also exemplified by the extensive dependence on a cross-talk between germ cells themselves, and between the differentiating germ cells and their surrounding somatic cells, i.e. Sertoli cells in the testis or granulosa cells in the ovarian follicle. Finally, the complexity of the meiotic process is depicted by the differences between males and females, regarding both the outcome of the meiotic division (four basically similar post meiotic round spermatids in the male versus one functional egg and three polar body cells that degenerate in the female), and its kinetics (a continuous process in the male versus an in-continuous process in the female). It is, therefore, absolutely crucial that the very many different molecular pathways operating during meiosis be tightly concerted and regulated. However, Virginia Hughes, in a paper published in Nature medicine (2008), stated that: "So far, scientists have identified nearly 300 DNA mutations in man with reproductive defects", implying that our understanding of the meiotic molecular network is still very limited, although significant progress has been made since 2008.

Various techniques were applied during the years to study the role of different genes during meiosis. These include: 1) developing spermatogenic cell culture systems and studying the effect of over-expressing / silencing specific genes on entry into and progressing through meiosis *in-vitro* (Farini et al. 2005; Feng et al. 2002; Nayernia et al. 2006); 2) developing genetically modified animal models, mainly mice, (including Knockout models) to study the effect of modification or deletion of a specific gene on the meiotic process *in*-vivo (review in Jamsai & O'Bryan, 2011); 3) utilizing complementation approaches to detect genes with new

*Corresponding author

meiotic functions, such as Aym1 (Malcov et al. 2004); and 4) utilizing spermatogonial cell transplantation approaches in testicular repopulation studies (Brinster 2002; Brinster & Zimmermann 1994; McLean 2005). These studies contributed greatly to understanding the role of specific genes during meiosis, but it was not until the emergence of the microarray technology and the development of sophisticated bioinformatics tools that large scale studies on meiotic molecular networks and regulation could be executed. Indeed, several microarray studies on meiotic genes were performed (Chalmel et al. 2007; Schlecht et al. 2004; Schultz et al. 2003; Shima et al. 2004; Yu et al. 2003), yielding a huge amount of new information. However, the biological significance of the transcriptomic data obtained in these experiments, in terms of understanding the molecular program of meiosis, is still an ongoing challenge.

Using mouse spermatogenesis as a model system, we recently performed a comprehensive meiotic microarray study (Waldman Ben-Asher et al., 2010). This study was based on the known developmental schedule of the first spermatogenic wave (Bellve et al. 1977; Malkov et al. 1998). According to this developmental schedule, until post-natal age of 7 days (pn d7), the seminiferous tubules within the testis contain only pre-meiotic spermatogonia cells, along side with the somatic Sertoli cells. By pn d10, spermatocytes from the first spermatogenic wave enter prophase I of the meiotic division, and by pn d12 zygotene spermatocytes first appear. At pn d14 and 17, these cells reach the early and late pachytene stage, respectively. At pn d21, post meiotic round spermatids are found and at pn d24 and d27 elongating and elongated haploid spermatids are present in the testis, respectively. Testes from pn d35 mice are expected to contain the entire spermatogenic lineage. Thus, in our microarray study we compared the testicular transcriptomes of pups at: pn d7, pn d10, pn d12, pn d14, and pn d17. In these experiments we were able to clearly define six apparent patterns of gene expression throughout meiosis (Figure 1). Given this as a starting point, we will describe in this chapter the use of several bioinformatic approaches to ascribe biological significance to our results, thus getting new insights into the molecular program of meiosis.

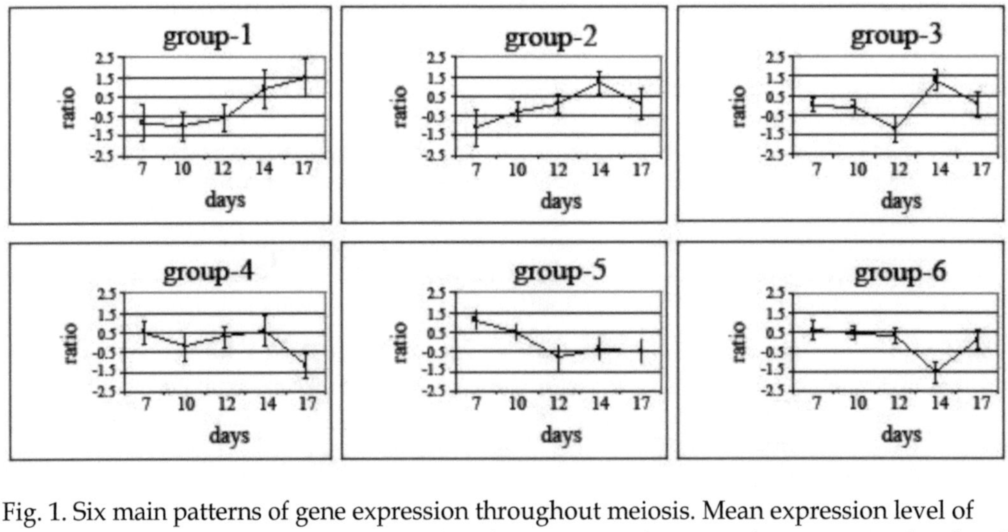


Fig. 1. Six main patterns of gene expression throughout meiosis. Mean expression level of the genes within each group is expressed as the mean ratio between the expression level and the geometric average for each developmental stage. (reproduced with permission from Waldman Ben-Asher et al., 2010).

## 2. Regulating meiotic gene expression

### 2.1 Chromosomal localization of genes as an expressional regulatory factor

One of the intriguing findings we have noticed in analyzing our microarray results was that genes from the different expressional groups are not randomly distributed throughout the genome. There are specific chromosomes that preferentially harbor genes from specific expressional groups, whereas other chromosomes are preferentially depleted of genes from specific expressional groups (Waldman Ben-Asher et al., 2010). For this analysis, we first determined, bioinformatically, the chromosomal location of each of the genes within each of the six expression groups that were obtained, and calculated the percentage of genes within each group that appear on a specific chromosome. This, was then, compared to the percentage of annotated genes from the entire mouse genome that are located on each specific chromosome. The statistical significance of the differences between the distribution of the meiotic genes within each group and that of the genes of the entire genome on each chromosome was determined using the confidence interval test, with $p<0.05$ indicating statistically significant differences. To address the randomness of the chromosomal location of genes that are specifically up-regulated or suppressed during the various meiotic stages, 1000 random lists from the entire genome, consisting of the same number of genes as in each of our six expression groups (6,000 lists altogether), were created and the mean distribution of all 1000 randomly sampled lists in each group (expressed as percentage of genes on each chromosome), ±SD, was calculated. We found that the obtained results were basically identical to those obtained with the whole genome distribution, with very small SDs. These results indicated that the distribution of annotated genes from the entire mouse genome along the chromosomes resembles random distribution, rendering the deviations in chromosomal distribution among meiotic genes, statistically and functionally significant. Our results, which are summarized in table 1, indicate that genes from group 1 are enriched on chromosome 11 and on chromosome 17, and are under represented on chromosome X. Genes from group 2 are enriched in chromosomes 3 and 15, and genes from group 3 are enriched in chromosome 11 whereas chromosome 13 is almost completely depleted of genes from this group. The distribution of genes from group 4, do not deviate significantly from the whole genome distribution. Genes from group 5 are under-represented in chromosome 4 and over-represented in chromosome 8, and group 6 genes are over-represented in chromosomes 1 and 6 and under represented in chromosome 15. Furthermore, an in-depth examination of the results in this analysis revealed a mirror-like patterns of expression of groups 2 and 6, with over and under representation on chromosome 15, respectively. This might point at chromosome 15 as containing genes that are especially required for the pachytene stage at day 14. A similar mirror-like patterns of expression exist also in groups 1 and 5 with over and under representation on chromosome 11, respectively (under representation of group 5 genes on chromosome 11 was just above the $p<0.05$ limit), suggesting that this chromosome contains meiotically-regulated genes that are not activated during the first steps of spermatogenesis, but only later, as cells enter and proceed through meiosis (p.n. days 12-17). The functional conclusion from this gene location analysis is that chromosomal location seems to be a factor in regulating gene expression during meiosis.

| | Group 1 | Group 2 | Group 3 | Group 4 | Group 5 | Group 6 |
|---|---|---|---|---|---|---|
| Chromo. 1 | | | | | | + 10% vs. 6% |
| Chromo. 3 | | + 9% vs. 4% | | | | |
| Chromo. 4 | | | | | - 1% vs. 7% | |
| Chromo. 6 | | | | | | + 9% vs. 5% |
| Chromo. 8 | | | | | + 10% vs. 5% | |
| Chromo. 11 | + 15% vs. 8% | | + 17% vs. 8% | | | |
| Chromo. 13 | | | - 0.1% vs. 4% | | | |
| Chromo. 15 | | + 9% vs. 3% | | | | - 1% vs. 3% |
| Chromo. 17 | + 9% vs. 5% | | | | | |
| Chromo. X | - 0.5% vs. 4% | | | | | |

Table 1. Summary of deviations in distribution of meiotic genes from the six expressional groups, along chromosomes, compared to whole genome/random distribution. All indicated deviations are statistically significant ($p<0.05$). Over-representation is denoted by (+), under-representation is denoted by (-). Percent of meiotic genes versus percent of whole genome genes are indicated. For example, 15% of group 1 genes are located on chromosome 11 versus 8% of whole genome/random distribution.

In an attempt to take the chromosomal location analysis one step forward, we asked, to what extend does genes from the same expressional group that are located on the same chromosome are clustered in the vicinity of each other. The rational for this analysis was that such clustering might enable co-regulation of expression by sharing overall chromatin organization that favors either transcription or silencing. For this analysis we used the DAVID program, a program that identifies functional groups of genes that are enriched in a given dataset compared with their representation in the entire genome (Huang et al., 2009a; Huang et al., 2009b). We, therefore, looked for genes that were clustered to specific cytobands. As shown in table 2, in four of the six groups we found only small clusters (2-5 genes), within specific cytobands, that were statistically significant compared to random distribution along the specific chromosome ($p<0.05$). This suggests that clustering to specific chromosomal regions (cytobands) might, at the most, contribute to regulation of expression at the local level but does not contribute significantly (if at all) to the overall co-regulation of expression within each group.

| Group | Cytoband | No. of genes | p-value | Gene symbol | Gene name |
|---|---|---|---|---|---|
| 1 | 10 D3 | 3 | 0.04 | DDIT3 | DNA-damage inducible transcript 3 |
| | | | | slc16a7 | solute carrier family 16 (monocarboxylic acid transporters), member 7 |
| | | | | USP15 | ubiquitin specific peptidase 15 |
| 2 | 17 B1 | 2 | 0.01 | Ppt2 | palmitoyl-protein thioesterase 2 |
| | | | | MSH5 | mutS homolog 5 (E. coli) |
| 2 | 15 A1 | 2 | 0.01 | GHR | growth hormone receptor |
| | | | | Lifr | leukemia inhibitory factor receptor |
| 2 | 3 F2.1 | 3 | 0.02 | PEX11B | peroxisomal biogenesis factor 11 beta |
| | | | | TCHH | trichohyalin |
| | | | | ANP32E | acidic (leucine-rich) nuclear phosphoprotein 32 family, member E |
| 2 | 15 D3 | 3 | 0.04 | Gml | GPI anchored molecule like protein |
| | | | | Hemt1 | hematopoietic cell transcript 1 |
| | | | | LRRC6 | leucine rich repeat containing 6 (testis) |
| 5 | 5 C3.1 | 2 | 0.01 | pgm1 | phosphoglucomutase 1 |
| | | | | UGDH | UDP-glucose dehydrogenase |
| 6 | 4 C3 | 2 | 0.01 | TYRP1 | tyrosinase-related protein 1 |
| | | | | Ptprd | protein tyrosine phosphatase, receptor type, D |
| 6 | 11 D | 5 | 0.02 | PPY | pancreatic polypeptide |
| | | | | utp18 | UTP18, small subunit (SSU) processome component, homolog (yeast) |
| | | | | NT5C3L | 5'-nucleotidase, cytosolic III-like |
| | | | | copz2 | coatomer protein complex, subunit zeta 2 |
| | | | | igfbp4 | insulin-like growth factor binding protein 4 |
| 6 | 13 A3.3 | 3 | 0.02 | LOC636537 | Signal sequence receptor 4 |
| | | | | dsp | desmoplakin |
| | | | | TXNDC5 | thioredoxin domain containing 5 |
| 6 | 7 F5 | 2 | 0.03 | Lsp1 | lymphocyte specific 1 |
| | | | | TSPAN3 | tetraspanin 32 |
| 6 | 3 G3 | 3 | 0.04 | Gm11295 or ELOVL6 | ELOVL family member 6 |
| | | | | TMEM56 | transmembrane protein 56 |
| | | | | NPNT | nephronectin |

Table 2. Summary of genes, from the different expressional groups, that are clustered at specific cytobands on the different chromosomes. Cytobands are denoted by the chromosome number followed by the specific cytoband location symbol. The p-value, as calculated by the DAVID program, represents the statistical significance of the clustering, compared to random distribution of the genes along the specific chromosome. Only clusters with $p<0.05$ were considered in this analysis.

### 2.2 Common cis-regulatory sequence elements within each expressional group

Unique cis-regulatory elements common to genes within a transcriptional group, if found, may explain co-regulation and similar expression patterns. To address this issue, regarding our six expression groups, we first created a file for each expression group, containing all of the gene promoter sequences in Fasta format. The length of the promoter region was defined as 1200 bp consisting of 1000 bp upstream to the transcription Initiation Site (TIS) and 200 bp downstream the TIS. The promoter region was extracted from the UCSC database, using the table application (NCBI37/mm9 assembly). Next, we used these lists as input in the Genomatix-MatInspector application (Cartharius et al., 2005) to search for matches against transcription factor (TF) recognition motifs. MatInspector is a software tool that utilizes a large library of matrix descriptions for transcription factor binding sites to locate matches in DNA sequences. The output of this application was a list of transcription factor families whose DNA recognition motifs are common to the promoters of the different expression groups. We defined a common TF family binding site as a motif which is

| TF | Group1 | Group2 | Group3 | Group4 | Group5 | Group6 |
|---|---|---|---|---|---|---|
| NKXH | | | * | * | * | * |
| ETSF | * | * | * | * | * | * |
| HOXF | * | | * | * | * | * |
| CREB | * | * | * | * | * | * |
| TBPF | | | * | | | |
| GATA | | | * | * | | |
| FKHD | * | | * | | * | * |
| NR2F | * | * | * | * | * | * |
| EVI1 | * | | * | * | * | |
| MZF1 | | | * | | | |
| PAX6 | | * | * | | | |
| CLOX | | | * | * | | |
| SORY | * | | | | | |
| ZBPF | | * | | | * | * |
| MYT1 | | | | * | | |
| RXRF | * | * | | * | * | * |
| SP1F | * | * | | * | * | * |
| EGRF | * | * | | * | | * |
| MYBL | * | | | * | | * |
| MAZF | | | | * | | * |
| E2FF | * | * | | * | | * |

Table 3. Common TF binding motifs in promoter sequences of genes within each expression group. An asterisk represents the presence of the specific transcription factor target sequence in at least 90% of the genes in that group. In yellow – TF common to all groups. In red - TF common to only one group.

represented in at least 90% of the promoter sequences of each specific group (Table 3). We noticed that three transcription factor families, ETSF (Human and murine ETS1 factors), CREB (cAMP-responsive Element Binding proteins) and NR2F (nuclear receptor subfamily 2 factor), were common to all groups, suggesting they are unlikely to be responsible for the differential expression pattern of any individual group. Of special interest were four TF families which appeared only in one group: TBPF (TATA-binding protein factors) in group 3, MZF1 (Myeloid Zinc Finger 1 factors) also in group 3, SORY (Sox/Sry-sex/testis determining and related HMG box factors) in group 1 and MYT1 (MYT1 C2HC zinc finger protein) in group 4. TATA box binding protein (TBP) is a general transcription factor that plays an important role in transcription initiation of many genes. Various members of the TBP family have been identified, such as the TBP-related factors (TRFs) as well as numerous tissue-specific homologs of TBP-associated factors (TAFs) (Hochheimer & Tjian, 2003). TRF2 (known also as TLP or TRP) has a testis-specific form which is first detectable at pn d14 mouse testis and its level is increased at later stages of testicular development (Sugiura et al., 2003). Our microarray results showed a rather similar pattern of expression for TRF2 (Figure 2 - green line). Interestingly, four other genes of the TBP family (TBP, TAF1b, TAF9( 2 probes) ,MED20) were present in our microarray list of meiotic regulated genes, all having the same pattern of increased level of expression from pn d12 (Figure 2). The similar expression pattern of these transcription factors through pn days 12-17 may suggest that they work together through the meiotic phase, and might account, at least in part, for the expression pattern of group 3.

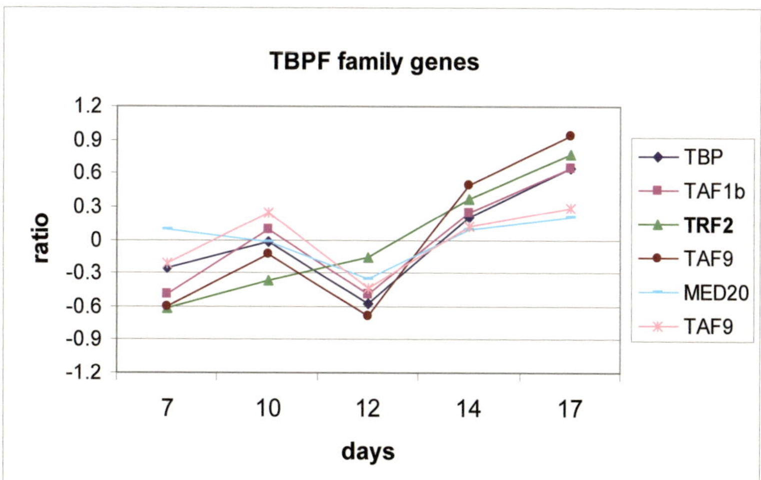


Fig. 2. Expression pattern of members of the TBPF family of transcription factors during meiosis, as obtained in our microarray analysis.

The specific binding motif for the myelin transcription factor 1 (Myt1) family appeared in the promoter sequences of more then 90% of genes of group 4. This family of transcription factors is comprised of three zinc finger genes: Myt1 (known also as Nzf2), Myt1L (known also as Png1), and Myt3 (known also as Nzf3 or St18). These transcription factors belong to the structurally unique CCHHC class, that are expressed predominantly in the developing Central Nervous System, CNS (Romm et al., 2005). Nonetheless, in rat cells, Myt1 was reported to interact with Sin3b, a protein that mediates transcriptional repression by binding to histone deacetylases (HDACs) (Romm et al., 2005). In our microarray results, the second member of the family, Myt1L, showed an increase in its expression between days 12 to 14, suggesting the potential involvement in regulating the characteristic transcriptional repression seen in group 4 between d14 and d17.

The SORY TF family consists of high mobility group (HMG) genes from two subfamilies: HMGA and HMGB. This family includes the SRY gene as well as various SOX genes, all of which function as transcriptional activators. Some of these genes were reported to play a role during spermatogenesis. For example, Sox3 expression was shown to be restricted to type A spermatogonia and to be required for spermatogenesis through a pathway that involves Ngn3 (Raverot et al., 2005). Sox7 and Sox17 were reported to function synergistically in the transcription of the Mouse laminin-α1 gene during differentiation of mouse F9 embryonal carcinoma cells into parietal endoderm cells (Niimi et al., 2004), and Hager et al. (2005) showed that laminin-α chains are vital for spermatogenesis. Notwithstanding, the expression pattern of some members of this family of transcription factors during meiosis, as depicted in our microarray analysis, do not intuitively favor specific involvement in transcriptional regulation of group 1 genes. Nevertheless, further analysis is required before definite conclusions are drawn.

The MZF1 family represents the Myeloid zinc finger protein 1 (also known as Znf42, Mzf2, Zfp98, or Zfp121). It belongs to the Krüppel family of zinc finger proteins, and it was found to play a key role in regulating transcription during differentiation along the myeloid lineage (Yan et al., 2006). These authors also demonstrated that over-expression of MZF1 repressed the ERCC1 promoter activity upon cisplatin exposure, suggesting that MZF1 might be a repressor of ERCC1 transcription. ERCC1 is a critical gene within the nucleotide excision repair pathway and only recently it was shown to play an essential role in DNA damage repair during spermatogenesis related recombination. Deficiency of this gene results in the production of abnormal sperm (Hsia et al., 2003; Paul et al., 2007). Our analysis revealed that only group 3 promoters met the limit of 90% representation of the Mzf1 TF binding site. The Mzf1 expression pattern itself was not revealed by our microarray analysis since it did not pass the stringent selection for genes exhibiting at least two-fold change in expression, compared to the geometric average, at any of the meiotic stages that were tested (Waldman Ben-Asher et al., 2010). However, it is still very well possible that Mzf1 indeed plays a role in repressing expression of meiosis-related genes, such as those of group 3.

Finally, it is, of-course, possible that the differential pattern of expression in each group is a result of a combinatorial co-regulation by several transcription factors. In this context it is noteworthy that none of the expressional groups share the same distribution of common TF motifs in their promoters (Table 3).

## 3. Functional analysis of gene networks – Apoptosis as a test case

Following the expression kinetics of genes, within specific gene networks, throughout meiosis, enables an insight as to how specific processes are operated and regulated during meiosis. In this study, we used apoptosis as a test case for such an analysis. Apoptosis plays a crucial role during spermatogenesis in general and meiosis in particular. It determines overall testicular cell load, balancing the proportion of the different cell types within the seminiferous tubules, and it plays a role in the removal of aberrantly differentiated meiotic spermatocytes and spermatids during and after meiosis (review in Print & Loveland, 2000).

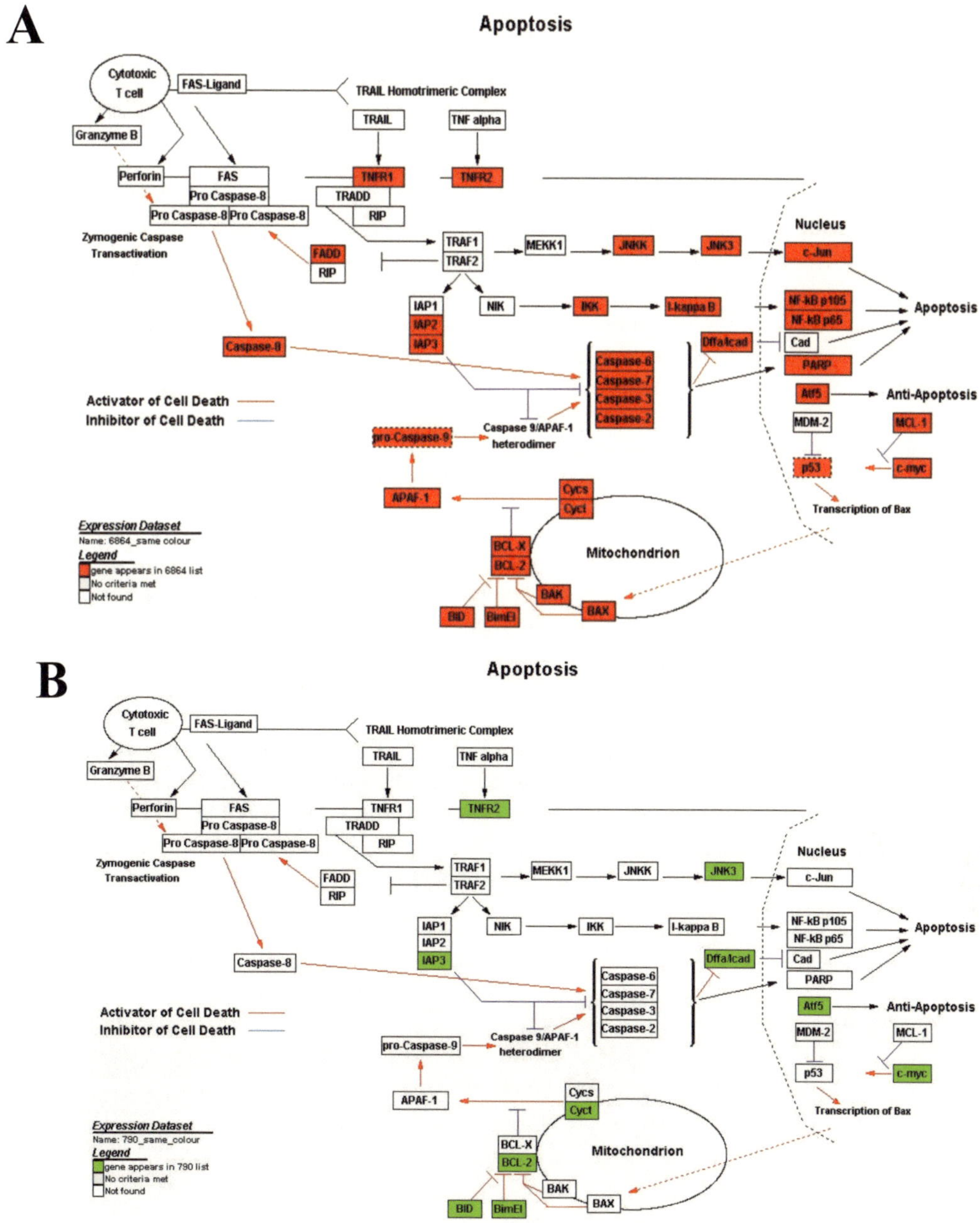


Fig. 3. Apoptotic expression maps highlighting in red genes that appear in our 6864 present sequences (A), and in green genes that appear in our 790 regulated sequences (B). These maps were obtained by applying the "Gene Map Annotator and Pathway Profiler" program to our microarray results.

Moreover, spermatocytes are unique in the sense that they "voluntarily" give up DNA integrity and undergo massive DNA breaks to enable synapsis of homologous chromosomes and crossing-over between them during meiosis. This puts conflicting requirements on the cell. On the one hand, a situation in which each and every chromosome harbors several double strand breaks (DSB) favors activation of the apoptotic pathway. On the other hand, these breaks are physiologically induced and the cells must not be sentenced to death unless breaks are not properly repaired or chromatin is not properly organized. To get an insight as to how these conflicting requirements are balanced, we applied the "Gene Map Annotator and Pathway Profiler" program to our microarray results to characterize the apoptotic pathway during meiosis. Two expression maps were used: one representing the 6864 present sequences (genes whose expression was detected in our microarray analysis but did not pass the two-fold change selection), and the other representing the 790 regulated sequences (Figure 3). 33 genes from our "present" sequences, and 10 genes from the regulated list, lighted-up using this program (Figure 3A-B). These 10 genes included TNFR2, Bid, BimEl, c-Myc and CytCt (a testis specific isoform of cytochrome C), which have a generally accepted pro-apoptotic function, and IAP3, Bcl-2, Dffa and ATF5 generally known as anti-apoptotic genes. The tenth gene, JNK3, is part of the more general MAP kinase signal transduction pathway that can either promote apoptosis or survival through activation of c-Jun (Ham et al., 2000; Kennedy & Davis, 2003). Following the specific expression pattern of these 10 regulated genes (Figure 4), it is apparent that towards the zygotene stage (pn d12), the caspase inhibitor IAP3 is up-regulated, whereas CytCt level is low, a pattern that restricts apoptosis. It is also apparent that at early pachytene (pn d14) the anti-apoptotic gene, Bcl-2, is up-regulated together with the anti apoptotic factor Dffa (Inhibitor of Caspase Activated DNase - ICAD), and BimEl, a mild negative regulator of Bcl-2. In contrast, as a mirror image, the pro-apoptotic genes Bid, which negatively regulates Bcl-2, and TNFR2, together with the anti-apoptotic transcription factor ATF5 (known also as ATFx), JNK3, and the caspase inhibitor IAP3 are down-regulated. This pattern is reversed by day 17. Thus, Bcl-2, Dffa and BimEl are down-regulated whereas Bid, TNFR2, IAP3, JNK3 and ATF5 are up-regulated. Note also that CytCt is up-regulated between pn d12 and pn d17.

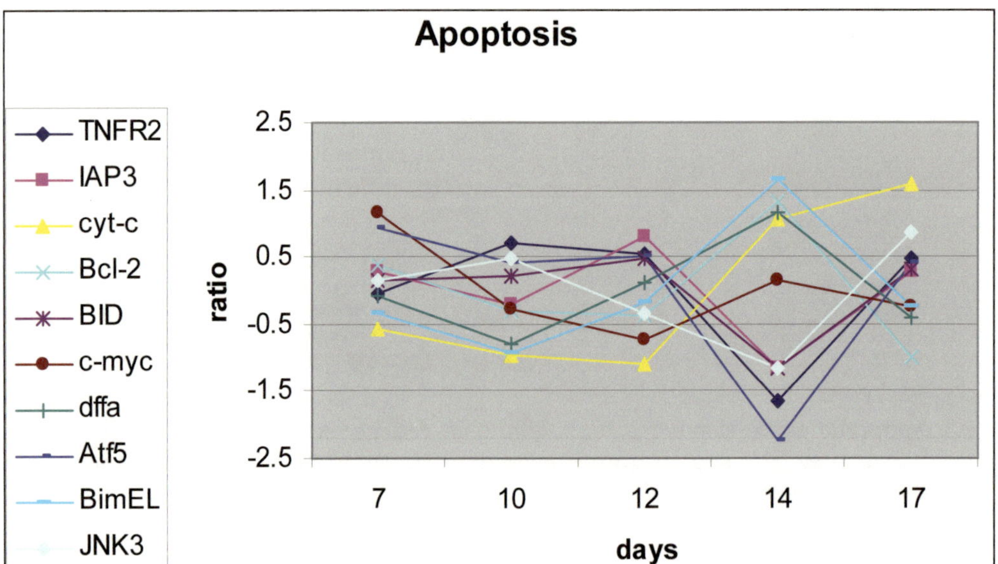


Fig. 4. Specific expression patterns of the ten genes that were highlighted in the apoptotic expression map of the 790 regulated sequences.

By drawing two maps, one for the 6864 present sequences and one for the 790 regulated sequences, we could determine two groups of apoptotic genes, the operational background genes and the actively regulated genes. The operational background genes are those whose transcript level does not change much as meiosis proceeds, but if needed, are available to execute apoptosis. The actively regulated genes are those pro and anti apoptotic genes whose transcript levels fluctuate significantly during the various meiotic stages and create a delicate balance between apoptosis and survival. DSB first appear just before zygotene, between pn d10 and pn d12, to enable synapsis of homologous chromosomes and crossing-over (review in Hochwagen & Amon, 2006). At this stage, elevated levels of the caspase inhibitor, IAP3, and low levels of CytCt seem to restrict apoptosis. As cells progress to early pachytene, high levels of Bcl2 and Dffa, together with low levels of the negative regulator of Bcl2, Bid, seem to protect cells from apoptosis and facilitate crossing-over, subsequent repair and chromatin organization. At this stage CytCt increases, IAP3 decreases, and elevated c-myc might put cells on stand-by to execute apoptosis if something goes wrong. By pn d17, representing late pachytene, DSB are repaired, and any un-repaired cell must undergo apoptosis. This is reflected by the mirror image where high CytCt , elevated Bid, TNFR2 and ATF5 together with down regulation of Bcl2 and Dffa are apparent. These results suggest that during meiosis, a delicate interplay between anti and pro-apoptotic genes and their relative abundance in a given cell determine its fate to life or death.

## 4. Comparing transcriptomes - A lesson to be learned

One way to ascribe biological significance to microarray results is to compare data obtained in parallel experiments on different differentiative systems sharing common molecular processes. Given that B-cell differentiation and meiosis both share DNA rearrangement processes (V(D)J recombination and meiotic recombination, respectively) we reasoned that novel insights could be obtained by comparing our meiosis microarray results to a B-cell differentiation database. Hoffmann et al. (2003) have classified the differentially expressed genes during murine B cell development into 20 clusters according to their expression pattern along the 5 differentiative stages: Pre-BI, Large Pre-BII, Small Pre-BII, Immature B and Mature B cells, and used this cluster classification to compare gene expression between parallel developmental stages of B cells and T cells. We focused our attention on genes that were highly expressed in either Pre BI cells (clusters 1, 2, 3 and 5, in Hoffmann et al, 2003), which undergo V(D)J recombination of the heavy chain (especially V to DJ rearrangement), or in small Pre BII and immature B cells (clusters 9, 10, 11, 12, 16 and 17, in Hoffmann et al, 2003) undergoing a second wave of rearrangement of the light chain ($V_L$ to $J_L$). These genes were compared to meiotic genes up-regulated towards early pachytene (d14) when meiotic recombination occurs (groups 1, 2 and 3, in this study). For the comparison, the accession numbers of the 390 sequences contained within the three relevant meiotic clusters, as well as of the 955 sequences consisting of the relevant B-cell differentiation clusters (obtained from supplementary data provided by the authors in Hoffmann et al, 2003), were all translated to new Affymetrix accession numbers to form a common identification base. Following this analysis, 11 genes emerged from the cross between the meiotic genes and the Pre BI specific genes, and additional 10 genes from the comparison between the meiotic genes and the genes up-regulated in small Pre BII and immature B cells (Figure 5). A more in-depth observation at some of these genes raises interesting insights as to some of the molecular pathways operating in these processes.

### 4.1 Rad54l and HOP2

Up-regulation of Rad54 and Hop2 (genes characteristic of the homologous recombination DNA repair pathway) during meiosis was not unexpected since the heterodimer Hop2-Mnd1, as well as Rad54, are known to physically interact with the recombinases Rad51 or Dmc1 during meiotic recombination and to stimulate their activity by facilitating the DNA-strand-invasion step, a key step in the homologous recombination process (Petukhova et al, 2005; Sung & Klein, 2006). On the other hand, V(D)J recombination during B-lymphocyte differentiation is thought to occur through the Non-Homologous End Joining (NHEJ) pathway, and hence up-regulation of these genes was less expected. Moreover, Essers et al., (1997) showed that RAD54-/- mice are viable and exhibit apparently normal V(D)J and immunoglobulin class-switch recombination. Nevertheless, up-regulation of these genes specifically during V(D)J recombination suggests that they might indeed play some role in NHEJ processes, and that in the absence of Rad 54 there might be compensating genes that function. If this is the case, Rad54 joins other homologous recombination DNA repair genes, such as the MRN complex (Mre11, Rad50 and Nbs1) and BRCA1, that were found to play a role in the NHEJ pathway as well (Durant & Nickoloff, 2005; Sancar et al, 2004).

### 4.2 Mog1 and Ranbp5

These two genes are involved with Ran-GTP-dependent nuclear / cytoplasmic transport of proteins. Mog1 is a nuclear protein that stimulates the release of GTP from Ran, forming a Mog1-Ran complex which stabilizes Ran in a nucleotide-free form thereby modulating nuclear levels of RanGTP (Steggerda & Paschal, 2000; Baker et al, 2001). Ranbp5 is an importin β related protein (also known as importin β3) that acts in a nucleocytoplasmic transport pathway that is distinct from the importin-alpha-dependent import of proteins (Deane et al, 1997). Both genes were previously reported to be expressed during spermatogenesis (Li et al, 2005; Loveland et al, 2006) but the fact that both are up-regulated during DNA rearrangement processes might hint that their target proteins for nucleocytoplasmic transport are involved with DNA rearrangement.

### 4.3 p107

One process that a cell undergoing DNA rearrangement must avoid is cell division. It is, therefore, expected that during physiological rearrangement processes cells would repress cell cycle promoting genes. p107, a member of the Rb pocket protein family of cell cycle regulators, forms repressive complexes with either E2F4 or E2F5 (Iaquinta & Jacqueline, 2007). Such complexes have been detected by ChIP analyses in many E2F-responsive promoters of G0 cells, ensuring they do not divide. Moreover, recruitment of HDACs (histone deacetylases) to these complexes further ensures that these important cell cycle genes stay silent (Cobrinik, 2005). Up-regulation of p107 in differentiating meiotic and B-cells, might, therefore, play a role in silencing cell division genes until DNA rearrangement processes has been successfully completed.

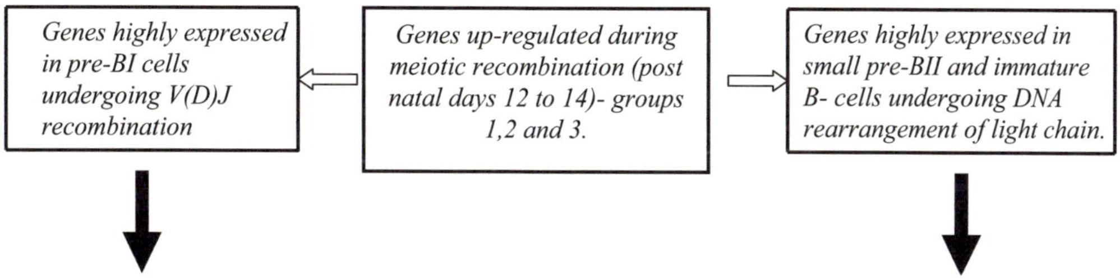


| Gene symbol | Gene name |
|---|---|
| Hop2 | Homologous pairing 2 |
| Rad54l | RAD54 like |
| Mogl | Ran binding protein |
| Ranbp5 | Ran binding protein 5 |
| Smc4l1 | Structural maintenance of chromosome 4-like 1 |
| C1qbp | Complement component 1,q-subcomponent binding protein |
| Tuba7 | Tubulin α7 |
| Pebp1 | Phosphatidylethanolamine Binding protein |
| Rbl1 | Retinoblastoma-like protein 1 (p107) |
| Anp32e | Acidic (leucin-rich) nuclear phosphoprotein 32 family, member E |
| Mpeg1 | Macrophage expressed gene 1 |

| Gene symbol | Gene name |
|---|---|
| Cxcr4 | Chemokine (C-X-C motif) receptor 4 |
| B4galnt1 | Beta-1,4-N-acetyl-galactosaminyl transferase |
| Prtn3 | Proreinase 3 |
| Fech | Ferrochelatase |
| β2AR | β-2-adrenergic receptor |
| Acyp1 | Acylphosphatase1, erythrocyte (common) type |
| Igh-6 | Immunoglobulin heavy chain 6 (heavy chain of IgM) |
| Slc2a3 | Solute carrier family 2(facilitated glucose transporter member 3) |
| Trim11 | Tripartite motif protein 11 |
| HSP70.2 | Mouse heat-shock-like protein 70.2 |

Fig. 5. Comparison between genes up-regulated towards the early pachytene stage (pn d14) where spermatocytes undergo meiotic recombination (groups 1, 2 and 3 in this study), and genes up-regulated in pre-BI or in small pre-BII and immature B-cells, undergoing V to DJ rearrangement of the heavy chain and $V_L$ to $J_L$ rearrangement of the light chain, respectively, during B-cell differentiation. The "B-cell differentiation" data was obtained from microarray data sets and clustering as reported by Hoffmann et al. (2003).

### 4.4 SMC4

In eukaryotes, the Structural Maintenance of Chromosome (SMC) proteins constitute a family of six highly conserved members of chromosomal ATPases, involved in chromosomal structural dynamics (review in Hirano, 2006). These SMC proteins form different complexes based on three SMC heterodimers. SMC1 and SMC3 form a heterodimer that, together with two other non-SMC subunits, form the cohesion complex which keeps sister chromatids together from S-phase until anaphase, when they are separated into two daughter cells. SMC2 and SMC4, form a heterodimer that together with three other non-SMC subunits compose the condensin complex, which plays an important role in mitotic/meiotic chromosomes condensation, as well as in non-mitotic chromatin condensation processes. A third pair of SMC subunits, SMC5 and SMC6, is thought to be essential for genomic integrity and DNA damage response (Hirano, 2006; De Piccoli et al., 2009). These latter SMC sub-units were reported to be highly expressed in the testes of mammals, together with a recently identified meiosis-specific SMC1 related protein (SMC1β) that was suggested to be crucial for completion of meiosis in mammals (Revenkova et al, 2004; Hirano, 2006). It is therefore interesting that among all SMC proteins, it is the SMC4 related protein that was identified in our comparison. This might suggest that SMC4, as part of the condensin complex is important for the DNA rearrangement processes. Indeed, some DNA repair roles have recently been attributed to cohesins and condensins, in addition to their traditional function, with condensins being involved specifically with single-strand break repair (Coldecott 2008; De Piccoli, 2009). This might imply that although DNA rearrangement consists basically of double strand breaks, single-strand break repair processes might also take place during rearrangement. Alternatively, condensins might play a role in DNA repair processes other then that of single-strand breaks. It is also possible, of-course, that SMC4 plays an as yet unknown role that has not been characterized to date.

### 4.5 Cxcr4

This gene encodes the chemokine receptor 4, a G-protein-coupled receptor for the CXCL12 chemokine (known also as SDF-1). Upon activation, this receptor mediates several biological activities, among which are the migration of primordial germ cells to the gonads (Molyneaux et al, 2003; Stebler et al, 2004), retention of primordial follicles in an un-activated state in the neonatal mouse ovary (Holt et al, 2006), and the retention of differentiating B cells in the bone marrow until maturation (Palmesino et al, 2006). Upon stimulation, CXCR4 has also been reported to induce the MAP-kinase cascade and the PI3/PKB pathway, which may elicit an anti-apoptotic response (Palmesino et al, 2006). The activated expression of Cxcr4 in both differentiating B lymphocytes in the bone marrow and during meiosis in the testis might suggest the intriguing possibility that it plays a somewhat similar role in the testis, i.e. retention of spermatocytes within the seminiferous epithelium until maturation (completion of meiosis and spermiogenesis) has been completed. Alternatively, it is also possible that it acts as a survival factor during meiosis.

### 4.6 β-2-adrenergic receptor (β2AR)

A disturbing unresolved discrepancy exists between the important role ascribed to the follicle-stimulating hormone (FSH) during spermatogenesis and the apparent lack of phenotype seen in FSH KO mice (review in Huhtaniemi, 2006). FSH binds to and activates the FSH receptor (FSHR) on Sertoli cells, which in turn utilize the cAMP / PKA signaling pathway to activate the CREB transcription factor. CREB activation is crucial for the ability of Sertoli cells to nurture primary spermatocytes and to support their survival. Expression of a dominant negative form of CREB in Sertoli cells resulted in apoptosis of spermatocytes (review in Don & Stelzer, 2002). Our results regarding the expression of β2AR, might provide at least a partial explanation to this discrepancy. On the one hand the β2AR was shown to activate the cAMP- PKA- CREB pathway in B-cells (Kin & Sanders, 2006). On the other hand, it was reported to be expressed in Sertoli cells of immature rats (Jacobus et al, 2005), although there are no data available as to its expression in Sertoli cells of mature animals. Our results demonstrating up-regulation of β2AR during meiosis suggest it might activate the cAMP- PKA- CREB pathway in Sertoli cells and hence compensate, at least partially, for the absence of FSH in the KO models. This hypothesis must, however, be experimentally tested.

In conclusion, the comparison between genes activated during B-cell differentiation and meiotic differentiation has focused our attention on several common genes, some of which shed light on novel molecular aspects of spermatogenesis in general, and of meiosis in particular.

## 5. Conclusions

The microarray technology has revolutionized the area of gene expression research by providing enormous amounts of transcriptome / proteome / phosphoproteome data, and enabling comparison between data sets representing the same tissue in different organisms, different tissues within the same organism or different treatments or conditions within a specific tissue or cell-type. The challenge in analyzing such experiments is to put these data in order and to extract the biological significance of it. In this study we used various bioinformatics tools in an attempt to ascribe biological significance to our microarray results, comparing the transcriptome of the mouse testis at five post-natal developmental ages representing different meiotic stages of the first spermatogenic wave. We found that chromosomal location of genes (but not clustering within a specific chromosome) could be a factor in determining specific patterns of gene expression during meiosis. Furthermore, we determined the distribution of common TF binding motifs in promoter sequences of genes within each of the six expressional groups that were determined (representing six major patterns of expression), pointing at specific transcription factors (or combination of transcription factors) that might contribute to the co-regulation of gene expression within each group. Expression kinetic analysis of gene networks is an important way of ascribing biological significance to microarray results. Using apoptosis as a test case we demonstrated herein how by a timely interplay between pro and anti apoptotic genes the delicate balance between the need to enable DNA breaks for pairing and recombination and the need to discard cells that their DNA has not been properly repaired, is kept. Finally, by comparing genes that are up-regulated during meiotic recombination, to genes up-regulated during DNA rearrangement in differentiating B-cells, we were able to get some new ideas regarding genes and molecular pathways operating during meiosis. Nevertheless, we have described only the tip of the iceberg of what could be concluded from our data, as well as from data obtained in corresponding studies executed by other groups, and most importantly, by the combined analyses of all these data sets. Further analysis and interpretations must await further studies.

## 6. References

Baker, R.P., Harreman, M.T., Eccleston, J.F., Corbett, A.H., & Stewart, M. (2001). Interaction between Ran and Mog1 is required for efficient nuclear protein import. *Journal of Biological Chemistry* 276, 41255-41262.

Bellve, A.R., Cavicchia, J.C., Millette, C.F., O'Brien, D.A., Bhatnagar, Y.M., & Dym, M. (1977). Spermatogenic cells of the prepuberal mouse. Isolation and morphological characterization. *Journal of Cell Biology* 74, 68-85.

Brinster, R.L. (2002). Germline stem cell transplantation and transgenesis. *Science* 296, 2174-2176.

Brinster, R.L., & Zimmermann, J.W. (1994). Spermatogenesis following male germ-cell transplantation. *Proceedings of the National Academy of Sciences USA* 91, 11298-11302.

Cartharius, K., Frech, K., Grote, K., Klocke, B., Haltmeier, M., Klingenhoff, A., Frisch, M., Bayerlein, M., & Werner, T. (2005). MatInspector and beyond: promoter analysis based on transcription factor binding sites. *Bioinformatics* 21, 2933-2942.

Chalmel, F., Rolland, A.D., Niederhauser-Wiederkehr, C., Chung, S.S., Demougin, P., Gattiker, A., Moore, J., Patard, J.J., Wolgemuth, D.J., Jégou, B., & Primig, M. (2007). The conserved transcriptome in human and rodent male gametogenesis. *Proceedings of the National Academy of Sciences USA* 104, 8346-8351.

Cobrinik, D. (2005). Pocket proteins and cell cycle control. Oncogene 24, 2796-2809.

Coldecott KW (2008) Single-strand break repair and genetic disease. *Nature Reviews Genetics* 9, 619-631.

Deane, R., Schafer, W., Zimmermann, H.P., Mueller, L., Gorlich, D., Prehn, S., Ponstingl, H., & Bischoff, F.R. (1997). Ran-binding protein 5 (RanBP5) is related to the nuclear transport factor importin-beta but interacts differently with RanBP1. *Molecular and Cellular Biology* 17, 5087-5096.

De Piccoli, G., Torres-Rosell, J., & Aragon, L. (2009). The unnamed complex: what do we know about Smc5-Smc6? *Chromosome Research* 17, 251-263.

Don, J., & Stelzer, G. (2002). The expanding family of CREB/CREM transcription factors that are involved with spermatogenesis. *Molecular and Cellular Endocrinology* 187, 115-124.

Durant, S.T., & Nickoloff, J.A. (2005). Good timing in the cell cycle for precise DNA repair by BRCA1. *Cell Cycle* 4, 1216-1222.

Essers, J., Hendriks, R.W., Swagemakers, S.M.A., Troelstra, C., deWit, J., Bootsma, D., Hoeijmakers, J.H.J., & Kanaar, R. (1997). Disruption of mouse RAD54 reduces ionizing radiation resistance. *Cell* 89, 195-204.

Farini, D., Scaldaferri, M.L., Iona, S., La Sala, G., & De Felici, M. (2005). Growth factors sustain primordial germ cell survival, proliferation and entering into meiosis in the absence of somatic cells. *Developmental Biology* 285, 49-56.

Feng, L.X., Chen, Y., Dettin, L., Pera, R.A., Herr, J.C., Goldberg, E., & Dym, M. (2002). Generation and *in vitro* differentiation of a spermatogonial cell line. *Science* 297, 392-395.

Hager, M., Gawlik, K., Nystrom, A., Sasaki, T., & Durbeej, M. (2005). Laminin alpha 1 chain corrects male infertility caused by absence of laminin alpha 2 chain. *American Journal of Pathology* 167, 823-833.

Ham, J., Eilers, A., Whitfield, J., Neame, S.J., & Shah, B. (2000). c-Jun and the transcriptional control of neuronal apoptosis. Biochem. Pharm. 60, 1015-1021.

Hirano T. (2006) At the heart of the chromosome: SMC proteins in action. *Nature Reviews Molecular Cell Biology* 7, 311-322.

Hochheimer, A., & Tjian, R. (2003). Diversified transcription initiation complexes expand promoter selectivity and tissue-specific gene expression. *Genes & Development* 17, 1309-1320.

Hochwagen, A., & Amon, A. (2006). Checking your breaks: Surveillance mechanisms of meiotic recombination. *Current Biology* 16, R217-R228.

Hoffmann, R., Bruno, L., Seidl, T., Rolink, A., & Melchers, F. (2003). Rules for gene usage inferred from a comparison of large-scale gene expression profiles of T and B lymphocyte development. *Journal of Immunology* 170, 1339-1353.

Holt, J.E., Jackson, A., Roman, S.D., Aitken, R.J., Koopman, P., & McLaughlin, E.A. (2006). CXCR4/SDF1 interaction inhibits the primordial to primary follicle transition in the neonatal mouse ovary. *Developmental Biology* 293, 449-460.

Hsia, K.T., Millar, M.R., King, S., Selfridge, J., Redhead ,N.J., Melton, D.W., & Saunders, P.T.K.(2003). DNA repair gene Ercc1 is essential for normal spermatogenesis and oogenesis and for functional integrity of germ cell DNA in the mouse. *Development* 130, 369-378.

Huang, D.W., Sherman, B.T., & Lempicki, R.A. (2009a). Systematic and integrative analysis of large gene lists using DAVID Bioinformatics Resources. *Nature Protocols* 4, 44-57.

Huang, D.W., Sherman, B.T., & Lempicki, R.A. (2009b). Bioinformatics enrichment tools: paths toward the comprehensive functional analysis of large gene lists. *Nucleic Acids Research*. 37, 1-13.

Hughes, V. (2008). Geneticists crack the code of infertility. *Nature Medicine* 14, 1174.

Huhtaniemi, I. (2006). Mutations along the pituitary - gonadal axis affecting sexual maturation: Novel information from transgenic and knockout mice. *Molecular and Cellular Endocrinology* 254, 84-90.

Iaquinta, P.J., & Jacqueline, A.I. (2007). Life and deathdecisions by the E2F transcription factors. *Current Biology* 19, 649-657.

Jacobus, A.P., Rodrigues, D.O., Borba, P.F., Loss, E.S., & Wassermann, G.F. (2005). Isoproterenol opens K+ (ATP) channels via a beta(2)-adrenoceptor-linked mechanism in sertoli cells from immature rats. *Hormone and Metabolic Research* 37, 198-204.

Jamsai, D., & O'Bryan, M.K. (2011). Mouse models in male fertility research. *Asian Journal of Andrology* 13, 139-151.

Kennedy, N.J., & Davis, R.J. (2003). Role of JNK in tumor development. *Cell Cycle* 2, 199-201.

Kin, N.W., & Sanders, V.M. (2006). It takes nerve to tell T and B cells what to do. *Journal of Leukocyte Biology* 79, 1093-1104.

Li, B., Nair, M., Mackay, D.R., Bilanchone, V., Hu, M., Fallahi, M., Song, H., Dai, Q., Cohen, P.E., & Dai, X. (2005). Ovol1 regulates meiotic pachytene progression during spermatogenesis by repressing Id2 expression. *Development* 132, 1463-1473.

Loveland, K.L., Hogarth, C., Szczepny, A., Prabhu, S.M., & Jans, D.A. (2006). Expression of nuclear transport importins beta 1 and beta 3 is regulated during rodent spermatogenesis. *Biology of Reproduction* 74, 67-74.

Malcov, M., Cesarkas, K., Stelzer, G., Shalom, S., Dicken, Y., Naor, Y., Goldstein, R.S., Sagee, S., Kassir, Y., & Don, J. (2004). Aym1, a mouse meiotic gene identified by virtue of its ability to activate early meiotic genes in the yeast *Saccharomyces cerevisiae*. *Developmental Biology* 276, 111-123.

Malkov, M., Fisher, Y., & Don, J. (1998). Developmental schedule of the postnatal rat testis determined by flow cytometry. *Biology of Reproduction* 59, 84-92.

McLean, D.J. (2005). Spermatogonial stem cell transplantation and testicular function. *Cell and Tissue Research* 322, 21-31.

Molyneaux, K.A., Zinszner, H., Kunwar, P.S., Schaible, K., Stebler, J., Sunshine, M.J., O'Brien, W., Raz, E., Littman, D., Wylie, C., & Lehmann, R. (2003). The chemokine SDF1/CXCL12 and its receptor CXCR4 regulate mouse germ cell migration and survival. *Development* 130, 4279-4286.

Nayernia, K., Nolte, J., Michelmann, H.W., Lee, J.H., Rathsack, K., Drusenheimer, N., Dev, A., Wulf, G., Ehrmann, I.E., Elliott, D.J., Okpanyi, V., Zechner, U., Haaf, T., Meinhardt, A., & Engel, W. (2006). *In vitro*-differentiated embryonic stem cells give rise to male gametes that can generate offspring mice. *Developmental Cell* 11, 125-132.

Niimi, T., Hayashi, Y., Futaki, S., & Sekiguchi, K. (2004). SOX7 and SOX17 regulate the parietal endoderm-specific enhancer activity of mouse laminin alpha 1 gene. *Journal of Biological Chemistry* 279, 38055-38061.

Palmesino, E., Moepps, B., Gierschik, P., & Thelen, M. (2006). Differences in CXCR4-mediated signaling in B cells. *Immunobiology* 211, 377-389.

Paul, C., Povey, J.E., Lawrence, N.J., Selfridge, J., Melton, D.W., & Saunders, P.T. (2007). Deletion of genes implicated in protecting the integrity of male germ cells has differential effects on the incidence of DNA breaks and germ cell loss. *PLoS. ONE.* 2, e989.

Petukhova, G.V., Pezza, R.J., Vanevski, F., Ploquin, M., Masson, J.Y., & Camerini-Otero, R.D. (2005). The Hop2 and Mnd1 proteins act in concert with Rad51 and Dmc1 in meiotic recombination. *Nature Structural & Molecular Biology* 12, 449-453.

Print, C.G., & Loveland, K.L. (2000). Germ cell suicide: new insights into apoptosis during spermatogenesis. *Bioessays* 22, 423-430.

Raverot, G., Weiss, J., Park, S.Y., Hurley, L., & Jameson, J.L. (2005). Sox3 expression in undifferentiated spermatogonia is required for the progression of spermatogenesis. *Developmental Biology* 283, 215-225.

Revenkova, E., Eijpe, M., Heyting, C., Hodges, C.A., Hunt, P.A., Liebe, B., Scherthan, H., & Jessberger, R. (2004). Cohesin SMC1 beta is required for meiotic chromosome dynamics, sister chromatid cohesion and DNA recombination. *Nature Cell Biology* 6, 555-562.

Romm, E., Nielsen, J.A., Kim, J.G., & Hudson, L.D. (2005). Myt1 family recruits histone deacetylase to regulate neural transcription. *Journal of Neurochemistry* 93, 1444-1453.

Sancar, A., Lindsey-Boltz, L.A., Unsal-Kacmaz, K., & Linn, S. (2004). Molecular mechanisms of mammalian DNA repair and the DNA damage checkpoints. *Annual Review of Biochemistry* 73, 39-85.

Schlecht, U., Demougin, P., Koch, R., Hermida, L., Wiederkehr, C., Descombes, P., Pineau, C., Jegou, B., & Primig, M. (2004). Expression profiling of mammalian male meiosis and gametogenesis identifies novel candidate genes for roles in the regulation of fertility. *Molecular Biology of the Cell* 15, 1031-1043.

Schultz, N., Hamra, F.K., & Garbers, D.L. (2003). A multitude of genes expressed solely in meiotic or postmeiotic spermatogenic cells offers a myriad of contraceptive targets. *Proceedings of the National Academy of Sciences U S A* 100, 12201-12206.

Shima, J.E., McLean, D.J., McCarrey, J.R., & Griswold, M.D. (2004), The murine testicular transcriptome: characterizing gene expression in the testis during the progression of spermatogenesis. *Biology of Reproduction* 71, 319-330.

Stebler, J., Spieler, D., Slanchev, K., Molyneaux, K.A., Richter, U., Cojocaru, V., Tarabykin, V., Wylie, C., Kessel, M., & Raz, E. (2004). Primordial germ cell migration in the chick and mouse embryo: the role of the chemokine SDF-1/CXCL12. *Developmental Biology* 272, 351-361.

Steggerda, S.M., & Paschal, B.M. (2000). The mammalian Mog1 protein is a guanine nucleotide release factor for Ran. *Journal of Biological Chemistry* 275, 23175-23180.

Sugiura, S., Kashiwabara, S., Iwase, S., & Baba, T. (2003). Expression of a testis-specific form of TBP-related factor 2 (TRF2) mRNA during mouse spermatogenesis. *The Journal of Reproduction and Development* 49, 107-111.

Sung, P., & Klein, H. (2006). Mechanism of homologous recombination: mediators and helicases take on regulatory functions. *Nature Reviews Molecular Cell Biology* 7, 739-750.

Waldman Ben-Asher, H., Shahar, I., Yitzhak, A., Mehr, R., & Don, J. (2010). Expression and Chromosomal Organization of Mouse Meiotic Genes. *Molecular Reproduction and Development* 77, 241-248.

Yan, Q.W., Reed, E., Zhong, X.S., Thornton, K., Guo, Y., & Yu, J.J. (2006). MZF1 possesses a repressively regulatory function in ERCC1 expression. *Biochemical Pharmacology* 71, 761-771.

Yu Z., Guo, R., Ge, Y., Ma, J., Guan, J., Li, S., Sun, X., Xue, S., & Han, D. (2003). Gene expression profiles in different stages of mouse spermatogenic cells during spermatogenesis. *Biology of Reproduction* 69, 37-47.

# Part 3

# Molecular and Cytogenetic Studies of Plant Meiosis

# 16

# Quantifying Meiosis: Use of the Fractal Dimension, $D_f$, to Describe and Predict Prophase I Substages and Metaphase I

Cynthia Ross Friedman[1] and Hua-Feng Wang[2]
[1]*Department of Biological Sciences, Thompson Rivers University,*
[2]*Beijing Urban Ecosystem Research Station,*
[2]*State Key Laboratory of Urban and Regional Ecology,*
[2]*Research Center for Eco-Environmental Sciences, Chinese Academy of Sciences,*
[1]*Canada*
[2]*China*

## 1. Introduction

### 1.1 Meiosis – Plants do it!

Plants undergo meiosis as a part of their life cycle, a fact that is sometimes forgotten and often misunderstood. Plants have a sporic life cycle wherein the living organism alternates between haploid and diploid states. Consequently, this cycle is also known as the "alternation of generations" (Gilbert, 2000). The generalization that states, "meiosis produces haploid gametes" is not technically true with respect to the intrepid members of Kingdom Plantae. Unlike the case in animal cells, the diploid plant (the sporophyte or "spore-producing plant") possesses "germ-line" cells (sporocytes) that undergo the reductive division of meiosis I followed by meiosis II to produce haploid spores. The spores then undergo mitosis, growing into a haploid "organism", which, in the flowering plants, is a small "gametophyte" (gamete-producing plant) housed within the confines of the original spore. In flowering plants, the female gametophyte (megagametophyte) held within the female spore (megaspore) inside the flower produces the egg, while the male gametophyte (microgametophyte) develops within the male spore (microspore). The microspore is better known as an immature pollen grain, and upon maturity, formation of the microgametophyte within the pollen effectively generates sperm. Ultimately, the pollen containing the sperm is released to find or "pollinate" the flower containing the egg, and two sperm are released from the pollen, one of which fertilizes the egg, forming a zygote and thus the next diploid sporophyte (Gilbert, 2000). The intricacies of flowering plant reproduction will not be described here: suffice it to say that plant sex is not quite as simple as the preceding story (for example, in flowering plants, a second fertilization event occurs, which forms a nutritive tissue called the endosperm). While leading to spores rather than gametes, meiosis the process in plant cells is *de facto* similar to that in animals.

### 1.2 Meiosis – A discrete continuum?

Meiosis, regardless of the organism in which it is occurring, is most often described as a series of discrete stages, even though it is really a continuum of events that flow from one to the next in a typically seamless and apparently effortless *pas de deux*. As will be described elsewhere in this book in more detail, the two meiotic divisions, meiosis I and meiosis II, are each conveniently subdivided into the familiar stages of prophase, metaphase, anaphase, and telophase, I and II, respectively. The most prolonged and intricate stage of meiosis is prophase I, which is highly regulated and concludes with the regimented alignment of homologous pairs along the equator at metaphase I (Alberts *et al.*, 2002).

During prophase I, replicated homologous pairs find each other in a process called "synapsis"; the synapsed homologues are often referred to as bivalents or tetrads, as a bivalent/tetrad has two chromosomes and four chromatids (Snustad & Simmons, 2008). DNA is exchanged between homologous chromosomes, usually resulting in chromosomal crossover. As prophase I is so protracted and complicated, it is usually described in five substages: leptotene, zygotene, pachytene, diplotene, and diakinesis.

The first stage of prophase I is the leptotene stage, also known as leptonema, from Greek words meaning "thin threads" (Snustad & Simmons, 2008), and is typically very short. Individual chromosomes—each consisting of two sister chromatids—change from the diffuse state they exist in during the cell's period of growth and gene expression, and condense into visible strands within the nucleus. However, the two sister chromatids are tightly bound to and hence indistinguishable from one another.

The zygotene stage, also known as zygonema, from Greek words meaning "paired threads", occurs as the chromosomes approximately line up with each other into homologous chromosome pairs in the initiation of synapsis (Snustad & Simmons, 2008). This is also called the "bouquet" stage because of the way the telomeres (chromosome "ends") cluster at one end of the nucleus. Pairing is brought about by a zipper like fashion and may start at any point along the chromosomes. While the initial alignment is approximate, the pairing is highly specific and exact, and complete by the end of zygotene.

The pachytene stage, also known as pachynema, from Greek words meaning "thick threads", is the stage when chromosomal crossover ("crossing over") occurs (Snustad & Simmons, 2008). In this process, nonsister chromatids of homologous chromosomes randomly exchange segments over regions of homology. The actual act of crossing over is not perceivable through the microscope, however, and pachytene is physically similar to zygotene, although the chromosomes are more condensed than in the previous stages.

During the diplotene stage, also known as diplonema from Greek words meaning "two threads", the homologous chromosomes separate from one another a little (Snustad & Simmons, 2008). The chromosomes themselves also uncoil a bit, allowing some transcription of DNA. However, the homologous chromosomes of each bivalent remain tightly bound at chiasmata, the regions where crossing-over occurred. The chiasmata remain on the chromosomes until they are severed in anaphase I.

In diakinesis, named from Greek words meaning "moving through", chromosomes condense further, and reaching maximum condensation (Snustad & Simmons, 2008). This is the first point in meiosis where the four chromatids of the tetrads are actually visible. Sites of crossing over entangle together, effectively overlapping, making chiasmata clearly visible. Diakinesis closely resembles prometaphase of mitosis: the nucleoli disappear, the nuclear membrane disintegrates into vesicles, and the meiotic spindle begins to form. Bivalents begin to migrate to the equator, guided by the spindle. When the bivalents reach the equator, the cell is said to be in metaphase I.

Thus, the chromosomes of any organism become increasingly condensed as they proceed through the substages of prophase I (Page & Hawley, 2003). Essentially, the chromosomes develop into "patches" in a "nucleoscape" before the metaphase I stage is reached. Could a method used to quantify the patchiness of chromosomal condensation provide a numerical predictor for metaphase I? Could the continuum of meiosis, or at least aspects of the continuum, be quantified?

### 1.3 Quantifying patchiness: Traditional methods versus the fractal dimension, $D_f$

The detection and quantification of spatial pattern, including the degree of patchiness of a landscape, is frequently undertaken in ecological studies. Methods to detect and measure special heterogeneity and patchiness calculate various multidimensional configurational indices that consider size, shape, patch density, and connectivity, to name a few variables (Gustafson, 1998). However, these typical "go-to" methods for detecting patchiness in landscape ecology are scale-dependent: simply stated, magnification of a patch results in the loss of the patchy pattern over the landscape, as one essentially "enters" the patch (or non-patch region), which then becomes the new prevalent, homogeneous environment (Kenkel & Walker, 1993). Likewise, what seem like large patches at one scale might appear like random bits of noise with a more distant perspective. This problem of scale is relevant to the idea of quantifying chromosomal patchiness: magnification with a microscope would also obscure patterns of patchiness. And what magnification is ideal for patch detection and measurement? Any measure of chromosomal patchiness must not depend on the scale.

Conveniently, the fractal dimension, $D_f$, is scale-independent (Julien & Botet, 1987). A fractal is an object or quantity that displays self-similarity on all scales. The object need not exhibit exactly the same structure at all scales, but the same "type" of structures must appear on all scales. The prototypical example for a fractal is the length of a coastline measured with different rulers of different lengths (Mandelbrot, 1967). A shorter ruler measures more of the sinuosity of bays and inlets than a larger one, so the estimated length continues to increase as the ruler length decreases. Plotting the length of the ruler versus the measured length of the coastline on a log-log plot gives a straight line, the slope of which is the fractal dimension of the coastline, $D_f$. In familiar Euclidean space, a line has 1 dimension, a plane has 2, and a cube, 3. However, the dimension of a fractal "line" in a two-dimensional surface has value of $1 \leq D_f \leq 2$ (Julien & Botet, 1987; Kenkel & Walker, 1993). A $D_f$ that approaches 1 implies that the particular object of interest (be it a landscape feature or chromosomal material) is found in patches and is less space-filling, whereas a $D_f$ that approaches 2 suggests the measured feature is space-filling and dispersed, so that the overall landscape (or nucleoscape!) is not patchy (Sugihara & May, 1990).

The fractal dimension $D_f$ has been used to quantify patchiness in landscapes, and often in digital landscape maps such as Landsat images (*e.g.*, Lam, 1990; Milne, 1992), which, as will become evident, is relevant to the work described in this chapter. In analyzing digital landscape maps, a useful calculation is the "mass dimension", which describes the number of grains or digital pixels of a given type occurring within a square window of size *LxL* (Julien & Botet, 1987; Milne, 1992; Kenkel & Walker, 1993). A series of windows of size *LxL* can be "slid" across the map, centring one on each pixel of the map that represents the object of interest. Within each window, the number of pixels of the object of interest ($n$) is then counted. The procedure is repeated across a range of length scales. Because large windows will be limited by the extent of the map, only the data sampled by all window sizes can be included. These measures can then be used to quantify the statistical behaviour of the pattern. From the geometric measures described, a probability density function, $P(n,L)$, can be defined, which describes the probability of finding $n$ pixels in a window of size (length) $L$. This probability function is analogous to a standard statistical distribution. The first moment of the probability distribution, $M(L)$, equivalent to mass dimension, is determined for increasing values of L; the slope of the plot of log $M(L)$ vs. log ($L$) represents $D_f$.

Could $D_f$ be used to measure patchiness in a nucleoscape? A role for $D_f$ in the quantification of meiosis seems possible: the $D_f$ of nuclei in early prophase I, in leptotene, should approach 2, as the chromosomal material would be relatively dispersed. The $D_f$ of nuclei progressing through zygotene, pachytene, diplotene, and diakinesis should decrease and approach 1as the chromosomal material becomes more condensed, reaching maximal condensation at diakinesis. Furthermore, some value of $D_f$ near 1would likely be a quantitative indicator for the onset of metaphase I, especially as the alignment of chromosomes along the equator would be more organized, and essentially represent one giant cluster or "super-patch". One of the authors of this chapter has done preliminary work toward this end (Ross 2005), and the results were promising enough to warrant the larger-scale study presented here.

### 1.4 Megasporogenesis and microsporogenesis in three flowering plants as the systems for study

Megasporogenesis in flowering plants, the process by which a megasporocyte undergoes meiosis to produce spores -- typically of which only one goes on to produce the megagametophyte and egg -- provides a useful system for studying meiosis, particularly the prolonged and complicated prophase I. *Arceuthobium americanum* Nutt. ex Englm., the lodgepole pine dwarf mistletoe, is a particularly interesting organism and one that will provide a system in which to examine $D_f$ as a measure of megasporocyte meiosis. The genus *Arceuthobium* comprises 42 species of economically-significant flowering plants that parasitize members of Pinaceae and Cupressaceae throughout North America, Central America, Asia, and Africa (Hawksworth *et al.*, 2002; Jerome & Ford, 2002). *Arceuthobium americanum* is found in North America, where it has the widest geographical range of any North American *Arceuthobium* species (Jerome & Ford, 2002), and can be found growing on two principal hosts, lodgepole pine (*Pinus contorta* var. *latifolia*) and jack pine (*Pinus banksiana*). The plant is dioecious, having female (Fig. 1A) and male flowers (Fig. 1B) on separate individuals (Hawksworth & Wiens, 1996), and a diploid number of 28 (2n = 28) chromosomes (Wiens, 1964). Notably, prophase I in the megasporocyte *A. americanum* female flower is especially protracted: the megasporocyte enters prophase I (leptotene) at the end of one summer, goes into a resting period over the winter, and resumes prophase I (zygotene) in the next year's growing season before proceeding into metaphase I and the rest of meiosis (Hawksworth & Wiens, 1996; Ross & Sumner, 2004; Ross, 2005). As prophase I is so prolonged, the ability to predict metaphase I within days is a considerable challenge, and hence presents the perfect opportunity to test the ability of $D_f$ to do so.

Two other species, similar to each other but decidedly different from *Arceuthobium americanum* should also be studied in order to capture more variability. The two species ideal for study are *Decaisnea insignis* (Fig. 1C) and *Sargentodoxa cuneata* (Fig. 1D), members of the Lardizabalaceae found in China and other Southeast Asian countries. Both are "winter bud" species that undergo megasporogenesis over three weeks (typically the last three in November) in the late fall (Wang *et al.*, 2009a, 2009b, & unpubl. data).

*Decaisnea* is a monotypic genus, with the species, *Decaisnea insignis* (Griffith) Hook. f. & Thomson, widely distributed from central to south-western China, extending into Bhutan, Myanmar, Nepal, Sikkim and north-eastern India (Chen & Tatemi, 2001). The plant is nicknamed 'dead man's fingers', as it possesses racemes of striking deep purplish-blue elongated fruits (follicles). The plant is economically important, as it is readily cultivated as an ornamental, and its fruits are deemed a delicacy. Plants are polygamo-monoecious, as individuals possess female flowers, male flowers and bisexual flowers (Wang *et al.*, 2009b). *Decaisnea insignis* has a diploid number of 30 (2n = 30) chromosomes (Wu, 1995).

Like *Decaisnea, Sargentodoxa,* is also generally agreed to be a monotypic genus of the Lardizabalaceae (Rehder & Wilson, 1913; Chen & Tatemi, 2001; Soltis *et al.*, 2000; Angiosperm Phylogeny Group [APG], 2003), consisting of the single species, *Sargentodoxa cuneata* (Oliver) Rehder and E. H. Wilson. It has a wide distribution in China, and can also be found in Laos and Vietnam. The plant has ethnobotanical significance, having been used in folklore and medicine as a treatment for anemia and numerous human parasites, among other ailments (Huang et al., 2004). Both male and bisexual flowers are found on the same individual, and thus the species is considered both dioecious and monoecious (Shi *et al.*, 1994). The functionally unisexual flowers are morphologically bisexual, at least developmentally, and the diploid number is 22 (2n = 22) chromosomes (Wu, 1995).

Microsporogenesis, the process by which immature haploid pollen grains are formed by meiosis of the microsporocyte, is another useful process in which to study meiotic events, including the substages of prophase I. In fact, karyotypes for many plants are derived from studies of microsporocyte meiosis (*e.g.*, Wiens, 1964). Microsporocytes are technically much easier to harvest from flowers than megasporocytes, and as such, $D_f$ can be determined for microsporocytes from several plant species undergoing prophase I and reaching metaphase I. *Arceuthobium americanum* also presents itself as a useful organism for study in this capacity, as microsporocytes in the male flower undergo meiosis rather rapidly over about three weeks at the end of the summer (Sereda, 2003). The resultant microspores (immature pollen) initiate microgametogenesis, but then overwinter prior to being released as mature pollen in the spring of the following year. The rapidity of meiosis in the microsporocytes should provide interesting fodder for comparison with the sluggish process in the *A. americanum* megasporocytes. Due to relative ease of obtaining microsporocytes, *Decaisnea insignis* (Fig. 1C) and *Sargentodoxa cuneata* (Fig. 1D) can also be mined for microsporocytes and $D_f$ calculation. As with megasporogenesis, these species undergo microsporogenesis in the late fall, in the last three weeks in November (Wang *et al.*, 2009a, 2009b, & unpubl. data).

### 1.5 Aims and concerns

The objective of this work is to (1) calculate $D_f$ for megasporocytes and microsporocytes from *Arceuthobium americanum, Decaisnea insignis,* and *Sargentodoxa cuneata* throughout prophase I and upon the onset metaphase I; (2) to assess the ability of $D_f$ to characterize the subphases of prophase I; (3) to evaluate the ability of $D_f$ to predict the onset of metaphase I; and (4) to compare $D_f$ between microsporogenesis and megasporogenesis amongst the three species, where informative. The ultimate goal will be to see if there is a universal value for $D_f$ for either or both processes at some point, or across the species.

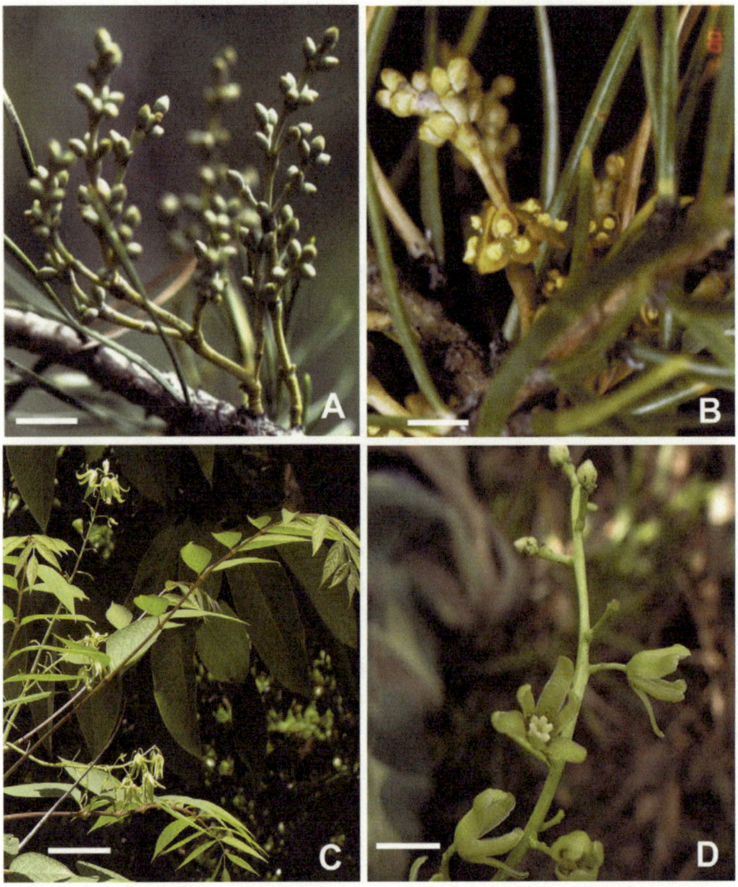


Fig. 1. Species used in this study. A) *Arceuthobium americanum* (female plant). B) *Arceuthobium americanum* (male plant). C) Portion of *Decaisnea insignis* shrub with inflorescences. D) *Sargentodoxa cuneata* inflorescence showing female flowers borne above the male. Scale bar = 15 mm in A, 5mm in B, 15 cm in C, and 9mm in D.

## 2. Materials and methods

### 2.1 Collection and preparation for microscopy

*Arceuthobium americanum* female flowers were collected daily from 1 March (prior to resumption of prophase I) until 1 May (when metaphase I has been reached or surpassed) in 2000 and 2001 from a stand of heavily infested jack pine in Belair, Manitoba, Canada as described in Ross (2005). Male *A, americanum* flowers were collected daily from August 14 until August 31 from infested lodgepole pine in Stake Lake, British Columbia, Kamloops.

Male and female flowers of *Decaisnea insignis* were collected daily from Taibai Mountain in Shaanxi Province, China 1 March 2005 to 1 May 2006 in order to obtain a range of developmental stages, although further work pinpointed the time of both megasporogenesis and microsporogenesis to about a three-week period at the end of November. Special attention was paid to when prophase I and metaphase I occurred. Only unisexual flowers were examined, even though the species sports bisexual flowers as well. Likewise, male and bisexual flower of *Sargentodoxa cuneata* were collected daily from the Nanchuan district of Chongqing city, China from 1 March 2006 to 1 May 2007, and as in *D. insignis*, further work pinpointed the time of both megasporogenesis and microsporogenesis to a three-week period at the end of November. Again, the occurrence of prophase I and metaphase I was noted. Only female components of the bisexual flowers were examined.

Flowers/buds for studies of megasporogenesis were fixed in formaldehyde/acetic acid/ethyl alcohol (FAA). Ovules were dissected from the ovaries, cleared in "4½" clearing solution (Herr, 1971) and mounted directly in Hoyer's medium on glass slides (Alexopoulos & Benke, 1952). Flowers/buds for the study of microsporogenesis were fixed in 1:3 acetic acid/ethanol, and the microsporocytes were spread directly on to glass slides with a dissecting needle. No staining was used, and the specimens were viewed with phase-contrast microscopy and consistent illumination. At least 5 megasporocytes and 5 microsporocytes were examined from each species per day.

### 2.2 Calculation of $D_f$

Whole megasporocytes or microsporocytes were digitized as binary (pure black and white) raster images with Adobe Photoshop® (resolution of 2400 dots per inch). Each image was cropped to include only the nucleus (nucleolus, if present, was ignored) and exported through NIH Image (Ross 2005) or Image J (Version 1.38) as a text file (black pixel=1, white pixel=0). This effectively converted chromosomes into black pixels, and any other nuclear material into white ones. Methods for the calculation of $D_f$ were as described in Ross (2005).

### 2.3 Data management and statistical analyses

All statistical work was done with Minitab®. The mean value of $D_f \pm$ standard error was calculated for the ~5 megasporocyte nucleoscapes for each day, considering each species individually, and, in the case of *A. americanum*, separately for its two sampling years (first reported in Ross, 2005). Likewise, the mean value of $D_f \pm$ standard error was calculated for the ~5 microsporocyte nucleoscapes for each day, also individually for each of the three species. A two-tailed student's *t*-test (was used to compare the mean value of $D_f$ from one day to the next, separately for each cell type (megasporocyte or microsporocyte) and species, to determine if the change in $D_f$ was significant or not. A two-tailed student's *t*-test was also used to compare the values of *A. americanum* megasporocyte $D_f$ between the two sampling years for days where the $D_f$ values appeared similar but needed statistical verification.

To compare amongst all datasets, a one-way analysis of variance ANOVA was performed across the datasets for the start and end mean values of $D_f$. Then, to fairly assess how similar the $D_f$ value was during the time period in which $D_f$ was changing significantly across the species and cell types, that time period was standardized (day number/total days of significant change), and a one-way ANOVA was performed for values of $D_f$ across all datasets for each standardized time.

## 3. Results

### 3.1 $D_f$ for megasporogenesis and microsporogenesis in each species

As was described in Ross (2005) but reinterpreted here, megasporocyte nucleoscapes from *A. americanum* were examined daily from 1 March to 1 May in both 2000 and 2001; thus the examination period was 66 days for each year. The mean $D_f$ for the 5 *A. americanum* megasporocyte nucleoscapes from the first date of sampling (1 March) was 1.903 (±0.004) in 2000 and 1.900 (±0.003) in 2001 (Fig. 2); these values are not significantly different (p>0.95). Visually, the chromosomal material appeared to be in leptotene and was relatively dispersed, (Fig. 3A), as would be anticipated for a mean $D_f$ that approached 2. Mean $D_f$ remained constant (±0.003, 2000 and 2001 values equivalent, p>95%) over the next 9 days in 2000 and over the next 13 days in 2001 (Fig. 2). However, mean $D_f$ then made a significant drop (p<5%) to 1.614 (±0.002) on 11 March 2000 and 1.606 (±0.003) on 15 March 2001 (Fig. 2); the "drop" values for 2000 and 2001 are equivalent (p>95%), and the drop corresponded with the chromosomal condensation associated with the resumption of prophase I, likely zygotene (Fig. 3B). The mean $D_f$ continued to decline significantly (p<5%) each day over the next 38 days in 2000 (until 18 April) and over the next 32 days in 2001 (until 16 April), reaching statistically-similar (p>99%) values of 1.352 (±0.002) in 2000 and 1.354 (±0.002) in 2001. At that time, the chromosomes were highly condensed but not yet at the equator, and were likely at diakinesis (Fig. 3B). The mean $D_f$ continued to decline significantly (p<5%) for the next 3 days until 21 April in 2000 (a total of 42 days of change) and for the next 3 days until 19 April in 2001 (total 36 days of change) to reach what would be a low of 1.332 (±0.001) in 2000 and 1.331 (±0.001) in 2001 (Fig. 2); values equivalent (p>95%). At the end of this period of change, the chromosomes were at the equator and cells were in metaphase I. The average period of change between the two years was thus 39 days. After metaphase I was attained, the mean $D_f$ did not change significantly (p>99%) over the remainder of the examination period. Therefore, a $D_f$ (both years considered) of about 1.353(±0.003) corresponded with diakinesis, which predicted metaphase I in *A. americanum* megasporocytes by 3 days in both study years, and $D_f$ at metaphase I was the lowest stable value of about 1.332 (±0.002), both years considered.

Mean $D_f$ for 5 megasporocyte nucleoscapes from *D. insignis* and *S. cuneata* (Fig. 4) as well as 5 microsporocyte nucleoscapes from these two species (Fig. 5) were determined each day from a period 13 November to 30 November (2005 for *D. insignis*, 2006 for *S. cuneata*); a total examination period of 18 days for each species. Similarly, mean $D_f$ for 5 *A. americanum* microsporocyte nucleoscapes were determined each day from 14 August to 31 August 2010 (Fig. 6), also 18 days of study. The results were startlingly uniform across the abovementioned species and the cell types. The mean $D_f$ at the beginning of the examination period ranged between 1.902 and 1.909 (±0.008) for these species and cells, and reached a low of 1.330 to 1.332 (±0.003) when the cells were in metaphase I (Figs. 4 to 6). The period in which mean $D_f$ was changing was 9 days. In all cases, when the mean $D_f$ had reached 1.355 to 1.360 (±0.006), the cells were apparently in diakinesis, and metaphase I occurred the day after diakinesis was reached. Notably, the high values, diakinesis values, and low values were all statistically similar to each other, respectively, and also to the values for *A. americanum* megasporocytes (Fig. 2) described previously (p>90%).

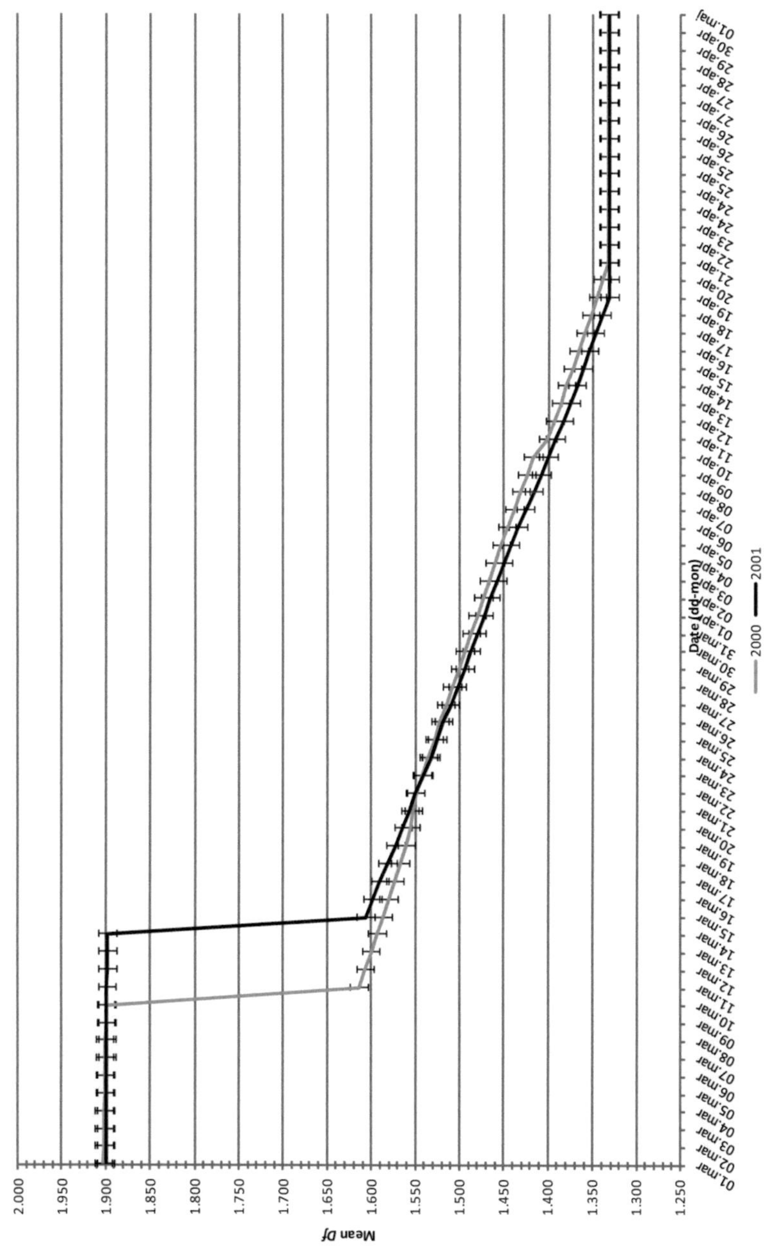


Fig. 2. Daily value of mean $D_f$ from 1 March to 1 May in 2000 and 2001 for *Arceuthobium americanum* megasporocytes undergoing prophase I. Mean $D_f$ makes a significant drop ($p<5\%$) to 1.614 (±0.002) on 11 March (2000) and 1.606 (±0.003) on 15 March (2001), continues to decline significantly ($p<5\%$) each day over the next 41 days in 2000 (until 21April) and next 35 days in 2001 (until 19April), to reach a stable low value of 1.332 (±0.001) in 2000 and 1.331 (±0.001) in 2001. There were thus 39 average total days of change.

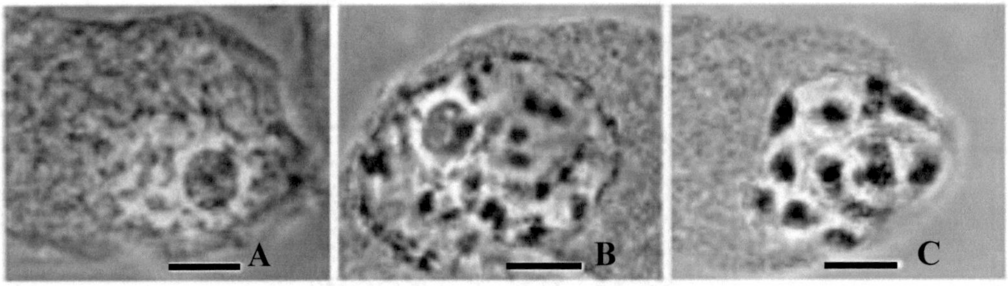


Fig. 3. Phase-contrast light micrographs of meiotic nuclei in megasporocytes of the dwarf mistletoe, *Arceuthobium americanum*. A) Nucleus sampled prior to the resumption of prophase I (near leptotene). B) Nucleus sampled when prophase I resumes (zygotene), chromosomal condensation commences, and the value of the fractal dimension, $D_f$, begins to drop. C) Chromosomes are maximally condensed, cell is in diakinesis. Metaphase I will occur in 3 days, and $D_f$ will reach its lowest value. Scale bar = 10 μm in A, B, C. (Used with permission from Ross (2005) and the *International Journal of Biological Sciences* ISSN 1449-2288).

Specifically, mean $D_f$ in both *D. insignis* and *S. cuneata* megasporocytes made a significant drop (p<5%) to 1.592 (±0.002) on 19 November (Day 7) and to 1.594 (±0.001) on 16 November (Day 4), respectively, and then continued to decrease significantly over the next 7 days, at which time diakinesis was achieved, with the mean $D_f$ becoming 1.357 (±0.002) on 26 November (Day 14) in *D. insignis* and 1.355 (±0.002) on 23 November (Day 11) in *S. cuneata* (Fig. 4). Chromosomal condensation from leptotene (Fig. 7A) to diakinesis (Fig. 7B) was accordingly evident in the megasporocytes (Fig. 7 shows an example from *D. insignis*). The next day, 27 November (Day 15) in *D. insignis* and 24 November (Day 12) in *S. cuneata,* the lowest mean $D_f$ was reached in both species (1.331 ±0.002 for *D. insignis* and 1.330±0.001 for *S. cuneata*), and the megasporocytes had reached metaphase I (Fig. 4). Thus, the period of change for mean $D_f$ was, as mentioned 9 days (inclusive).

Similarly, mean $D_f$ in *A. americanum, D. insignis,* and *S. cuneata* microsporocytes made a significant drop (p<5%) to 1.595 (±0.003) on 18 August (Day 5), to 1.597 (±0.002) on 17 November (also Day 5), and to 1.595 (±0.001) on 18 November (Day 6), respectively, and then continued to decrease significantly for the next 7 days, reaching diakinesis on 25 August (Day 12), 24 November (also Day 12), and 25 November (Day 13) with mean $D_f$ values of 1.358 (±0.003), 1.360 (±0.002), and 1.357 (±0.003), respectively (Figs. 5 and 6). As in the megasporocytes, according chromosomal condensation from leptotene (Fig. 8A) to diakinesis (Fig. 8B) was evident in the microsporocytes (Fig. 8 shows an example from *S. cuneata*). The day after diakinesis occurred, microsporocytes in *A. americanum, D. insignis,* and *S. cuneata* reached metaphase I, specifically 26 August (Day 13), 25 November (also Day 13) and 26 November (Day 14), respectively, with respective lowest mean $D_f$ values (Figs. 5 and 6) of 1.330 (±0.001), 1.329 (±0.002), and 1.332 (±0.002). Again, as was the case for *D. insignis* and *S. cuneata* megasporocytes, $D_f$ decreased over a 9-day period in the microsporocytes for all three species examined.

### 3.2 Comparing $D_f$ over a standard time frame: Have we some universal values?

The time frame for the progression of prophase I into metaphase I in *Arceuthobium americanum* megasporocytes was much longer than in its microsporocytes and longer than the period in both the megasporocytes and microsporocytes of *Decaisnea insignis* and *Sargentodoxa cuneata*. Specifically, the period for which mean $D_f$ experiences significant daily drops in *A. americanum* megasporocytes averaged 39 days, but was only 9 days for the others. However, it is patently clear that $D_f$ has statistically-significant similar value and meaning for meiosis across the cells and species studied here. Furthermore, when the time frame of mean $D_f$ is standardized for each cell type and species, the values are all statistically equivalent (p>95%). This similarity is also evident in Fig. 9, which depicts the change in $D_f$ for both cells and all species studied. Most notably, the slope of the regression line for the averaged values is -0.289, and the Y intercept for the regression line (the value at which mean *Df* begins to drop) is 1.602. It is this slope which could likely be used to predict substages of prophase I and metaphase I. Other key predictive values of $D_f$ are given in Table 1.

| **Mean $D_f$ ± Standard Error** | **Event** |
|---|---|
| 1.904 ±0.009 | Prophase I (leptotene) |
| 1.599 ±0.008 | Prophase I (zygotene) |
| 1.356 ±0.003 | Prophase I (diakinesis) |
| 1.331 ±0.004 | Metaphase I |

Table 1. Mean $D_f$ averaged across megasporocytes and microsporocytes in *Arceuthobium americanum*, *Decaisnea insignis*, and *Sargentodoxa cuneata* as predictors (all were statistically similar, p>95%).

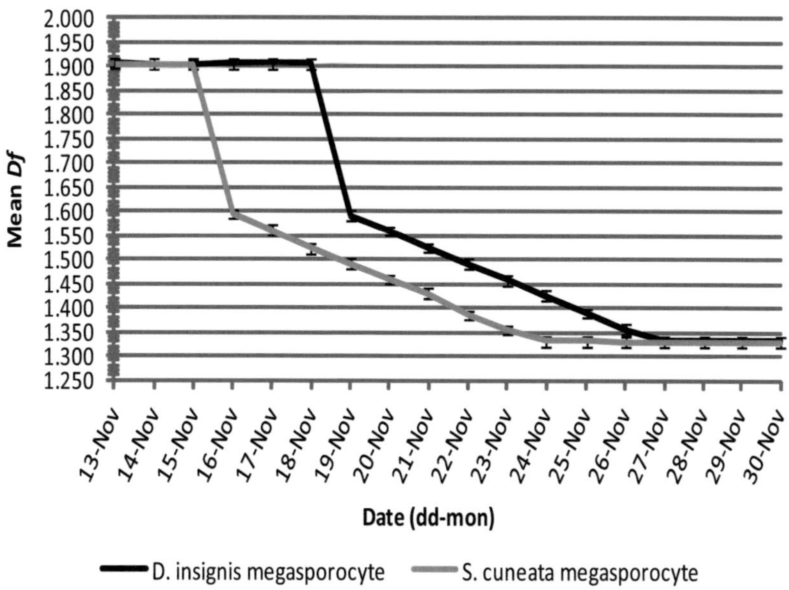


Fig. 4. Daily value of mean $D_f$ from 13 November to 30 November for *Decaisnea insignis* (2005) and *Sargentodoxa cuneata* (2006) megasporocytes undergoing prophase I. Mean $D_f$ makes a significant drop (p<5%) to 1.592 (±0.002) on 19 November (*D. insignis*) and to 1.594 (±0.001) on 16 November (*S. cuneata*), continues to decline significantly (p<5%) each day over the next 8 days in both species (until 27 November and 24 November, respectively), to reach a stable low value of 1.331 (±0.002) and 1.330 (±0.001), respectively (total 9 days of change).

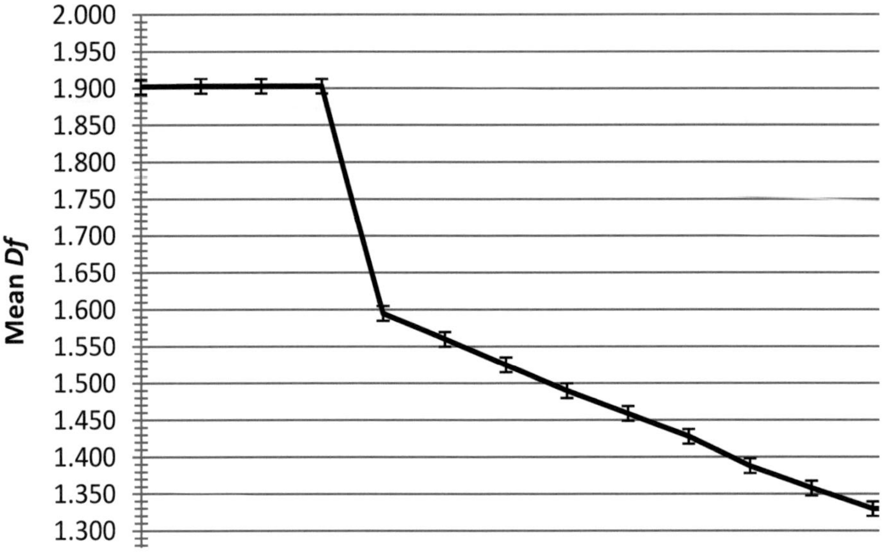


Fig. 5. Daily value of mean $D_f$ from 14 August to 31 August in 2010 for *Arceuthobium americanum* microsporocytes undergoing prophase I. Mean $D_f$ makes a significant drop (p<5%) to 1.595 (±0.003) on 18 August, continues to decline significantly (p<5%) each day over the next 9 days (until 26 August), to reach a stable low value of 1.330 (±0.001), 9 days of changing $D_f$.

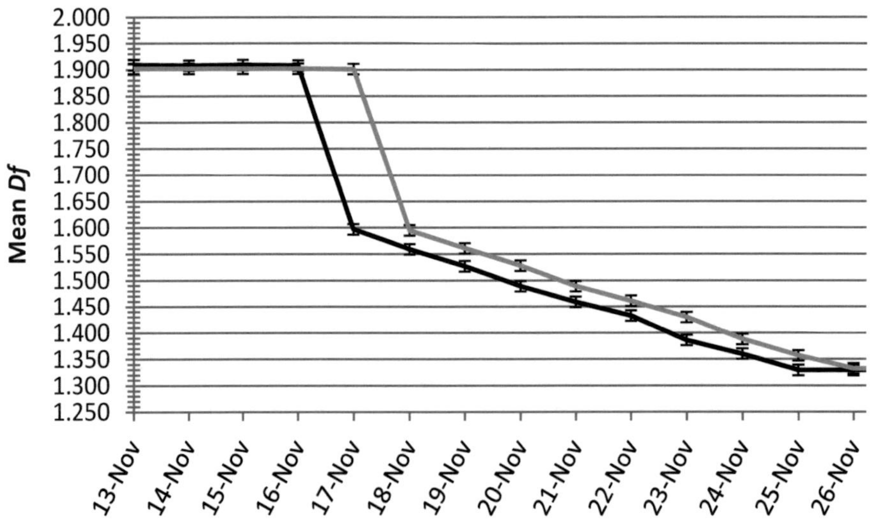


Fig. 6. Daily value of mean $D_f$ from 13 November to 30 November for *Decaisnea insignis* (2005) and *Sargentodoxa cuneata* (2006) microsporocytes undergoing prophase I. Mean $D_f$ makes a significant drop (p<5%) to 1.597 (±0.002) on 17 November (*D. insignis*) and to 1.595 (±0.001) on 18 November (*S. cuneata*), continues to decline significantly (p<5%) each day over the next 8 days in both species (until 25 November and 26 November, respectively), to reach a stable low value of 1.329 (±0.002) and 1.332 (±0.002), respectively (total 9 days of change).

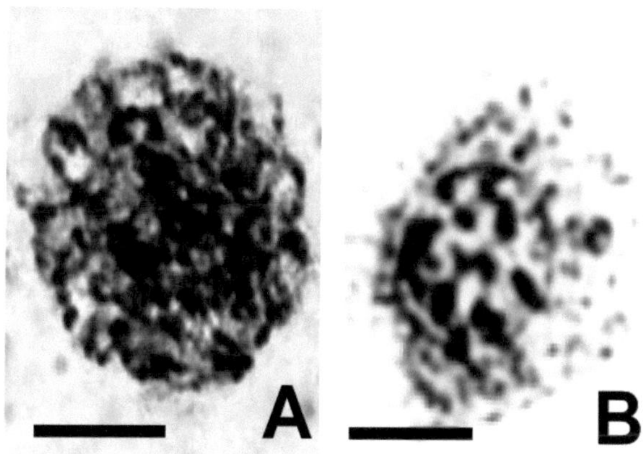


Fig. 7. Phase-contrast light micrographs of meiotic nuclei in the megasporocytes *Decaisnea insignis*. A) Nucleus sampled prior to the resumption of prophase I (near leptotene). B) Nucleus sampled when prophase I resumes (zygotene), chromosomal condensation commences, and the value of the fractal dimension, $D_f$, begins to drop. Metaphase I will occur in 1 day, and $D_f$ will reach its lowest value. Scale bar = 15 μm in A, 30 μm in B.

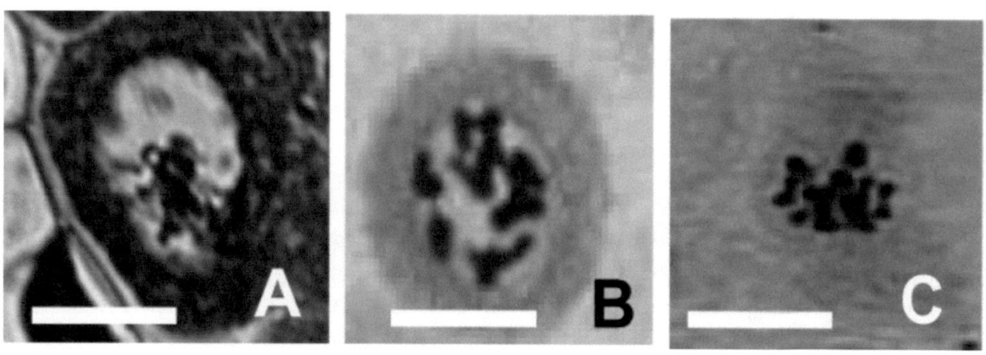


Fig. 8. Phase-contrast light micrographs of meiotic nuclei in the microsporocytes of *Sargentodoxa cuneata*. A) Nucleus sampled prior to the resumption of prophase I (near leptotene). B) Chromosomes are maximally condensed, cell is in diakinesis, and the value of the fractal dimension, $D_f$, has reached a low value that predicts metaphase I by one day. C) Nucleus is in metaphase I, one day after diakinesis was reached, and $D_f$ has reached its stable, lowest value. While chromosomes are maximally condensed in B, their position along the equator drove $D_f$ to its lowest value. Scale bar = 30 μm in A, B, C.

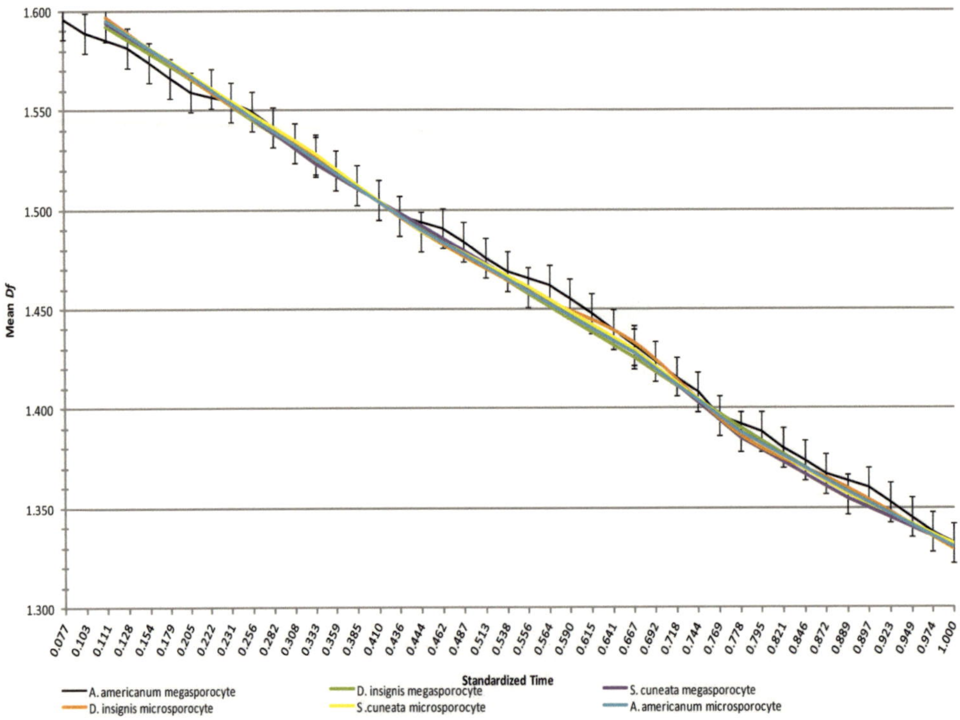


Fig. 9. Daily value of mean $D_f$ over the standardized period of change (day number/total days of significant change) for *Arceuthobium americanum*, *Decaisnea insignis*, and *Sargentodoxa cuneata* megasporocytes and microsporocytes undergoing prophase I. Values for *A. americanum* megasporocytes were averaged over the two years of study (2000 and 2001). The values follow a statistically-similar linear trendline. Slope of the regression line = -0.289; Y intercept = value at which mean $D_f$ begins to drop = 1.602 for the regression line.4.

## 4. Discussion

In the work done here with *Arceuthobium americanum*, *Decaisnea insignis*, and *Sargentodoxa cuneata* megasporocytes and microsporocytes undergoing meiosis, the fractal dimension $D_f$ described the relative degree of chromosomal condensation in prophase I to metaphase I more sensitively and quantitatively than microscopic observation alone. Across all species and cell types, a $D_f$ of 1.904 ±0.009 described leptotene of prophase I, $D_f$ of 1.599 ±0.008 delimited zygotene of prophase I, and Df of 1.356 ±0.003 characterized diakinesis. A $D_f$ approaching 1 is consistent with a nucleoscape made patchy with highly condensed chromosomal material, as would be the case for patches in a landscape (Sugihara & May, 1990). Even though the timing was different with respect to the *A. americanum* megasporocytes, the values across all species and both cell types were statistically similar. Interestingly, the timing of prophase I and the onset of metaphase I in microsporocytes across the three species as well as the timing of the same stages in the megasporocytes in *D. insignis* and *S. cuneata* was astonishingly similar: prophase seemed to occur in 9 days in all of these. One might have thought that the disparities amongst the species, particularly regarding microsporogenesis between *A. americanum* and the two members of Lardizabalaceae, would have resulted in different timing. However, it might be that these three species have similar amounts of DNA, as nuclear DNA content is known to be important factors determining or affecting the duration of male meiosis (Bennett *et al.*, 1973). These workers found that the timing of microsporogenesis and, to a certain extent, megasporogenesis, was similar in *Triticum aestivum* L. (wheat), *Hordeum vulgare* L. (barley), and *Secale cereale* L. (rye).

A mean $D_f$ 1.331 ±0.004 quantified metaphase I, which was also predicted by the $D_f$ measured for diakinesis. In *A. americanum* megasporocytes, metaphase I occurred 3 days after reaching diakinesis, and in the remaining cells and species examined, it occurred one day after diakinesis. "Fractally speaking", a low value of 1.331 ±0.004 make sense as a descriptor of metaphase I: while the chromosomes are as about as condensed as they are in diakinesis, their clustering at the equator contributes to the patchiness, which in turn is captured in the calculation of $D_f$ by the probability-density function. Ross (2005) described slightly different results for the same data, but had erroneously identified metaphase I as diakinesis. In other species not studied here, the timing might be different, but perhaps the the values of $D_f$ calculated for these stages (Table 1) can be predictive.

One might argue that the mere occurrence of diakinesis could just as effectively predict metaphase I without the calculation of $D_f$, but is should be stressed that the rate of change of mean $D_f$ as determined by the slope and determined within a few days during the decrease, one would be able to predict diakinesis as well as metaphase I! In other words, once $D_f$ begins to drop (i.e., the Y-intercept value), one could easily calculate the slope of the line (which this study showed to be consistent across all species and both cell types at around -0.289) with a few days' worth of data, then estimate when the consistent metaphase I low of 1.331 ±0.004 will be reached. This is extremely powerful.

This study has shown that meiotic timing and events amongst different species can be compared quantitative fashion that will eliminate the subjectivity inherent in qualitative descriptions. The method for harvesting nuclei and extracting $D_f$ is relatively simple, much more so than embedding and staining tissues, so time may be saved if many metaphase I slides are required. As prophase I is always prolonged relative to metaphase I, regardless of the organism, some value of $D_f$ should be predictive in any species examined. The method as described here will work particularly well in other species with relatively long meiotic divisions, such as peonies, genus *Paeonia* (Shamrov, 1997). In commercially important plants such as these, predicting when meiotic events occur can be particularly important and could streamline the culture of zygotic embryos. The examination and calculation of $D_f$ in other species and other stages of meiosis should be tackled.

Use of this technique should also allow for the quantification of *mitosis* (the equational nuclear division) along with the prediction of mitotic metaphase. As for meiosis, quantification of mitosis will facilitate objective comparisons of mitotic events amongst cells, tissues, individuals, and species. Notably, a quantification of mitosis could prove considerably valuable for another reason; if $D_f$ values can be determined for normal tissues, it is likely that deviations in $D_f$, either in absolute value or rate of change, could signal abnormalities in the cell cycle that might be correlative to precancer events in animals.

Fractal analysis and chaos theory have been used to describe the histological texture of tumours (Mattfeldt, 1997), and so the work described in our study seems like it would be applicable to systems beyond the study of meiosis.

## 5. Conclusion

Key values of the fractal dimension ($D_f$) is *Arceuthobium americanum, Decaisnea insignis,* and *Sargentodoxa cuneata* megasporocytes and microsporocytes undergoing meiosis were able to describe leptotene, zygotene, diakinesis, and metaphase I. When $D_f$ began to drop, the rate of change across all species and both cell types was consistent (slope = - 0.289), and this slope could be used as a predictor for the abovementioned stages. The results are novel and exciting, and we hope they will be re-examined and extrapolated to other cells, species, processes, and systems.

## 6. Acknowledgements

Cynthia is grateful to Dr. M.J. Sumner for his supervision during her Ph.D., from which some of this work was derived. She fully acknowledges Dr. Norman C. Kenkel and Dr. David J. Walker for their guidance and suggestions with the initial research approach. Finally, she thanks Dr. D.R. McQueen for preparation of some of the samples, and Dr. D. Punter for his advice and expertise with the dwarf mistletoes. Hua-Feng is grateful to Mr. Cheng Guo, Mr. Zhengyu Liu, and Mr. Mingbo Ren for field work assistance and also thanks Professor Yi Ren at the Shaanxi Normal University for providing us with some material. We thank Dr Qing Cai, Ms. Jie Wen, Mr. Yinhou Xiao, and Dr. Shengxiang Yu for technical assistance in the laboratory. This work was supported by a Natural Sciences and Engineering Research Council of Canada Discovery Grant (grant number 164375 provided to C.R.F.) and by the National Basic Research Program of China (grant 2006CB403207).

## 7. References

Alberts, B.; Johnson, A.; Lewis, J.; Raff, M.; Roberts, K. & Walter, P. (2002). *Molecular Biology of the Cell* (4th edition), Garland Science, ISBN-10: 0-8153-3218-1, New York, USA

Alexopoulos, C.J. & Benke, E.S. (1952). *Laboratory Manual for Introductory Mycology,* Burgess Publishing Co., Minneapolis, USA

Angiosperm Phylogeny Group, APG (2003). An update of the angiosperm phylogeny group classification for the orders and families of flowering plants: APG II. *Botanical Journal of the Linnean Society,* Vol. 141, No. 4 (November 2003), pp. 399-436, ISSN 0024-4074

Bennett, M.D.; Finch, R.A.; Smith, J.B. & Rao, M.K. (1973). The time and duration of female meiosis in wheat, rye and barley. *Proceeding of the Royal Society of London Series B,* Vol. 183, No. 1072 ( May 1973), pp. 301-319, ISSN 0962-8452

Chen, D.-Z. & Tatemi, S. (2001). Lardizabalaceae. In: *Flora of China,* C.-Y. Wu, (Ed.), Vol. 6., 440-454, Missouri Botanical Garden Press, ISBN 1-930723-25-3, St. Louis, USA

Gilbert, S. F. (2000). *Developmental Biology* (6th edition), Sinauer Associates, ISBN-10: 0-87893-243-7, Sunderland, USA.

Gustafson, E.J. (1998). Quantifying landscape spatial pattern: what is the state of the art? *Ecosystems,* Vol. 1, No. 2 (February 1998), pp. 143-156, ISSN 14329840

Hawksworth, F.G & Wiens, D. (1996). *Dwarf Mistletoes: Biology, Pathology, and Systematics, United States Department of Agriculture Forest Service Handbook Number 709*, US Government Printing Office, ISBN 0788142011, Washington, USA

Hawksworth, F.G.; Wiens, D. & Geils B.W. (2002). *Arceuthobium* in North America. In: *Mistletoes of North American Conifers, United States Department of Agriculture Rocky Mountain Research Station Forest Service Center General Technical Report 98,* B.W. Geils, J. Cibrián Tovar & B. Moody, (Tech. Coords.), Chapter 4, 29-56, Government Printing Office, OCLC 51521345, Washington, USA

Herr, J.M. Jr. (1971). A new clearing-squash technique for the study of ovule development in angiosperms. *American Journal of Botany,* Vol. 58, No. 8 (August 1971), pp. 785-790, ISSN 0002-9122

Huang, J.; Pei, S.-J. & Long, C.-L. (2004). An ethnobotanical study of medicinal plants used by the Lisu people in Nujiang, northwest Yunnan, China. *Economic Botany,* Vol. 58, Supplement (Winter 2004), pp. S253-264, ISSN 0013-0001

Jerome, C.A. & Ford, B.A. (2002). The discovery of three genetic races of the dwarf mistletoe *Arceuthobium americanum* (Viscaceae) provides insight into the evolution of parasitic angiosperms. *Molecular Ecology,* Vol. 11, No. 3 (March 2002), pp. 387-405, ISSN 0962-1083

Julien, R. & Botet, R. (1987). *Aggregation and Fractal Aggregates,* World Scientific Publishing Co., ISBN 9971502488, Singapore

Kenkel, N.C. & Walker, D.J. (1993). Fractals and ecology. *Abstracta Botanica,* Vol. 17, No. 1, (1993), pp. 53-30, ISSN 0133-6215

Lam, N. S.-N. (1990). Description and measurement of Landsat TM images using fractals. *Photogrammetric Engineering and Remote Sensing,* Vol. 56, No. 2 (February 1990), pp. 187-95, ISSN 0099-1112

Mandelbrot, B. (1967). How long is the coast of Britain? Statistical self-similarity and fractional dimension. *Science,* New Series, Vol. 156, No. 3775 (May 1967), pp. 636-638 doi:10.1126/science.156.3775.636, ISSN 0036-8075

Mattfeldt, T. (1997). Spatial Pattern Analysis using Chaos Theory: A Nonlinear Deterministic Approach to the Histological Texture of Tumours, In: *Fractals in Biology and Medicine, Volume II,* G.A. Losa, D. Merlini, T.F Nonnenmacher & E.R. Weibel (Eds.), 50-72, Birkhäuser, ISBN 3-7643-5715-0, Basel, Boston, Berlin

Milne, B.T. (1992). Spatial aggregation and neutral models in fractal landscapes. *The American Naturalist,* Vol. 139, No. 1 (January 1992), pp. 32-57, ISSN 00030147

Page, S.L. & Hawley, R.S. (2003). Chromosome choreography: the meiotic ballet. *Science,* Vol. 301, No. 5634 (August 2003), pp. 785-789, ISSN 0036-8075

Rehder, A. & Wilson, E.H. (1913). Lardizabalaceae. In: *Plantae Wilsonianae,* C.S. Sarge, (Ed.), 334-352, Arnold Arboretum of Harvard University, ISBN 9781171493068, Cambridge, USA

Ross, C.M. & Sumner, M.J. (2004). Development of the unfertilized embryo sac and pollen tubes in the dwarf mistletoe *Arceuthobium americanum* (Viscaceae). *Canadian Journal of Botany,* Vol. 82, No. 11 (November 2004), pp. 1566-1575, ISSN 0008-4026

Ross, C.M. (2005). A new way of thinking about meiosis: using the fractal dimension to predict the onset of metaphase I. *International Journal of Biological Sciences,* Vol. 1, No. 3 (August 2005), pp. 123-125, ISSN 1449-2288

Sereda, K.Y. (2003). *Phenology of Anther Development of Dwarf Mistletoe (Arceuthobium americanum Nutt. Ex Englem.): An Anatomical Investigation of Microsporogenesis and Microgametogenesis.* Department of Botany, University of Manitoba. Winnipeg, Manitoba, M.Sc. Thesis

Shamrov, I.I. (1997). Ovule and seed development in *Paeonia lactiflora* (Paeoniaceae). *Botanicheskii Zhurnal,* Vol. 82, No. 6, (June 1997), pp. 24-46, ISSN 0006-8136

Shi, J.-X.; Ren, Y. & Di, W.-Z. (1994). Taxonomic studies on Sargentodoxaceae. *Acta Botanica Boreali-Occidentalia Sinica,* Vol. 14, No. 5 (May 1994), pp. 99-103, ISSN 1000-4025

Snustad, D.P. & Simmons, M.J. (2008). *Principles of Genetics* (5th edition), John Wiley & Sons, ISBN 9780470388259, New York, USA

Soltis, D.E.; Soltis, P.S.; Chase, M.W; *et al.* (2000). Angiosperm phylogeny inferred from 18 s rDNA and atpB sequence. *Botanical Journal of the Linnean Society,* Vol. 133, No. 4 (August 2000), pp. 99-118, ISSN 0024-4074

Sugihara, G. & May, R.M. (1990). Applications of fractals in ecology. *Trends in Ecology and Evolution,* Vol. 5, No. 3 (March 1990), pp. 79-86, ISSN 0169-5347

Wang, H.-F.; Kirchoff, B.K.; Qin, H.-N. & Zhu, Z.-X. (2009a). Reproductive morphology of *Sargentodoxa cuneata* (Lardizabalaceae) and its systematic implications. *Plant Systematics and Evolution,* Vol. 280, No., 4, (November 2009), pp. 207-217, DOI: 10.1007/s00606-009-0179-3, ISSN 0378-2697

Wang, H.-F.; Ross Friedman, C.M.; Zhang, Z-X. & Qin, H-N. (2009b). Early reproductive developmental anatomy in *Decaisnea* (Lardizabalaceae) and its systematic implications. *Annals of Botany,* Vol. 104, No. 6 (September 2009), pp. 1243-1253, doi:10.1093/aob/mcp232, ISSN 0003-4754

Wiens, D. (1964). Chromosome numbers in North American Loranthaceae (*Arceuthobium, Phoradendron, Psittacanthus, Struthanthus*). *American Journal of Botany,* Vol. 51, No. 1 (January 1), pp.1-6, ISSN 0002-9122

Wu, Z.-M. (1995 ). Cytological studies on some plants of woody flora in Huangshan, Anhui Province. *Journal of Wuhan Botanical Research,* Vol. 13, No. 2 (May 1995), pp. 107-112, ISSN 1000-470X (in Chinese).

# 17

# Haploid Independent Unreductional Meiosis in Hexaploid Wheat

Filipe Ressurreição, Augusta Barão, Wanda Viegas and Margarida Delgado
*CBAA, Instituto Superior de Agronomia,*
*Technical University of LisbonTapada da Ajuda,*
*Portugal*

## 1. Introduction

Polyploidy correspond to the presence of more than two complete sets of chromosomes and is considered a major plant evolutionary force connected with adaptive plasticity (review in Comai, 2005). Within angiosperms it is estimated that at least 50% of its members have suffered one or more rounds of polyploidization (Wendel, 2000). Formation of functional unreduced gametes (2n) due to meiotic abnormalities is considered the key event associated with chromosome doubling and has been described in several dicot and monocot plant species (Ramanna and Jacobsen, 2003, Fawcett and Van de Peer, 2010). While autopolyploids are a direct result of duplication thus having multiple chromosome sets of the same origin, allopolyploids result from interspecific or intergeneric hybridization associated or followed by chromosome doubling, allowing for the emergence of new sexually reproduced species. Among sexual polyploids are many of the most important crops worldwide as it is the case of bread wheat (*Triticum aestivum* L.).

*Triticum aestivum* L. is an allohexaploid with 3 genomes designated A, B and D (2n = 6x = 42, AABBDD). It is believed that the formation of hexaploid wheat has occurred about 8000 years ago (Huang et al., 2002) through the cross between *Aegilops tauschii* Coss. (2n = 2x = 14) donor of genome D, and *Triticum turgidum* L. (2n = 4x = 28; AABB) (McFadden and Sears, 1946). By its turn *Triticum turgidum* L. (durum or macaroni wheat) is an allotetraploid resulting from the hybridization between *Triticum urartu* Tumanian (2n = 2x = 14) and *Aegilops speltoides* Tausch (2n = 2x = 14) the diploid donors of the genomes A and B, respectively (Dvorak et al., 1993). Since wheat progenitor species are close related, pairing can occur between corresponding (homoeologous) chromosomes of the distinct genomes. This phenomenon is however suppressed by the *Pairing homoeologous* gene (*Ph 1*) mapped in the long arm of chromosome 5B (Riley and Chapman, 1958). The presence of *Ph 1* results in a diploid-like meiosis both in tetra- and hexaploid wheat and is believed to have arisen by mutation at the time of the tetraploid formation (Riley and Chapman, 1958; Jauhar, 2007).

It is accepted that formation of unreduced gametes is the most important mechanism for fertile allopolyploid formation. Two main pathways are associated with meiotic restitution according with the composition of the duplicated meiotic products: First Division Restitution (FDR) and Second Division Restitution (SDR). FDR and SDR correspond in *sensu lato* to the omission of the first division or the second meiotic division respectively, this is failure of either homologous chromosome segregation or sister chromatid segregation (Ramanna and Jacobsen, 2003). Meiotic restitution corresponding FDR has been described in *Triticeae* as a haploid-dependent process and repeatedly addressed through the use of intergeneric hybrids (between wheat and related species) and wheat polyhaploids (recovered from hybridization with maize) (Islam and Shepherd, 1980; Balatero and Darvey, 1993; Jauhar, 2007; Matsuoka and Nasuda, 2004; Shamina, 2011).

In summary it has been shown that the haploid dependent meiotic restitution trait is genetically controlled and is only present in some wheat genotypes. When meiotic restitution trait is present, unreduced gametes result from lack of univalent segregation at meiosis I and subsequent sister chromatid disjunction at anaphase although the level of penetrance is generally very low. Analysis of microtubule cytoskeleton revealed that haploid unreductional meiosis depends on the bipolar attachment of univalents (Cai et al., 2010). In addition, it was also recently shown that even in genotypes with meiotic restitution, formation of unreduced gametes is obstructed by the occurrence of some level of homologous pairing (Wang et al., 2010).

So far, in wheat meiotic restitution was only described for haploid genotypes in which asynapsis results from the absence of homologous chromosome pairs. Here we investigated the influence of induced asynapsis in the progression of meiosis in a diploid context. For this purpose we took advantage of aneuploid hexaploid wheat line nulisomic for 5D and tetrassomic for 5B (N5DT5B) derived from cv Chinese Spring that display inducible asynapsis. This phenotype is associated with the lack of *Low temperature pairing* (*Ltp*) gene mapped in the long arm of chromosome 5D. N5DT5B plants are fertile with regular diploid-like meiosis when grown at temperatures ranging from 19 to 29°C, however for temperatures lower than 15°C or higher than 30°C meiocytes are asynaptic (Bayliss and Riley, 1972a). Moreover it has been established that the sensitive state for asynapis is the last interphase prior to meiosis and not the meiotic division itself (Bayliss and Riley, 1972b).

## 2. Material and methods

### 2.1 Plant material and growth conditions

We analyzed the chromosome and cytoskeleton behaviour during male meiosis in aneuploid lines N5DT5B and N5DT5A derived from hexaploid wheat (*Triticum aestivum* L.) cv Chinese Spring. Plants were continuously grown at 22°C or exposed to 10°C for 15-20 days prior to meiosis (Queiroz et al, 1991). Under the low temperature regime N5DT5B line is completely asynaptic while N5DT5A line displays a low level of asynapsis (Riley et al., 1966, Bayliss and Riley, 1972a). In these lines all chromosmes are present as homologues pairs with exception of chromosome 5B or 5A that are present in four copies in N5DT5B and N5DT5A, respectively. Wheat x rye F1 hybrid between hexaploid wheat cv. Chinese Spring and Portuguese rye (*Secale cereale* L.) landrace Centeio do Alto continuously grown at 22°C was also analyzed corresponding to an haploid-dependent asynaptic genotype.

### 2.2 Cytological analysis of meiocytes

Anthers selected for all meiotic stages were fixed in 4% (w/v) formaldehyde in MTSB (50 mM piperazine-N,N-bis(2-ethanesulfonic acid), 5 mM MgSO4.7H2O, 5 mM EGTA, pH 6.9) for 45 min at room temperature, and then rinsed twice in MTSB. Meiocytes were processed for subcellular localization of microtubules (MT) by indirect immunofluorescence. Briefly, fixed anthers were dissected permitting meiocyte dispersal in multiwall slides coated with aminopropyltriethoxysilane (Sigma) and left to air dry. The cells were then permeabilized in 0.5% Triton X-100 in MTSB for 15 min and rinsed prior to labeling. MT were localized with mouse monoclonal antibody against alpha-tubulin DM1A (Serotec) diluted 1 : 100 in MTSB, which recognizes alpha-tubulin a component of MT. Indirect detection of DM1A was performed with a secondary antibody conjugated with fluorescein isothiocyanate, diluted 1 : 300 in MTSB. DNA was counterstained 4_,6-diamidino-2-phenylindole hydrochloride (DAPI) in Citifluor antifade buffer (AF1; Agar Scientific, Stansted, U.K.).

Immunofluorescence was recorded using an epifluorescence microscope Zeiss Axioskop2 equipped with a Zeiss AxioCam MRc 5 digital camera. Images were captured using the appropriate excitation and emission filters and composited using Adobe Photoshop 7.0 (Adobe Systems Inc.) software. For N5DT5B and N5DT5A in both growth conditions and for wheat x rye F1 hybrid several plans were analyzed and at least 100 meiocytes were scored at each stage (prophase I, metaphase I, anaphase/telophase I, prophase II and anaphase/telophase II).

## 3. Results

N5DT5B and N5DT5A lines grown t 22°C have a regular meiotic chromosome behaviour as previously described (Bayliss and Riley, 1972a). Also the microtubule dynamics follows the typical *Triticeae* meiotic pattern (Shamina, 2005, Cai et al., 2010). During the first meiotic division prophase a perinuclear ring is formed, from which microtubules emanate into the nuclear area with progression of prophase (Figure 1 a). Metaphase I and anaphase I are characterized by the presence of a spindle where microtubules converge at two polar foci forming a clear fusiform spindle responsible for homologous chromosome segregation (Figure 1 b and c, respectively). At telophase I a prominent fragmoplast is formed resulting in cytokinesis and formation of two reduced dyads (Figure 1 d). In the second meiotic division in each dyad following a brief prophase a spindle is observed at metaphase/anaphase leading to sister chromatid segregation and a fragmoplast is formed at telophase producing a tetrad with four haploid microspores (Figure 1 e and f).

As previously described (Bayliss and Riley, 1972a), in N5DT5B plants exposed to 10°C prior to meiosis asynapsis is induced. Under these asynaptic conditions at first meiotic division 81.6% of the meiocytes present a low level of bivalent formation (3-6 bivalents per cell). In these cases a spindle is formed although major disturbances such as twisted spindles are common. Syntetelical orientation to the spindle (monopolar attachment) of sister kinetochores is observed for both bivalents and univalents (Figure 2 a). This results in the gathering of bivalents at the metaphase plate and their correct segregation while univalents are dispersed and randomly segregated. Progression into meiosis II occurs with sister chromatid segregation and cytokenesis with consequent uneven meiotic products and high level of micronuclei (Figure 2 d, left).

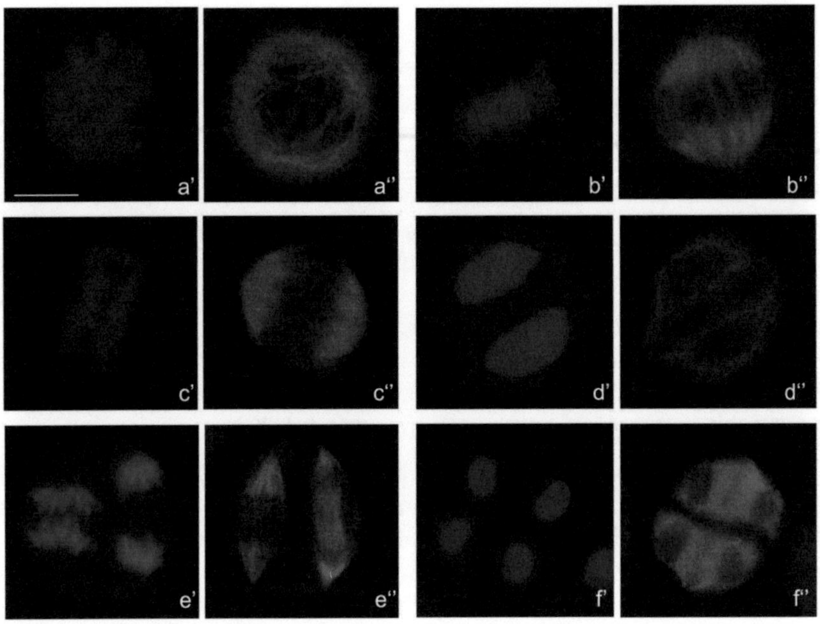


Fig. 1. Regular meiosis of the aneuploid line N5DT5B derived from hexaploid wheat cv Chinese Spring grown at 22ºC. a. prophase I, b. metaphase I, c. anaphase I; d. telophase I, e. anaphase II, f. telophase II. Chromosome DAPI staining is shown in blue (a′, b′, c′, d′, e′ and f′) and microtubule cytoskeleton in green (a′′, b′′, c′′, d′′, e′′ and f′′). All images have identical magnification, bar = 10µm.

However, a significant proportion of the meiocytes (18.4%) present complete asynapsis. These cells undergo sister chromatid separation with tendentially equational chromatid segregation originating diads that further progress to interphase with a cytoskeleton organization characteristic of young pollen grain (Figure 2 d, right). Interestingly, the level of micronuclei in dyads is much low than in tetrads indicating high probability of balanced division. This results in the formation of unreduced gametes what is also supported by the fact that dyads nuclei are considerably larger than those of tetrads although the compaction level of chromatin is similar (Figure 2 d). At this stage, a high proportion (27%) of dyads are observed although simultaneously with tetrads, triads and other highly unbalanced meiotic products since unreductional division only occurs in some meiocytes within the same anther.

In the N5DT5B line under asynaptic condition we found that unreductional division can occur by two distinct pathways (Figure 2 b and c). (i) Segregation of chromatids during the first division and blockage of second division. In this case sister kinetochores orient amphitelically to the spindle (bipolar attachment) and chromosome arm cohesion is lost. At anaphase sister chromatids are pulled to opposite poles although one ore two lagging chromosomes can occur (Figure 2 b). (ii) Failure of first division with formation of a restitution nucleus encaging all univalents coincident with chromosome decondensation (Figure 2 c). The monads formed undergo to second division where sister chromatids are segregated.

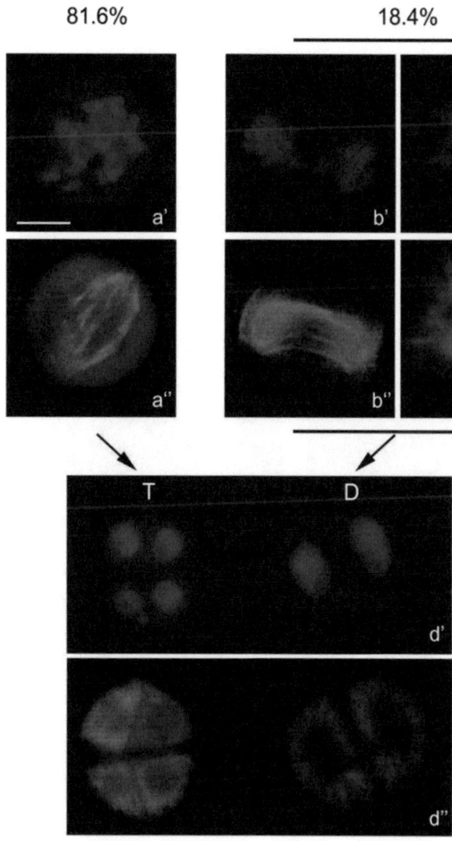


Fig. 2. Aspects of asynaptic meiosis in the aneuploid line N5DT5B due to exposure to 10°C prior to meiosis. a. Univalents at metaphase I (a') with bipolar spindle (a'') corresponding to 81.6% of the meiocytes at this stage b. and c. The remaining 18.4% of meiocytes undergo unreductional meiosis either through segregation of sister chromatids (b') with formation of bipolar spindle (b'') or through nuclear restitution and (c') absence of spindle (c'').
d. Distinct meiotic products at the end of meiosis, a tretrad on the left (T) and a dyad on the right (D) are simultaneously observed in a single microscopic field. All nuclei show identical chromatin condensation but dyad nuclei are larger than tetrad nuclei, a micronulei is present in the tetrad (d'). Microtubule organization characteristic of young pollen grain stage is present in both cell sets (d''). All images have identical magnification, bar = 10μm.

The meiotic behaviour of N5DT5A line under asynaptic conditions differs from that of N5DT5B line in the level of asynapsis that is much lower. Only a small fraction of meiocytes display complete or nearly complete asynapsis (10% of meiocytes with less than 6 bivalents). Meiocytes with a low number of bivalents behave as described for N5DT5B, while the majority of meiocytes undergo regular meiotic division although with a high frequency of micronuclei.

In the hexaploid wheat x rye F1 hybrid asynapsis at 22°C occurs due to haploid condition. Meiosis progress with a high level of irregularities as previously described for other wheat hybrid genotypes. Metaphase I form irregular spindles that result from monopolar attachement of univalents and at anaphase/telophase I univalents are randomly segregated. Meiocytes progress into meiosis II with formation of highly unbalanced gametes (Figure 3 b). Importantly, the hybrid does not display any of the characteristic features of unreductional meiosis, although it has as female parent Chinese Spring wheat from which N5DT5B and N5DT5A are derived. Neither first division nuclear restitution or sister chromatid segregation are ever observed. Occasionally meiocytes (8,6% at metaphase I) present premature sister chromatid separation but in contrast with N5DT5B this is always associated with spindled collapse and consequently impairment of sister chromatids segregation (Figure 3 a).

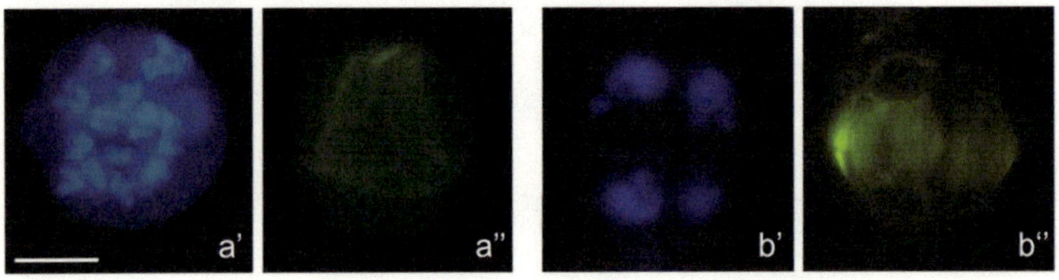


Fig. 3. Aspects of asynaptic meiosis in the hexaploid wheat cv Chinese Spring x rye Centeio do Alto F1 hybrid. a. Permature sister chromatid separation at first division (a') associated with spindle collapse (a''). b. Unbalance telophase II with several micronuclei. DAPI staining (b´) and microtubule cytoskeleton (b'') reflects the random univalent segregation at previous anaphase I since both nuclei on the left have very distinct size from those on the right and dyad cleavage divides left and right nuclei. All images have identical magnification, bar = 10μm.

## 4. Discussion

Our results show that unreductional meiosis occurs in the aneuploid wheat line N5DT5B with formation of 2n pollen grains. To our knowledge this is the first time that unreductional meiosis is described in a wheat line with homologous pairs for all chromosomes present. Formation of unreduced gametes has recurrently been reported as a characteristic of some wheat genotypes described as having meiotic restitution trait. However, this characteristic was always considered as a haploid dependent process occurring in either interspecific F1 hybrids (for review see Silkova at al., 2011) or in the polyhaploid plants (Jauhar, 2007, Cai et al., 2010). In the case of N5DT5B this phenomena is induced under low temperature conditions as the meiotic behaviour of this line is completely regular at 22ºC. N5DT5B was characterized by inducible asynapsis by low temperature exposure prior to meiosis due to the absence of the *Ltp* gene mapped in the in the long arm of chromosome 5D (Bayliss and Riley, 1972a).). This implies that in wheat asynapsis rather than haploid condition is the key feature for unreduced pollen grain formation. Supporting this hypothesis is the recent demonstration that the meiotic restitution phenotype observed in F1 hybrids between *T. turgidum* with diploid *Ae. tauschii* is completely abolished when tetraploid *Ae. tauschii* is used due to the formation of bivalents between the homologues chromosomes of *Ae. tauschii* (Wang et al 2010).

Distinct cytological processes leading to unreductional meiosis were described in distinct *Triticeae* genotypes using distinct terminology. First division restitution (FDR) was used to describe the lack of chromosome segregation at anaphase I followed by nuclear restitution and second meiotic division in hybrids between *T. turgidum* L. ssp. *durum* cultivars Langdon and Golden Ball and *S. cereale* L. cultivar Gazelle or *Ae. tauschii* Coss. (Xu and Joppa, 2000). More recently the designation unreductional meiotic cell division (UMCD) was used to describe this meiotic behavior (Cai and al., 2010). On the other hand, in very close related hybrids between *T. turgidum* L. ssp. *turgidum* and *Ae. tauschii* Coss., other authors described a single-division meiosis (SDM) characterized by a mitosis-like equational division with univalent sister chromatid segregation and blockage of second division (Zhang et al., 2007). The divergence in terminology reflects the lack of knowledge regarding the mechanisms that govern meiotic division in haploid genotypes. It should be emphasized that either nuclear restitution at meiosis I followed by regular meiosis II or sister chromatid segregation at anaphase I and absence of the second division have exactly the same genetic outcome, i.e. formation of two genetically identical unreduced microspores since cell division only involves sister chromatids segregation. Additionally, it has been shown that both types of division coexist with various frequencies depending on the genotype analysed (Xu and Joppa, 2000, Zhang et al., 2007, Silkova et al., 2011). In fact this is also the case observed here for the N5DT5B line under asynaptic conditions. This suggests that processes leading to the previously described haploid dependent formation of unreduced gametes in F1 hybrids or polyhaploids also occur when two homologous chromosomes are present if synapsis is inhibited.

Interestingly, when the wheat cv Chinese Spring, the genotype from which N5DT5B line is derived, is crossed with Portuguese rye Centeio do Alto, the F1 hybrid does not present meiotic restitution features since at meiosis I univalents are either randomly segregated or if sister chromatid cohesion is lost microtubule spindle collapses and therefore no segregation of chromatid is observed. Similarly, Zhang et al. (2007) found no evidence of meiotic restitution in the F1 hybrid between Chinese Spring wheat and a Chinese rye landrace or *Ae. variabilis*. On the other hand, analysis of polyhaploid lines derived from hexaploid wheat cv Chinise Spring showed that although meiotic restitution can occur with seed production (Jauhar, 2007) the level of seed set is much lower than that observed in polyhaploid lines derived from the tetraploid wheat Langdon, one of the most studied genotypes for its haploid dependent meiotic restitution trait (Cai et al., 2010). Together these observations indicate that hexaploid wheat cv Chinese Spring genotypes cannot be characterized as having haploid dependent meiotic restitution trait as previously assumed by Zhang et al. (2007). This does not exclude however that a high level of meiotic restitution can occur in some in wheat cv Chinese Spring interspecific hybrids as has been observed with *Hordeum vulgare* cv. Betzes (Islam and Shepherd, 1980) since this phenomenon is influenced by both parental genomes.

The present results show that meiotic restitution and unreduced gamete formation can occur in hexaploid wheat genotypes without meiotic restitution trait in a haploid independent manner in conditions of induced asynapsis. These observations raise the hypothesis that in some step of hexaploid wheat evolution interspecific hybridization could result from unreduced gamete fertilization.

Taken together, this challenges the widely accepted notion that interspecific hybridization has taken place prior to chromosome duplication in wheat evolution. Considering that formation of 2n gametes in sexual species is rare and highly dependent on environment

(Ramanna and Jacobsen, 2003), it is plausible that allopolyploidization results from fusion of unreduced gametes which in turn are the result of environmental conditions in established species sharing the same geographical niche. In fact, it has been proposed that this is the primarily process in the formation of neopolyploids in flowering plants (Ramsey and Schemske, 2002).

From the extensive data on wheat haploid-dependent meiotic restitution it is clear that this genetically controlled trait occurs in some genotypes of tetraploid wheat but not in others. If we consider that haploid dependent restitution is the genesis of wheat species it must be assumed that at least in some genotypes controlling gene(s) were conserved throughout wheat evolution, although only effective in the haploid condition. Based on our observations, we are proposing the alternative hypothesis that the haploid-dependent meiotic restitution trait has been acquired in some genotypes after allopolyploidization and that this acquired trait resulted from a loss or reduction in function of genes involved in promoting meiotic pairing.

Several genes promoting meiotic pairing have been identified in wheat (Feldman, 1966, Riley, 1974, Queiroz et al., 1991). The most well studied genes involved in wheat meiotic chromosome pairing are *Ph* (*Pairing homoeologous*) genes, which ensure that pairing is limited to homologous rather than between homoeologous chromosomes. We suggest that in genotypes without haploid-dependent meiotic restitution, promoting pairing genes allow transient chromosome synapsis and thus result in a dysfunctional meiosis. On the other hand, in genotypes with haploid-dependent meiotic restitution, reduced pairing capacity could lead to a situation similar to that observed in the N5DT5B line at low temperatures. In this case, absence of meiotic synapsis can be attributable to defective initiation of meiotic chromosome pairing therefore becoming reminiscent of a mitotic division.

Our hypothesis that haploid-dependent meiotic restitution in wheat evolved more recently is supported by phylogenetic evidence. Chromosome structure of Chinese Spring wheat, which does not have the haploid-dependent meiotic restitution trait, is more similar to the primitive tetraploid wheat than other wild tetraploids (Kawahara, 1988). Also significantly, a recent report showed that tetraploid wheat genotypes without haploid-dependent meiotic restitution have less meiotic abnormalities in conditions of heat stress than tetraploid genotypes with this trait, suggesting that haploid-dependent meiotic restitution is directly associated with less efficient meiotic control (Rezaei and Sayed-Tabatabaei, 2010). Taken together, we believe our results provide a novel and comprehensive view of wheat evolution.

## 5. Conclusion

Unreductional meiosis and formation of 2n gametes is the main mechanism in the emergence of sexual polyploids. Bread wheat (*Triticum aestivum* L.) is a natural allohexaploid with regular diploid-like meiosis resulting from two sequential events of hybridization associated with chromosome doubling. Several studies have addressed the question of chromosome duplication considering that this is a haploid-dependent process. We show here that unreductional meiosis occurs in hexaploid wheat genotypes where two homologues are present for each chromosome as an asynapsis dependent process controlled by a genotype-temperature mechanism. This is the first time that formation of 2n microspores is observed in wheat as a haploid independent process. The present results raise the hypothesis that wheat evolution could result from unreduced gamete fertilization challenging the generalized idea that wheat intergeneric hybridization occurred prior to chromosome duplication.

## 6. Acknowledgements

This work was funded by Pest-OE/AGR/UIO240/2011, FCT-Portugal

## 7. References

Balatero CH, Darvey NL. 1993. Influence of selected wheat and rye genotypes on the direct synthesis of hexaploid triticale. *Euphytica* 66: 179-185

Bayliss MW, Riley R. 1972a. An analysis of temperature-dependent asynapsis in *Triticum aestivum*. *Genetical Research* 20: 93-200

Bayliss MW, Riley R. 1972b. Evidence of premeiotic control of chromosome pairing in *Triticum aestivum*. *Genetical Research* 20:201-212

Cai X, Xu SS, Zhu X. 2010. Mechanism of haploidy-dependent unreductional meiotic cell division in polyploid wheat. *Chromosoma* 119:275–285

Comai L. 2005. The advantages and disadvantages of being polyploid. *Nat Rev Genet.* 6:836-846.

Dvorak J, DiTerlizzi P, Zhang H-B, Resta P. 1993. The evolution of poly- ploid wheats: identification of the A genome donor species. *Genome.* 36:21–31.

Fawcett JA, Van de Peer Y. 2010. Angiosperm polyploids and their road to evolutionary success. *Trends in Evolutionary Biology* 2:e3.

Feldman M. 1966 The effect of chromosomes 5B, 5D and 5A on chromosomal pairing in Triticum aestiuum. *Proc. Natl. Acad. Sci.* US. 55: 1447-1453.

Huang S, Sirikhachornkit A, Su X, Faris J, Gill B, Haselkorn R, Gornicki P. 2002. Genes encoding plastid acetyl-CoA carboxylase and 3-phosphoglycerate kinase of the Triticum/Aegilops complex and the evolutionary history of poly- ploid wheat. *Proc Natl Acad Sci* USA. 99:8133–8138.

Islam AKMR, Shepherd KW. 1980. Meiotic Restitution in Wheat-Barley Hybrids. *Chromosoma* 79:363-372

Jauhar P. 2007. Meiotic Restitution in Wheat Polyhaploids (Amphihaploids): A Potent Evolutionary Force. *Journal of Heredity* 98:188–193

Kawahara T. 1988. Confirmation of primitive chromosome structure in the hexaploid wheats. *Theor Appl Genet* 75: 717-719.

Matsuoka Y, Nasuda S. 2004. Durum wheat as a candidate for the unknown female progenitor of bread wheat: an empirical study with a highly fertile F1 hybrid with *Aegilops tauschii* Coss. *Theor Appl Genet* 109:1710–1717

McFadden ES, Sears ER. 1946. The origin of *Triticum spelta* and its free threshing hexaploid relatives. *J Hered.* 37:81–89.

Queiroz A, Mello-Sampayo T, Viegas W. 1991. Identification of low temperature stabilizing genes, controlling chromosome synapsis or recombination, in short arms of chromosomes from the homoeologous group 5 of *Triticum aestivum*. *Hereditas* 115: 37-41

Ramanna MS, Jacobsen E. 2003. Relevance of sexual polyploidization for crop improvement - A review. *Euphytica* 133: 3–18

Ramsey J, Schemske DW. 2002. Neopolyploidy in flowering plants. *Annu. Rev. Ecol. Syst.* 33:589–639

Rezaei M, Arzani A, Sayed-Tabatabaei B. E. 2010 Meiotic behaviour of tetraploid wheats (*Triticum turgidum* L.) and their synthetic hexaploid wheat derivates influenced by meiotic restitution and heat stress. *J. Genet.* 89, 401–407

Riley R. 1974. Cytogenetics of chromosome pairing in wheat. *Genetics* 78: 193-203

Riley R, Chapman V. 1958. Genetic control of the cytologically diploid behaviour of hexaploid wheat. *Nature*. 182:713–715.

Riley R, Chapman V., Young RB, Belfield AM. 1966. Control of meiotic chromosome pairing by the chromosomes of the homoeologous group 5 of *Triticum aestivum*. *Nature*. 212:1475–1477.

Silkova OG, Shchapova AI Shumny VK. 2011 Meiotic restitution in amphihaploids in the tribe *Triticeae*. *Russian Journal of Genetics*. 47:383–39.

Shamina NV. 2005. Formation of division spindles in higher plant meiosis. *Cell Biol Int.* 29:307-318.

Shamina NV. 2011."Bouquet arrest", monopolar chromosomes segregation, and correction of the abnormal spindle. *Protoplasma*. 2011 Jan 28. [Epub ahead of print]

Wang CJ, Zhang LQ, Dai SF, Zheng YL, Zhang HG, Liu DC. 2010. Formation of unreduced gametes is impeded by homologous chromosome pairing in tetraploid *Triticum turgidum* x *Aegilops tauschii* hybrids. *Euphytica* 175:323–329

Wendel JF. 2000. Genome evolution in polyploids. *Plant Mol Biol*. 42:225-249.

Xu SJ, Joppa LR. 1995.Mechanisms and inheritance of first division restitution in hybrids of wheat, rye, and Aegilops squarrosa. *Genome*. 38:607-15.

ZhangL-Q, Yen Y, Zheng Y-L, Liu D-C. 2007.Meiotic restriction in emmer wheat is controlled by one or more nuclear genes that continue to function in derived lines. *Sexual Plant Reproduction*. 20: 159-166

# 18

# Meiotic Behavior in Intra- and Interspecific Sexual and Somatic Polyploid Hybrids of Some Tropical Species

Maria Suely Pagliarini,
Maria Lúcia Carneiro Vieira and Cacilda Borges do Valle
*University of Maringá, Department of Cell Biology and Genetics,*
*University of Sao Paulo, College of Agriculture 'Luiz de Queiroz',*
*Department of Genetics, Embrapa Beef Cattle,*
*Brazil*

## 1. Introduction

Hybridization, as stated by the plant evolutionist G. Ledyard Stebbins, can be viewed as a reunion between differentiated genetic materials. Plant intra and interspecific hybridization is a common means of extending the range of variation beyond that displayed by the parental species. Hybridization is a strong evolutionary force which can potentially reshape the genetic composition of populations and create novel genotypes that facilitate adaptation to new environments (Stebbins, 1950).

Interspecific hybridization provides information on phylogenetic relationships between any two species giving clues with regard to evolutionary patterns. Often generation of such information is based on cross compatibility, chromosome association, and pollen fertility. Such information also helps in developing breeding strategies for introgression of genes from related species into economically useful species. As it creates genetic variation, it has great potential for plant improvement (Goodman et al., 1987; Choudhary et al., 2000; Sain et al., 2002).

For certain crops, plant breeders in the 20$^{th}$ century have increasingly used interspecific hybridization for gene transfer from a non-cultivated plant species to a crop variety in a related species. Goodman et al. (1987) presented a list of species in which gene transfer have been successful. Wild relatives may be sources of useful traits for the improvement of crops. From a plant breeding point of view it is desirable to document the possibility of transferring traits to a crop plant from its wild relatives through conventional sexual hybridization. Sexual exchanges between species as sources of genetic variability to improve crops have been made possible during the last century by the discovery of efficient ways to circumvent the natural barriers to genetic exchange (Goodman et al., 1987). However, inherent problems of specific introgression such as hybrid instability, infertility, non-Mendelian segregations, and low levels of intergenomic crossing-over can constitute important limitations (Stebbins, 1950). Moreover, features associated with polyploidy or ploidy dissimilarity between species may result in additional constraints for interspecific gene flow (Rieseberg et al., 2000).

After a hybrid plant has been successfully recovered, differences in the number or compatibility of parental chromosomes may cause sterility. Cytogenetic manipulations have been instrumental in obtaining stable gene transfers. Sterility may result from incomplete or unstable pairing of chromosomes during cell division. For a desired gene from the donor to be incorporated into a chromosome of the crop variety, recombination must take place. If the two species are closely related, natural pairing and recombination may occur (Goodman et al., 1987). High pairing affinity contributes so that once the barriers separating the species are overcome the gene pools of the two genera are interchangeable (Zwierzykowski et al., 1999).

Until recently, the results of interspecific hybridization could only be studied in a fairly indirect manner. One method was to analyze the phenotype of hybrids, such as the symmetry of morphological characters or the viability of pollen or seed. Alternatively, meiosis in hybrids could be studied by light microscopy and the degree of differentiation between hybridizing taxa estimated by analyses of chromosome pairing behavior and meiotic abnormalities (Rieseberg et al., 2000). Although both of these approaches have been extremely valuable, they can only provide glimpses into the complex interactions of alien genes and genomes following genetic recombination.

Cytological analyses are usually performed to evaluate the meiotic process in experimental hybrids. Species with close genetic affinity produce hybrids with regular chromosome pairing, while the hybrids of those more distantly related species have meiotic irregularities and are sterile (Marfil et al., 2006). In diploid interspecific hybrids, the meiotic analysis of chromosome association in the $F_1$ generation shows the genetic homology between the respective pairs of chromosomes. However, in interspecific tetraploid or hexaploid hybrids, chromosome pairing is affected by the number and similarity among genomes.

In this chapter, we will describe some examples of tropical species for which microsporogenesis was analyzed under light microscopy. Particularly, we will discuss the meiotic behavior in interspecific sexual tetraploid hybrids of *Brachiaria ruziziensis* x *B. brizantha* and in intraspecific sexual hexaploid hybrids of *B. humidicola*. The meiotic behavior of some artificial polyploids, namely somatic hybrids obtained through protoplast fusion in *Citrus* and *Passiflora* species will be discussed.

## 2. Some considerations about the *Brachiaria* genus

*Brachiaria* (Syn. *Urochloa* P. Beauv.), a genus of African origin, consists of about 100 species distributed across tropical and subtropical regions of the world, most of which are apomictic. It is the single most important grass genus for tropical pastures, widely adopted due to widespread adaptation to poor and acid soils commonly found in the tropics (Miles et al., 1996). Some *Brachiaria* species were introduced into South America during the second half of the $20^{th}$ century and are currently used over millions of hectares as pastures for both beef and dairy cattle (Boddey et al. 2004). In Brazil, there are ten registered cultivars listed on the National Service for Cultivar Protection. Among them, only one (cv. Mulato II) is a hybrid. The others are derived from selection of the natural variability found in the genus. *Brachiaria brizantha* and *B. decumbens* are considered pivotal species in the genus since the first contains accessions resistant to the major insect-pest, spittlebugs, and the second, although lacking resistance to the insect, is well adapted to infertile, acid soils generally found in tropical savannas (Keller-Grein et al., 1996). The gene pools in the genus *Brachiaria* are not yet well defined. A throrough taxonomic study of a large germplasm collection classified *Brachiaria brizantha, B. decumbens* and *B. ruziziensis* in the same taxonomic group together with four other species (Renvoize et al., 1996). These species are cross-compatible. *Brachiaria* breeding is difficult to accomplish because of differences in chromosome numbers among accessions and lack of sexuality in the most important species. The majority of accessions are polyploid, mainly tetraploid (Mendes-Bonato et al., 2002; 2006a; Utsunomiya et al., 2005; Risso-Pascotto et al., 2005; 2006; Pagliarini et al., 2008) and polyploidy in the genus is correlated with apomixis (Valle & Savidan, 1996).

The *Brachiaria* germplasm collection existing at Embrapa Beef Cattle Research Center (Campo Grande, Mato Grosso do Sul, Brazil) was collected in eastern and southeastern wild tropical African savannas in the mid-1980s by the International Center for Tropical Agriculture (CIAT, Colombia) and, after, introduced to Brazil by the Embrapa Genetic Resources & Biotechnology (Cenargen/Embrapa, Brasilia, DF, Brazil). After quarantine, the *Brachiaria* collection was transferred to Embrapa Beef Cattle to serve as the basis for the breeding program.

## 3. Hybridization in the genus *Brachiaria*

In the existing *Brachiaria* germplasm collected in Africa, considerable genetic variation is available and much more is presently being released using sexuality to access heterozygosity otherwise fixed by apomixis (Valle & Pagliarini, 2009). Until three decades ago, the genetic improvement of *Brachiaria* species depended entirely on selection among naturally existing germplasm. Apomixis among polyploid accessions made genetic recombination impossible to exploit (Valle & Savidan, 1996). Fully sexual genotypes have since then been found, either within the species themselves or among close relatives, but generally among diploids.

Artificial hybridization in *Brachiaria* has been tried at least since the early 1970s, when Ferguson and Crowder (1974) attempted to produce hybrids by pollinating diploid (2n = 18) sexual *B. ruziziensis* with pollen from a tetraploid (2n = 36) apomictic *B. decumbens*. This early attempt was unsuccessful, and the authors suggested duplication of the chromosome number to overcome the ploidy barrier. This indeed was the right direction in *Brachiaria* breeding when an obligate sexual tetraploid was produced by the colchicine treatment of a sexual diploid *B. ruziziensis* (Swenne et al., 1981). The Belgian material became the basis of breeding in *Brachiaria*. In Brazil, the first attempt at the interspecific hybridization using the Belgian material was undertaken in 1988 at Embrapa Beef Cattle, using tetraploid apomictic accessions of *B. brizantha* and *B. decumbens* as pollen donors (Valle & Savidan, 1996).

### 3.1 Interspecific hybrids

#### 3.1.1 *Brachiaria ruziziensis* (sexual, artificial tetraploid) *x B. decumbens* (apomictic, natural tetraploid)

Ndikunama (1985) reported the first successful interspecific hybridization done in Belgium, using the artificial tetraploid sexual genotype of *B. ruziziensis* as the female parent and apomictic accessions of *B. decumbens* and *B. brizantha* as pollen donors. New attempts were done by Lutts et al. (1991, 1994). They concluded that the hybrids produced significantly more seed when *B. ruziziensis* was pollinated by *B. decumbens* than when crossed to *B. brizantha* and the seedlings were also less vigorous. At Embrapa Beef Cattle (Brazil), several hybrids were also obtained from *B. ruziziensis* x *B. decumbens* crosses, but lack of spittlebug resistance among other undesirable phenotypic traits made them unfit as candidates for a new cultivar. Thus, efforts were not spent in the analysis of their microsporogenesis.

### 3.1.2 *Brachiaria ruziziensis* (sexual, artificial tetraploid) *x B. brizantha* (apomictic, natural tetraploid)

Several hybrids between *B. ruziziensis* x *B. brizantha* were selected to continue in the breeding program based on their phenotypical performance, including seed production to attend the Brazilian as well as the export market. Meiotic behavior was analyzed in 11 hybrids obtained from these crosses. The mean frequency of abnormalities in the hybrids was variable (Table 1). Only in one hybrid, the mean of abnormalities was low (18.2%) (Felismino et al., 2010). In the other hybrids, the mean of meiotic abnormalities ranged from 44.9% to 69.1% (Risso-Pascotto et al., 2005; Fuzinatto et al. 2007, Adamowski et al. 2008, Felismino et al. 2010; Felismino, 2011). The main meiotic abnormalities were those related to irregular chromosome segregation due polyploidy. Precocious migration of univalents to the poles at metaphase I (Fig. 1 c), lagging chromosomes at anaphase I, and micronuclei at telophase I (Fig. 1 d) were recorded in the first meiotic division of most hybrids. In the second division, abnormalities were the same; micronuclei at prophase II (Fig. 1 e), precocious migration of chromatids to the poles at metaphase II (Fig. 1 f), lagging chromatids at anaphase II (Fig. 1 g), that generated micronuclei at telophase II (Fig. 1 h), that, in some cases, remained in the tetrad (Fig. 1i) were recorded.

| Hybrids | Mode of reproduction | Mean of meiotic abnormalities | References |
|---|---|---|---|
| Hb S05 | Sexual | 67.4% | Risso-Pascotto et al., 2005 |
| Hb A14 | Apomictic | 65.1% | Risso-Pascotto et al., 2005 |
| HBGC076 | Sexual | 53.3% | Fuzinatto et al., 2007 |
| HBGC009 | Sexual | 50.9% | Fuzinatto et al., 2007 |
| HBGC014 | Sexual | 46.5% | Fuzinatto et al., 2007 |
| H34 | Sexual | 69.1% | Adamowski et al., 2008 |
| H27 | Sexual | 56.1% | Adamowski et al., 2008 |
| H17 | Apomictic | 44.9% | Adamowski et al., 2008 |
| HBGC313 | Sexual | 55.6% | Felismino et al., 2010 |
| HBGC315 | Sexual | 48.3% | Felismino et al., 2010 |
| HBGC324 | Sexual | 18.2% | Felismino et al., 2010 |
| HBGC325 | Apomictic | 46.1% | Felismino et al., 2010 |
| Hb 331 | Apomictic | 64.6% | Felismino, 2011 |
| Hb 336 | Sexual | 49.8% | Felismino, 2011 |

Table 1. Percentage of meiotic abnormalities recorded in interspecific *Brachiaria* hybrids

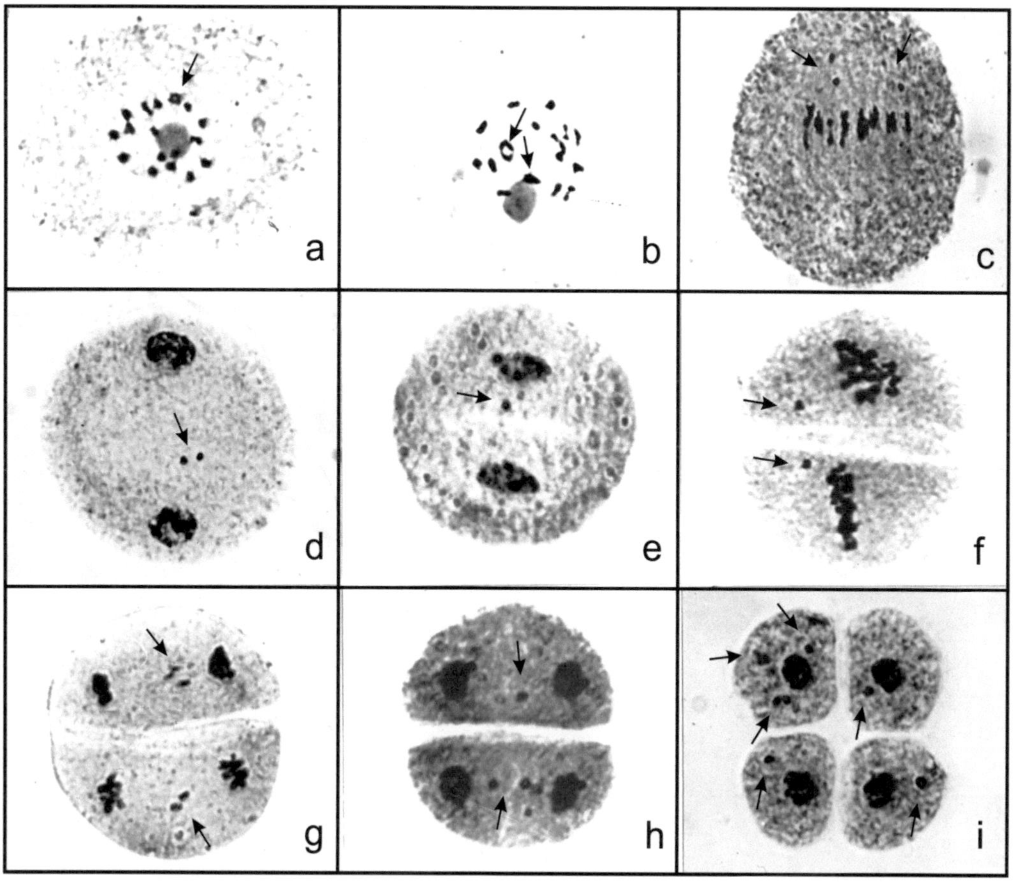


Fig. 1. Chromosome pairing and irregular chromosome segregation in interspecific *Brachiaria* hybrids. a, b) Meiocytes in diakinesis showing one (a) and two (b) quadrivalents (arrows). c) Metaphase I with precocious chromosome migration to one pole (arrows). d) Telophase I with two micronuclei (arrow). e) Early prophase II with a micronucleus (arrow). f) Metaphase II with precocious chromosome migration to one pole in both cells (arrows). g) Late anaphase II with laggard chromosomes in both cells (arrows). h) Telophase II with micronuclei in both cells (arrows). Tetrad of microspores with several micronuclei in the four microspores (i).

The meiotic behavior of micronuclei was variable among meiocytes and hybrids. In some cells, the micronuclei originated in the first meiotic division were separated by an abnormal cytokinesis, generating microcytes of different sizes and chromosome contents (Fig. 2 a - d) that entered the second division. At the end, the meiotic products depended on the number and the result of meiotic behavior of micronuclei in the first and in the second meiotic division. The end products were a tetrad with micronuclei in one, two, three or the four microspores (Fig. 2 e to g) up to a tetrad with several micronuclei in the microspores.

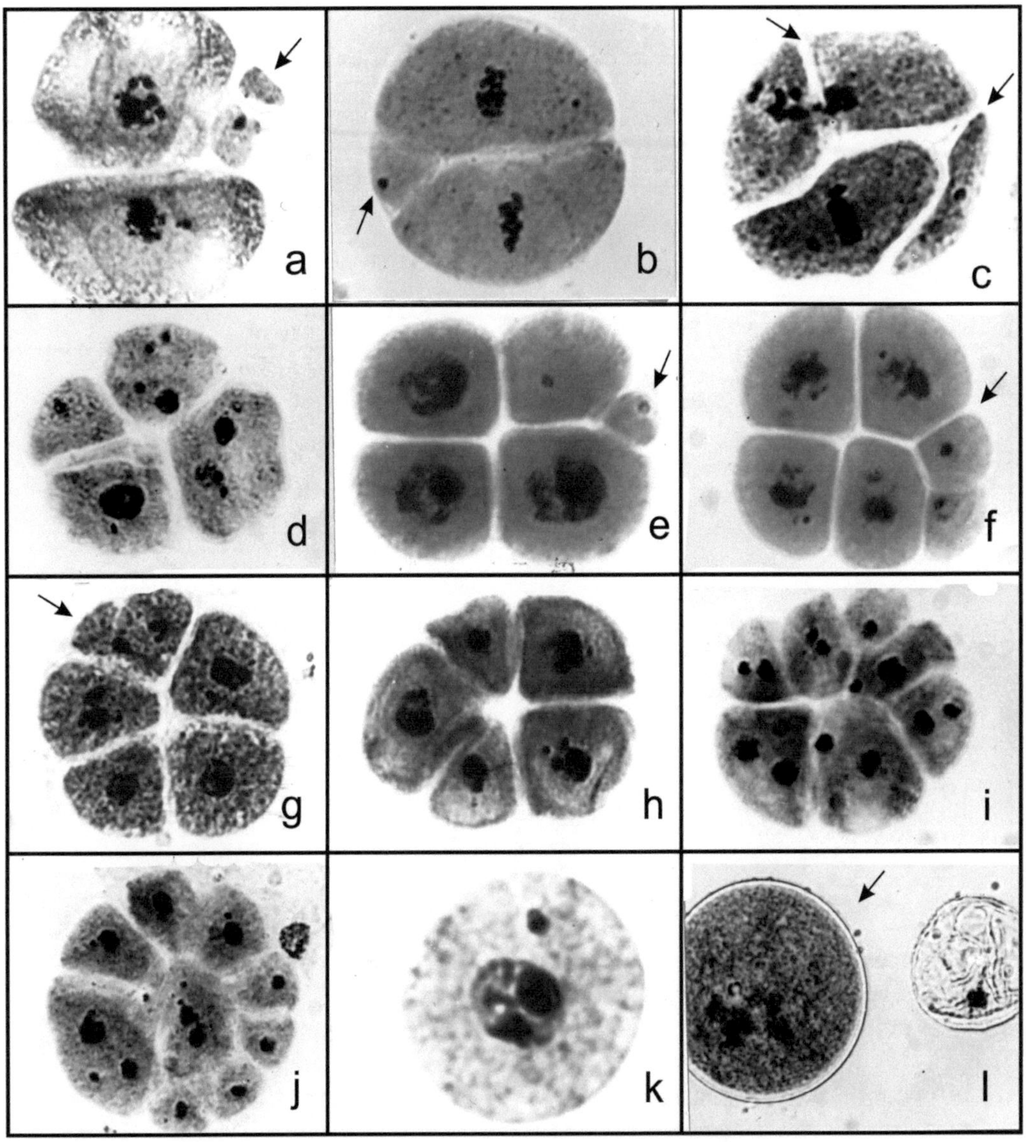


Fig. 2. Abnormal cytokinesis and the meiotic product formation in interspecific *Brachiaria* hybrids. a – c) Abnormal cytokinesis at the end of the first division leading to microcyte formation in prophase II (a) and metaphases II (b, c) (arrows) .d - g) Tetrads with micronuclei (d) and microcyte (e - g) (arrows). h) Pentad. i) Polyads with micronuclei and microcytes. k) Microspore with micronuclei (arrow). l) Viable (arrow) and sterile pollen grains.

Micronuclei were separated as microcytes with different amount of chromatin all the way to polyads with microspores and microcytes of different sizes (Fig. 2 h to j). The result was microspores of different sizes and with (Fig. 2 k) or without micronuclei. As these meiotic products are unbalanced, pollen sterility was high (Fig. 2 l).

### 3.1.3 *Brachiaria brizantha* (sexual, diploid) x *B. decumbens* (sexual, diploid) – tetraploidized hybrids

The first successful attempt in obtaining interspecific hybrids between *B. brizantha and B. decumbens* was recently accomplished and microsporogenesis was analyzed by Souza-Kaneshima et al. (2010). These constitute the two most widely used tropical forage species for cultivated pastures and support both beef and dairy cattle production in the tropics. Two apomictics cultivars - *B. brizantha* cv. Marandu and *B. decumbens* cv. Basilisk - cover more than 100 million hectares of cultivated pastures throughout Latin America and Southeast Asia. Artificial hybridization between two diploid (2n = 2x = 18) sexual accessions (*B. brizantha*, B105 x *B. decumbens*, D004) was performed in the greenhouse. Only three hybrids were recovered. One of them was treated with colchicine in tissue culture and two amphidiploid plants were obtained (Simioni & Valle, 2009).

The meiotic behavior was quite normal in the female (B105) and male (D004) genitors. In the diploid hybrid, genome separation was detected in a high number of cells since pachytene but chromosome association at diakinesis could not unfortunately be evaluated. At pachytene, both parental genomes were distantly positioned in the cytoplasm. The inability to share the same position inside the cell was also detected in metaphase I, when two metaphase plates were organized. In the following phases of meiosis, genome separation was not found among meiocytes, but polyads were recorded as meiotic products. These abnormalities increased the frequency of abnormal cells to 17.8% in the diploid F1 generation.

The same abnormalities recorded in the diploid hybrid were detected also in the amphidiploid hybrids CH4-8 and CH4-100, but in higher frequencies. In amphidiploids there was a predominance of bivalents at diakinesis, but one to three quadrivalents were recorded among meiocytes. Genome separation was also detected. Metaphase I with two metaphase plates and doubled anaphases I, giving rise to tetranucleated telophase I were recorded. In the second division, four cells, instead the two normal ones were observed. Polyads were also recorded among the meiotic products.

In the amphidiploid plants, however, another abnormality related to spindle organization was detected in high frequency. In the affected cells, meiosis was normal until diakinesis. From this phase on, chromosomes were chaotically dispersed in the cytoplasm because of absence of a spindle organizing center in the poles. In these cells, anaphase I did not occur and chromosomes, alone or in groups, generated several telophase nuclei of different sizes. In these cells, the first cytokinesis was abnormal, dividing the meiocyte in more than two cells. The plane of cytokinesis was apparently determined by the position of the telophase nuclei. In the second division, meiocytes with multiple spindles were abundantly recorded, generating multinucleated cells in telophase II. In both amphidiploid hybrids, meiotic products were highly abnormal, with several micronuclei and microcytes in the tetrads generating pollen grains of different sizes. The percentage of abnormal cells in the tetraploid progenies was similar, 49.2% in CH4-8 and 50.8% CH4-100.

## 4. Intraspecific *Brachiaria* hybrids

### 4.1 *Brachiaria humidicola* (sexual, natural hexaploid) x *B. humidicola* (apomictic, natural hexaploid)

Genetic variation and the means to manipulate it are the primary requirements in a breeding program. Interspecific *Brachiaria* hybrids between *B. ruziziensis* x *B. brizantha* have shown a considerable range of meiotic abnormalities which could impair pollen viability and seed production. In interspecific tetraploid hybrids within the genus, the problem can be compounded by the issues of genome affinity (Risso-Pascotto et al., 2005; Mendes-Bonato et al., 2006 b; Fuzinatto et al., 2007; Adamowski et al., 2008; Felismino et al., 2010; Souza-Kaneshima et al., 2010). Theoretically, intraspecific hybridization should produce fewer meiotic abnormalities than interspecific hybridization, thus efforts were directed at identifying sexually compatible genitors to be crossed to the natural apomicts within the same species. The discovery of a sexually reproducing, 36-chromosome accession of *B. humidicola* (H031, BRA005100) in Burundi (Africa) by Valle & Glienke (1991) opened new opportunities for the exploitation of genetic variability within this species. *Brachiaria humidicola* is adapted to poorly drained soils (Argel & Keller-Grein, 1996) and shows desirable agronomic characteristics. This accession was crossed with an apomictic cultivar (BRS Tupi) with the same ploidy level, originating from the same African region. BRS Tupi has excellent productivity, good nutritive value, and performance under grazing, and it is being released as a new *Brachiaria* cultivar for the tropics. From among 361 progeny obtained, 50 were selected based on vigor and overall suitability for further breeding work. In the female parent (H031), meiosis was somewhat irregular, with 16.3% of abnormal tetrads, whereas the male (cv. BRS Tupi) meiosis was very regular, with only 3.1% of abnormal tetrads. Among hybrids (sexual and apomictic), the percentage of abnormal tetrads ranged from 15.8% to 98.3%. Among the hybrids, high frequencies of meiotic abnormalities were unexpected both because they were intraspecific hybrids and because both parents' meioses were relatively stable.

The frequency of abnormalities at metaphase I in the hybrids was, in general, lower than that at metaphase II. The meiotic phases more affected by irregular chromosome segregation were anaphase II and telophase II. Metaphase II was affected by chromosomes outside the plate as well as anaphase II showing a great frequency of several lagging chromosomes. This suggests that the parental genomes did not display the same meiotic rhythm in the second division, generating several micronuclei in telophase II which remained in the tetrads. Problems related to differences in the meiotic rhythm have also been frequently recorded among interspecific tetraploid *Brachiaria* hybrids (Mendes-Bonato et al., 2006 b; Adamowski et al., 2008; Souza-Kaneshima et al., 2010). In general, the absence of genome affinity can result in chromosome elimination of one of the parents by asynchrony during meiotic phases.

## 5. Chromosome association and gene introgression

The knowledge about the similarity of the genomes in different species provides a means by which evolutionary relationships can be assessed. In addition, it offers an important starting point in alien introgression programs. According to King et al. (1999), the similarity of the genomes of the crop to those of related species is important as this permits an estimation of the frequency of recombination that will occur in interspecific hybrids. Thus, this information allows predictions to be made of the likelihood of transferring specific target genes from one species to another.

Multivalent chromosome association at diakinesis revealed genome affinity between both parental species in the hybrids, suggesting some possibility for gene introgression. Analyses of meiocytes at diakinesis in the 11 interspecific tetraploid *Brachiaria* hybrids showed that some chromosome association can occur among the parental genomes, but in low frequency.

No more than four quadrivalents were found in these hybrids (Fig. 1 a, b), but one tetravalent was the most common multiple chromosome association (Risso-Pascotto et al., 2005; Fuzinatto et al., 2007; Adamowski et al., 2008; Felismino et al., 2010; Felismino, 2011). The occurrence of quadrivalents among *B. ruziziensis* x *B. brizantha* shows that both species are closely related and their gene pools are interchangeable. Thus, we can assume that gene introgression can occur in the hybrids, but in low frequency. Recombination was expected in these hybrids because these species belong to the same taxonomic/genomic group - group 5 (Renvoize et al., 1996; Valle & Savidan, 1996). However, the occurrence of chromosome pairing per se does not ensure that the desirable genes are being introgressed into the hybrid because of the probability of the chromosomes involved containing such genes. According to Goodman et al. (1987), even when successful, interspecific hybrids generally present other problems: (1) even after several cycles of selection, the recombination will frequently not separate tightly linked genes, and undesirable traits may be carried along with the desirable one; (2) the inheritance and expression of the desirable introgressed gene may be unpredictable in the new genetic background.

## 6. Genome affinity

Genome separation and genome elimination are common among interspecific hybrids. Shwarzacher et al. (1992) reported several examples among plants where the phenomenon occurred. According to Luckens et al. (2006), the formation of natural allopolyploids requires the adaptation of two nuclear genomes within a single cytoplasm, which may involve programmed genetic changes during the first generation following genome fusion.

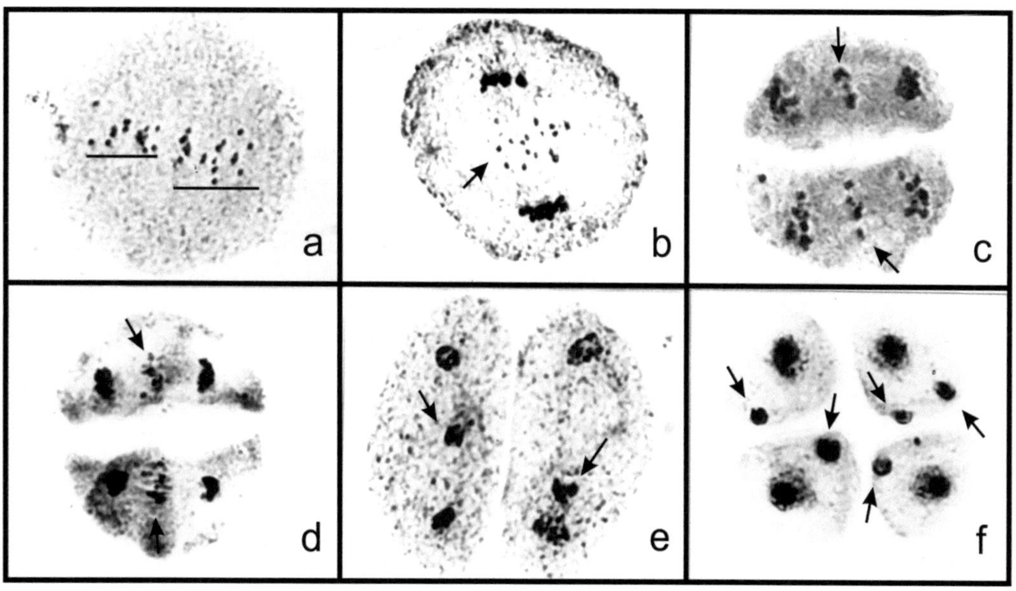


Fig. 3. Aspects of genome affinity and chromosome elimination observed in some interspecific hybrids. a) The parental genomes separated into two metaphase plates in the meiocyte. b) Meiocyte in anaphase I with a laggard genome (arrow). c, d) Meiocytes in anaphase II with a laggard genome (arrow). Meiocyte in telophase II with large micronuclei resulting from the laggard genome (arrow). f) Tetrad of microspores with large micronuclei (arrows).

Genome similarities in the genus *Brachiaria* were not studied from the cytogenetic point of view. Karyological studies in the genus were performed for a few species and accessions (Bernini & Marin-Morales, 2001), and genomes were not yet described. In the last decade, however, evaluation of the meiotic behavior in some hybrids between *B. ruziziensis* x *B. brizantha* (Risso-Pascotto et al., 2004; Mendes-Bonato et al., 2006b; Adamowski et al., 2008; Fuzinatto et al., 2007; Felismino et al., 2010; Felismino, 2011) has revealed that genomes of parental species not always show perfect affinity. Lacking of genome affinity during meiosis was revealed by asynchrony in the meiosis time (Fig. 3 b to f) (Risso-Pascotto et al., 2004; Adamowski et al., 2008) or separation of the two parental genomes into two metaphase plates (Fig. 3 a) (Mendes-Bonato et al., 2006b). The lack of genome affinity between *B. ruziziensis* and *B. brizantha* seems to be genotype-specific.

## 7. Artificial polyploids obtained through protoplast fusion, a case study involving *Passiflora* species

The genus *Passiflora* L. (Passifloraceae), which includes the commercial species of passionflowers, is a large and widespread genus consisting primarily of tropical species. Currently the taxonomy of the genus designates four subgenera *Astrophea* (with 57 species), *Deidamioides* (13) *Decaloba* (214) and *Passiflora* (236), in which are included the typical passion fruits (Ulmer & MacDougal, 2004). Most are vines, though some representatives are shrubs or trees. South America is the center of diversity for most of the *Passiflora* species; around 40 are indigenous to Asia and South Pacific Islands. Passion vines are evergreen climbers, grown for their edible fruits, and several species are cultivated for their unusual and beautiful flowers (Vanderplank, 1996).

Several species are important for their nutritional and pharmacological properties, but some of them are used as ornamental plants. Among all, about 50 species bear edible fruits but only the two forms of *Passiflora edulis,* i.e., the purple and the yellow ones are considered to be of value in international commerce. Although small-scale, the juice is manufactured to be exported to EU countries. The wide genetic variability, known to exist within and between *Passiflora* species can be exploited in breeding programs in order to obtain improved populations or to search for genes of interest. Commercial passion fruit varieties available are susceptible to a number of pests and diseases with considerable negative effects on production (for a review see Vieira & Carneiro, 2004; Zerbini et al., 2008). With the purpose of producing rootstocks resistant to soil-borne diseases, interspecific protoplast fusion was performed, and the hybrids between the yellow passion fruit, *P. edulis* f. *flavicarpa* and two wild species *P. amethystina* and *P. cincinnata*, all with 2n=2x=18 were obtained (Dornelas et al. 1995; Vieira & Dornelas, 1996). Briefly, all the hybrid cells were produced by PEG-mediated protoplast fusion and shoot regeneration occurred via indirect organogenesis. Selection was performed based on total protein and isoenzyme electrophoretic patterns at the callus stage (Vieira & Dornelas, 1996). After being acclimatized, the plantlets were transferred to the field where the vines grew to maturity and flourished, but did not set normal fruits, even when artificially crossed. In this section, we present the meiotic study of these somatic hybrids carried out in our laboratory (Barbosa & Vieira, 1997; Barbosa et al. 2007).

Firstly, we will discuss the meiotic behavior of the two parental diploid species, *P. edulis* f. *flavicarpa* (E) and *P. amethystina* (Am) and their four somatic hybrids denoted (E +Am) # 12, # 13, # 28 and # 35, each derived from different calli. Flower buds were collected from the vines, fixed, and slides were prepared using standard protocols. For segregation analysis, cells were studied in the diakinesis, and pollen viability (V) was determined according to Alexander (1980), which employs malachite green and fuchsinic acid.

As expected, the meiosis of the parental species showed nine bivalents (9II). In *P. edulis* f. *flavicarpa*, one or two bivalents were associated with the nucleolus in 33% or 67% of the cells, respectively, indicating the presence of two nucleolar organizing regions (NOR's). In *P. amethystina*, two bivalents were associated with the nucleolus in all cells analyzed. Chromosome pairing in the parental species was regular, although some laggard chromosomes and anaphase bridges were observed (less than 1%). The analysis of somatic hybrids showed 4x = 36 chromosomes, with four NOR's; no aneuploids were present. Meiosis was irregular with high frequencies of bridges and laggards in both divisions (Table 2). Interestingly, clear differences in the meiotic behavior among the hybrids were observed. The hybrids (E + Am) # 12 and # 28 had more regular meiosis than (E + Am) # 13 and # 35. Meiotic figures in hybrid cells display bivalents and a few univalent or multivalent. The configurations observed at diakinesis are presented on Table 2. At least 14 II were observed in 96.7% of the cells of the hybrids (E + Am) # 12 and # 35 meanwhile, the same minimum of bivalents was detected in 100% of the cells of the hybrids (E +Am) # 13 and # 28. As expected, the two sets of homologous chromosomes pair preferentially in the hybrids, reflecting the level of homology between the parental chromosomes. Moreover, the frequencies of cells with quadrivalents were 73.3% in (E + Am) # 13, 83.3% in # 12 and, 93.3% in (E + Am) # 28 and # 35.

Hybrid # 28 shows the lowest number of bridges in anaphase cells (I and II) and laggard chromosomes. The hybrid (E + Am) # 35 differs from the other three, by the largest number of cells with univalents (33.3%) which explains the high level of laggard chromosomes and chromatids in the subsequent division stages (Table 2). The present data support that recombination of the chromosomes of the two parental species occurred in the hybrids, mainly in the hybrid # 28 and # 35, since most of their cells showed the occurrence of quadrivalents. In view of the presence of quadrivalents in all hybrid genotypes analyzed, *P. edulis* f. *flavicarpa* and *P. amethystina* may possess some chromosome homoeology. Later on, we observed that *P. edulis* f .*flavicarpa* and *P. amethystina* show very similar karyotypes (Cuco et al., 2005).

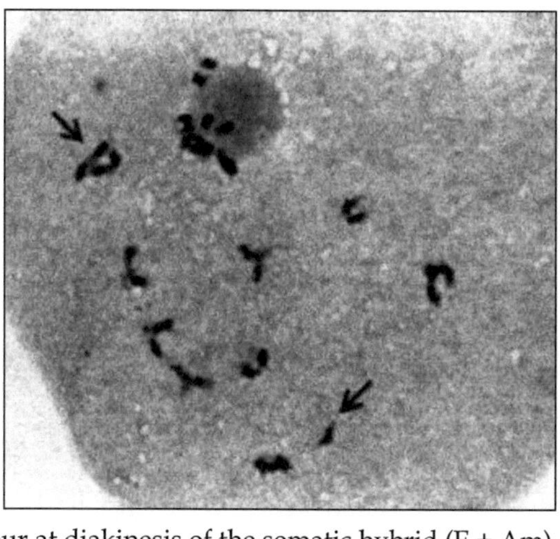

Fig. 4. Meiotic behaviour at diakinesis of the somatic hybrid (E + Am). Note the presence of bivalents, a quadrivalent (arrow) and a univalent (arrow).

| **Plant material** | **Diakinesis configurations**[1] | | | | | | | | **Laggards**[2] | | **Bridges** | **Laggards**[2] | | **Chromatid Bridges** |
|---|---|---|---|---|---|---|---|---|---|---|---|---|---|---|
| | 12II +4I +2IV | 13II +2I +2IV | 14II +4I +1IV | 14II +2IV | 15II +2I +1IV | 16II +1IV | 17II +2I | 18II | MI | AI | | MII | AII | |
| (E) | | – | – | – | | | | | 0.99 | 0.00 | 0.65 | 0.38 | 0.0 | 0.25 |
| (Am) | | – | – | – | | | | | 0.44 | 0.00 | 0.79 | 0.68 | 0.0 | 0.23 |
| (E+Am) #12 | 3.3 | 0.0 | 3.3 | 26.7 | 10.0 | 40.0 | 10.0 | 6.7 | 1.15 | 0.00 | 2.12 | 2.47 | 0.00 | 7.11 |
| (E+Am) #13 | 0.0 | 0.0 | 0.0 | 16.7 | 13.3 | 43.3 | 6.7 | 20.0 | 5.90 | 0.00 | 3.83 | 4.10 | 1.92 | 4.39 |
| (E+Am) #28 | 0.0 | 0.0 | 0.0 | 30.0 | 20.0 | 43.3 | 0.0 | 6.7 | 1.15 | 0.00 | 2.09 | 1.15 | 0.00 | 1.37 |
| (E+Am) #35 | 0.0 | 3.3 | 0.0 | 40.0 | 23.3 | 26.7 | 6.7 | 0.0 | 8.11 | 7.57 | 12.37 | 13.16 | 3.95 | 16.05 |

[1]Number of cells analyzed = 30; [2]MI and MII, first and second metaphase, respectively, AI and AII, first and second anaphase, respectively.

Table 2. Meiotic behavior (in percentages) in *P. edulis* f. *flavicarpa* (E), *P. amethystina* (Am) and their four somatic hybrids (E+Am). Modified from Barbosa & Vieira (1997).

On average, all the materials analyzed presented high levels of pollen viability, ranging from 72.9% up to 88.2%. The hybrid showing the lowest mean viability is the one that presents the higher percentage of meiotic irregularities. In contrast, the high levels of mean viability found for the parental species (>95%) and the remaining hybrid plants were related to the low percentage of meiotic irregularities observed (Table 2). The correlations between pollen viabilities and meiotic irregularities were high and negative.

Similarly, the meiotic behavior of four somatic hybrids were examined and compared with their corresponding diploid fusion parents, *P. edulis* f. *flavicarpa* (E) and *P. cincinnata* (C).The meiotic behavior revealed relatively high stability, with most of the hybrid cells showing 18 bivalents. Some instability, such as a quadrivalent configuration was also recorded which has been interpreted as an interchange that occurred in the progenitors more than as a result of *in vitro* culture or chromosome reorganization in the new genome. Even in low frequencies, the occurrence of univalents resulted in misdivision, laggard and micronucleus formation. High values of pollen viability (>70%) were found in the diploid parents as well as in the hybrid plants. As expected, the course of meiosis was regular in the parental cells. Some chromosome bridges and laggards were observed, possibly as a consequence of the formation of univalents, though they were not actually recorded. These abnormalities occurred at a very low frequency, i.e. <2% of the cells.

As expected, the meiosis of the parental species showed nine bivalents (9II), two of them were attached to the nucleolus in 67% of the cells at diakinesis. In *P. cincinnata*, this percentage was higher (73%).The four hybrid plants were 4x=36; the hybrid cells *per se* were not variable in number, i.e. no aneuploid cells occurred, at least within the sample cells analyzed.

A certain frequency of laggards and anaphase bridges in both divisions was observed in all hybrid plants (Table 3). However, differences amongst them were noted: (E+C) #07 and (E+C) #25 had a more irregular meiotic behavior than (E+C) #14 and (E+C) #26, but in the second division, the configuration changed, and the hybrids #25 and #26 had more irregular behavior. The frequency of bivalents at diakinesis in the hybrids varied from 55% to 78.5%. These percentages should be associated with the presence of a quadrivalent, which was found in 30.0% and 32.5% of the cells of the hybrids #07 and #26, respectively, and in 17.1% and 13.3% of the cells of the hybrids #14 and #25, respectively. The disassociation of those quadrivalents should explain the laggards and the chromosome bridges observed at division II. The hybrids #07 and #25 showed higher percentages of univalents, which were also the plants that had cells with higher proportions of laggards at meiosis I and II. The occurrence of univalents varied from 4.2% in (E+C) #14 up to 15% in (E+C) #07 and #25, being correlated with other meiotic alterations and as well bivalent frequency at diakinesis. In the plant (E+C) #25 with 15% of diakinesis cells showing univalents, they appeared as laggards at metaphase I (12.3%) and underwent centromere misdivision (2.3%). Moreover, the results suggest that chromosomes that suffered longitudinal division at meiosis I underwent centromere misdivision at meiosis II (Table 3).

| Plant material | Diakinesis configurations | | | Laggards[1] | | Bridges | Laggards[1] | | Chromatid bridges | No. cells analyzed |
|---|---|---|---|---|---|---|---|---|---|---|
| | 17II +2I | 16II +1IV | 18II | MI | AI | | MII | AII | | |
| (E) | – | – | – | 1.0 | 0.0 | 0.6 | 0.4 | 0.0 | 0.2 | 40 |
| (C) | – | – | – | 1.3 | 0.0 | 0.2 | 0.0 | 0.8 | 0.6 | 40 |
| (E+C) #07 | 15.0 | 30.0 | 55.0 | 19.9 | 28.8 | 1.2 | 15.8 | 16.0 | 1.8 | 40 |
| (E+C) #14 | 4.2 | 17.1 | 78.5 | 7.1 | 28.2 | 5.0 | 13.0 | 4.0 | 10.6 | 70 |
| (E+C) #25 | 15.0 | 13.3 | 71.6 | 12.3 | 26.9 | 2.3 | 15.5 | 7.6 | 16.1 | 60 |
| (E+C) #26 | 7.5 | 32.5 | 60.0 | 15.3 | 15.5 | 2.1 | 13.4 | 13.4 | 13.3 | 40 |

[1]MI and MII, first and second metaphase, respectively, AI and AII, first and second anaphase, respectively.

Table 3. Meiotic behavior (in percentages) in *P. edulis* f. *flavicarpa*(E), *P. cincinnata*(C) and their four somatic hybrids (E+C). Modified from Barbosa et al. (2007).

The frequency of microspores with micronuclei was relatively low (6.4% up to 23.2%) considering the abnormalities found at all the meiotic stages. Probably, many laggards forming bridges at anaphase I and II were included in telophase nuclei. Certainly, a fraction of these laggards was included as entire chromosomes. The frequency of laggards in metaphase II cells was somewhat the same in metaphase I (3). However, misdivision was five times more frequent at metaphase II, although laggards were found in a reduced frequency (three times less), suggesting that almost all the chromosomes that underwent longitudinal division at first division did undergo misdivision at meiosis II. Laggards in (E+C) #25 were observed in 7.6% of the anaphase II cells and did result in a micronucleus in 8.7% of the tetrad cells. Those chromosomes that went through longitudinal division at first meiosis underwent misdivision because they were attached to the centromeres, while laggards at anaphase II were eliminated.

Parental pollen viability values were 96%. In the hybrid plants, on average, all values were high, ranging from 71.6% up to 82.1%. For the meiotic analyses, one can first state that the two bivalents attached to the nucleolus of the parental cells correspond to the smallest chromosomes, i.e. 8 and 9. Our study on *Passiflora* using fluorescent *in situ* hybridization detected positive signals corresponding to 45S rDNA sites on the secondary constrictions of chromosome 8 and satellites of chromosome 9 of *P. edulis* f. *flavicarpa* and *P. cincinnata* (Cuco et al., 2005). In addition, chromomycin A3 bandings were found in regions corresponding to 45S rDNA sites, therefore, in two chromosome pairs. No other preferentially GC-rich regions were observed in these species. The nucleolar activity was also investigated by silver staining and four silver-positive signals were detected on the smallest chromosomes pairs.

Minimal differences are also reported between the karyotypes of *P.edulis* f. *flavicarpa* and *P. cincinnata* (Cuco et al., 2005). In addition, the DNA content amongst the *Passiflora* species (at least into the subgenus *Passiflora*) is slightly variable (Souza et al. 2004; Souza et al., 2008), and *P.edulis* f. *flavicarpa* and *P. cincinnata* are very close in terms of phylogenetics (Muschner et al. 2003; Cuco et al., 2005; Padua, 2004). Based on all those features, high chromosome stability is not expected for the somatic hybrids studied here. The presence of just a few univalents in the hybrid plants is expected considering the classical taxonomy (Killip, 1938) and the modern classification proposed for the genus *Passiflora* (Ulmer & Macdougal, 2004) that indicate the proximity of these species. Univalents and the various ways they behave throughout meiosis probably contributed to the formation of the micronuclei observed in the somatic hybrid microspores. The presence of univalents as micronuclei in tetrads was frequently associated with a reduction of vigor and fertility in hybrid plants (e.g. Cao et al., 2003) as above reported for the somatic hybrids between *P. edulis* f. *flavicarpa* and *P. amethystina*. Finally, the more irregular the meiotic behavior, the lower was the pollen viability. This correlation was also abovementioned for the previous set of hybrids (E+Am).

All species used as parents are auto-incompatible and when they were artificially crossed with the somatic hybrids (theoretically, $2n=2x=18 \times 2n=4x=36 \rightarrow 2n=3x=27$), few seeds were obtained. The hybrids were female-sterile and pollen producers. In practical terms, the levels of pollen viability and multivalent pairing in the two types of somatic hybrids suggest that these materials can be used as rootstocks due to their compatibility to *P. edulis* f. *flavicarpa* promoting resistance to soil diseases. The three *Passiflora* species investigated are closely related as they belong to the same subgenus (*Passiflora*), although *P. amethystine* belongs to the series *Lobatae*, and *P. edulis* and *P. cincinnata* are members of the series *Passiflora*. Most passionflowers are diploids, though aneuploidy and polyploidy have been reported as evolutionary mechanisms, and have symmetrical karyotypes that could be distinguished from each other by minor differences (Melo et al., 2001; Cuco et al., 2005; Souza et al., 2008).

Intriguingly, newly formed polyploids show genetic and cytological alterations. Consequently, an interest in studies aiming at understanding these genetic events involved in artificial allopolyploid formation increased in recent years, also for *Citrus*, another important fruit species (Chen et al., 2004). In the case of the interspecific allotetraploid somatic hybrids, 'Hamlin' sweet orange + 'Rough Lemon' and 'Key'lime + 'Valencia' sweet orange, meiotic analysis revealed that <20% of the meiocytes exhibited normal tetrad formation in somatic hybrid plants, and irregular chromosome behavior with univalent or multivalent pairing also occurred. Moreover, meiotic abnormalities such as chromosome bridges, chromosomes orientated away from the equatorial plate, especially lagging chromosomes, which resulted in different sizes of pollen grains, were frequently observed in both somatic hybrids. Comparing to passionflowers hybrids, pollen germinability was very low (<15%), intermediate between their corresponding *Citrus* fusion parents. Concluding, the meiotic behavior of *Citrus* somatic hybrids provided valuable information for their practical utilization, particularly for intergenomic recombination, and increased the germplasm available for interploid crosses in *Citrus* triploid seedless breeding programs.

## 8. Conclusion

The meiotic analysis of polyploidy hybrids is an important element in taxonomic and evolutionary studies of plants. It also provides an important starting point in alien introgression programs and permits an estimation of the frequency of recombination that will occur in interspecific hybrids. Chromosome pairing is the most used method of assessing genomic relationships between species. This information allows predictions to be made of the likelihood of transferring specific target genes from one species to another. From accumulated results obtained through cytological studies in hybrids, it is evident that cytogenetic analyses are of prime importance in determining which genotypes can continue in the process of cultivar development and which can be successfully used in breeding programs.

## 9. References

Adamowski EV, Pagliarini MS, Valle CB. (2008). Meiotic behavior in three interspecific three way hybrids between *Brachiaria ruziziensis* and *B. brizantha* (Poaceae: Paniceae). *Journal of Genetics*, 87, 33-38

Alexander MP. (1980). A versatile stain for pollen from fungi, yeast and bacteria. *Stain Technology*, 55, 13-18

Argel PJ, Keller-Grein G. (1996). Regional experience with *Brachiaria*: Tropical America - Humid lowlands, In: *Brachiaria: biology, agronomy, and improvement*, Miles JW, Maass BL, Valle CB (eds), 205-224, CIAT/Embrapa, Cali

Barbosa LV, Vieira MLC. (1997). Meiotic behavior of passion fruit somatic hybrids, *Passiflora edulis* f. *flavicarpa* Degener + *P. amethystina* Mikan. *Euphytica*, 98, 121-127

Barbosa LV, Mondin M, Oliveira CA, Souza AP, Vieira MLC. (2007). Cytological behavior of the somatic hybrids *Passiflora edulis* f. *flavicarpa* + *P. cincinnata*. *Plant Breeding*, 126, 323-328

Bernini C, Marin-Morales MA. (2001). Karyotype analysis in *Brachiaria* (Poaceae) species. *Cytobios*, 104, 157-171

Boddey RM, Macedo R, Torres RM, Ferreira E, Oliveira O, Cantaruti RB, Perreira JM, Alves BJR, Urquiaga S. (2004): Nitrogen cycling in *Brachiaria* pastures: the key to understanding the process of pasture decline. Agriculture and Ecosyst.em Environment ,103, 389-403.

Cao M., Bughrarab SS, Sleper DA. (2003). Cytogenetic analysis of *Festuca* species and amphiploids between *Festuca mairei* and *Lolium perenne*. *Crop Science* 43, 1659-1662

Chen CL, Guo WW, Yi HL, Deng XX. (2004). Cytogenetic analysis of two interspecific *Citrus* allotetraploid somatic hybrids and their diploid fusion parents. *Plant Breeding*, 123, 332-337

Choudhary BR, Joshi P, Ramarao S. (2000). Interspecific hybridization between *Brassica carinata* and *Brassica rapa*. *Plant Breeding*, 119, 417-420

Cuco SM, Vieira MLC, Mondin M, Aguiar-Perecin MLR. (2005). Comparative karyotype analysis of three *Passiflora* L. species and cytogenetic characterization of somatic hybrids. *Caryologia*, 58, 220-228

Dornelas MC, Tavares FCA, Oliveira JC, Vieira MLC. (1995). Plant regeneration from protoplast fusion in *Passiflora* spp. *Plant Cell Reports*, 15, 106-110

Felismino MF, Pagliarini MS, Valle CB. (2010). Meiotic behavior of interspecific hybrids between artificially tetraploidized sexual *Brachiaria ruziziensis* and tetraploid apomictic *B. brizantha* (Poaceae). *Scientia Agricola*, 67, 1-8

Felismino MF. (2011). Microsporogenesis in interspecific *Brachiaria* hybrids. Ph. D Thesis, University of Maringá, Brazil.

Ferguson JE, Crowder LV. (1974). Cytology and breeding behaviour of *Brachiaria ruziziensis*. *Crop Science*, 14, 893-895

Fuzinatto VA, Pagliarini MS, Valle CB. (2007). Microsporogenesis in sexual *Brachiaria* hybrids (Poaceae). *Genetics and Molecular Research*, 6, 1107-1117

Goodman RM, Hauptti H, Crossway A, Knauf VC. (1987). Gene transfer in crop improvement. *Science*, 236, 48-54

Keller-Grein G, Mass BL, Hanson F. (1996). Natural variation in *Brachiaria* and existing germplasm collection, In: *Brachiaria: biology, agronomy, and improvement*, Miles JW, Maass BL, Valle CB (eds), 16-42, CIAT/Embrapa, Cali

Killip EP. (1938). The American species of Passifloraceae. *Field Museum Natural History, Botanical Series*, 19, 1-613

Luckens LN, Pires JC, Leon G, Vogelzang R, Oslack L, Osborn T. (2006). Patterns of sequence loss and cytosine methylation within a population of newly resynthesized *Brassica napus* allopolyploids. *Plant Physiology*, 140, 336-348

Lutts S, Nidikumana J, Louant BP. (1991). Fertility of *Brachiaria ruziziensis* in interspecific crosses with *Brachiaria decumbens* and *Brachiaria brizantha*: meiotic behavior, pollen viability and seed set. *Euphytica*, 57, 267-274

Lutts S, Ndikumana J, Louant BP. (1994). Male and female sporogenesis and gametogenesis in apomictics *Brachiaria brizantha, Brachiaria decumbens* and $F_1$ hybrids with sexual colchicine induced tetraploid *Brachiaria ruziziensis. Euphytica*, 78, 19-25.

Marfil CF, Masuelli RW, Davison J, Comai L. (2006). Genomic instability in *Solanum tuberosum* x *Solanum kurtzianum* interspecific hybrids. *Genome*, 49, 104-113.

Melo NF, Cervi AC, Guerra M. (2001). Karyology and cytotaxonomy of the genus *Passiflora* L. (Passifloraceae). *Plant Systematics Evolution*, 226, 69-84

Mendes-Bonato AB, Pagliarini MS, Forli F, Valle CB, Penteado MIO. (2002). Chromosome number and microsporogenesis in *Brachiaria brizantha* (Gramineae). *Euphytica*, 125, 419-425

Mendes-Bonato AB, Pagliarini MS, Risso-Pascotto C, Valle CB. (2006a). Chromosome number and meiotic behavior in *Brachiaria jubata* (Gramineae). *Journal of Genetics*, 85, 83-88

Mendes-Bonato AB, Risso-Pascotto C, Pagliarini MS, Valle CB. (2006b). Cytogenetic evidence for genome elimination during microsporogenesis in interspecific hybrid between *Brachiaria ruziziensis* and *B. brizantha* (Gramineae). *Genetics and Molecular Biology*, 29, 711-714

Miles, J. W., B. L. Maass, and C. B. Valle, 1996: *Brachiaria*: Biology, Agronomy, and Improvement. CIAT/Embrapa, Cali

Muschner V C, Lorenz AP, Cervi AC, Bonatto SL, Souza-Chiez TT, Salzano FM, Freitas LB. (2003). A first molecular phylogenetic analysis of *Passiflora* (Passifloraceae). *American Journal of Botany*, 90, 1229-1238

Ndikumana J. (1985). Etude de l'hybridation entre espèces apomictiques et sexuées dans le genre *Brachiaria*. Ph.D. dissertation, Université Catholique de Louvain. Belgium

Padua JG. (2004). Análise genética de espécies do gênero *Passiflora* L. com base em abordagens filogenéticas, morfométricas e em marcadores microssatélites, *PhD Thesis*, Universidade de São Paulo, Brazil

Pagliarini MS, Risso-Pascotto C, Souza-Kaneshima AM, Valle CB. (2008). Analysis of meiotic behavior in selecting potential genitors among diploid and artificially induced tetraploid accessions of *Brachiaria ruziziensis* (Poaceae). *Euphytica*, 164, 181-187

Renvoize SA, Clayton WD, Kabuye CHS. (1996). Morphology, taxonomy, and natural distribution of *Brachiaria* (Trin.) Griseb, In: *Brachiaria: biology, agronomy, and improvement*, Miles JW, Maass BL, Valle CB (eds), 1-15, CIAT/Embrapa, Cali

Rieseberg LH, Baird SJE, Gardner KA. (2000). Hybridization, introgression, and linkage evolution. *Plant Molecular Biology*, 42, 205-224

Risso-Pascotto C, Pagliarini MS, Valle CB, Jank L. (2004) Asynchronous meiotic rhythm as the cause of selective chromosome elimination in an interspecific *Brachiaria* hybrid. *Plant Cell Reports*, 22, 945-950

Risso-Pascotto C, Pagliarini MS, Valle CB. (2005). Meiotic behavior in interspecific hybrids between *Brachiaria ruziziensis* and *Brachiaria brizantha* (Poaceae). *Euphytica*, 145, 155-159

Risso-Pascotto C, Pagliarini MS, Valle CB. (2006). Microsporogenesis in *Brachiaria dictyoneura* (Fig. & De Not.) Stapf (Poaceae: Paniceae). *Genetics and Molecular Research*, 5, 837-845

Sain RS, Joshi P, Satry EVD. (2002). Cytogenetic analysis of interspecific hybrids in genus *Citrullus* (Cucurbitaceae). *Euphytica*, 128, 205-210

Schwarzacher T, Heslop-Harrison JS, Anamthawat-Jónsson K. (1992). Parental genome separation in reconstructions of somatic and premeiotic metaphases of *Hordeum vulgare* x *H. bulbosum*. *Journal of Cell Science*, 101, 13-24

Simioni C, Valle CB do. (2009). Chromosome duplication in *Brachiaria* (A.Rich.) Stapf allows intraspecific crosses. *Crop Breeding and Applied Biotechnology*, 9, 328 - 334.

Souza MM, Palomino G, Pereira TNS, Pereira MG, Viana PA. (2004). Flow cytometric analysis of genome size variation in some *Passiflora* species. *Hereditas*, 141, 31-38

Souza MM, Pereira TNS, Vieira MLC. (2008). Cytogenetic studies in some species of *Passiflora* L. (Passifloraceae): A review emphasizing Brazilian species. *Brazilian Archives of Biology and Technology*, 51, 247-258

Souza-Kaneshima AM, Simioni C, Felismino MF, Mendes-Bonato AB, Risso-Pascotto C, Pessim C, Pagliarini MS, Valle CB. (2010). Meiotic behavior in the first interspecific hybrid between *B. brizantha* and *B. decumbens*. *Plant Breeding*, 129, 186-191

Stebbins GL. (1950). Variation and evolution in plants. Columbia University Press, New York

Swenne A, Louant BP, Dujardin M. (1981). Induction par la colchicine de formes autotétraploïdes chez *Brachiaria ruziziensis* Germain et Evrard (Gramínée). *Agronomia Tropicale*, 36, 134-141

Ulmer T, Macdougal JM. (2004). *Passiflora* Passionflowers of the World, Timber Press, Portland

Utsunomiya KS, Pagliarini MS, Valle CB. (2005) Microsporogenesis in tetraploid accessions of *Brachiaria nigropedata* (Ficalho & Hiern) Stapf (Gramineae). *Biocell*, 29, 295-301

Valle CB, Glienke C. (1991). New sexual accession in *Brachiaria. Apomixis Newsletter*, 7, 42-43

Valle CB, Savidan Y. (1996). Genetics, cytogenetics, and reproductive biology of *Brachiaria*, In In: *Brachiaria: biology, agronomy, and improvement*, Miles JW, Maass BL, Valle CB (eds), 147-163, CIAT/Embrapa, Cali

Valle CB, Pagliarini MS. (2009). Biology, cytogenetics, and breeding of *Brachiaria* In: *Genetic resources, chromosome engineering, and crop improvement,* Singh RJ (ed) 103-151, CRC Press, Boca Raton

Vanderplank J. (1996). *Passion flowers*, Cambridge Press, London

Vieira MLC, Dornelas MC. (1996). Regeneration of plants from protoplasts of *Passiflora* species (Passion Fruit). In: *Plant Protoplasts and Genetic Engineering VII, Biotechnology in Agriculture and Forestry*, Bajaj YPS (ed), 38, 108-119, Springer Verlag, Berlin

Vieira MLC, Carneiro MS. (2004). Passifloraceae *Passiflora* spp. Passionfruit. In: *Biotechnology of fruit and nut crops,* Litz R (ed), 436-453, CAB International, Oxfordshire

Zerbini FM, Otoni, WC, Vieira MLC. (2008). Passionfruit. In: *Compendium of transgenic crop plants: transgenic tropical and subtropical fruits and nuts,* Kole C, Hall T. (org.), Blackwell Publishing, Oxford, 5, 213-234

Zwierzykowski Z, Lukaszewski AJ, Naganowska B, Lesniewska A. (1999). The pattern of homologous recombination in triploid hybrids of *Lolium multiflorum* with *Festuca pratensis. Genome*, 40, 720-726

# 19

# Meiotic Irregularities in Interspecific Crosses Within Edible Alliums

Agnieszka Kiełkowska
*University of Agriculture in Krakow, Poland*

## 1. Introduction

The economically most important edible alliums are onion (*Allium cepa* L.), Japanese bunching onion (*A. fistulosum* L.), leek (*A. apmleroprasum* spp. *porrum* L.), and garlic (*A. sativum* L.). These species are mostly used as condiments, but also have medicinal value (Keusgen, 2002). Onion and garlic are grown worldwide, leek is predominantly grown in Europe, and Japanese bunching onion in East Asia (Kik, 2002). Hybridization of certain genotypes, increasing genetic variability, is the predominant breeding method used for onion, leek and Japanese bunching onion. Garlic breeding is accelerated by clonal selection (Etoh & Simon, 2002).

Interspecific hybridization within the genus *Allium* has a long history, and has been an important tool for increasing genetic variation. It was used for creating new varieties as well as for transferring agronomically useful traits from wild relatives (Brewster, 1994; Kiełkowska & Adamus, 2010; Kik, 2002). However, techniques of sexual hybridization very often have been accompanied by several difficult to overcome pre- and post-fertilization barriers, resulting in a limited number of obtained F1 hybrids, as well as difficulties with back-crossing. Meiotic studies of hybrids and back-cross progenies within *Allium* revealed interesting information about the nature of alien introgression and improved our understanding of "foreign" chromatin transmission into cultivated species (Kik, 2002; van Heusden et al., 2000).

The purpose of the present paper is to give a concise review of meiosis in pollen mother cells (PMC) and pollen fertility in *Allium cepa* and its crosses with *A. fistulosum, A. ampeloprasum*, and *A. sativum*.

## 2. Chromosome number and meiosis

Most alliums are diploids (2n=2x), with basic chromosome numbers x=7 (North America), x=8 (Eurasia and Mediterranean basin), or x=9 (Eurasia) (Havey, 2002; Ved Brat, 1965a). Polyploids such as triploids (*A. rupestre, A. scordoprasum*), tetraploids (*A. ampeloprasum, A. chinense, A. nutans*), pentaploids (*A. splendens*), hexaploids (*A. lineare*), and octoploids (*A. nutans*) also occur (Jones R.N., 1990; Jones R.N & Rees, 1968; Ved Brat, 1965a).

Accessory chromosomes (B-chromosomes, supernumerary) have been documented (Bougourd and Plowman 1996). Their size and centromere position is variable within species (Ved Brat, 1965a, 1965b). B-chromosomes found in *A. paniculatum* never undergo pairing with other chromosomes during meiosis, however, occurrence of chiasmata associations among B-chromosomes in *A. schoenoprasum* was observed (Bougourd & Parker 1979).

The majority of species within the genus carry meta- or submetacentric chromosomes (Ved Brat, 1965a). Levan (1932, 1935) noted that species with x=7 had larger chromosomes than those with x=8 or x=9 and that arm-length asymmetry was more frequent in the "16" and "18"-chromosomes types and that the "14"-chromosome types were the most primitive. Ved Brat (1965a) estimated, that 40% of the forms within the genus possessing eight chromosomes had varying number of asymmetrical chromosomes, often carrying the nucleolar organizer regions (NOR), whereas remaining 60% had symmetrical chromosomes. Reports about differences in telomeric sequences in *Allium* (Fuchs et al., 1995) and stabilization of chromosome ends by highly repetitive satellites and rDNA (Pich et al., 1996) were also published.

Length of the alliums chromosomes also varies; the shortest (~7 μm) chromosomes were found in *A. yunnanense* (x=8), the longest (~22 μm) in *A. fragrans* (x=9) (Levan 1935). Investigation of the nuclear DNA content revealed that evolution of alliums was associated with variation in DNA amounts. Nuclear DNA content was proportional to chromosome 'volume' in the cell, and changes in the DNA amount were distributed between chromosomes within complements (Jones R.N. & Rees, 1968). *Alliums* with n=8 have in general the lowest; mean 28,9 pg/2C nuclear DNA amounts, while those with n=9, the highest; mean 42,2 pg/2C (Bennett & Leitch, 2010).

Breeding systems in alliums are variable; some are reproduced sexually as outbreeders or inbreeders, some asexually with vivapory or apomixis and some are vegetatively propagated (Ved Brat, 1965b). An overwhelming majority of the genus is propagated sexually, which allows for gene exchange and, in consequence, more genetic variability. However, in the vegetatively reproduced *A. sativum* the main source of variation is the occurrence of alterations in the number and morphology of chromosomes in somatic cells of the clone (Konvička & Levan, 1972).

Meiosis in alliums was reviewed by Levan (1931, 1935). In prophase I of the diploid forms chiasmata are visible at early diakinesis. Terminalization of chiasmata causes a decrease in their number from 10-15 to 2-3 in each conjugating pair. The most common types of chromosome shape in metaphase are rings and rods. In some cases i.e. *A. nutans*, pairing in meiosis is incomplete in certain chromosome pairs (Levan, 1931). During meiosis in the polyploid forms, associations of chromosomes are common. Appearance of trivalents in *A. nutans* was reported (Levan, 1935). Observed trivalents had different forms, i.e V-shaped trivalents with one rod on each arm or with two rods on one arm. In anaphase I trivalents are distributed randomly, usually twelve to the pole, however, formation 8 to one pole and 16 to other was also observed (Levan, 1931). Occurrence of lagger chromosomes developing micronuclei, as well as formation of unreduced gametes was reported in triploids (Ved Brat, 1967). Quadrivalents were formed in meiosis I in the PMC of *A. schoenoprasum* and *A. porrum*. The most frequent types of quadrivalents were rings and chains (Levan, 1935). In polyploid *A. oleraceum* (2n=24, 32, 40) elimination of chromosomes during meiosis was observed, thus pollen grains with 13, 15, 17, and other number of chromosomes were noted (Levan, 1931).

### 2.1 *A. cepa*

*Allium cepa* L. belongs to the genus *Allium*, subgenus *Rhizirideum*, section *Cepa* (Mill.) (Fritsch & Friesen, 2002). It is a diploid (2n=2x=16) and possesses one of the largest genomes among cultivated plants (Havey, 2002). The nuclear genome of onion contains 35,8 pg per 2C (Labani & Elkington, 1987), which is reflected by very large chromosomes. Onion has a complement of eight pairs of metacentric and submetacentric chromosomes including one set of terminal satellite chromosomes. Meiosis in onion is regular with eight bivalents (R.N. Jones, 1990). Chiasmata during metaphase I in PMC in onion are distributed at random in each bivalent and by the mid-metaphase they become terminal or sub-terminal and either rod or ring bivalents are formed (Fig. 1 & Fig. 2) (Emsweller & H.A. Jones, 1945; Levan, 1936). The cross-over points are therefore located mainly in distal and interstitial regions of the chromosome arms (Koul & Gohil, 1970; Levan, 1933). There is no information about localized chiasmata in onion (Emsweller & H.A. Jones, 1945).

### 2.2 Hybrids with introgression from *A. fistulosum*

*Allium fistulosum* L. (Japanese bunching onion, Welsh onion) is a diploid species (2n=2x=16). *A. fistulosum,* similarly to onion, belongs to section *Cepa* of the genus *Allium* (R.N. Jones, 1990). Nuclear DNA content is 26,3 pg (2C), what is about 20% less than in onion (R.N. Jones & Rees, 1968).

During meiosis I in *A. fistulosum* eight bivalents are formed. Bivalents are held together by two chiasmata, one on each side of the centromere, thus in the metaphase plate they appear like a cross (Fig. 2). Chiasmata in the bivalent are usually localized proximally, adjacent to the centromere, however, occasional formation of more interstitial and randomized chiasmata were observed (R.N. Jones, 1990; Levan, 1933; Maeda, 1937).

Progenies from generative hybridization of onion with *A. fistulosum* have been studied most extensively among all interspecific crosses in the genus *Allium*. Those two species can be easily hybridized in the greenhouse and the success rate can be enhanced by the use of embryo-rescue in tissue cultures (Doležel et al., 1980). First hybrids between *A. cepa* and *A. fistulosum* were reported in 1935 by Emsweller and Jones. Meiotic studies showed that in early prophase I the hybrid chromosomes appear to be single threads, like in the parents. Abnormalities in the cell division start at late prophase, what was confirmed by Maeda (1937). In pachytene, single threads are doubled and chiasmata are visible between some conjugating partners, whereas other chromosomes probably just overlapped each other at entire length of the arms. When the bivalents were formed by chromosomes of different length, they sometimes separated in association long plus long chromatid, as well as long plus short chromatid. Emsweller and Jones (1935b) observed extension of long arm of conjugated chromosomes well beyond the end of the other. That condition depends on the arrangement of chiasmata at the ends of a bivalent (Emsweller & H.A. Jones, 1935a). In diakinesis, chromosomes were usually well-separated and their configuration could be easily determined. In *A. cepa,* chiasmata are predominantly terminal, in *A. fistulosum* chiasmata are localized near the centromere region (Fig. 1). The hybrids have chiasmata localized randomly (Emsweller & H.A. Jones, 1945; Maeda, 1937). Hybrids had high frequency of complete bivalent pairing, but unpaired chromosomes were also observed (Emsweller & H.A. Jones, 1935a, 1938). In anaphase I, when the separations of chromosomes occur, occasional chromosome bridges were present (Emsweller & H.A. Jones, 1938).

Emsweller and Jones (1935a, 1935b, 1938) as well as Peffley (1986) and Maeda (1937) reported regular bivalentization (Fig. 2) in about 70% of tested cells, whereas Levan (1941) reported regular bivalent formation in only 2% of the tested PMC in his *A. cepa* x A. *fistulosum* hybrids. Early stages of meiosis in that plant material showed a number of unpaired threads, the maximal pairing was found before diplotene. Few pachytene chromosomes had threads longer than their pairing partner, what in consequence lead to occurrence of loop shape formations. Loops were localized on one side of the pairing complex, but in some cases the longer thread folded and paired with itself. Ring (Fig. 2.) and chromosome configurations with three chiasmata were also found (Levan, 1935). Inter-chromosomal differences, resulting in pairing of more than two chromosomes were observed. Levan (1941) observed frequent trivalents (14%), forming rings in metaphase. Seldom quadrivalents, pentavalents, hexavalents, were reported (Emsweller & H.A. Jones, 1935b, 1938; Levan, 1936; Peffley, 1986). However, Maeda (1937) reported absence of associations higher than bivalents in his hybrids. Abnormalities observed by Peffley (1986) in anaphase I included bridge formation in 28% and lagging chromosomes in 10% of the cells. Deficiencies, translocations, and inversions were reported (Emsweller & H.A. Jones, 1938; Levan, 1935, 1941; Peffley, 1986). Presence of heteromorphic pairing in $F_1$ interspecific hybrids was observed (Emsewller & H.A. Jones, 1935b; Maeda, 1937). Peffley (1986) suggested that heteromprphic bivalents were the consequence of pairing between chromosomes with translocation or inversion at the centromeric region.

The above-described discrepancies in meiotic events in F1 *A. cepa x A. fistulosum* hybrids may be explained by a different origin of *A. cepa* and *A. fistulosum* used in the discussed studies. Maeda and Emsweller and Jones used the same variety of *A. cepa* (Yellow Danvers) and *A. fistulosum* in Japanese form (Nebuka, Hidanegi), whereas Levan mentioned the use of a commercial onion variety 'Braunschweiger' and as a source of *fistulosum* points one of the European botanical gardens. Peffley (1986) used onion cv. 'Yellow Grano' and ten different accessions of *A. fistulosum* supplied by International Plant Breeders. Thus, it can be concluded that the cytological behavior during meiosis in F1 interspecific hybrids seems to be accession-specific. Moreover, chromosomal variants (multivalents) and changes in the chromosome structure (bridges) offer an explanation of the low pollen fertility of the $F_1$ hybrids (H.A. Jones & Mann, 1963; Levan, 1941; Peffley, 1986).

Using GISH (Genomic *In Situ* Hybridization) Stevenson et al. (1998) detected reciprocal crossover events in $F_1$ interspecific hybrids. The frequencies of crossovers detected as label exchanges in anaphase I chromosomes were about 20% higher than metaphase I chiasma frequencies. Since the synaptonemal complex (SC) is responsible for transmission of the interference, discontinuities in SC may cause that crossover occur in much closer proximity than they normally would with uninterrupted SCs (Sybenga, 1996). Albini and Jones (1990) reported incomplete synapsis in the centromeric region and other irregularities in the SC in the *A. cepa* x *A. fistulosum* hybrids. The failure of synapsis might explain differences in chiasmata frequencies reported by Stevenson et al. (1998). Additionally, Albini and Jones (1990) suggested, that DNA differences between *A. cepa* and *A. fistulosum* chromosomes were localized in the centromeric region, which prevented regular synapsis or progression of synapsis and possible proximal chiasma formation.

The $F_1$ hybrids between *A. cepa* and *A. fistulosum* can be easily produced, but have low pollen fertility, often not exceeding 10% (H.A. Jones & Mann, 1963; Levan, 1941; Maeda, 1937; Peffley, 1986; van der Valk et al., 1991b). Additionally Emsweller and Jones (1938) reported occurrence of egg sterility of the $F_1$ hybrids. Successful production of $F_2$ progenies was reported by Levan (1941). The $F_2$ plants were exclusively polyploids (tri- and tetraploids). Analysis of meiosis showed frequent disturbances, such as chromatin bridges and micronuclei in dyads and tetrads. Random distribution of chiasmata was dominant.

Cytological analysis of tetraploid forms revealed that they were amphidiploids built up from 2 *cepa* and 2 *fistulosum* genomes. Morphology of the tetraploids was intermediate between the parents, while their pollen fertility varied. One tetraploid was sterile, the other had moderate (50%) pollen fertility. In the triploid form, the frequency of trivalents was high (80-90%). In about 33% of tested cells micronuclei and chromosomal bridges were observed. Pollen fertility was low; not exceeding 10% (Levan, 1936, 1941).

Levan's (1941) attempts to backcross (BC) $F_1$ hybrid *A. cepa* x *A. fistulosum* to *cepa* were unsuccessful. The studies of van der Valk et al. (1991a) showed that difficulties in this type of cross were due to pre-fertilization barrier, as the growth of onion pollen tubes in the style of the hybrid was disturbed. Maeda (1937) backcrossed $F_1$ to *A. fistulosum* and obtained viable seeds. Emsweller and Jones (1945) obtained several BC progenies, but only when the hybrid was used as the pollen source.

In $BC_1$, the most common meiotic configuration were eight bivalents and eight univalents. Both randomized and localized chiasmata were observed (Emsweller & H.A. Jones, 1935b). Multivalents (quadrivalents, pentavalents) were observed in about 40% of the meiocytes. A ring univalent, lagging chromosomes, and chromosomal bridges were also observed (Peffley & Mangum, 1990). Analysis of the structural differences of chromosomes revealed presence of at least three paracentric inversions and one translocation, producing changes in gene order (Ulloa et al., 1994). Emsweller and Jones (1945), using $F_1$ as a pollen source, backcrossed them to both *A. cepa* and *A. fistulosum*. On average 44% of PMC in population backcrossed to *A. cepa* showed regular chromosome pairing, additionally those plants segregated with regard to male fertility; some individuals after self-pollination yielded in few seeds, and some were complete sterile. The first backcross to *A. fistulosum* possessed both randomized and localized chiasmata, however the second backcross had a high frequency of localized chiasmata (Fig. 1). This increase of localized chiasmata in subsequent backcrosses was correlated with pollen fertility.

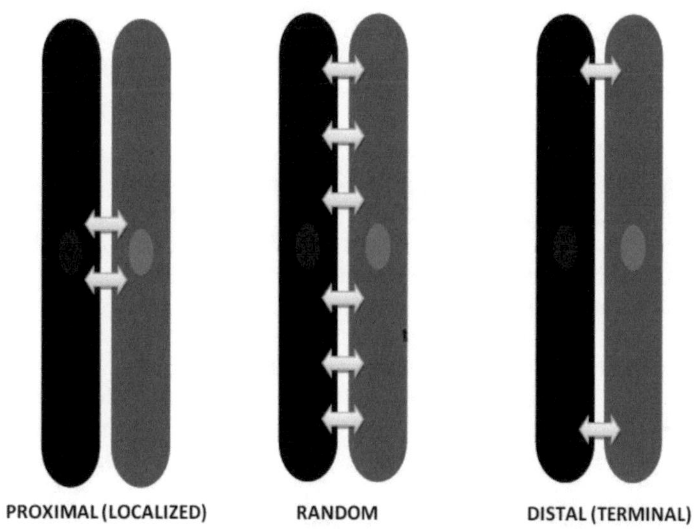


Fig. 1. Diagram showing the types of chiasmata distribution in the interspecific F1 hybrids within edible alliums.
Arrows indicating possible position of chiasmata between two homologous chromosomes in bivalent.

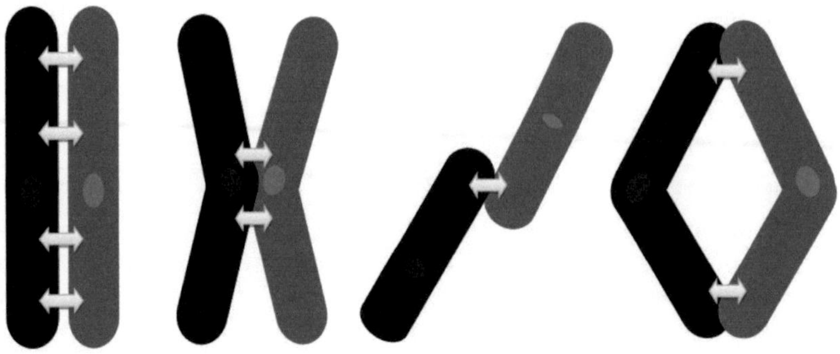


Fig. 2. Diagram showing configurations of bivalents observed in metaphase I of interspecific F1 hybrids within edible alliums.
Arrows indicating position of chiasmata between two homologous chromosomes in bivalent.

The fertile $BC_2$ plants had localized chiasmata and their morphology was similar to *A. fistulosum*, while sterile plants had mostly randomized chiasmata and morphologically were in the *A. cepa* type. Hou and Peffley (2000) examined 16 $BC_3$ plants and observed very high pollen fertility (90-92%) of the plants with eight bivalents at metaphase I. Those plants had low percentage of chromosomal aberrations such as bridges, laggards, or micronuclei. One male sterile plant had recombinant chromosomes. Thirteen among sixteen chromosomes in PMCs of the sterile plant gave strong hybridization signals at telomeres when *A. fistulosum* was used as a genomic DNA. Similar GISH patterns were reported by Khrustaleva and Kik (1998), suggesting differences in heterochromatin distribution at the telomeres between two parental species.

Khrustaleva and Kik (1998) introgressed genes from *A. fistulosum* to *A. cepa* using *A. roylei* as a bridge in crossing. Multi-colour GISH was performed to analyze genome organization of the hybrid. Results showed 8 *cepa* chromosomes, 1 metacentric chromosome from *roylei*, and 7 recombinant chromosomes. Recombination between *A. roylei* and *A. fistulosum* took place in distal and interdistal regions of hybrid chromosomes, centromeric regions originated from *roylei*. Meiosis in PMC of the first generation bridge-cross hybrid [*A. cepa* x (*A. fistulosum* x *A. roylei*)] was rather regular, about 53% of tested cells possessed 8 ring bivalents (Fig. 2), however occasional presence of univalents was noted. No multivalents were observed. Some of the bivalents were heteromorphic, indicating homologous pairing and chiasmata formation during prophase I. Pollen viability of the hybrid was about 50-60%. Detailed analysis of meiosis in the second generation hybrid (*A. cepa* x first generation bridge cross) showed that recombination between three genomes was frequent and that chiasmata were randomly distributed (Fig. 1) (Khrustaleva & Kik, 2000). Keeping in mind that chiasmata are located adjacent to the centromere in *A. fistulosum* and randomly distributed in *A. cepa* and *A. roylei* (Emsweller and H.A. Jones, 1935b; Levan, 1933, de Vries et al., 1992) in the bridge-cross hybrid random chiasmata prevailed over the *fistulosum* type. Translocations of *roylei-fistulosum* segment and deficiencies (absence of *roylei* segment) were also reported (Khrustaleva & Kik, 2000). Pollen fertility of the second generation bridge-cross hybrid was variable, what might be caused by the use of CMS onions as the female parent and/or the lack of *roylei* chromosome segments containing male sexual reproduction genes (Khrustaleva & Kik, 2000; Ulloa et al., 1995).

Monosomic addition lines of *fistulosum* – *cepa* (Shigyo et al., 1998) and *cepa* – *fistulosum* (Hang et al., 2004; Peffley et al., 1985) were reported. These lines are valuable to study genome organization in *A. cepa* and *A. fistulosum*.

### 2.3 Hybrids with introgression from *A. ampeloprasum* spp. *porrum*

Leek is a tetraploid species (2n=4x=32). Nuclear DNA content is 52,7 pg per 2C (Bennett & Leitch, 2010). Leek belongs to the genus *Allium,* subgenus *Allium,* section *Allium* (Hirschegger et al., 2010).

Meiosis in the leek was first described by Levan in 1940, showing almost complete localization of chiasmata at prophase I. Khazanehdhari et al. (1995) reported frequent formation of quadrivalents at this stage. Further studies showed that those quadrivalents were resolved in to bivalents in metaphase I (G.H. Jones et al., 1996); however, occasional persistence of quadrivalents in this stage was also observed (Koul & Gohil, 1970; Levan, 1940). Formation of bivalents in metaphase I was due to proximal localization of chiasmata in leek (Stack & Roelofs, 1996). Usually, four chromosomes in tetrasome are clustered by chiasmata located immediately adjacent to and on either side of the median or sumbedian centromere. As pairing partner switches are unlikely to occur between two proximal chiasmata, thus quadrivalent fall apart into two bivalents having a characteristic cross-shape (Fig 2.) (G.H. Jones et al., 1996; Khazanehdhari et al., 1995). Occurrence of univalents in the PMC of the leek was also reported (G.H. Jones et al., 1996; Khazanehdhari & G.H. Jones, 1997).

Interspecific hybrids between *Allium cepa* and *A. ampeloprasum* were generated with the aim of introduction of the S-cytoplasm from onion into leek. Few attempts of sexual hybridization of onion and leek failed, suggesting that this strategy to create F1 progeny may be difficult (Doležel et al., 1980; Currah, 1986). Peterka et al. (1997) used *in vitro* culture to rescue the $F_1$ embryos at the early stages of development (7-14 days after pollination); as a result they obtained seven hybrid plants, which were triploids with 24 chromosomes. Authors reported presence of three chromosomes with satellites and two with intercalary pseudosatellites. Onion carries two chromosomes with satellites (Kalkmam, 1984; Taylor, 1925), leek has four, and additionally leek has four chromosomes with intercalary pseudosatellites (Murin, 1964). GISH with onion DNA as a probe, showed hybridization of eight chromosomes of the hybrid plant, the remaining 16 did not hybridized, which enabled identification of onion and leek chromosomes. Further studies of meiosis in the interspecific hybrids showed presence of eight leek bivalents and eight onion univalents in the prophase I (Peterka et al., 2002). The leek bivalents in the hybrids had localized chiasmata (Fig. 1). During late metaphase and early anaphase, in some of the observed cell the onion univalents were arrested at the periphery of the nucleus, while the leek chromatids moved to the poles. The onion chromatids, due to their retarded movement, were frequently excluded from the daughter nuclei in the form of micronuclei observable in the dyad or tetrad stage (Schrader et al., 2000).

Peterka et al. (2002) investigated chromosome composition of the backcross progenies. Their $BC_1$ plants always possessed eight onion chromosomes and from 30 to 33 leek chromosomes. Only in one tested hybrid a recombinant chromosome was identified. In the $BC_2$ and $BC_3$ decreased transmission rate of univalent onion chromosomes were observed, resulting in the production of alloplasmic leek plants in the third backcross.

Buiteveld et al. (1998a, 1998b) reported the symmetric fusion of protoplasts isolated from suspension cultures of *A. ampeloprasum* and leaf mesophyll protoplasts of onion, resulting in somatic hybridization of onion and leek. Analysis of chromosome composition of somatic hybrids was performed using GISH. All obtained hybrids were identified as hexaploids. In eight tested hybrids, chromosome number varied from 41 to 45. Authors found differences among hybrids with regard to the number of parental chromosomes. Some hybrids carried eight onion and less than 32 leek chromosomes, other possessed 12 onion and 30 leek chromosomes. Flow cytometry measurements showed that the suspension culture used for the fusion was of a mixture of aneuploid (hypotetraploid) and normal tetraploid cells of leek. Since aneuploid leek protoplasts were used for the fusion, it is possible that the hybrids resulted from fusions with leek protoplasts with different chromosome numbers, which might explain the differences in the number of leek chromosomes in the hybrids. Loss of the onion chromosomes may be a consequence of spontaneous chromosome elimination after the fusion. Moreover, recombinant chromosomes in cells of leek and onion somatic hybrids were also reported. Two of those chromosomes were of a reciprocal translocation type and one was an interstitial translocation type (Buiteveld, 1998a).

### 2.4 Hybrids with introgression from *A. sativum*

*A. sativum L.* is a diploid with (2n=2x=16) with nuclear DNA content 32,5 pg per 2C (Bennett & Leitch, 2010). The DNA content of garlic is the most similar to onion among the discussed species. Garlic belongs to the genus *Allium*, subgenus *Allium*, section *Allium* (Hirschegger et al., 2006; Keller et al., 1996).

The majority of garlic cultivars are sterile, which preclude to use them as a partner in sexual crossing, however occurrence of fertile garlic plants was also reported (Hong et al., 1997; Kik, 2002). Flowering in some garlic clones is often associated with presence of bulbils formed in the place of aborted flowers. Bulbils are used as a source material for vegetative reproduction (R.N. Jones, 1990; Kik, 2002).

To study meiosis in the garlic, Konvička and Levan (1972) used two fertile clones named OH and LH. The clone OH formed medium size bulbils and normal flowers in the inflorescence. The clone LH had an abundance of flowers together with many small bulbils, moreover this clone formed original chromosome ring at meiosis (amphibivalent) (Levan, 1936). Majority of tested meiocytes in the clone OH formed eight bivalents at meiosis I; however presence of spherical chromatic bodies outside the spindle was observed. Produced pollen grains differ in size. The first meiotic division in the clone LH proceeded regularly, but two out of four bivalents formed an ring consisting of four chromosomes. This structure could be observed from diplotene through diakinesis and metaphase I. In metaphase I authors observed ring configurations in the majority of the cells; only in one of them an open ring was present. The formation of rings caused occurrence of lagging chromosomes observable during the first anaphase. The second division was usually normal, but in few cells chromatin body outside the spindle was present. Two satellite chromosome pairs were noted in cells of both tested clones. The clones had their own characteristic pattern of meiotic abnormalities, what is in contrary to results presented by Koul and Gohil (1970) where in three tested fertile clones meiosis was completely regular. Differences in chromosome length, positions of NOR or arm ratios were variable among garlic clones (R.N. Jones, 1990). Such differences may partially develop after the loss of sexual propagation and changes occurring in the somatic cells of vegetatively propagated garlic.

*Allium cepa* and *A. sativum* for a long time have not been hybridized sexually because of the narrow pool of fertile garlics and a large genetic distance (Kik, 2002; Keller et al., 1996). The first interspecific hybrids between onion and garlic were reported by Ohsumi et al. in 1993. Authors performed reciprocal crosses of onion and garlic, but embryos were formed only when onion was the female parent. Embryos were rescued in tissue culture. Regenerated hybrids possessed 16 chromosomes in somatic cells, with clearly distinguishable two satellite chromosomes. Since onion cv. 'Sapporoki' used in the study did not possess satellite chromosomes, those chromosomes were inherited from *A. sativum*. Chromosome elimination was not observed in the study. The pollen viability of the obtained hybrid vas very low (2%).

Worth mention is work of Yanagino et al. (2003) with aim of increasing fertility in garlic through sexual hybridization with leek. Success of this cross was accelerated, since both leek and garlic belong to the subgenus *Allium*. Leek was used as the female partner. Interspecific hybrids were obtained with the use of the embryo-rescue technique. Hybrids were triploids and possessed 24 chromosomes (16 from onion and 8 from garlic), however meiosis in PMC was not examined. Obtained hybrids were almost completely sterile.

Somatic hybrids of onion and sterile garlic were reported by Yamashita et al. (2002). Onion and garlic have sixteen chromosomes, however obtained hybrids were classified as aneuploids with total number of chromosomes 40 or 41. In the tested somatic cells of the hybrids authors noted presence of two subtelocentric chromosomes and three intercalary satellite chromosomes, inherited from both parents. GISH analysis revealed 17 garlic and 20 or 21 onion chromosomes and three chromosomes consisting of chromosomal regions from both parents. Presence of chimeric chromosomes in the somatic hybrids originated from translocation between chromosomes or chromosome fusions.

## 3. Conclusions and future directions

Pre- fertilization barriers in distant crosses, such as failure in pollen germination, slow pollen tube growth, or foreign pollen tube arrest in the style have been reported in different species (Kiełkowska & Adamus, 2006; Manickam & Sarkar, 1999b) including alliums (Gonzalez & Ford-Lloyd, 1987; Ohsumi et al., 1993; van der Valk et al., 1991a). Post-fertilization barriers are related to abnormalities in the development of the zygote, absence or abnormal development of the endosperm which causes embryo starvation and abortion (Zenkteller, 1990). Within the discussed species, the embryos developed regularly in the hybrids with introgression from *A. fistulosum*, or had to be rescued on the early stages of the development in hybrids with the leek and garlic introgression. Cytological studies showed reproductive abnormalities in F1 hybrids and their progenies. Irregularities of chromosome pairing and occurrence of a range of structural changes in meiotic chromosomes resulted in unbalanced chromosome complements in the gametes, often causing lowered fertility or even sterility of the $F_1$ hybrids (Khush & Brar, 1992; Peffley, 1986; van der Valk et al., 1991a).

A. *fistulosum* carries resistance genes for fungal, bacterial, and viral diseases (Rabinowitch, 1997). Moreover *fistulosum* has several agronomically important traits such as high dry-matter content, winter-hardiness, high pungency and earlier flowering as compared to onion (van der Meer & van Bennekom, 1978). Hence, hybrids between onion and *A. fistulosum* as well as several backcross progenies were deeply studied, with *A. cepa* as either the female parent (Emsweller & H.A. Jones, 1935a, 1935b; Levan, 1941; Van der Meer and Van Benekom, 1978) or pollen parent (Peffley, 1986; Peters et al., 1984; van der Valk et al. 1991a). Cytological studies have shown that chromosome pairing is highly variable in the $F_1$ hybrid depending on the parental combination (Emsweller & H.A. Jones, 1935a, 1953b; Peffley, 1986; Ulloa et al., 1994). Presence of heteromorphic pairing was reported in each of the discussed studies, showing evidence for recombination of genetic material between homologous chromosomes in the F1 hybrid between *A. cepa* and *A. fistulosum* (Emsweller & H.A. Jones, 1935a, 1935b; Peffley & Mangum, 1990; van der Meer & Van Benekom, 1978), and when the hybrid was backcrossed to *A. cepa* (Hou & Peffley, 2000). Khrustaleva and Kik (1998, 2000) showed that gene exchange is possible even in the three-way (*cepa* x (*fistulosum* x *roylei*)) hybrid, resulting in partially fertile progenies. Nucleo-cytoplasmic incompatibility interactions reported between these two species may also reduce fertility of $F_1$ hybrids (Ulloa et al., 1994).

Although pollen sterility of hybrids is a major barrier to gene introgression, occurrence of fertile F1 hybrids able to produce further progenies and introduce them into the breeding process, was also reported. Jones and Clarke (1942) reported obtaining of amphidiploid arose by spontaneous doubling from unreduced gamete of $F_1$ *A. cepa x A. fistulosum* hybrid. At metaphase I of the hybrid, there were 16 bivalents with localized and non-localized chiasmata and meiosis was regular. The obtained plant was fertile, vigorous, and resistant to several diseases. This amphidiploid is known as 'Beltsville Bunching' and was released in the United States in 1950, and sold on the market as green bunching onion (H.A. Jones & Mann, 1963). Many years of research resulted in the release of the several other hybrids grown as vegetatively propagated onions in *fistulosum* type or sexually reproduced bulb onions resistant to pink root (*Phoma terrestris*) (for review see Kik, 2002).

In the leek, the main problem concerning sexual hybridization lies in the high (98%) occurrence of chiasmata localized near the centromere (Levan, 1940). Such localized chiasmata prevent formation of multivalents during meiosis (metaphase I) and prevents recombination on the distal ends of chromosomes (Khazanehdari & G.H. Jones 1997). The localization of chiasmata in this near-centromeric section prevents association of more than two chromosomes during leek meiosis, which may be beneficial for its capacity to form fertile gametes. However, if the pairing behavior in metaphase I is different between sexually hybridized components that may lead to infertility of the hybrids (Brewster, 1994). Peterka et al. (2002) reported complete sterility of onion x leek hybrids.

Morphology and hybrid status of progenies from a cross between *A. cepa* x *A. sativum* were reported (Ohsumi et al., 1993), however, meiotic chromosomes behavior in the hybrids as well as their pollen fertility have not been deeply investigated. Broadening genetic diversity in garlic is very desired. It can be achieved with the use of protoplast cultures, which offers a large spectrum of possibilities with regard to selection of components for the fusion. Sexual hybridization is rather difficult in garlic, due to high seed sterility of the clones. However, utilization of wild relatives and search for novel fertile accessions like the one found in South America (Hirschegger et al., 2006) is very important for increasing available germplasm pool.

During the years of studies researchers attempted to develop techniques helping to overcome barriers between incompatible species for successful production of hybrid seeds.

Worthy mentioning is bridge crossing (Dionne, 1963; McCoy & Echt 1993), use of exogenous plant growth regulators, i.e. gibberelic acid, dichloro-acetic acid (Brock, 1954; Manickam & Sarkar, 1999a), mixed pollen technique (Asano & Myodo, 1977), use of the 'mentor' pollen (Sastri & Shivanna, 1976; Settler, 1968), *in vitro* fertilization (De Verna et al., 1987; Zenkteller et al., 2005), embryo rescue (Sukno et al., 1999; Williams et al., 1982), and somatic cell hybridization (Kirti et al., 1991; Smith, 1976).

Embryo rescue promotes the development of an immature or weak embryo into a viable plant. The most commonly used procedure is careful excision of hybrid embryos and placing directly onto the culture medium. Sometimes when there are difficulties with embryo excision or embryos are very small, whole ovules (ovule culture, *in ovolo*) or ovaries are put to the culture (Bridgen, 1994). Embryo rescue has been widely used for producing hybrid plants in onions. *Alliums* hybrid embryos were usually cultured on a phytohormone-free medium (Amagai et al., 1995; Gonzalez & Ford-Lloyd, 1987; Nomura & Makara, 1993; Umehara et al., 2006). Whole ovary culture supported maturation of viable seeds in hybrids of *A. cepa* x A. *sphaerocephalon* (Bino et al., 1989) or *A. fistulosum* x *A. schoenoprasum* (Umehara et al., 2007). Keller et al. (1996) adopted ovary culture and obtained many hybrids between onion and other distant species. This technique was used in the crosses between onion and *A. fistulosum* (Doležel et al., 1980; van der Valk, 1991a), onion and leek (Peterka et al., 1997), onion and garlic (Ohsumi et al., 1993), rakkyo (*A. chinense*) and *A. fistulosum* L. (Nomura et al., 1994; Nomura & Makara, 1993), Welsh onion and chives (*A. schoenoprasum*) (Umehara et al., 2006) and many others (Gonzalez & Ford-Lloyd, 1987; Nomura et al., 2002; Nomura & Oosawa, 1990; Yanagino et al., 2003). Application of protoplast cultures for obtaining interspecific crosses in edible alliums (Buiteveld et al., 1998a, 1998b; Shimonaka et al., 2002; Yamashita et al., 2002) was also reported. Genomic *in situ* hybridization enabled the identification of genomes in the interspecific and intergeneric hybrids together with direct detection of genetic recombination (Friesen et al., 1997; Schwarzacher et al., 1989; Thomas et al., 1994). It seems that studies on the interspecific crosses in alliums employed a wide range of different biotechnological and cytogenetical tools to facilitate obtainment and characterization of hybrid, however one issue still remains unsolved and problematic. Many authors pointed low pollen fertility of generated hybrids what in consequence significantly decreased the number of obtained seeds and narrowed the pool of accessions for cytogenetic studies (H.A. Jones & Mann, 1963; Peffley, 1986; van der Valk et al., 1991a, 1991b). Most of the hybrids from crosses of *A. cepa* with *A. fistulosum* (Doležel et al., 1980; Emsweller & H.A. Jones 1935a, 1935b; Maeda, 1937), leek (Doležel et al, 1980), garlic (Ohsumi et al., 1993), as well as with *A. galanthum* (Kiełkowska & Adamus, 2010), *A. oschaninii* or *A. pskemense* (McCollum, 1971) were reported as sterile.

Possibly, restoration of fertility of interspecific hybrids can be achieved by chromosome doubling (R.N. Jones, 1983). Chromosomes are doubled by treating the plant tissue with antimitotic agents such as colchicine (Blakslee, 1939; Blakslee & Avery, 1937). McCollum (1980) reported fertile amphidiploid of *A. cepa* x *A. galanthum* obtained by colchicine treatment. Autotetraploids in *A. cepa* and *A. fistulosum* were obtained by soaking germinating seeds in aqueous colchicine solution, but the recovery of tetraploids was low (2%) (Toole & Clarke, 1994). Song et al. (1997) treated calli form $F_1$ hybrids of *A. fistulosum* x *A. cepa* with 0.1 and 0.2% colchicine and regenerated tetraploids. It seems that the potential is promising and the recovery of fertile plants from colchicine-treated $F_1$ hybrids has been reported in other species (Eigsti & Dustin 1955; Orton & Steidl, 1980). The optimum concentration and duration of treatment has to be determined empirically as it strongly affects the success in doubling and the survival of the treated plant material (Eikenberry, 1994; Hansen & Andersen 1996; Klima et al., 2008; Wan et al., 1989). In the literature concerning doubled haploids, authors mention use of trifluraline, oryzaline or amiprophos methyl (Hansen and Andersen, 1996; Zhao & Simmonds, 1995) which are considered less toxic and may be beneficial for fertility restoration in onion interspecific hybrids.

The state of knowledge about meiosis in $F_1$ hybrids and further generations from crossings of onions with *A. fistulosum* was deeply investigated, however meiotic studies of hybrids between onion and garlic and leek is limited. The change of the status is needed, because the understanding of meiotic process in crucial for further research on the reproduction, fertility, genetics and breeding of discussed species.

## 4. References

Albini , S.M. & Jones G.H. (1990) Synaptotemal complex spreading in *Allium cepa* and *Allium fistulosum*. III. The Hybrid. *Genome,* Vol. 33, pp. 854-866

Amagai, M.; Ohashi K. & Kimura S. (1995). Breeding of interspecies hybrid between *Allium fistulosum* and *A. tuberosum* by embryo culture. *Bull Tochigi Agr Exp Stn,* Vol. 43, pp. 87–94

Asano, Y. & Myodo H. (1977). Studies on crosses between distantly related species of lilies for the intrastyllar pollination technique. *J Jpn Soc of Hort Sci,* Vol. 46, pp. 59-65

Bennett, M.D. & Leitch, I.J. (2010). Plant DNA C-values Database (release 5.0, December 2010) http://data.kew.org/cvalues/

Bino, R.J.; Janssen M.G.; Franken, J. & de Vries, J.N. (1989). Enhanced seed development in the interspecific cross *Allium cepa* x *A. sphaerocephalon* through ovary culture. *Plant Cell Tiss and Org Cult,* Vol. 16, pp. 135-142

Blakeslee, A. & Avery A. (1937). Methods of inducing doubling of chromosomes in plants by treatment with colchicine. *J Hered,* Vol. 28, pp. 393–411

Blakeslee, A. (1939). The present and potential service of chemistry to plant breeding. *Am J Bot,* Vol. 26, pp. 163–172

Bougoud, S.M. & Plowman A.B. (1996). The inheritance of B chromosomes in *Allium schoenoprasum* L. *Chromosome Res,* Vol. 4, pp. 151-158

Bougourd, S.M. & Parker J.S. (1979). The B-chromosome system of *Allium schoenoprasum. Chromosoma,* Vol. 75, pp. 369-383

Brewster, J.L. (1994). The genetics and Plant breeding of *Allium* crops. In: *Onions and other vegetable alliums.* Brewster J.L., pp. 41-61, CAB International, ISBN 0581995101,UK

Bridgen, M.P. (1994). A review of plant embryo culture. *HortScience,* Vol. 29, pp. 1243–1246

Brock, R.D. (1954). Hormone induced pear-apple hybrids. *Heredity,* Vol. 8, pp. 421-429

Buiteveld, J.; Kassies W.; Geels R.; van Lookeren Campagne M.M., Jacobsen E. & Creemers-Molenaar J. (1998b). Biased chloroplast and mitochondrial transmission in somatic hybrids of *Allium ampeloprasum* L. and *Allium cepa* L. *Plant Sci,* Vol. 131, pp. 219-228

Buiteveld, J.; Suo Y.; van Lookeren Campagne M.M. & Creemers-Molenaar J. (1998a). Production and characterization of somatic hybrid plants between leek (*Allium ampeloprasum* L.) and onion (*Allium cepa* L.). *Theor Appl Genet,* Vol. 96, pp. 765-775

Currah, L. (1986). Leek breeding: a review. *J Hortic Sci,* Vol. 61, pp. 407-415

De Verna, J.W.; Myers J.R. & Collins G.B. (1987). Bypassing prefertilization barriers to hybridization in *Nicotiana* using *in vitro* pollination and fertilization. *Theor Appl Genet,* Vol. 73, pp. 665-671

de Vries, J.N.; Wietsma W.A.; & Appels M. (1992). Direct and *Allium roylei* mediated transfer of *A. fistulosum* genes to onion. *Allium Improvement Newsletter,* Vol. 2, pp. 9-10

Dionne, L.A. (1963). Studies on the use of *Solanum acaule* as a bridge between *Solanum tuberosum* and species in the *Bulbocastana, Cardiophylla* and Pinnatisecta. *Euphytica,* Vol. 12, pp. 263-269

Doležel, J.; Nowak F.J. & Lužny J. (1980). Embryo development and *in vitro* culture of *Allium cepa* and its interspecific hybrids. *Z. Pflanzenzüchtg,* Vol. 85, pp. 177-184

Eigsti, D.I. & Dustin P. Jr (1955). Spindle and cytoplasm. In: *Colchicine in agriculture, medicine, biology and chemistry,* pp. 65-139, The Iowa State University College Press, ISBN 9780598806932, Ames

Eikenberry, E. (1994). Chromosome doubling of microspore- derived canola using trifluralin. *Cruciferae Newsletter,* Vol. 16, pp. 51–52

Emsweller, S.L. & Jones H.A. (1935a). An interspecific hybrid in *Allium. Hilgardia* Vol. 9, pp. 265-273

Emsweller, S.L. & Jones H.A. (1935b). Meiosis in *A. fistulosum, A. cepa* and their F1 hybrid. *Hilgardia* Vol. 9, pp. 277-294

Emsweller, S.L. & Jones H.A. (1938). Crossing-over, fragmentation, and formation of new chromosomes in an *Allium* species hybrid. *Botanical Gazette,* Vol. 99, pp. 729-772

Emsweller, S.L. & Jones H.A. (1945). Further studies on the chiasmata of the *Allium cepa* x *A. fistulosum* hybrid and its derivatives. *American Journal of Botany,* Vol. 32, pp. 370-379

Etoh, T. & Simon P.W. (2002). Diversity, fertility and seed production of garlic. In: *Allium Crop Science: recent advances,* Rabinowitch H.D. & Currah L., pp. 101-117, CABI Publishing, ISBN 0851995101, UK

Friesen, N.; Fritsch R. & Bachman K. (1997). Hybrid origin of some ornamentals of Allium subgenus *Melanocrommyum* verified with GISH and RAPD. *Theor Appl Genet,* Vol. 95, pp. 1229-1238

Fritsch, R.M. & Friesen N. (2002). Evolution, domestication and taxonomy. In: *Allium Crop Science: recent advances.* Rabinowitch H.D. & Currah L., pp. 5-30, CABI Publishing, ISBN 0851995101, UK

Fuchs, J.; Brandes A. & Schubert I. (1995). Telomere sequences localization and karyotype evolution in higher plants. *Plant systematic and Evolution,* Vol. 196, pp. 227-241

Gonzalez, L.G. & Ford-Lloyd B.V. (1987). Facilitation of wide crossing through embryo rescue and pollen storage in interspecific hybridization of cultured *Allium* species. *Plant Breed,* Vol. 98, pp. 318–322

Hang, T.T.M.; Shigyo M.; Yamaguchi N. & Tashiro Y. (2004). Production and characterization of alien chromosome addition in shallot (*Allium cepa* L. Aggregatum group) carrying extra chromosome(s) of Japanese bunching onion (*A. fistulosum* L.). *Genes Genet Syst,* Vol. 79, pp. 263-269

Hansen, N.J.P. & Andersen S.B. (1996). *In vitro* chromosome doubling potential of colchicine, oryzalin, trifluralin, and APM in *Brassica napus* microspore culture. *Euphytica,* Vol. 88, pp. 156–164

Havey, M.J. (2002). Genome organization in *Allium.* In: *Allium Crop Science: recent advances.* Rabinowitch H.D. & Currah L., pp. 59-79, CABI Publishing, ISBN 0851995101, UK

Hirschegger, P.; Galmarini C. & Bohanec B. (2006). Characterization of novel form of fertile great headed garlic (*Allium* sp.). *Plant Breed,* Vol. 125, pp. 635-637

Hirschegger, P.; Jakše J.; Trontelj P. & Bohanec B. (2010). Origins of *Allium ampeloprasum* horticultural groups and a molecular phylogeny of the section *Allium* (*Allium: Alliaceae*). *Molecular Phylogenetics and Evolution,* Vol. 54, pp. 488-479

Hong, C.; Etoh T.; Landry B. & Matsuzoe N. (1997). RAPD markers related to pollen fertility in garlic (*Allium sativum* L.) *Breeding science,* Vol. 74, pp. 359-362

Hou, A. & Peffley E.B. (2000). Recombinant chromosomes of advanced backcross plants between *Allium cepa* L. and *A. fistulosum* L. revealed by *in situ* hybridization. *Theor Appl Genet,* Vol. 100, pp. 1190-1196

Jones, G.H.; Khazanehdhari K.A & Ford-Lloyd B.V. (1996). Meiosis in leek (*Allium porrum* L.) revisited. II. Metaphase I observations. *Heredity,* Vol. 76, pp. 186-191

Jones, H.A. & Clarke A.E. (1942). A natural amphidiploid from an onion species hybrid *Allium cepa* x *Allium fistulosum* L. *Heredity,* Vol. 33, pp. 25-32

Jones, H.A. & Mann L.K. (1963). Onions and Their Allies - Botany, Cultivation, and Utilization. Interscience Publishers Inc., ISBN 100249388731, New York3.

Jones, R.N. & Rees H. (1968) Nuclear DNA variation in *allium. Heredity,* Vol. 23, pp. 591-605

Jones, R.N. (1983). Cytogenetic evolution in the genus *Allium.* In: *Cytogenetic of crop plants.* Swaminathan M.S.; Gupta P.K. & Sinha V., pp. 516-554, Macmillan Press Ltd, ISBN 0333904230, India

Jones, R.N. (1990). Cytogenics. In: *Onions and Allied crops. Vol I. Botany, physiology and genetics,* Rabinowitch H.D. & Brewster J.L., pp. 199-214, CRC Press, ISBN 0849363004, Florida

Kalkman, E.R. (1984). Analysis of the C-banded karyotype of *Allium cepa* L. Standard system of nomenclature and polymorphism. *Genetica,* Vol. 65, pp. 141-148

Keller, R.J.; Schubert I.; Fuchs J. & Meister A. (1996). Interspecific crosses of onion with distant *Allium* species and characterization of the presumed hybrids by means of flow cytometry, karyotype analysis and genomic *in situ* hybridization. *Theor Appl Genet,* Vol. 92, pp. 417-424

Keusgen, M. (2002). Health and *Alliums.* In: *Allium Crop Science: recent advances.* Rabinowitch H.D. & Currah L., pp. 537-379, CABI Publishing, ISBN 0851995101, UK

Khazanedhari, K.A. & Jones G.H. (1997). The causes and consequences of meiotic irregularity in the leek (*Allium ampeloprasum* spp. *Porrum*); implications for fertility, quality and uniformity. *Euphytica,* Vol. 93, pp. 313-319

Khazanehdhari, K.A.; Jones G.H. & Ford-Lloyd B.V. (1995). Meiosis in the leek (*Allium porrum* L.) revisited. I. Prophase I pairing. *Chromosome Research,* Vol. 3, pp. 433-439

Khrustaleva L.I. & Kik C. (2000) Introgression of *Allium fistulosum* into *A. cepa* mediated by *A. roylei. Theor Appl Genet,* Vol. 100, pp. 17–26

Khrustaleva, L.I. & Kik C. (1998) Cytogenetical studies in the bridge cross *Allium cepa* x (*A. fistulosum x A. roylei*). *Theor Appl Genet,* Vol. 96, pp. 8–14

Khush, G.S. & Brar D.S. (1992). Overcoming the barriers in hybridization. In: *Distant hybridization of crop plants,* Monographs on Theoretical and Applied Genetics. Vol 16., Kaloo G. & Chowdhury J.B., pp. 47-61, Springer Verlag, ISBN 3540531734, Berlin

Kiełkowska, A. & Adamus A. (2006). Growth of pollen tubes from foreign species in carrot (*Daucus carota* L.) pistils. In: *Haploids and doubled haploids in genetics and plant breeding*. Adamski T. & Surma M., pp. 193-197, Prodruk, ISBN 8389887444, Poland

Kiełkowska, A. & Adamus A. (2010). Morphological, cytological and molecular evaluation of interspecific F1 (*A.galanthum* x *A.cepa)* hybrids. *Biotechnologia*, Vol. 2(89), pp. 146-155

Kik, C. (2002). Exploitation of wild relatives for the breeding of cultivated *Allium* species. In: Allium Crop Science: recent advances. Rabinowitch H.D. & Currah L., pp. 81-100, CABI Publishing, ISBN 0851995101, UK

Kirti, P.B., Prakash S. & Chopra V.L. (1991). Interspecific hybridization between *Brassica juncea* and *B. spinescens* through protoplast fusion. *Plant Cell Rep*, Vol. 9, pp. 639-642

Klima, M.; Vyvadilov□ M. & Kučera V. (2008). Chromosome doubling effects of selected antimitotic agents in *Brassica napus* microspore culture. *Czech J Genet Breed*, Vol. 44, pp. 30-36

Konvička, O. & Levan A. (1972). Chromosome studies in *Allium sativum*. Hereditas, Vol. 72, pp. 129-148

Koul, A.K. & Gohil R.N. (1970). Cytology of the tetraploid *Allium ampeloprasum* with chiasma localization. *Chromosoma*, Vol. 29, pp. 12-19

Labani, R. & Elkington T. (1987). Nuclear DNA variation in the genus *Allium* L. (*Liliaceae*). *Heredity*,Vol. 59, pp. 119-128

Levan, A. (1931). Cytological studies in Allium. A preliminary note. Hereditas, Vol.15, pp. 347-356

Levan, A. (1932). Cytological studies in *Allium* II. Chromosome morphological contribution. *Hereditas*, Vol. 16, pp. 57-299

Levan, A. (1933). Cytological studies in *allium* IV. *Allium fistulosum*. *Svensk Bot Tids*, Vol. 27, pp. 211-232

Levan, A. (1935). Cytological studies in *Allium* V. The chromosome morphology of some diploid species of *Allium*. *Hereditas*, Vol. 20, pp. 289-330

Levan, A. (1936) Die zytologie von *Allium cepa* x *fistulosum*. *Hereditas*, Vol. 21, pp. 195-214

Levan, A. (1940). Meiosis of *Allium porrum*, a tetraploid species with chiasma localization. *Hereditas*, Vol. 26, pp. 454-462

Levan, A. (1941). The cytology of the species hybrid *Allium cepa* x *fistulosum* and its polyploidy derivatives. *Hereditas*, Vol. 27, pp. 253-272

Maeda, T. (1937). Chiasma studies in *Allium fistulosum*, *Allium cepa* and their F1, F2 and backcross hybrids. *Jap J Genet*, Vol. 13, pp. 146-159

Manickam, S. & Sarkar K.R. (1999a). Foreign pollen tube growth in maize after chemical treatments. *Indian J Gen & Plant Breed*, Vol. 59(1), pp. 53-58

Manickam, S. & Sarkar K.R. (1999b). Maize, pearl millet and sorghum pollen tube growth rate in maize silk. *Ann Agricult Research*, Vol. 20(2), pp. 216-219

McCollum, G.D. (1971). Sterility of some interspecific *Allium* hybrids. *J Am Soc Hort Sci*, Vol. 96, pp. 359-362

McCollum, G.D. (1980). Development of the amphidiploids of *A. galanthum x A. cepa*, J *Heredity*, Vol. 71, pp. 445-447

McCoy, T.J. & Echt C.S. (1993). Potential of trispecies bridge crosses and random amplified DNA markers for introgression of *Medicago daghestanica* and *M. pironae* germplasm in to alfalfa (*M. sativa*). *Genome,* Vol. 36, pp. 594-601

Murin, A. (1964). Chromosome study in *Allium porrum* L. *Caryologia* Vol, 17, pp. 575-578

Nomura, Y. & Makara K. (1993). Production of interspecific hybrids between Rakkyo (*Allium chinense*) and some other *Allium* species by embryo rescue. *Jpn J Breed,* Vol. 43, pp. 13–21

Nomura, Y. & Oosawa K. (1990). Production of interspecific hybrids between *Allium chinense* and *Allium thunbergii* by in ovulo embryo culture. *Jpn J Breed,* Vol. 40, pp. 531-535

Nomura, Y.; Kazuma T.; Makara K. & Nagai T. (2002). Interspecific hybridization of autumn-flowering *Allium* species with ornamental *Alliums* and characteristics of the hybrid plants. *Sci Hort,* Vol. 95, pp. 223-237

Nomura, Y.; Maeda M.; Tsuchiya T. & Makara K. (1994). Efficient production of interspecific hybrids between *Allium chinense* and edible *Allium* spp. through ovary culture and pollen storage. *Breed Sci*, Vol. 44, pp. 151-155

Ohsumi, C.A.; Kojima K.; Hinata K.; Etoh T. & Hayashi T. (1993). Interspecific hybrid between *Allium cepa* and *Allium sativum*. *Theor Appl Genet,* Vol. 85, pp. 969-975

Orton, T.J. & Steidl P.J. (1980). Cytogenetic analysis of plants regenerated from colchicine-treated callus cultures of an interspecific *Hordeum* hybrid. *Theor Appl Genet*, Vol. 57, pp. 89-95

Peffley, E.B. & Mangum P.D. (1990) Introgression of *Allium fistulosum* L. into *Allium cepa* L: cytogenetic evidence. *Theor Appl Genet,* Vol. 79, pp. 113-118

Peffley, E.B. (1986). Evidence for chromosomal differentiation of *A. fistulosum* and *A. cepa*. *J Am Soc Hort Sci,* Vol. 111, pp. 126-129

Peffley, E.B.; Corgan J.N.; Horak H.G. & Tanksley S.D. (1985). Electrophoretic analysis of *Allium* alien addition lines. *Theor Appl Genet,* Vol. 71, pp. 176-184

Peterka, H.; Budahn H. & Schrader O. (1997). Interspecific hybrids between onion (Allium cepa L.) with S-cytoplasm and leek (*Allium ampeloprasum* L.). *Theor Appl Genet*, Vol. 94, pp. 383-389

Peterka, H.; Budahn H.; Schrader O. & Havey M.J. (2002). Transfer of male-sterility-inducing cytoplasm from onion to leek (*Allium ampeloprasum*). *Theor Appl Genet*, Vol. 105, pp. 173-181

Peters, R.J.; Netzer D. & Rabinowitch H.D. (1984). A progress report: pink root resistance in *Allium cepa* x *Allium fistulosum L* hybrids and progeny. In: *Proc. 3rd Allium Eucarpia Symp.*, Wageningen, pp. 70-73, The Netherlands

Pich, U.; Fritsch R. & Schubert I. (1996) Closely related *Allium* species (*Alliaceae*) share a very similar satellite sequence. *Plant Systematics and Evol,* Vol. 202, pp. 255-264

Rabinowitch, H.D. (1997) Breeding alliaceous crops for pest resistance. *Acta Hort,* Vol. 433, pp. 223-246

Sastri, D.C. & Schivanna K.R. (1976). Attempts to overcome interspecific incompatibility in *Sesanum* by using of recognition pollen. *Ann Bot,* Vol. 40, pp. 891-893

Schrader, O.; Budahn H.; Ahne R. & Peterka H. (2000). Cytogenetic and molecular analysis of somaclonal variants in *Allium cepa* x *A. ampeloprasum* hybrid. *Vortr Pflanzenzuecht*, Vol. 47, pp. 53, ISSN 0723-7812

Schwarzacher, T.; Leith A.R.; Benett M.D. & Heslop-Harrison J.S. (1989). *In situ* localization of parental genomes in a wide hybrid. *Ann Bot* Vol. 64, pp. 315-324

Settler, R.F. (1968). Irradiated mentor pollen: Its use in remote hybridization of the cottonwood. *Nature,* Vol. 219, pp. 746-747

Shigyo, M.; Imamura K. Iino M.; Yamashita K., & Tashiro Y. (1998). Identification of alien chromosomes in a series of *Allium fistulosum – A. cepa* monosomic addition lines by means of genomic in situ hybridization. *Genes Genet Syst,* Vol. 73, pp. 311-315

Shimonaka, M.; Hosoki T.; Tomita M. & Yasumuro Y. (2002). Production of somatic hybryd plants between Japanese bunching onion (*A. fistulosum* L.) and bulb onion (*A. cepa* L.) *via* electrofusion. *J Jpn Soc Hort Sci,* Vol. 71, pp. 623-631

Smith, H.H.; Kao K.N. & Combatti N.C. (1976). Interspecific hybridization by protoplast fusion in *Nicotiana. The J Heredity,* Vol. 67, pp. 123-128

Song, P.; Kang W. & Peffley E.B. (1997). Chromosome doubling of *Allium fistulosum x A. cepa* interspecific F1 hybrids through colchicine treatment of regenerating callus. *Euphytica,* Vol. 93, pp. 257-262

Stack, S.M. & Roelofs D. (1996) Localized chiasmata and recombination nodules in the tetraploid onion *Allium porrum. Genome,* Vol. 39, pp. 770-783

Stevenson, M.; Armstrong S.J.; Ford-Lloyd B.V. & Jones G.H. (1998). Comparative analysis of crossover exchanges and chiasmata in *Allium cepa x fistulosum* after genomic in situ hybridization (GISH). *Chromosome Research,* Vol. 6, pp. 567-574

Sukno, S.; Ruso J.; Jan C.C; Melero-Vara J.M. & Fernandez-Martinez J.M. (1999). Interspecific hybridization between sunflower and wild perennial *Helianthus* species *via* embryo rescue. *Euphytica,* Vol. 106, pp. 69–78

Sybenga, J. (1996). Recombination and chiasmata: few but intriguing discrepancies. *Genome,* Vol. 39, pp. 473-484

Taylor, R.W. (1925). The chromosome morphology of *Velthemia, Allium* and *Cyrtanthus. Am J Bot,* Vol. 12, pp. 104-115

Thomas, H.M.; Morgan W.G.; Meredith W.G.; Humphreys M.W.; Thomas H. & Legget JM (1994). Identification of parental and recombined chromosomes in hybrid derivatives of *Lolium multiflorum* x *Festuca pratensis* by genomic *in situ* hybridization. *Theor Appl Genet,* Vol. 88, pp. 903-913

Toole, M.G. & Clarke A.E. (1994). Chromosome behavior and fertility of colchicine-induced tetraploids in *A. cepa* and *A. fistulosum. Herbertia,* Vol. 11, pp. 295-303

Ulloa, M.; Corgan J.N. & Dunford M. (1994). Chromosome characteristics and behavior differences in *Allium fistulosum* L., *A. cepa* L., their F1 hybrid, and selected backcross progeny. *Theor Appl Genet,* Vol. 89, pp. 567-571

Ulloa, M.; Corgan J.N. & Dunford M. (1995). Evidence for nuclear-cytoplasmic incompatibility between *Allium fistulosum* and *A. cepa. Theor Appl Genet,* Vol. 90, pp. 746-754

Umehara, M.; Sueyoshi T. & Shimomura K. (2006). Interspecific hybrids between *Allium fistulosum* and *Allium schoenoprasum* reveal carotene-rich phenotype. *Euphytica,* Vol. 148, pp. 295–301

Umehara, M.; Sueyoshi T.; Shimomura K.; Hirashima K.; Shimoda M. & Nakahara T. (2007) Production and characterization of interspecific hybrids between *Allium fistulosum* L. and *Allium schoenoprasum* L. *Bull of the Fukuoka Agric Res Center,* Vol. 26, pp. 25-30

van der Meer, Q.P. & van Bennekom J.L. (1978). Improving the onion crop (*Allium cepa* L.) by transfer of characters from *A. fistulosum. Biuletyn Warzywniczy,* Vol. 22, pp. 87-91 van der Valk P.; de Vries S.E.; Everink J.T.; Verstappen F. & de Vries J.N. (1991a). Pre- and post-fertilization barriers to backcrossing the interspecific hybrid between *Allium fistulosum* L. and *A. cepa* L. with *A. cepa*. *Euphytica*, Vol. 53, pp. 201-209

van der Valk, P.; Kik C.; Verstappen F.; Evernik J.T. & de Vries J.N. (1991b). Independent segregation of two isozyme markers and inter-plant differences in nuclear DNA content in the intespecific cross (*Allium fistulosum* L. x *A. cepa* L.) x *A. cepa* L. *Euphytica*, Vol. 55, pp. 151-156

van Heusden, A.W.; van Ooijen J.W.; Vrielink-van Ginkel M.; Verbeek W.H.J.; Wietsma W.A. & Kik C. (2000). A genetic map of an interspecific cross in *allium* based on amplified fragment length polymorphism (AFLP) markers. *Theor Appl Genet*, Vol. 100, pp. 118-126

Ved Brat, S. (1965a). Genetic systems in *Allium* I. Chromosome variation. *Chromosoma*, Vol. 16, pp. 486-49

Ved Brat, S. (1965b). Genetic systems in *Allium* III. Meiosis and breeding systems. *Heredity*, Vol. 20, pp. 325-339

Ved Brat, S. (1967). Genetic systems in *Allium* IV. Balance in hybrids. *Heredity*, Vol. 22, pp. 387-396

Wan, Y.; Petolino J.F. & Widholm J.M. (1989). Efficient production of doubled haploid plants through colchicine treatment of anther derived maize callus. *Theor Appl Genet*, Vol. 77, pp. 889-892

Williams, E.G.; Verry I.M. & Williams W. M. (1982). Use of embryo culture in interspecific hybridization. In: *Plant Improvement and Somatic Cell Genetics*. Vasil I.K.; Scowcroft W.R. & Frey K.J., pp. 119–128, Academic Press, ISBN 0127149805, New York

Yamashita, K.; Hisatsune Y.; Sakamoto T.; Ishizuka K. & Tashiro Y. (2002). Chromosome and cytoplasm analyses of somatic hybrids between onion (*Allium cepa* L.) and garlic (*A. sativum* L.). *Euphytica*, Vol. 125, pp. 163-167

Yanagino, T.; Sugawara E. & Watanabe M. (2003). Production and characterization of an interspecific hybrid between leek and garlic. *Theor Appl Genet* Vol. 107, pp. 1–5

Zenkteller, M. (1990) *In vitro* fertilization and wide hybridization in higher plants. *Plant Sci*, Vol. 9, pp. 267-279

Zenkteller, M.; Bagniewszka-Zadworna A. & Zenkteller E. (2005). Embryological studies on ovules of *Melandrium album* pollinated *in vitro* with *Lychnis coronaria* pollen grains. *Acta Biol Cracoviensia series Bot*, Vol. 47, pp. 135-138

Zhao, J. & Simmonds D.H. (1995). Application of trifluralin to embryogenic microspore cultures to generate doubled haploid plants in *Brassica napus*. *Physiol Plantarum*, Vol. 95, pp. 304–309

# 20

# Evaluation of Interspecific-Interploid Hybrids ($F_1$) and Back Crosses ($BC_1$) in *Hylocereus* Species (Cactaceae)

Aroldo Cisneros and Noemi Tel-Zur
*French Associates Institute for Agriculture and Biotechnology of Drylands, The Jacob Blaustein Institutes for Desert Research (BIDR), Ben-Gurion University of the Negev (BGU), Beer Sheva, Israel*

## 1. Introduction

### 1.1 Background - *Hylocereus* species

Vine cacti are night-blooming epiphytes plants, endemic to the Americas, and belong to Cactaceae, subfamily Cactoideae, tribe Hylocereeae (Br. and R.) Buxbaum (Barthlott & Hunt, 1993). According to the New Cactus Lexicon (Hunt, 2006), the genera *Hylocereus* (Berger) Br. and R., comprises 14 species, and they are widely distributed in tropical and subtropical regions of the Americas from Mexico to North Argentina (Mizrahi & Nerd, 1999; Merten, 2003). They inhabit a wide range of ecosystems, including coastal areas, high mountains and tropical rainforests (Ortiz, 1999). These species, known as pitahaya or Dragon fruit, are currently being marketed worldwide and have a high economic potential as exotic fruit crops in arid regions where water is scarce, since they use a Crassulacean acid metabolism (CAM) pathway and are exceptionally drought-tolerant (Raveh et al., 1998; Mizrahi & Nerd, 1999; Nobel & de la Barrera, 2004).

*Hylocereus* species are characterized by triangular stems, bearing large edible fruits (200-600 g) with broad scales and various peels and flesh colours (Lichtenzveig et al., 2000). These species have big flowers (25-30 cm) with large male and female reproductive organs, facilitating manual pollination and manipulation for breeding studies (e.g. the anthers can be easily removed to avoid contamination). The number of ovules per flower is very high, with ~7,200, 5,300 and 2,000 ovules per locule in *Hylocereus undatus* (Haw.) Britton et Rose, *H. monacanthus* (Lem.) Britton et Rose, and *H. megalanthus* (K. Schumann ex Vaupel) Bauer, respectively (Nerd & Mizrahi, 1997; Bauer, 2003; Tel-Zur et al., 2005). *H. megalanthus*, resembles *Hylocereus* in its vegetative appearance, but bears medium-sized (80-200 g) yellow fruit with a spiny peel and a white tasty pulp (Weiss et al., 1994). Seed viability varies among different *Hylocereus* species, as well as within the same species. The pollen donor has an effect on fruit weight, and a positive correlation was found between fruit weight and total seed number when self-pollinated fruit was compared with cross-pollinated fruit (Weiss et al., 1994; Lichtenzveig et al., 2000). *H. monacanthus* was reported to be self-incompatible (Weiss et al., 1994; Lichtenzveig et al., 2000), while *H. undatus,* under growing conditions in Israel, is self-compatible at the end of the season, yet its fruits are smaller than those obtained following cross-pollination. Because of the low yields obtained after self-pollination, hand-cross pollination is routinely carried out for both *H. monacanthus* and *H. undatus* (Mizrahi et al., 2004).

Over the past 20 years, in order to develop this crop to its full economic potential, a traditional breeding program has been developed at Ben-Gurion University of the Negev, focused on the production of superior hybrids in terms of fruit quality, though few of them currently grow at a commercial scale (Tel-Zur et al., 2004, 2005).

## 2. Polyploidy

Polyploidy is the state of having more than two full sets of homologous chromosomes. Polyploidization may have played a major role in the diversification and speciation of the plant kingdom, generating the genetic and epigenetic novelty that has resulted in the significant diversity observed today (Stebbins, 1971; Soltis & Soltis, 1993). Two forms of polyploidization are autopolyploidization and allopolyploidization. Allopolyploids result from the combination of two genetically and evolutionarily different (or homeologous) genomes. Allopolyploids originated from wide hybridization, as in the case of *Triticum turgidum* L. (Zhang et al., 2010). Enzymes encoded by both parents' alleles and novel enzymes that are encoded by new allelic combinations may be produced by allopolyploids, possibly contributing to their evolutionary success (Soltis & Soltis, 1993). Autopolyploids result from the combination of genomes from two individuals of the same species, producing multiple chromosome sets with similar (homologous) genomes. Autopolyploids can arise from a spontaneous, naturally occurring genome doubling, such as *Galax urceolata* (Soltis et al., 2007).

## 3. Meiosis and fertility of polyploids

The ploidy level refers to the number of sets of chromosomes (basic number) and is notated by an "$x$". The basic number is the haploid number of the diploid species, being the chromosome number in a polyploid series, divisible by its basic number (Ranney, 2000).

Both diploid and polyploid organisms can produce viable germ cells. Those of tetraploid organisms are diploid. Since four chromosomes are homologous, quadrivalents are frequently formed during meiosis. Their stability is much less than that of bivalents, leading to an increased ratio of mistakes and, therefore, to reduced fertility and, in extreme cases, even to gamete sterility. Some species have an undisturbed quadrivalent development, while, in others, it does not take place at all (Elliot, 1958).

Polyploid crop species include potatos, coffee, bananas, peanuts, tobacco, wheat, oats, sugarcane, plums, loganberries and strawberries (Stebbins, 1950). Frequently, polyploidization results in bigger organs and improved traits; thus, plant breeders have become interested in the artificial induction of polyploids. It must be pointed out that, in many seed crops, polyploidy lines have shown lower fertility rates than their diploid prototypes; also, in general, there is an optimum range of polyploidy, beyond which growth may be depressed along with increasing chromosome numbers (Elliot, 1958; Wolfe, 2001).

### 3.1 Meiosis of triploids

Triploids have generally been considered an evolutionary dead end because they have very low fertility and tend to produce aneuploid or unbalanced gametes (Ollitrault et al., 2008). Triploid formation is commonly caused by the fertilization of a haploid egg with diploid pollen or vice versa (Figure 1). During the meiosis of triploids, trivalents are frequently formed. During Anaphase I, the chromosomes are distributed onto both daughter cells. Only in rare cases does one of them receive exactly double the amount ($2n$) of the simple set ($1n$). Generally, both of them are equipped with incomplete sets (aneuploidy; Figure 1). This nearly always results in an imbalance of the chromosome composition, leading to lethality. Therefore, triploidy causes , with a few rare exceptions, sterility of the pollen (or strongly reduced fertility). However, triploids can produce haploid, diploid, or triploid gametes at low rates, which can lead to diploid, triploid, and tetraploid progenies (Otto & Whitton, 2000).

There have been numerous reports in the literature of meiotic behaviour in triploid plants, resulting in valuable cytogenetic information regarding the species investigated. Studies of *Solanum tuberosum* triploids have also provided evidence that the amount of lagging chromosomes is, more or less, proportional to the average number of univalents (Lange & Wagenvoort, 1973). In the case of the wild citrus 'Hong Kong' Kumquat (*Fortunella hindsii* Swing), early cytogenetic studies have described triploid meiosis, showing either trivalent pairing and some univalents (Longley, 1926) or the predominance of trivalents but, also, the presence of numerous bivalents and univalents, as well as great variation in the number of some genotypes (Frost & Soost, 1968).

In general, the triploid plants have failed to set seed with its own pollen; therefore, only in rare cases in citrus and only under controlled conditions was possible to obtain seeds (Ollitrault et al., 2008). In the case of citrus, the seeds obtained from the triploid plants were produced with pollen from diploid species (Ollitrault et al., 2008). Wakana et al. (1981) have shown that the formation of triploid embryos are associated with a pentaploid endosperm, which is a strong indication that triploid hybrids result from the fertilization of unreduced ($2n$) ovules by normal haploid ($1n$) pollen (Esen et al., 1979).

### 3.2 Meiosis of tetraploids

Polyploidy plays an important role in plant evolution, and it is known that the genomes of flowering plants, including many crop plants of worldwide importance, are polyploidy (Doyle et al., 2008; Leitch & Leitch, 2008).

The meiotic behaviour of plant chromosomes is affected by both genetic and environmental factors (Rezaei et al., 2010). Gametic viability is generally lower in autotetraploid genotypes that have multivalent chromosome association during meiosis than in allotetraploids that form bivalents, leading to equilibrated disomic segregation (Ollitrault et al., 2008). In citrus, it has been shown that the degeneration of pollen mother cells is more frequent in autotetraploids than in their diploid parental genotypes (Frost & Soost, 1968). These authors also observed a great variability in chromosome conjugation (quadrivalents, trivalents, bivalents, and univalents) during Metaphase I and showed that one third to one half of sporads have more than the normal number of four microspores (generally six or seven).

Meiotic restitution (working in functional unreduced female and male gametes) plays a predominant role in producing allopolyploids in flowering plants. This phenomenon, including first division restitution (FDR) and second division restitution (SDR), has been documented in cereal crops (Jauhar, 2003, 2007; Matsuoka & Nasuda, 2004; Zhang et al., 2007, 2010; Wang et al., 2010). It has been suggested that the unreduced gametes produced through meiotic restitution may have been a major mechanism for the widespread occurrence of polyploidy in nature (Jauhar, 2003, 2007; Ramanna & Jacobsen, 2003).

During the meiosis of tetraploids, trivalents and quadrivalents are formed. In Figure 1, the possible combination of balanced and unbalanced gametes in tetraploids during meiosis and in the following Anaphase I and the chromosome distribution onto both daughter cells are shown. Contrary to triploids, tetraploids frequently result with exactly double the amount ($2n$) of the simple set ($1n$).

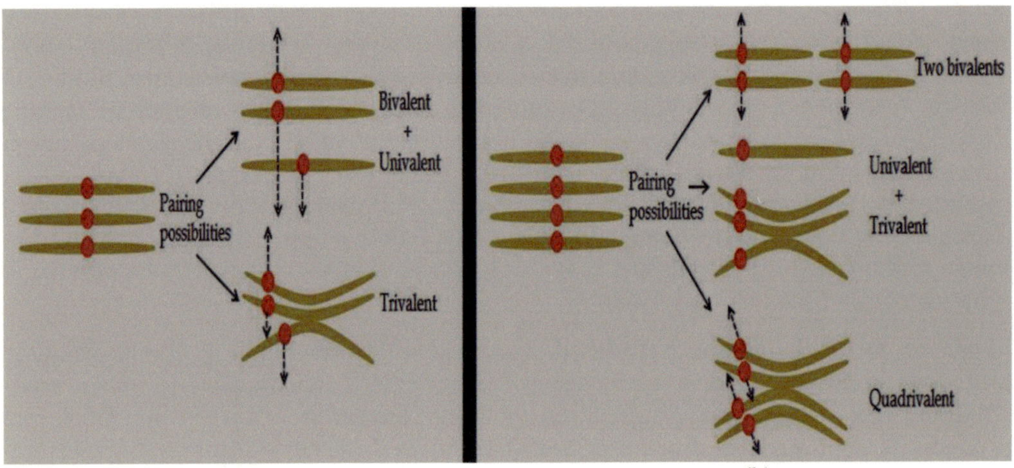


(a) (b)

Fig. 1. Production of balanced and unbalanced gametes in (a) triploids and (b) tetraploids during meiosis that may to lead balanced and unbalanced segregation and partitioning of chromosome sets.

## 4. Interspecific-interploid crosses

The following are crucial questions in allopolyploid research: what are the genetic and functional consequences of combining two genetic systems into a common nucleus (Huxley, 1942), and what are their ultimate effects on plant development (Steimer et al., 2004), flowering time (Simpson, 2004) and plant evolution (Kalisz & Purugganan, 2004). The critical period of allopolyploid formation seems to be immediately after fertilization, which probably involves intensive genetic, genomic and physiological changes (McClintock, 1984). In maize, for example, reciprocal interploidy crosses resulted in very small and largely infertile seeds with defective endosperms (Pennington et al., 2008). In *Arabidopsis thaliana*, reciprocal crosses between diploid and tetraploid plants resulted in viable triploid seeds; however, the seed development pattern and, in particular, the endosperm were abnormal (Scott et al., 1998). Additionally, Bushell et al. (2003), working with interspecific-interploid crosses between the diploid *A. thaliana* (2n = 2x = 10) as the seed parent and the tetraploid *A.*

*arenosa* (2n = 4x = 32) as the pollen donor, produced fruits with aborted seeds, while the reciprocal cross failed to produce fruits, and the flowers collapsed one day after pollination. Several theories have been developed to explain the success or failure of such crosses. Müntzing (1930) postulated that any deviation from the 2:3:2 maternal:endosperm:embryo genome ratios would result in seed failure, but his theory was widely disproved. Von Wangenheim (1957) proposed that seed failure in interploid crosses is caused by shifts in the initial quantity of cytoplasm per nuclear chromosome set, a theory later refuted by Lin (1982). Johnston et al. (1980) put forward the endosperm balance number (EBN) theory, which stated that hybrid success is based on an effective maternal:paternal genome ratio that must be 2:1 for normal endosperm development. This simplified theory was useful for plant breeders for predicting the success of a cross, especially among *Solanum* species (Carputo et al., 1997), but it failed to predict crossing success in other plant species. Haig & Westoby (1989) pointed out that the effect of "parental conflict of interests" on the growth of offspring suggested that maternal and paternal growth-promoting genes would be expressed differentially. Nowack et al. (2006) found that endosperm development is initiated by fertilizing the egg cell only and not the central cell with a mutant of the *A. thaliana* Cdc2 homolog CDC2A (cdc2a mutant pollen produces one sperm cell instead of two), suggesting that a positive signal for proliferation of the central cell triggered endosperm formation following egg fertilization. Nowack et al. (2007) showed that endosperm, exclusively derived from maternal origin, is able to sustain complete embryo development. These findings support Strasburger's (1900) hypothesis that, during evolution, the female gametophyte was reduced to the central cell of modern angiosperms and that fusion of the second sperm is used as a trigger to start endosperm development.

The fertilization process includes the fusion of the gametic membranes and the uptake of sperm cytoplasm by the female gametes, after which the fertilized egg is covered by a cell wall; thus, the endosperm and embryo develop in parallel to form a mature seed.

Crosses between the tetraploid *Hylocereus megalanthus* as the female parent and the diploid *H. undatus* or *H. monacanthus* as the male parent yielded pentaploid, hexaploid and 6x-aneuploid hybrids, while the reciprocal cross, using *H. monacanthus* as the female parent, yielded triploid and 3x-aneuploid hybrids (Tel-Zur et al., 2003). In *H. monacanthus* × *H. megalanthus* crosses, a higher number of truth hybrids were found about 92 %, of them were 3x while the reciprocal cross resulted in 5 % of truth hybrids with a ploidy level higher than expected (Tel-Zur et al., 2003, 2004). Endosperm breakdown is widely believed to be the cause of seed failure; however, seed abortion in vine cactus was probably due to a genomic imbalance between the seed parent and the embryo, rather than the maternal:paternal genome ratio in the endosperm (Tel-Zur et al., 2005) (Table 1). Endosperm dysfunction was the primary reason for hybrid abortion in a range of Angiosperm families (Brink & Cooper, 1947). Nowack et al. (2010) showed that the fertilized egg transmits a signal for development, but it cannot continue without the fertilization of the central cell. On the basis of this hypothesis, Cisneros et al. (2011) postulate, for vine cacti, that: 1) double fertilization happened but the zygote aborted, resulting in empty seeds due to post-zygotic barriers; 2) endosperm formation is necessary (and double fertilization is required) for normal seed coat development, but the presence of an embryo is not essential for the development of a normal black seed coat; and 3) increased genome dosage in the polyploid results in reduced seed viability, which may be attributable to a maternal/paternal imbalance or a lack of double fertilization.

Hybridization is an important source of improved genotypes for cultivation. Hybrids have been produced recently in our laboratory, following interspecific-interploidy crosses among *Hylocereus* species, setting fruits with a range of 5 to 15 % of unviable seed/fruit. The number of the unviable seeds was higher than that observed in the diploid *Hylocereus* species and lower than that observed in the female parent (S–75 or 12-31), suggesting that the triploid and tetraploid level of the hybrids result in a better seed viability. Few of the interspecific-interploidy hybrids set small fruits with a low seed number.

| | Seed parent ploidy | Pollen parent ploidy | Predicted seedling ploidy | Predicted endosperm ploidy (m:p) | Seedling ploidy (m:p) | Average seed weight (mg ± SE) |
|---|---|---|---|---|---|---|
| Homoploid crosses | 2x | 2x | 2x | 3x (2m:1p) | 2x (1m:1p) | 2.44 ± 0.05 |
| | 4x | 4x | 4x | 6x (4m:2p) | 4x (2m:2p) | 7.73 ± 0.39 |
| Paternal excess | 2x | 4x | 3x | 4x (2m:2p) | 3x (1m:2p) | 4.37 ± 0.19 |
| Maternal excess | 4x | 2x | 3x | Unreduced female gamete[1] | | |
| | | | | 9x (8m:1p) and not 5x (4m:1p) | 5x (4m:1p) | 3.1 to 5.9 |
| | | | | Chromosome doubling[2] | | |
| | | | | 5x (4m:1p) | 6x (4m:2p) | 3.1 to 5.9 |
| | | | | Aborted seeds[3] | | |
| | | | | 5x (4m:1p) | 3x (2m:1p) | <3.0 |

[1]Assuming that all the embryo sac cells (including the egg cell) are a result of unreduced meiosis, since megasporogenesis occurs before megagametogenesis.
[2]Ploidy in the embryo sac cells was assumed as remaining normal, while the hexaploid hybrids are probably a result of chromosome doubling (*see* Tel-Zur et al., 2003).
[3]Triploid hybrids were obtained in this cross direction using embryo rescue (*see* Cisneros, 2009).
(m:p): maternal to paternal genome ratios.
2x: *Hylocereus* species, 4x: *H. megalanthus*.

**The results presented in this table are a composite of unpublished and previously published data in Tel-Zur et al. (2005).*

Table 1. Outcome of homoploid and interspecific-interploid crosses in species of vine cacti*

## 5. Phenotypic and genomic evaluation

At the beginning of the 90s, there was very little scientific information available on the cultivation and the biological background of vine cacti. As of now in contrast to the early 90s, investigations in both horticultural and physiological aspects of climbing cacti have been covered and published in the professional literature; beginning with its reproductive biology (Weiss et al., 1994; Nerd & Mizrahi, 1997), shading requirements (Raveh et al., 1998), and fruit development, ripening, and post-harvest handling (Nerd & Mizrahi, 1998; Nerd et al., 1999; Ortiz, 1999).

Phenotypic and genomic characterization of the vine cactus core collection was reported by Tel-Zur et al. (2011), showing a high level of variability for most of the traits studied.

Although the heritability of these traits has yet to be studied, and some are likely to have a substantial environmental component, the levels of variation reported strongly suggested to us that vine cacti have high potential for breeding programs as exotic fruit crops, intrinsically adapted to dry areas (Tel-Zur et al., 2011).

Morphological traits, such as fruit shape, peel and flesh colour, stem size or height, often have one to one correspondence with the genes controlling the traits. In such cases, the morphological characters (the phenotypes) can be used as reliable indicators for specific genes that can be linked with quantitative trait loci (QTL), amplified fragment length polymorphism (AFLP), simple sequence repeat (SSR), among others and must be used to build the genetic linkage map of the vine cacti.

### 5.1 Phenological characterization

Morphological characteristics have not only been used for formal taxonomical overviews of large germplasm collections, but also for studying geographical patterns, as was done for durum wheat (Yang et al., 1991), bread wheat (Börner et al., 2005), barley (Tolbert et al., 1979) and triticale (Furman et al., 1997). Large variations in morphological characteristics were reported in garlic (Baghalian et al., 2006), different species of onions (Ozodbek et al., 2008; Zammouri et al., 2009), bananas (Uma et al., 2004) and pomegranates (Zamani et al., 2007).

Morphological traits are considered easy to observe, and it is possible to screen and categorize large amounts of genotypes at a low cost, which is a great advantage when managing large germplasm collections (Diederichsen, 2008). However, the optimal utilization of morphological descriptors involves the evaluation of agronomic performance in the farm (Zammouri et al., 2009). The exploitation of such traits increases our knowledge of the genetic variability available and strongly facilitates breeding for wider geographic adaptability, with respect to biotic and abiotic stresses (Diederichsen, 2004).

The vine cacti plants grow up tree trunks and are anchored by aerial roots. The fruits have red, purple or yellow peels, while the colour of the flesh can range from white to red or magenta. The skin is covered with bracts or "scales", hence the name dragon fruit. The seeds are small and are consumed with the fruit. The fruit can weigh up to 900 grams, but the average weight is between 350 and 450 grams (Mizrahi & Nerd, 1999; Merten, 2003). The weight depends on pollination management as well as the genotype (Weiss et al., 1994; Nerd & Mizrahi, 1997). The fruits are most often consumed fresh. In some parts of South America, the pulp is used to prepare drinks (Ortiz, 2001).

One of the major problems in cultivating vine cacti under desert conditions is their sensitivity to both low and high temperatures (Mizrahi & Nerd, 1999). Since variability in these characteristics exist among genotypes, and since there is no genetic barrier among species and even genera, breeding may solve these problems (Lichtenzveig et al., 2000; Tel-Zur, 2001). Another important problem with these fruits that might be solved with breeding is the poor taste of the red pitahayas, *H. monacanthus* and *H. undatus* (Mizrahi et al., 2002). The delicious yellow pitahaya, *H. megalanthus*, can tolerate high temperatures better than the other species, but the fruits are smaller (Mizrahi et al., 2002; Dag & Mizrahi, 2005).

The initial interploid crosses between the diploid *H. monacanthus* as a female parent and the tetraploid *H. megalanthus* as a male parent resulted in the release of two triploid hybrids (named S–75 and 12–31) to growers (Tel-Zur et al., 2004). These hybrids offered better taste than their diploid female parent and larger fruits than their tetraploid male parents, but, still, their spiny peel (a dominant trait), which is characteristic of *H. megalanthus*, was a limitation to further cultivation.

Recently, we performed an evaluation of 109 hybrids for three consecutive years; of this number, 40 were interspecific interploid $F_1$ (IH) hybrids (among the triploids S–75 or 12–31 and the diploid species *H undatus*), and 69 were first-back crosses ($BC_1$) between the triploids (S–75 and 12–31) and their parental lines. The morphological and agronomical fruit traits from the interspecific interploid $F_1$ hybrids, as well as the $BC_1$, under study are presented in Table 2, while the characteristics of the parental line were summarized in Tel-Zur et al. (2004, 2005). Variations in fruit form from round to elongated ellipse were observed in the basis of the dissimilarities of the fruit shape index (lower values were shown in hybrids not listed in the Table 2).

The number of flowers per hybrid per year was evaluated in 78 hybrids that set fruits. Among them, a wide range was observed, from one for BC–022 (not listed in Table 2) to 21 for IH–052 (Table 2). The weight of the fruits ranged from 119 to 273 grams and was intermediate between the fruit weights of the parental lines. Comparing these results with the parental genotypes, the majority of the hybrids were intermediate or lower than those of the parents, indicating partial dominance or co-dominance, similar to that described by Tel-Zur et al. (2004).

The potential yield per plant, a very important agricultural trait and a target trait in breeding programs, was calculated on the basis of the number of flowers per year and mean fruit weight (Tel-Zur et al., 2011). Two accessions demonstrated high potential yield, IH–003 and IH–052 with 3.25 and 3.72 kg/plant/year, respectively (Table 2). This trait was probably underestimated and will increase when the plants are older. Tel-Zur et al. (2005) reported the fruit weight in the female parent (hybrids S–75 and 12–31) to be between 192 to 267 grams, depending on the pollen donor used. This trait was intermediate between the parents, indicating partial dominance or co-dominance, as was previously described for others hybrids (Tel-Zur et al., 2004, 2011).

The number of viable seeds/fruit was quantified in several hybrids studied, showing a very high percentage of viable seeds (more than 85%), and their total number did not affect fruit size. In general, the phenotype of the seeds was similar to that described in tetraploids vine cacti (Cisneros et al., 2011); thus, we assume that this is a characteristic inherited from *H. megalanthus*.

The flowering season of the $F_1$ hybrids and $BC_1$ was from August to November. The time to full ripeness was extremely variable among the studied plants. The results showed variation within hybrids belonging to the same cross and ranged from 52 days in IH–011 (12–31 × *H. undatus*) to 156 days in IH–057 (12–31 × *H. undatus*), while in $BC_1$ (S–75 × *H. monacanthus* or *H. megalanthus*), the variation was lower but more similar to that reported in *H megalanthus*. The ripening time was found to be a genotype-specific trait with considerable variability among *H. megalanthus* accessions (Dag & Mizrahi, 2005). Mizrahi & Nerd (1999); later, Tel-Zur et al. (2004, 2011) reported that flowers of *H. megalanthus* that bloomed in early autumn matured in 90 days while those that bloomed later (November and December) matured in 160 days. Thus, this characteristic had an intermediate behaviour, implying that its inheritance was co-dominant and that the influence of low temperature was minimal.

| Plant code[1] | Flowers/ plant/year | Fruit shape index (FL/FW) ± SE | Fruit weight (g) ± SE | Flesh/Peel ratio ± SE | Potential yield/plant (kg)* | Ave. days to ripening |
|---|---|---|---|---|---|---|
| IH-001 | 8 | 1.9 ± 0.04 | 131 ± 18 | 0.88 ± 0.11 | 1.05 | 58 |
| IH-002 | 5 | 1.9 ± 0.08 | 273 ± 33 | 2.36 ± 0.36 | 1.36 | 92 |
| IH-003 | 16 | 1.8 ± 0.03 | 203 ± 15 | 1.39 ± 0.14 | 3.25 | 75 |
| IH-004 | 12 | 1.8 ± 0.04 | 119 ± 10 | 1.74 ± 0.22 | 1.43 | 67 |
| IH-005 | 6 | 1.8 ± 0.06 | 199 ± 27 | 1.23 ± 0.19 | 1.19 | 83 |
| IH-006 | 12 | 1.8 ± 0.05 | 169 ± 14 | 2.12 ± 0.29 | 2.03 | 85 |
| IH-007 | 8 | 1.8 ± 0.05 | 231 ± 25 | 1.68 ± 0.24 | 1.85 | 88 |
| IH-008 | 9 | 1.9 ± 0.04 | 203 ± 26 | 1.25 ± 0.23 | 1.83 | 86 |
| IH-009 | 13 | 2.0 ± 0.07 | 197 ± 17 | 1.39 ± 0.16 | 2.56 | 82 |
| IH-011 | 11 | 1.6 ± 0.06 | 203 ± 10 | 2.22 ± 0.19 | 2.23 | 52 |
| BC-026 | 10 | 1.7 ± 0.08 | 170 ± 25 | 1.82 ± 0.21 | 1.70 | 81 |
| BC-027 | 7 | 1.7 ± 0.13 | 204 ± 26 | 2.61 ± 0.32 | 1.43 | 101 |
| BC-028 | 12 | 1.9 ± 0.05 | 220 ± 17 | 1.85 ± 0.17 | 2.64 | 90 |
| BC-029 | 10 | 1.8 ± 0.03 | 150 ± 14 | 1.87 ± 0.23 | 1.50 | 87 |
| BC-036 | 8 | 1.9 ± 0.04 | 180 ± 16 | 1.47 ± 0.06 | 1.44 | 85 |
| BC-045 | 11 | 1.8 ± 0.04 | 171 ± 12 | 2.04 ± 0.20 | 1.88 | 81 |
| BC-047 | 10 | 2.0 ± 0.06 | 158 ± 24 | 1.39 ± 0.17 | 1.58 | 78 |
| BC-049 | 8 | 1.9 ± 0.05 | 200 ± 21 | 1.20 ± 0.16 | 1.60 | 88 |
| IH-050 | 16 | 1.8 ± 0.03 | 181 ± 24 | 1.81 ± 0.16 | 2.90 | 94 |
| IH-051 | 12 | 1.9 ± 0.04 | 176 ± 9 | 1.86 ± 0.13 | 2.12 | 88 |
| IH-052 | 21 | 1.9 ± 0.03 | 177 ± 13 | 1.43 ± 0.10 | 3.72 | 63 |
| IH-057 | 8 | 1.6 ± 0.04 | 153 ± 32 | 1.11 ± 0.15 | 1.23 | 156 |
| BC-066 | 7 | 1.9 ± 0.09 | 149 ± 29 | 1.59 ± 0.30 | 1.04 | 103 |
| IH-070 | 10 | 1.7 ± 0.09 | 134 ± 19 | 2.03 ± 0.25 | 1.34 | 94 |
| IH-074 | 6 | 1.8 ± 0.06 | 177 ± 24 | 2.09 ± 0.31 | 1.06 | 82 |
| BC-075 | 9 | 1.9 ± 0.09 | 169 ± 23 | 1.78 ± 0.21 | 1.52 | 80 |
| BC-077 | 6 | 1.9 ± 0.05 | 228 ± 28 | 1.69 ± 0.24 | 1.37 | 91 |
| BC-098 | 8 | 1.8 ± 0.07 | 152 ± 17 | 1.90 ± 0.18 | 1.22 | 61 |
| IH-106 | 6 | 1.8 ± 0.07 | 177 ± 19 | 1.64 ± 0.46 | 1.06 | 72 |
| IH-107 | 7 | 1.9 ± 0.08 | 191 ± 19 | 1.70 ± 0.28 | 1.33 | 78 |

[1] Plant codes refer to IH: Interspecific-interploid cross and BC: Back crosses

* Potential yield per plant was calculated as a number of flowers/year × mean fruit weight

Table 2. $F_1$ and $BC_1$ characterization: flowers per plant, fruit shape index (fruit length/fruit width), fresh/peel ratio, fruit weight, potential yield and average number of days until ripening

### 5.2 Genome size analyses and ploidy estimation

Estimating genome size and ploidy level in putative hybrids is the first step in evaluating the success of the interploid cross. Two methods are generally used: chromosome count and flow cytometry. Flow cytometry is a technique of genome quantification, initially developed for biomedical research and adapted for genetic plant analysis (Segura et al., 2007), that provides an accurate method to estimate ploidy level by measuring the proportions of cells in the G1, S and G2/M stages of the cell cycle (Doležel et al., 1989). The nuclear phase status is, by convention, indicated using the letter "n". The designations (meiotically) reduced and non-reduced, or haplophasic and diplophasic, are preferable to haploid and diploid, respectively, because their meaning is unambiguous. "n" indicates the meiotically reduced chromosome number, 2n the non-reduced number (Greilhuber et al., 2005; Murray, 2005).

Determining the intra- and inter-specific variation of DNA content is important to prove the success of the hybridization event, as well as for breeding programs and for genetic manipulation (Doležel et al., 1994; Doležel & Bartoš, 2005). These data can also be used to calculate cell cycle times, which are needed in genetic studies, and are useful for analysis of plant growth and development (Loureiro et al., 2007).

There are many examples of correlations between C-value variation between species and cellular parameters, such as the duration of the mitotic and meiotic cell cycle and the sizes of cells. From a taxonomic standpoint, intraspecific C-value variation is probably the most significant indicator that proves the presence of more than one genome combined within a species (Bennett, 1972; Murray, 2005; Záveský et al., 2005). The nuclear replication status ($G_1$ for non-replicated, S for replicating, $G_2$ for replicated) leads to DNA content changes expressed in terms of 'C'. For instance, 1C can be the DNA content of a young pollen cell nucleus just after meiosis, and 2C the content of a Telophase root tip nucleus (Moscone et al., 2003; Greilhuber et al., 2005).

Bennett & Leitch (2005) developed a Plant DNA C-values database that currently contains data for 7,058 plant species. It combines the DNA C-values database from the Angiosperm, Gymnosperm, the Pteridophyte, and the Bryophyte, together with the addition of the Algae DNA C-values database. Also included in the database are two Cactaceae species, *Opuntia microdasys* (1C = 2.24 pg) and *Rebutia albiflora* (1C = 1.91 pg), and a number of succulent species from the families Asparagaceae, Bromeliaceae, Crassulaceae, Apocynaceae, Xanthorrhoeaceae and a small number of genera in Asteraceae, in which the 2C-DNA values ranged from 1.11 to 16.85 pg. Segura et al. (2007) reported four different ploidy levels of 23 *Opuntia* species determined by flow cytometry, and the amounts of 2C-DNA ranged from 4.17 pg in *Opuntia incarnadilla* Griffiths to 6.53 pg in *Opuntia heliabravoana* Scheinvar.

A flow cytometric analysis was used to determine chromosome numbers and ploidy in *Consolea* species (Cactaceae). Compared to the base number, the mitotic and meiotic counts indicated hexaploid (2n = 66) and octoploid (2n = 88) species and no diploids, with the 2C-DNA values ranging from 4.88 to 9.50 pg (Negron-Ortiz, 2007). The 2C-DNA content was studied for species of *Hylocereus, Selenicereus* and *Epiphyllum,* showing a diploid level for all the species studied, except for two cases of a tetraploid level in *H. megalanthus* and *S. vagans* (Bgek.) Britton et Rose (Tel-Zur et al., 2011). The range of the 2C-DNA content varied from 3.21 pg for *S. grandiflorus* spp. *grandiflorus* (L.) Britton et Rose to 8.77 pg for *H. megalanthus* (Tel-Zur et al., 2011).

2C-DNA content and ploidy estimation was studied in the 109 $F_1$ and $BC_1$ of vine cacti using flow cytometry (Table 3). Table 3 shows a random sample chosen from all of them. The 2C-DNA amount in these hybrids ranged from 3.30 pg for IH–051 to 11.67 pg for BC–031 (Table 3), comparable with that reported in different *Hylocereus* and *Selenicereus* species (Tel-Zur et al., 2011) and in other cacti species (Negron-Ortiz, 2007; Segura et al., 2007). These results showed that the ploidy level of the hybrids were diploid, triploid, tetraploid and

| Plant code[1] | Nuclear DNA content pg/ 2C ± SD | Genome size 1C (Mbp) | Ploidy analyzed* | Ploidy estimated |
|---|---|---|---|---|
| **IH-001** | 8.52 | 4166 | N.D | 4x |
| **IH-002** | 6.67 | 3300 | N.D | 3x |
| **IH-003** | 8.42 | 4044 | N.D | 4x |
| **IH-004** | 8.43 | 4122 | N.D | 4x |
| **IH-005** | 6.62 | 3237 | N.D | 3x |
| **IH-006** | 8.22 | 4068 | N.D | 4x |
| **IH-011** | 4.38 | 2141 | N.D | 2x |
| **BC-016** | 8.52 | 3921 | N.D | 4x |
| **BC-017** | 8.66 | 4234 | N.D | 4x |
| **BC-018** | 4.04 | 1975 | N.D | 2x |
| **BC-019** | 6.80 | 3325 | N.D | 3x |
| **BC-020** | 8.08 | 4469 | N.D | 4x |
| **BC-021** | 6.55 | 3281 | N.D | 3x |
| **BC-023** | 11.44 | 5594 | N.D | 6x |
| **BC-025** | 7.67 | 4528 | 44 | 4x |
| **BC-026** | 6.03 | 3041 | N.D | 3x |
| **BC-027** | 6.20 | 3022 | N.D | 3x |
| **BC-028** | 4.22 | 2063 | N.D | 2x |
| **BC-029** | 3.80 | 1858 | N.D | 2x |
| **BC-031** | 11.67 | 5706 | 66 | 6x |
| **BC-032** | 8.51 | 4811 | N.D | 4x |
| **BC-033** | 5.72 | 2934 | N.D | 3x |
| **BC-034** | 8.00 | 3735 | N.D | 4x |
| **BC-035** | 6.22 | 2997 | 33 | 3x |
| **BC-036** | 7.25 | 3545 | N.D | 4x |
| **BC-037** | 6.98 | 3413 | N.D | 3x |
| **BC-045** | 6.87 | 3359 | 29 - 33 | 3x or mix |
| **IH-050** | 3.40 | 1662 | N.D | 2x |
| **IH-051** | 3.30 | 1613 | N.D | 2x |
| **IH-052** | 4.53 | 2215 | N.D | 2x |
| **IH-057** | 9.00 | 4401 | N.D | 4x |
| **IH-062** | 4.33 | 2117 | N.D | 2x |
| **IH-106** | 4.57 | 2234 | N.D | 2x |

[1] Plant codes refer to IC: Interspecific-interploid cross and BC: Back crosses

* Ploidy analyzed was based on the number of chromosomes counted using acetocarmine stain

Table 3. Genome size and ploidy estimation in $F_1$ and $BC_1$.

hexaploid, with only one exception, BC-045, that was triploid or aneuploid (Table 3). In different species of *Hylocereus* and *Selenicereus*, diploid and tetraploid were reported (Tel-Zur et al., 2011). In the $BC_1$, we expected to find ploidy levels ranging from 2x to 4x, according to the ploidy of the parents, [for example, the cross between the female triploid S-75 or 12-31 (2n=3x=33) and the diploid male parent *H. monacanthus* (2n=2x=22) or the tetraploid *H. megalanthus* (2n=4x=44)], but never 6x, as was obtained for the BC-023 (12-31 × *H. monacanthus*) and BC-031 (S-75 × *H. monacanthus*). In these cases, we assumed that the genome was duplicated following a fertilization event with an unreduced (2*n*) female gamete from the triploid female parent (S–75 or 12–31) and a normal reduced (*n*) male gamete from the diploid *H. monacanthus*. Cisneros (2009) reported analogous unexpectedly high ploidy levels (6x) obtained in similar interspecific-interploid crosses between the triploid S–75 and the tetraploid *H. megalanthus* accession 96-667. Ploidy levels higher than 3x, observed in the hybrids under study, were probably due to unreduced gametes produced by the mother plant or by the pollen donor.

## 6. Cytology of chromosome non-disjunction

One of the major routes for polyploidization involves gametic "non-reduction" or "meiotic nuclear restitution" during microsporogenesis and megasporogenesis, resulting in unreduced 2*n* gametes. Non-reduction could be due to meiotic non-disjunction, failure of cell wall formation or formation of gametes by mitosis instead of meiosis (Elliot, 1958; Grant, 1981). Unreduced gametes (2*n*) are recognized as a common mechanism of origin of most polyploids in plants (Sang et al., 2004; Otto, 2007; Matthew et al., 2009). Generally, 2*n* gametes originate due to deviating meiosis in plants. Deviations can occur in plants with normal chromosome pairing, as well as in those with disturbed chromosome pairing as, for example, in distant interspecific hybrids or synaptic mutants. The process that leads to the formation of 2*n* gametes is called meiotic nuclear restitution and occurs either during micro- or megasporogenesis (Ramanna & Jacobsen, 2003).

Cytological disturbances may lead to sterility or reduced seed viability. Cytological disturbances and anomalous behaviours, such as heavy-walled coenocytes, uncoiled chromosomes, supernumerary chromosomes, production of cross-bridges at second division and the occurrence of globular structures in the microsporocytes, were reported for several species and are strongly associated with a high level of sterility in polyploids, e.g., in the triploid hybrid of *Gossypium hirsutum-herbaceum* (Beasley, 1940), in the allohexaploid of *Phleum pratense* (Nath & Nielsen, 1961) and in the tetraploids of *Brachiaria decumbens* (Simioni & Borges do Valle, 2011).

Winge (1917) proposed a theory of "hybridization followed by chromosome doubling" as a mechanism enabling the survival and development of the hybrid zygote by providing each chromosome with a homologue with which to pair. Despite the lack of well-documented evidence, generations of biologists believed that polyploids were generated by somatic doubling (zygotic or meristematic). Conversely, Harlan & de Wet (1975) listed 85 plant genera known to produce 2*n* or "unreduced" gametes (pollen or egg cells carrying the somatic chromosomal numbers), which reinforced the theory of Karpechenko (1927) and of Darlington (1956) that sexual polyploidization, resulting from 2*n* gamete fusion, is the driving force behind the origin of polyploid species. Currently, most of the evidence attributes polyploid formation to: (1) sexual polyploidization through fusion of 2*n* gametes; (2) somatic mutations in meristematic cells, namely, chimera (Morgan et al., 2001; Karle et al., 2002); (3) somatic polyploidization by nuclear fusion (Baroux et al., 2004); or (4) polyspermy, the fertilization of an egg by more than one sperm (Virfusson, 1970).

There is, however, some scientific evidence supporting the occurrence of "hybridization followed by chromosome doubling", the best known example being that of *Primula "kewensis"*, a first-generation hybrid between *P. floribunda* and *P. verticillata* (Newton &

Pellew, 1929). For some unknown reason, the chromosomes in one branch of the plant had spontaneously doubled (somatic doubling), a process that apparently restored fertility by providing each chromosome with an identical partner with which to pair. Other examples are the spontaneous appearance of the tetraploid *Oenothera lamarckiana* Ser. (Gates, 1924) and the amphidiploids *Nicotiana glutinosa* L. and *N. tabacum* L. (Clausen & Goodspeed, 1925), which provide empirical evidence for polyploidization, presumably, by chromosome doubling. Furthermore, corn plants exposed to heat shock after pollination produced diploid, tetraploid and octaploid seedlings. The latter two states of polyploidy seem to be the result of somatic doubling in the zygote or young embryo (Müntzing, 1933). Nath & Nielsen (1961) reported that the origin of the hexaploid level in *Phleum pratense* was due to the trebling of the diploid genome complement from the *P. nodosum* species.

Lately, evidence supporting Winge's theory has been reported by Tel-Zur et al. (2003) in vine cacti crosses between the tetraploid *Hylocereus megalanthus* as the female parent and the diploid *H. undatus* or *H. monacanthus* as the male parent, yielding several hybrids with an unexpectedly high ploidy level, always higher than that of the female parent. Since unreduced gametes were not observed in the diploid *Hylocereus* species (Tel-Zur et al., 2003), the origin of 6x is still not clear, and could be the result of chromosome doubling following interspecific-interploid crosses. Cisneros (2009) found similar results following interspecific-interploid crosses by using the embryo rescue technique, in which only one hybrid out of 22 tested showed the expected (3x) ploidy level that was lower than the ploidy of the female parent.

Univalents and multivalents were observed in the pollen mother cells (PMCs) of the tetraploid *H. megalanthus* at Metaphase I, even though chromosome disjunction at Anaphase I was very balanced (Lichtenzveig et al., 2000). The large pollen grains observed in this species, about 12% of the sample, were probably unreduced gametes formed due to meiotic irregularities during Anaphase II (Tel-Zur et al., 2003). Therefore, the pentaploid hybrids reported were probably the result of a fertilization event between an unreduced egg cell (from the tetraploid *H. megalanthus*) and a reduced pollen grain (from the diploid *H. undatus* or *H. monacanthus*). However, the hexaploid and 6x-aneuploid hybrids are an exceptional case, since the diploid *H. undatus* and *H. monacanthus* showed a regular chromosome disjunction at Anaphase I and a uniform pollen diameter, and all the interspecific-homoploid (2x) *Hylocereus* × *Hylocereus* hybrids were diploids, which strongly indicated insignificant or null production of unreduced gametes (Lichtenzveig et al., 2000; Tel-Zur et al., 2003, 2004).

Consequently, the hexaploid hybrids obtained as a result of the interspecific-interploid cross occurred at a frequency much higher than that expected for a possible fusion of $2n$ gametes from both egg and pollen donor parents. In interspecific-interploidy triploid and 3x-aneuploid hybrids, rod and ring bivalents were observed in the PMCs at Metaphase I. The frequency of the ring bivalents was much lower than that of the rod bivalents, followed by a balanced segregation in Anaphase I (Tel-Zur et al., 2005). Abnormal spindle geometry during Metaphase I (parallel and tripolar) and lagging chromosomes were also observed (Figure 2). Therefore, the relatively high percentages of functional female and male gametes (9.8 - 18.6% of viable pollen and 6.0 - 35.5% of viable seeds) produced by 3x hybrids are most likely the result of balanced chromosome segregation during meiosis (Tel-Zur et al., 2005). Moreover, all the hybrids were fertile or partially fertile, indicating that pre- and post-zygotic barriers are not a major factor blocking the development and viability of hybrids among vine cacti species (Tel-Zur et al., 2003, 2004, 2005).

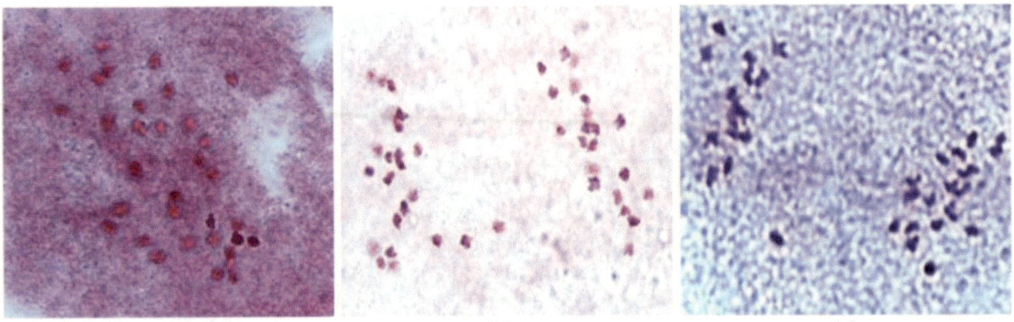

(a) (b) (c)

Fig. 2. Meiotic abnormalities observed in interspecific-interploid hybrids. (a) Hybrid BC–045 (3x aneuploid): Prophase I showing 32 chromosomes. (b) Hybrid BC–025 (4x): later Anaphase I showing balanced chromosome disjunction and lagging chromosomes. (c) Hybrid BC–035 (3x): later Anaphase I showing unbalanced chromosome disjunction and a lagging chromosome.

## 7. Cytomixis

Cytomixis was defined as the migration of chromatin between adjacent cells through a cytoplasmic connection channel, i.e., chromatin migration between meiocytes, and was reported for the first time in the PMCs of *Crocus sativus* by Körnicke in 1901 (as cited in Bellucci et al., 2003). Cytomixis has been extensively studied in a great number of species; however, its origin and significance are still unclear, and its role in evolution, as well as its genetic control, remains speculative and controversial. Cytomixis is now considered to be a cytological phenomenon, though infrequent, and not an artefact that occurred during slide preparations (Bellucci et al., 2003). This phenomenon was observed more frequently during microsporogenesis, mostly during Prophase of the meiotic division, but can occur in all stages of the meiosis, especially in genetically unbalanced genotypes such as haploids, triploids, aneuploids, mutants and hybrids (de Nettancourt & Grant, 1964; Gottschalk, 1970; Salesses, 1970; Mantu & Sharma, 1983). Usually, a few cells (two to four) participated in the process, while a large numbers of PMCs were involved (Malallah & Attia, 2003).

The process of chromatin transference occurs mainly from the donor to the recipient cell and could include a small part of the chromatin material or the whole genome of the donor cell. Negron-Ortiz (2007) reported, in *Consolea* species, the occurrence of cytomixis, and the number of cells involved varied from two to nine, depending on the species, resulting, occasionally, in the establishment of empty microsporocytes after a total chromatin migration. The meiocytes with no chromatin were lost during the meiotic division, and those with abnormal genome size formed unbalanced gametes.

Previous reports indicated a genetic control of the cytomixis process (Omara, 1976; Morikawa & Legget, 1996), which can be affected by extremely high temperatures (Mantu & Sharma, 1983), herbicides (Bobak & Herich, 1978), or by pathological agents (Bell, 1964).

During observations of immature anthers of the $F_1$ and $BC_1$ vine cacti, multiple chromatin bridges between microsporocytes were observed at Prophase I; such bridges allow chromatin transfer between cells (Figure 3). These observations of PMCs showed that the cytomixis process detected during the Prophase of the meiosis was more frequent in some of the interspecific interploid hybrids between the allotriploid S-75 as the mother parent, and the diploid *H. undatus*, as the pollen donor. Most likely, this phenomenon took place in these hybrids because of the convergence of three different genomes (*H. monacanthus, H. megalanthus* and *H. undatus*), and may thus imply selective DNA elimination as a response to the allopolyploidization process. The number of cells involved in the phenomenon varied from two to four. Completely empty microsporocytes were not observed. In some PMCs' donor, the remark of some chromosomes indicated that the migration to its attached recipient cell was not complete (Figure 3). Another interesting phenomenon observed was the formation of vesicle-like objects in the walls of the PMCs (Figure 3). Chromosome segments were observed in some of those vesicles and around them, which seems to be a way to remove DNA from the PMCs before the meiotic division. To the best of our knowledge, no previous reports were found in the literature addressing similar vesicle-like formation.

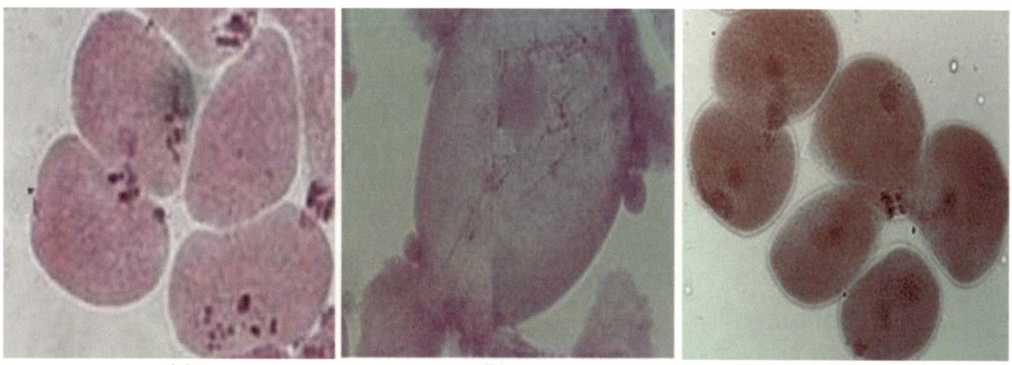

(a) (b) (c)

Fig. 3. Cytomixis process in PMCs in vine cacti. (a) Cytoplasmic connections in IH-006. (b) Vesicle-like formation with DNA material during Prophase in BC-023. (c) Prophase showing chromosomes that were not involved in the migration process in BC-032.

The ability of cytoplasmic channels to penetrate the callus walls, which are usually formed around microsporocytes at the end of Prophase, determines the beginning of the cytomixis process. Still unknown are the trigger that induces the PMCs to develop a connection channel with its neighbour; what points are involved in the process of recognizing the potential receptor cell; and if this process is a result of the genetic instability and/or incompatibility due to the combination of different genomes in a single cell.

## 8. Conclusions

Classical breeding methods can be defined as a set of tools that allows researchers to improve and characterize plants or living organisms. Several technologies, such as fluorescent activated cell sorting (FACS), molecular markers [e.g., random amplified polymorphism (RAP), amplified fragment length polymorphism (AFLP) and fluorescent *in situ* hybridization (FISH)], marker assistant selection (MAS), and quantitative trait loci (QTL) are currently extensively used for the purpose of plant evaluation and characterization. Combining these technologies with phenotypic, genomic and cytological evaluations has given us a model system by which to associate the agronomical trait with the gene controlling its expression and making it possible to infer the inheritance. Additionally, this model system provides an excellent research tool to elucidate the pathways of polyploid formation and seed development following interspecific-interploid hybridization and to solve critical hypotheses related to the origin of vine cacti species, contributing to the new discoveries of improved nutritional value, potential yield enhancement, breaking the self-incompatibility of the diploid lines and improving resistance to abiotic factors.

Two major basic mechanisms are most likely involved in polyploidization in vine cacti: (1) unreduced ($2n$) gametes, mostly arising from the nuclear division restitution during the meiosis of the micro- or megasporegenesis that can produce hybrids with a ploidy level higher than that of the parents in triploid × diploid and triploid × tetraploid hybridizations; and (2) duplication of the chromosomes after hybridization that gives rise to polyploidy.

In general, the meiocytes resulting from the meiosis in triploids and tetraploids can display more than one possible pairing association (*see* Figure 1); thus, the probability to produce unreduced ($2n$, $3n$ or $4n$) and unbalanced gametes is high.

The results summarized here provide experimental support to the hypothesis of polyploidization through somatic chromosome doubling or due to meiotic non-disjunction, although both the timing of the polyploidization event and the nature of the trigger remain unclear, as does the entire process leading to genome doubling. Further work on this topic will be directed to elucidate this phenomenon.

## 9. Acknowledgments

The authors thank Zin Scholarship Kreitman School and A. Katz International School for Desert Studies (BGU) for partial support of this work with a doctoral fellowship granted to A. Cisneros. This research was supported by Research Grant No. IS-4017-07 from BARD, the United States—Israel Binational Agricultural Research and Development Fund. We extend our gratitude to Mr. J. Mouyal and to the late Dr. B.Schneider for valuable assistance.

## 10. References

Baghalian, K., Sanei, M.R., Naghavi, M.R., Khalighi, A. & Naghdi, B.H. (2006). Post-culture evaluation of morphological divergence in Iranian garlic ecotypes. *Scientia Horticulturae,* 107: 405–410.

Baroux, C., Pecinka, A., Fuchs, J., Schubert, I. & Grossniklaus, U. (2007). The triploid endosperm genome of *Arabidopsis* adopts a peculiar, Parental-Dosage-Dependent chromatin organization. *The Plant Cell,* 19: 1782–1794.

Barthlott W, Hunt DR (1993) Cactaceae. In: Kubitzki K (ed) *The families and the genera of vascular plants*, Vol. 2, Springer, Berlin, pp. 161–196.

Bauer, R. (2003). A synopsis of the tribe Hylocereeae. F. Buxb. Cactaceae System. *Initiatives* 17: 3–63.

Beasley, J.O. (1940). The production of polyploids in *Gossypium*. Journal of Heredity, 30: 39–48.

Bellucci, M., Roscini, C. & Mariani, A. (2003). Cytomixis in Pollen Mother Cells of *Medicago sativa* L.. Journal of Heredity, 94: 512–516.

Bennett, M.D. (1972). Nuclear DNA content and minimum generation time in herbaceous plants. *Proc. R. Soc. Lond. B.*, 181: 109–135.

Bennett, M.D. & Leitch, I.J. (2005). Plant DNA C-values database, In: Release 5.0, December 2010, Available from http://www.rbgkew.org.uk/cval/homepage.html

Bobak, M. & Herich, R. (1978). Cytomixis as a manifestation of phatological changes after the application of Trifuraline. *Nucleus,* 21: 22–26.

Börner, A., Schäfer, M., Schmidt, A., Grau, M. & Vorwald, J. (2005). Associations between geographical origin and morphological characters in bread wheat (*Triticum aestivum* L.). *Plant Genetic Resource*, 3: 360–372.

Brink, R.A. & Cooper, D.C. (1947). The endosperm in seed development. *The Botanical Review*, 13: 423–541.

Bushell, C., Spielman, M. & Scott, R.J. (2003). The basis of natural and artificial postzygotic hybridization barriers in *Arabidopsis* species. *Plant Cell*, 15: 1430–1442.

Carputo, D., Barone, A., Cardi, T., Sebastiano, A., Frusciante, L. & Peloquin, S.J. (1997). Endosperm balance number manipulation for direct *in vivo* germplasm introgression to potato from a sexually isolated relative (*Solanum commersonii* Dun.). *Proceeding of National Academy of Science*, USA, 94: 12013–12017.

Cisneros, A. (2009). Seed development following interespecific-homoploid and interespecific-interploid crosses in species of vine cactus. In: *Thesis submitted in partial fulfilment of the requirements for the degree of Master of Science*, (April 2009), pp. 9–46, Ben-Gurion University of the Negev, Beer Sheva, Israel.

Cisneros, A., Benega Garcia, R. & Tel-Zur, N. (2011). Ovule morphology, embryogenesis and seed development in three *Hylocereus* species (Cactaceae). *Flora*206 (12): 1076- 1084, ISSN 0367-2530.

Clausen, R. E. & Goodspeed, T.H. (1925). Interspecific hybridization in *Nicotiana*. II. A tetraploid *glutinosa-tabacum* hybrid, an experimental verification of Winge's hypothesis. *Genetics*, 10: 278–284.

Dag, A. & Mizrahi, Y. (2005). Effect of pollination method on fruit set and fruit characteristics in the vine cactus Selenicereus megalanthus ("yellow pitaya"). J *Hortic. Sci. Biotechnol.*, 80: 618–622.

Darlington, C.D. (1956). *Chromosome botany*, Allen & Unwin, London, England.

de Nettancourt, D. & Grant, W.F. (1964). La cytogenetique de *Lotus (leguminosae)* III. Un cas de cytomixie dans un hybride interspecifique. *Cytologia*, 29: 191–195.

Diederichsen, A. (2004). Case studies for the use of infraspecific classifications in managing germplasm collections of cultivated plants. *Acta Horti*culturae, 634: 127–139.

Diederichsen, A. (2008). Assessments of genetic diversity within a world collection of cultivated hexaploid oat (*Avena sativa* L.) based on qualitative morphological characters. *Genetic Resources and Crop Evolution*, 55: 419–440.

Doležel, J. & Bartoš, J. (2005). Plant DNA flow cytometry and estimation of nuclear genome size. *Annal of Botany*, 95: 99–110.

Doležel, J., Binarová, P. & Lucretti, S. (1989). Analysis of nuclear DNA content in plant cells by flow cytometry. *Biol. Plant.*, 31: 113–120.

Doležel, J., Doleželová, M. & Novák, F.J. (1994), Flow cytometric estimation of nuclear DNA amount in diploid bananas (*Musa acuminata* and *M. balbisiana*). *Biol. Plant.*, 36: 351–357.

Doyle, J.J., Flagel, L.E., Paterson, A.H., Rapp, R.A., Soltis, D.E., Soltis, P.S. & Wendel J.F. (2008). Evolutionary genetics of genome merger and doubling in plants. *Annu. Rev. Genet.*, 42: 443–461.

Elliot, F.C. (1958). *Plant breeding and cytogenetics*. McGraw Hill Book Co., pp. 10–178, New York, USA.

Esen, A., Soost, R. K. & Geraci, G. (1979). Genetic evidence for the origin of diploid megagametophytes in Citrus. *Journal of Heredity*, 70: 5–8.

Frost, H.B. & Soost, R.K. (1968). Seed reproduction: Development of gametes and embryos. In: *The citrus industry*, W. Reuther, L.D. Batchelor, and H.B. Webber (eds.), Univ. California Press, Vol. 2, pp. 290–324.

Furman, B.J., Qualset, C.O., Skovmand, B., Heaton, J.H., Corke, H. & Wesenberg, D.M. (1997). Characterization and analysis of North American triticale genetic resources. *Crop Science*, 37: 1951–1959.

Gates, R. R. (1924). Polyploidy. *Brit. J. Exp. Biol.*, 1: 153–182.

Gottschalk, W. (1970). Chromosome and nucleus migration during microsporogenesis of *Pisum sativum*. *Nucleus*, 13: 1–9.

Grant, V.P. (1981). *Polyploidy*, Columbia University Press, pp. 283-352, New York, USA.

Greilhuber, J., Doležel, J., Lysák, M.A. & Bennett, M.D. (2005). The origin, evolution and proposed stabilization of the terms 'Genome Size' and 'C-Value' to describe nuclear DNA contents. *Annal of Botany*, 95: 255–260.

Haig, D. & Westoby, M. (1989). Parent-specific gene-expression and the triploid endosperm. *Am. Nat.*, 134: 147–155.

Harlan, J.R. & de Wet, J.M.J. (1975). On Ö. Winge and a prayer: The origins of polyploidy. *The Botanical Review*, 41: 361–390.

Hunt, D. (2006). Hunt, D. (2006). *The New Cactus Lexicon*. Remous Ltd., ISBN 0953813444, Milborne Port, England.

Huxley, J. (1942). *Evolution: the modern synthesis*, Harper and Brothers, London, England.

Jauhar, P.P. (2003). Formation of 2*n* gametes in durum wheat haploids: sexual polyploidization. *Euphytica*, 133: 81–94.

Jauhar, P.P. (2007). Meiotic restitution in wheat polyhaploid (amphihaploids): a potent evolutionary force. *Journal of Heredity*, 98: 188–193.

Johnston, S.A., den Nijs, T.P.M., Peloquin, S.J. & Hanneman, R.E. (1980). The significance of genetic balance to endosperm development in interspecific crosses. *Theoretical and Applied Genetics*, 57: 5–9

Kalisz, S.M. & Purugganan, M.D. (2004). Epialleles via DNA methylation: consequences for plant evolution. *Trends in Ecology and Evolution*, 19: 309–314.

Karle, R., Parks, C.A., O'Leary, M.C. & Boyle, T.H. (2002). Polyploidy-induced changes in the breeding behavior of *Hatiora xgraeseri* (Cactaceae). *J. Am. Soc. Hort. Sci.*, 127: 397–403.

Karpechenko, G.D. (1927). The production of polyploid gametes in hybrids. *Hereditas*, 9: 349–368.

Lange, W. & Wagenvoort, M. (1973). Meiosis in triploid *Solanum tuberosum* L. *Euphytica*, 22: 8–18.

Leitch, A.R. & Leitch, I.J. (2008). Genomic plasticity and the diversity of polyploid plants. *Science,* 320: 481–483.

Lichtenzveig, J., Abbo, S., Nerd, A., Tel-Zur, N. & Mizrahi, Y. (2000). Cytology and mating systems in the climbing cacti Hylocereus and Selenicereus. *American Journal of Botany,* 87: 1058–1065.

Lin, B.Y. (1982). Association of endosperm reduction with parental imprinting in maize. *Genetics,* 100: 475–486.

Longley, A.E. (1926). Triploid *Citrus. J. Wash. Acad. Sci.,* 16: 543–545.

Loureiro, J., Rodriguez, E., Doležel, J. & Santos, C. (2007). Two new nuclear isolation buffers for plant DNA flow cytometry: A test with 37 species. *Annal of Botany,* 100: 875–888.

Malallah, G.A. & Attia, T.A. (2003). Cytomixis and its possible evolutionary role in a Kuwaiti population of *Diplotaxis harra* (Brassicaceae). *Botanical Journal of the Linnean Society* 143: 169–175.

Mantu, D.E. & Sharma, A.K. (1983). Cytomixis in pollen mother cell of an apomitic ornamental *Ervatamia divaricata* (Linn) Alston. *Cytologia* 48: 201–207.

Matsuoka, Y. & Nasuda, D.S. (2004). Durum wheat as a candidate for the unknown female progenitor of bread wheat: an empirical study with a highly fertile F1 hybrid with *Aegilops tauschii* Coss. *Theoretical and Applied Genetics,* 109: 1710–1717.

Matthew, N.N., Mason, A.S., Castello, M.C., Thomson, L., Yan, G. & Cowling, W.A. (2009). Microspore culture preferentially selects unreduced (2n) gametes from an interspecific hybrid of *Brassica napus* L. × *Brassica carinata* Braun. *Theoretical and Applied Genetics,* 119: 497–505.

McClintock, B. (1984). The significance of responses of the genome to challenge. *Science,* 226: 792–801.

Merten, S. (2003). A review of *Hylocereus* production in the United States. *J PACD,* 5: 98–105.

Mizrahi, Y. & Nerd, A. (1999). Climbing and columnar cacti: New arid land fruit crops. In: *Perspective in new crops and new uses,* J. Janick (ed.), ASHS Press, Alexandria, VA, pp: 358–366.

Mizrahi, Y., Nerd, A. & Sitrit, Y. (2002). New fruits for arid climates. In: *Trends in new crops and new uses,* J. Janick and A. Whipkey (eds.), ASHS Press, Alexandria, VA, pp: 378–384.

Mizrahi, Y., Mouyal, J., Nerd, A. & Sitrit, Y. (2004). Metaxenia in the vine cacti *Hylocereus polyrhizus* and *Selenicereus* spp. *Annal of Botany,* 93: 469–472.

Morgan, W.G., King, I.P., Koch, S., Harper, J.A. & Thomas, H.M. (2001). Introgression of chromosomes of *Festuca arundinacea* var. glaucescens into *Lolium multiflorum* revealed by genomic in situ hybridisation (GISH). *Theoretical and Applied Genetics,* 103: 696–701.

Morikawa, T. & Leggett, J.M. (1996). Cytological variations in wild populations of *Avena canariensis* from the Canary Islands. *Genes Genet. Syst.,* 71: 15–21.

Morisset, P. (1978). Cytomixis in the pollen mother cells of Ononis (Leguminosae). *Can. J. Genet. Cytol.,* 20: 383–388.

Moscone, E.A., Baranyi, M., Ebert, I., Greilhuber, J., Ehrendorfer, F. & Hunziker, A.T. (2003). Analysis of nuclear DNA content in Capsicum (Solanaceae) by flow cytometry and feulgen densitometry. *Annal of Botany,* 92: 21–29.

Müntzing, A. (1930) Uber chromosomenvermehrung in *Galeopsis* - Kreuzungen und ihre phylogenetische Bedeutung. *Hereditas,* 14: 153–172.

Müntzing, A. (1933). Hybrid incompatibility and the origin of polyploidy. *Hereditas*, 18 (1-2): 33–55.

Murray, B.G. (2005). When does intraspecific C-value variation become taxonomically significant?, *Annal of Botany*, 95: 119–125.

Nath, J. & Nielsen, E.L. (1961). Cytology of plants from self and open-pollination of *Phleum pratense*. *American Journal of Botany*, 48 (9): 772–777.

Negron-Ortiz, V. (2007). Chromosome numbers, nuclear DNA content, and polyploidy in Consolea (Cactaceae), an endemic cactus of the Caribbean islands. *American Journal of Botany*, 94: 1360–1370

Nerd, A. & Mizrahi, Y. (1997). Reproductive biology of cactus fruit crops. *Hort. Rev.*, 18: 321–346.

Nerd, A. & Mizrahi, Y. (1998). Fruit development and ripening in yellow pitaya. *J. Amer. Soc. Hortic. Sci.*, 123: 560–562.

Nerd, A., Guttman, F. & Mizrahi, Y. (1999). Ripening and postharvest behaviour of fruits of two *Hylocereus* species (Cactaceae). *Postharvest Biol. Technol.*, 17: 39–45.

Newton, W.C.F. & Pellew, C. (1929). *Primula kewensis* and its derivatives. *Journal of Genetics*, 20 (3): 405–467.

Nobel, P.S. & de la Barrera, E. (2004). $CO_2$ uptake by the cultivated hemiepiphytic cactus, *Hylocereus undatus*. *Ann. Appl. Biol.*, 144: 1–8.

Nowack, M.K., Grini, P.E., Jakoby, M.J., Lafos, M., Koncz, C. & Schnittger, A. (2006). A positive signal from the fertilization of the egg cell sets of endosperm proliferation in angiosperm embryogenesis. *Nature Genet.*, 38: 63–67.

Nowack, M.K., Shirzadi, R., Dissmeyer, N., Dolf, A., Endl, E., Grini, P.E. & Schnittger, A. (2007). Bypassing genomic imprinting allows seed development. *Nature*, 447: 312–316.

Nowack, M.K., Ungru, A., Bjerkan, K.N, Grini, P.E. & Schnittger, A. (2010). Reproductive cross-talk, seed development in flowering plants. *Bioch. Soc. Trans.*, 38: 604–612.

Ollitrault, P., Dambier, D., Luro, F. & Froelicher, Y. (2008). Ploidy Manipulation for Breeding Seedless Triploid Citrus. In: *Plant Breeding Reviews*, J. Janick (ed), Vol. 30, pp: 323–353, John Wiley & Sons Inc., Hoboken, NJ, USA. doi:10.1002/9780470380130.ch7

Omara, M.K. (1976). Cytomixis in *Lolium perenne*. *Chromosoma*, 55: 267–271.

Ortiz, Y.D.H. (1999). Pitahaya a new crop for Mexico. Editorial Limusa, S.A. de C.V. Grupo Noriega Edit., pp: 35–58, ISBN 968-18-5775-5.

Ortiz, Y.D.H. (2001). Hacia el conocimiento y conservacion de la pitahaya (*Hylocereus* spp.). In: *IPN-SIBEJ-CONACYT-FMCN*, Oaxaca, Mexico.

Otto, S.P. & Whitton, J. (2000). Polyploid incidence and evolution. *Annu. Rev. Genet.*, 34: 401–437.

Otto, S.P. (2007). The evolutionary consequences of polyploidy. *Cell*, 131: 452–462.

Ozodbek, A.A., Svetlana, S.Y. & Reinhard, M.F. (2008). Morphological and embryological characters of three middle Asian *Allium* L. species (Alliaceae). *Bot. J. Lin. Soc.*, 137 (1): 51–64.

Pennington, P.D., Costa, L.M., Gutierrez-Marcos, J.F., Greenland, A.J. & Dickinson, H.G. (2008). When genomes collide: Aberrant seed development following maize interploidy crosses. *Annal of Botany*, 101: 833–843.

Ramanna, M.S. & Jacobsen, E. (2003). Relevance of sexual polyploidization for crop improvement–a review. *Euphytica*, 133: 3–18.

Ranney, T.G. (2000). Polyploidy: From Evolution to Landscape Plant Improvement. *Proceedings of the 11th Metropolitan Tree Improvement Alliance (METRIA)*. Gresham - Oregon, USA, August 23–24, 2000.

Raveh, E., Nerd, A. & Mizrahi, Y, (1998). Responses of two hemiepiphytic fruit-crop cacti to different degrees of shade. *Scientia Horticulturae*, 73 (2, 3): 151–164.

Rezaei, M., Arzani, A. & Sayed-Tabatabaei, B.E. (2010). Meiotic behaviour of tetraploid wheats (*Triticum turgidum* L.) and their synthetic hexaploid wheat derivates influenced by meiotic restitution and heat stress. *J. Genet.*, 89: 401–407.

Salesses, G. (1970). Sur le phenomene d cytomixie chez des hybrids triploides de prunier. Consequences genetiques possibles. *Annales del amerioration des plantes*, 20: 383–440.

Sang, T., Pan, J., Zhang, D., Ferguson, D., Wang, C., Hong, D.Y. & Pan, K.U. (2004). Origins of polyploids: an example from peonies (Paeonia) and a model for angiosperms. *Biol. J. Linn. Soc.*, 82: 561–571.

Scott, R.J., Spielman, M., Bailey, J. & Dickinson, H.G. (1998). Parent-of-origin effects on seed development in *Arabidopsis thaliana*. *Development*, 125: 3329–3341.

Segura, S., Scheinvar, L., Olalde, G., Leblanc, O., Filardo, S., Muratalla, A., Gallegos, C. & Flores, C. (2007). Genome sizes and ploidy levels in Mexican cactus pear species *Opuntia* (Tourn.) Mill. series *Streptacanthae* Britton et Rose, *Leucotrichae* DC., *Heliabravoanae* Scheinvar and *Robustae* Britton et Rose. Genet. Resour. *Genetic Resources and Crop Evolution*, 54: 1033–1041.

Simioni, C. & Borges do Valle, C. (2011). Meiotic analysis in induced tetraploids of *Brachiaria decumbens* Stapf. *Crop Breed. App. Biotech.*, 11: 43–49.

Simpson, G.G. (2004). The autonomous pathway: epigenetic and post-transcriptional gene regulation in the control of *Arabidopsis* flowering time. *Current Opinion in Plant Biology*, 7: 570–574.

Soltis, D.E. & Soltis, P.S. (1993). Molecular data and the dynamic nature of polyploidy. *Crit. Rev. Plant Sci.*, 12: 243–273.

Soltis, D.E., Soltis, P.S., Schemske, D.W., Hancock, J.F., Thompson, J.N., Husband, B.C. & Judd, W.S. (2007). Autopolyploidy in angiosperms: have we grossly underestimated the number of species. *Taxon*, 56: 13–30.

Stebbins, G.L. (1950). *Variation and Evolution in plants*. Columbia University Press, New York, USA.

Stebbins, G.L. (1971). *Chromosomal evolution in higher plants*. Columbia University Press, New York

Steimer, A., Schob, H. & Grossniklaus, U. (2004). Epigenetic control of plant development: new layers of complexity. *Current Opinion in Plant Biology*, 7: 11–19.

Strasburger, E. (1900). *Handbook of practical botany*. The Macmillan Co, New York, USA, pp: 294–315.

Tel-Zur, N. (2001) Genetic relationships between vine-cacti of the genera Hylocereus and Selenicereus. In: *Ph.D. Thesis*, Ben-Gurion University of the Negev, Beer-Sheva, Israel.

Tel-Zur, N., Abbo, S., Bar-Zvi, D. & Mizrahi, Y. (2003). Chromosome doubling in vine cacti hybrids. *Journal of Heredity*, 94: 329–333.

Tel-Zur, N., Abbo, S., Bar-Zvi, D. & Mizrahi, Y. (2004). Genetic Relationships among *Hylocereus* and *Selenicereus* Vine Cacti (Cactaceae): Evidence from Hybridization and Cytological Studies. *Annal of Botany*, 94: 527–534.

Tel-Zur, N., Abbo, S. & Mizrahi, Y. (2005). Cytogenetics of semi-fertile triploid and aneuploid intergeneric vine cacti hybrids. *Journal of Heredity*, 96: 124–131.

Tel-Zur, N., Mizrahi, Y., Cisneros, A., Mouyal, J., Schneider, B. & Doyle, J.J. (2011). Phenotypic and genomic characterization of vine cactus collection (Cactaceae). *Genetic Resources and Crop Evolution*, 58: 1075–1085. ISSN 1573-5109.

Tolbert, D.M., Qualset, C.O., Jain, S.K. & Craddock, J.C. (1979). A diversity analysis of a world collection of barley. *Crop Science*, 19:789–794.

Uma, S., Sudha, S., Saraswathi, M.S., Manickavasagam, M., Selvarajam, R., Dukai, P., Sathiamoorthy, S. & Siva, S.A. (2004). Analysis of genetic diversity and phylogenetic relationships among and exotic Silk (AABB) group of bananas using RAPD markers. *J. Hort. Sci. Biotechnol.*, 79: 523–527.

Vigfusson, E. (1970). On polyspermy in the sunflower. *Hereditas*, 64: 1–52.

Von Wangenheim, K.H. (1957). Untersuchungen uber den Zusammenhang swischen. Chromosomenzahl und Kreuzbarkeit bei *Solanum*-Arten. *Z. induckt. Abstamm. u. Vererb. Lehre*, 88: 21–37.

Wakana, S., Iwamasa, M. & Uemoto, S. (1981). Seed development in relation to ploidy of zygotic embryo and endosperm in polyembryonic citrus. *Proc. Int. Soc. Citric*, 1: 35–59.

Wang, C.J., Zhang, L.Q., Dai, S.F., Zheng, Y.L., Zhang, H.G. & Liu, D.C. (2010). Formation of unreduced gametes is impeded by homologous chromosome pairing in tetraploid *Triticum turgidum* × *Aegilops tauschii* hybrids. *Euphytica*, 175: 323–329.

Weiss, J., Nerd, A. & Mizrahi, Y. (1994). Flowering behavior and pollination requirements in climbing cacti with fruit crop potential. *HortScience*, 29: 1487–1492.

Winge, O. (1917). The chromosomes. Their numbers and general significance. *Compt. Rend. Lab. Carlsberg*, 13: 131–275.

Wolfe, K.H. (2001).Yesterday's polyploids and the mystery of diploidization. *Nat. Rev. Genet.*, 2 (5): 333–341.

Yang, R.C., Jana, S. & Clarke, J.M. (1991). Phenotypic diversity and association of some potentially drought-responsive characters in durum wheat. *Crop Science*, 31: 1484–1491.

Zamani, Z., Sarkhosh, A., Fatahi, R. & Ebadi, A. (2007). Genetic relationships among pomegranate genotypes studied by fruit characteristics and RAPD markers. *J. Hort. Sci. Biotechnol.*, 82: 11–18.

Zammouri, J., Arbi, G. & Neffati, M. (2009). Morpho-phenological characterization of *Allium roseum* L. (Alliaceae) from different bioclimatic zones in Tunisia. *African J. Agricul. Res.*, 4 (10): 1004–1014.

Záveský, L., Jarolímová, V. & Štěpánek, J. (2005). Nuclear DNA Content Variation within the Genus *Taraxacum* (Asteraceae). *Folia Geobotanica*, 40: 91–104.

Zhang, L.Q., Liu, D.C., Zheng, Y.L., Yan, Z.H., Dai, S.F., Li, Y.F,, Jiang, Q., Ye, Y.Q. & Yen, Y. (2010). Frequent occurrence of unreduced gametes in *Triticum turgidum–Aegilops tauschii* hybrids. *Euphytica*, 172: 285–294.

Zhang, L.Q., Yen, Y., Zheng, Y.L. & Liu, D.C. (2007). Meiotic restriction in emmer wheat is controlled by one or more nuclear genes that continue to function in derived lines. *Sex. Plant. Reprod.*, 20: 159–166.

# 21

# Embryology of Flowering Plants Applied to Cytogenetic Studies on Meiosis

Jorge E. A. Mariath et al*
*Plant Anatomy Laboratory, Biosciences Institute,*
*Electron Microscopy Centre, Federal University of Rio Grande do Sul-RS,*
*Brazil*

## 1. Introduction

The present chapter has three specific goals: (1) to discuss the incongruencies in terminology applied to meiosis and to pollen grains, (2) to describe cellular and subcellular aspects of plant meiosis and pollen, and (3) to review cytogenetic studies in plant meiosis involving embryological approaches.

The life cycle of plants is constituted by two generations: sporophytic and gametophytic. Gametophytic generation is the sexual generation. Differently from meiosis in animals, which gives rise to gametes, meiosis in plants originates spores. Heterospory occurs in some pterydophytes and in seed plants. This consists of the formation of two types of spores in separate sporangia (androsporangium and gynosporangium). In angiosperms, when meiosis occurs in anther sporangia, the spores are called androspores. When it occurs in seminal rudiment sporangia, they are called gynospores. The sporogenesis develops in a complete endosporic manner. In the case of gynospores formed, generally only one is viable in each sporangium. The viable spore germinates and, after three mitotic divisions, forms the female gametophyte, which develops in the sporangium tissue - the nucellus. During the development of the male gametophyte, the first mitosis occurs inside the sporangium, the other ones may occur after male gametophyte release. The androgametophyte is called pollen grain and the gynogametophyte is called embryo sac. The two sperm cells formed in the second mitosis of the male gametophyte, are the male gametes. They are present in the tricellular pollen grain or after mitosis of the generative cells during the pollen tube germination. The female gametes are called egg cell and central cell. In this way, sexual

* André L. L. Vanzela[2], Eliane Kaltchuk-Santos[3], Karen L. G. De Toni[4], Célia G. T. J. Andrade[5], Adriano Silvério[1], Erica Duarte-Silva[1], Carlos R. M. da Silva[2], Juca A. B. San Martin[1], Fernanda Nogueira[5] and Simone P. Mendes[6]
[1]*Plant Anatomy Laboratory, Biosciences Institute,*
*Electron Microscopy Centre, Federal University of Rio Grande do Sul-RS, Brazil*
[2]*Biodiversity and Ecosystems Restorations Laboratory, State University of Londrina-PR, Brazil*
[3]*Cytogenetic Laboratory, Biosciences Institute, Brazil*
*Federal University of Rio Grande do Sul-RS, Brazil*
[4]*Botanical Garden of Rio de Janeiro- RJ, Brazil*
[5]*Electron Microscopy and Microanalyses Laboratory, State University of Londrina-PR, Brazil*
[6]*National Museum- Federal University of Rio de Janeiro-RJ, Brazil*

generation in flowering plants is reduced to few cells and nutritionally dependent on the sporophyte. All the structures of the plant body, except the pollen grain and the embryo sac belong to the sporophytic generation.

We must not confuse or mix the different plant generations based on Hofmeister's alternation of generations (1851). When we analyze meiosis we are analyzing the reproductive results of the sporophyte, with the genetic recombinations present in the spores. No relation with sexuality was needed to obtain the expected result from a sporophytic generation - only SPORITY - androspores or gynospores, maintaining the reference to its localization in the androceum or gynoeceum in the word etymology, but without a sexuated connotation.

On the other hand SEXUALITY is present in the gametophytes, a generation that produces the male and female gametes, in individuals that are separate and thus unisexuated. They form, through fertilization, the new sporophytic generation (embryo) and the xenophytic generation (endosperm). The xenophyte is an accessory generation responsible for nourishing the embryo that is being formed, not directly connected to the reproductive cycle, since it never manages to produce its own reproductive structures.

In this chapter we will discuss the terminology applied to meiosis and to pollen grains, in accordance with the spority and sexuality of generations, the cellular and subcellular aspects of these structures, and cases of cytogenetic studies involving embryological approaches.

## 2. Terminology applied to meiosis in plants and pollen grains

The scientific investigation of plant sexuality began in the 17th century with Rudolph Camerarius (1694) in his work De Sexu Plantarum Epistola. Camerarius was the first to prove the existence of sex in plants. His discovery was a Copernicus-like event for Botany, and for several fields of biology (Zàrsky & Tupy 1995). According to Cocucci (1969), Camerarius work was preceded by Nehemiah Grew (1682) that described the pollen, and Marcello Malpighi (1687) that described ovary and ovules, nowadays, known as seminal rudiment. Camerarius mistakenly identified sexuality in sporophytic structures, since he established that the stamina and pistils were male and female "organs". Carolus Linnaeus established a classification system that includes two basic principles: the use of Latinized or Latin words to name groups of organisms, as well as the use of categories that distribute the organisms from large to limited groupings. Linnaeus (1810) created the "Sexual System" positioning the plants with flowers in twenty-four classes based on the number of stamina and pistils. According to Quammen (2007) descriptions of flowers were compared to sexual relations among human beings, causing polemic and scandal in the society of his time. The *Fuchsia* flower, for instance, was classified in this system containing eight male stamina around a female pistil, belonging to class 8, described as 'eight men in the nuptial chamber of only one woman'.

In 18th century, Hedwig (1784) thought the antheridia of mosses to be equivalent to anthers (Wagenitz 1999). In the 19th century, Hofmeister (1851) published the theory of alternation of generations, accepting that there could be two generations for briophytes and pterydophytes, one of them sporophytic and the other gametophytic.

Darwin (1877) was the first to discuss the presence of different floral types in plants of the same species, and called the flower hermaphrodites, female and male. The terminologies adopted by Darwin, attributing sexuality to flowers, are used in biology even today, in a large part of scientific production. (Richards 1997; Ainsworth 1999; Barrett 2002; Mitchell & Diggle 2005; Karasawa 2009).

The Hofmeister's work, considered as genial as that of Mendel or Darwin, was not widely disseminated in scientific circles (Kaplan & Cooke 1996). Scholars in the field of biology, taking Darwin as their primordial, guiding assumption (Cohen 2010), commonly observe a flower from the perspective of Camerarius and Linnaeus, as a sex organ, attributing sexuality to the sporophyte. The terms female flower and male flower are wrong, since they include both sporophytically originated structures, to which no sex is ascribed (calyx, corolla, androecium and gynoecium), and gametophytic structures that express sexuality such as the female gametophyte (embryo sac) and the male one (pollen grain). Further criticism of the term hermaphrodict is that every gametophyte in angiosperms and gymnosperms is unisexual, and in turn, hermophroditism is a condition present until isospore pterydophytes along the evolutionary scale of plants, in which a single spore gives rise to a prothallus with male and female gametangia. (Cocucci 1969; 1973; 1980; Cocucci & Hunziker 1994; Cruden & Lloyd 1995; Cocucci & Mariath 1995).

The terms 'female', 'male' and 'hermaphrodite' (Camerarius 1694; Linnaeus 1754, 1810; Darwin 1877) should be replaced by "imperfect pistillate", "imperfect staminate" and "perfect", respectively (Cocucci & Mariath 1995; Cocucci 1980; Greyson 1994; Cruden & Lloyd 1995). These terms are utilized by the APG (2007). This is due to the fact that the flower constitutes a sporophytic structure holding one or two gametophytes that depend nutritionally from the sporophyte (Coccuci 1973).

Based on these assumptions, Cocucci & Mariath (1995) propose to name flowers as: "monosporic" when only one kind of sporangium developed, producing androspores or gynospores; and "bisporic", when the flower presents the two types of sporangia, producing androspores and gynospores. The present study adopts the terms perfect flower, imperfect pistillate and imperfect staminate, due to their frequent use in current scientific literature, avoiding an inappropriate sexual connotation.

Despite the conceptual issue of considering flowers as a structure that includes tissues of the sporophytic and gametophytic generation, studies on their evolution have developed greatly, and are currently one of the topics discussed in the fields of evolution, ecology and genetics. Charles Darwin (1877) recognized that plants with seeds have an incredible diversity of reproductive systems, a 'sexual diversification' that is determined by ecological and genetic factors that are one of the core problems of evolutionary biology. The integration of phylogeny, ecology and studies on population genetics has supplied new ideas regarding the selection mechanisms that are responsible for the greatest evolutionary transitions between the modes of reproduction (Barrett 2002).

However, in our view, this so-called 'sexual diversity' is actually the expression of the 'spority' of the antophytes, a diversification that includes flowers with different morphologies, and may carry both functional sporangia, androgynosporangiates (perfect flower), or only one of these two types, androsporangiate (androic) or gynosporangiate (ginoic), or other combinations of these sporangia (monoic, dioic, trimonoic, andromonoic and gynomonoic).

As regards the gametophytic generation, based on the heterospored pterydophytes, the gametophytes are always unisexuate, and they are never hermaphrodite or bisexuate. Cocucci & Mariath (1995) and Cocucci (2006), within the sphere of studies on plant reproduction and improvement, propose to limit the sexual terminology to the gametophytes, erradicating the sexual terminology applied to sporophytes.

## 3. Meiosis and pollen grain: Cellular and subcellular aspects

The life cycle of plants consists of two generations: a sporophytic, diploid, and a gametophytic, haploid (Hofmeister 1851; Cocucci 1969; Cocucci & Mariath 1995). In seeds plants, gametophytic and thus sexuated generation begins from a spore that develops a multicellular structure called gametophyte through mitotic divisions. If this process occurs in the androecium, the male gametophyte is called androgametophyte, microgametophyte, androphyte or pollen grain. If it occurs in the gynoecium, the female gametophyte is called gynogametophyte, megagametophyte, gynophyte or embryo sac. Therefore, in the seed plants, the gametophytic sexuated generation is small and depends nutritionally on the sporophyte, and the morphological structures, except the embryo sac and the pollen grains, belongs to the sporophytic generation (Cocucci 1969; Cocucci & Hunziker 1994; Cocucci & Mariath 1995).

As a case study we shall analyze *Passiflora elegans* Master (Passifloraceae), a species of passion flower native to Brazil, regarding aspects of the development of androsporogenesis and androgametogenesis, divided into four stages described below.

Stage I - Sporangium and archesporial cells. The completely formed young anther has four sporangia, two of them in the ventral-lateral regions and the other ones in the dorsal-lateral regions (Figure 1 A). The epidermal cells, as well as the endothecium and middle layers, present vacuolated cells with conspicuous nuclei (Figure 1B). The epidermis and endothecium are indifferentiated at this stage. The middle layers present nuclei with portions of condensed chromatin and small vacuoles in the cytoplasm. The tapetal cells are radially elongated, multinucleated, their nuclei have conspicuous nucleoli, the cytoplasm is dense, with the presence of small vacuoles (Figure 1B). The archesporial cells are the largest cells of the sporangium, the nuclei are hyaline, with conspicuous nucleoli, and few portions of condensed chromatin, the cytoplasm presents storage lipids granules (Figure 1B) which, through their oxidation, ensure the energy needed to trigger the meiotic process.

Stage II - Meiosis and the end of sporophytic generation. Concomitantly, when meiosis begins, deposition of a callose wall begins on the inner side of the primary wall of the androspore mother cell. Individual isolation of the young androspores occurs through the formation of a callose wall, only after the tetranucleated phase, thus characterizing cytokinesis as being of the simultaneous type (Figure 2A-H). The tetrads present a tetrahedric spatial arrangement (Figure 2E,G-H). The sporoderm begins to be deposited around the future androspores, already in the tetrad phase, through the formation of the primexine that is initially internal to the callose wall. This wall is constituted by polysaccharide and protein.

The deposition of sporopollenin inside the tetrad occurs after the primexine wall is formed, and it was confirmed with Auramine O (Figure 2G). The reticulated aspect of the future exine is noted when it is submitted to analysis with differential interference contrast. (Figure 2H).

In monocotyledons, the most common cytokinesis is of the successive type, as demonstrated in *Pitcairnia encholirioides* (Bromeliaceae) (Figure 3A-C). After telophase I, the androspore mother cell gives rise to a dyad of androspores (Figure 3B). A callose wall is syntethized between the dyad of androspores. Meiosis II takes course forming the androspore tetrads, mostly with an isobilateral arrangement (Figure 3C).

Stage III - Beginning of the gametophytic phase (unicellular gametophyte). The young androspores are released from the tetrads inside the anther loculus and take on a spherical shape (Figure 2I). The androspores present a large hyaline nucleus, with a conspicuous

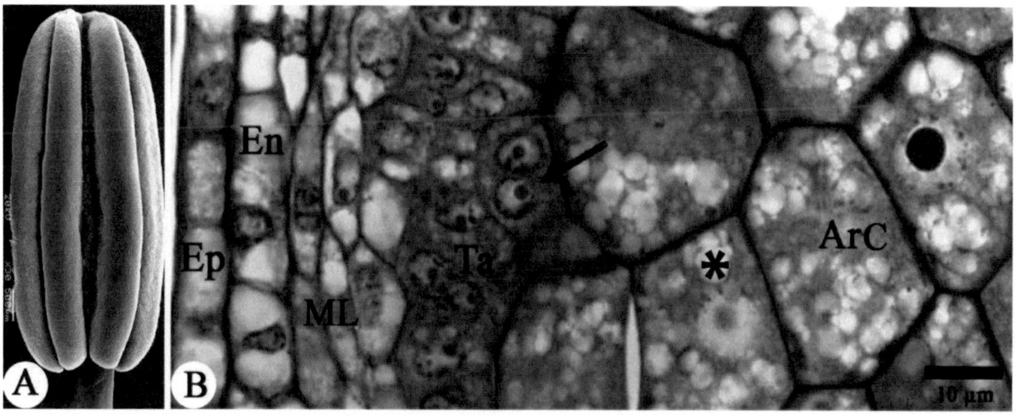


Fig. 1. Young anther of *Passiflora elegans* at the pre-meiotic stage. (A) Tetrasporangiated anther under scanning electron microscopy. (B) Cross-section of anther in pre-meiosis with archesporial cells. (Ep) epidermis; (En) Endothecium; (ML) middle layer; (ArC) Archesporial cell; (*) storage granules with lipidic nature.

nucleolus, and a large vacuole inside them (Figure 2I), signaling the beginning of gametogenesis. Sporoderm formation begins during the tetrad phase and in the free androspore phase the exine presents two stracta (ectexine and endexine) (Figure 4A). The ectexine, in *Passiflora elegans,* does not present a basal layer, so that the collumelae are plunged directly into the endexine. The intine, as well as the exine, are thick in *P. elegans* and are constituted by three chemically distinct pectic-proteic-cellulosic strata (Figure 4a). The cytoplasm presents a dense aspect and concentrates its largest volume at the polarized nucleus. After polarization, the androspore nucleus undergoes mitotic division forming the vegetative cell (VC), and the generative cell (GC) (Figure 4B). The tapetal cells, which previously were elongated and organized around the loculus, present irregular contours and degrade at the end of meiosis.

Stage IV - Bicellular pollen grain (bicellular gametophyte). Once the mitotic division has occurred, the central vacuole becomes smaller and the vegetative nucleus returns to the median portion of the cytoplasm, while the generative cell is kept in a parietal position. The wall separating the two cells is continuous with the intine. The vegetative cell includes the generative cell, acquiring a shape that ranges from lenticular to sickle-like (Figure 4B). From this phase on, the vegetative cells accumulates a large quantity of starch in their cytoplasm. This starch is distinctly hydrolyzed during the differentiation of pollen, so that different species can present pollen with or without starch during anthesis. In cases in which the starch is hydrolyzed, the cytoplasm is reactive to the PAS reaction while in the others, without hydrolysis, there is a weaker PAS reaction of the cytoplasm. The bicellular mature pollen grain, in cross-section, presents a hyaline vegetative nucleus, with a rounded shape and a conspicuous nucleolus. The generative cell is found immediately next to it and has an elongated shape (Figure 4B), in longitudinal section and a roundish cross-section, and a nucleus with portions of condensed chromatin (Figure 4B). Depending on the plant analyzed, the pollen grain is released in this bicellular form, completing the formation of gamete cells along the germinated pollen tube, as a result fo the mitosis of the generative cell (Figure 4D).

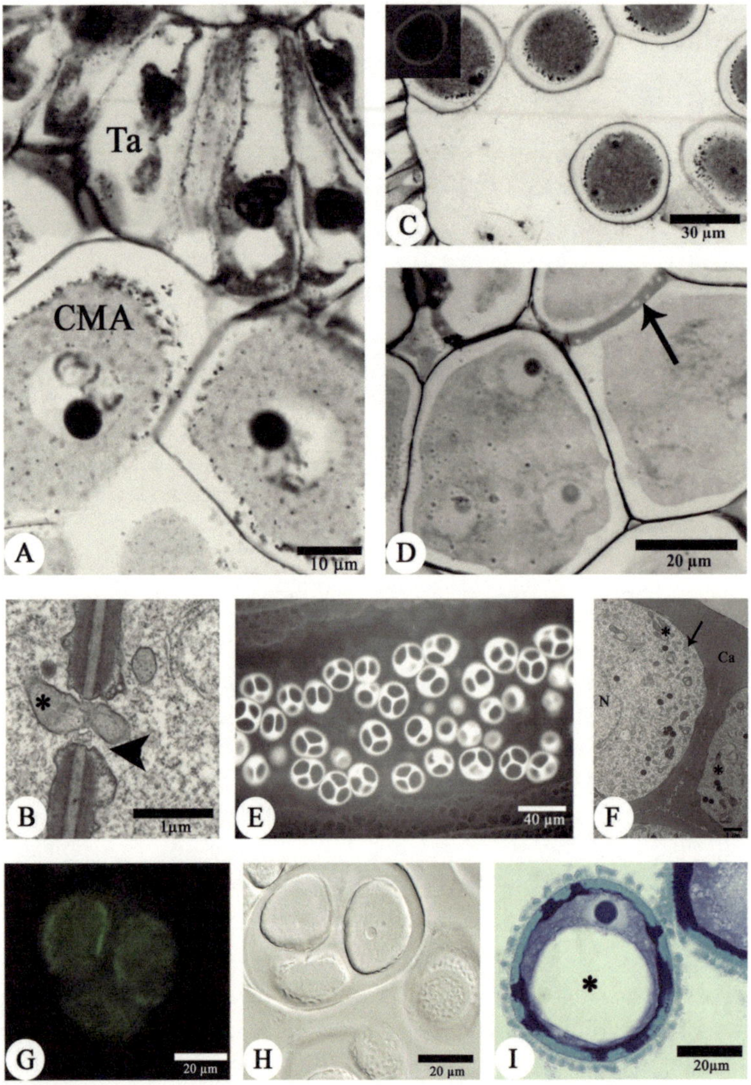


Fig. 2. Young anther of *Passiflora elegans* in meiotic and post-meiotic stage. (A) Androspores mother cells in prophase I. (B) Electron micrography of a cytomitic channel between androspores mother cells with the transit of plastids during meiosis. * means plastid, and arrowhead means cytomitic channel. (C) Meiocytes in telophase II. Insert reveals positive reaction to callosis with aniline Blue under fluorescence microscopy. (D) Cytomitic channels between meiocytes (arrow). (E) Tetrad after simultaneous cytokinesis, with callose between the androspores, marked with Aniline Blue under fluorescence microscopy. (F) Electron micrography of the callose wall involving the androspores in the tetrad. * means plastid, and arrow means mitochondria. (G) Androspores tetrad with exine deposited in the primexine, below the callose walls. Tetrad stained with Auramine O and observed under fluorescence microscopy. (H) Androspores tetrad in differential interference contrast, showing the reticulated aspect of the exine. (I) Androspore released from the tetrad in a vacuolated state (asterisk) stained with Toluidine Blue O.

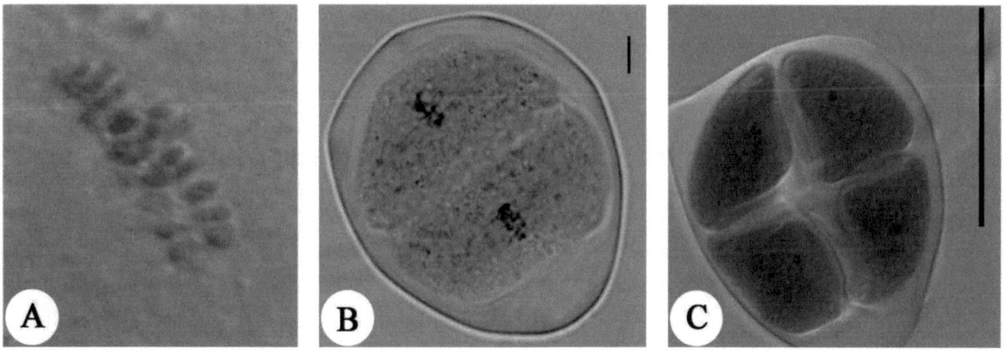


Fig. 3. Successive cytokinesis in *Pitcairnia encholirioides*. (A) Androspore mother cell, metaphase I (B) Androspores dyad in metaphase II . (C) Androspores tetrad at the end of meiosis. Scale: 3A-B =20μm; 3C=50μm.

## 4. Cytogenetic studies involving embryological approaches

### 4.1 Cytogenetic and embryological analyses of sporophytic sterility and gametophytic sterility, in flowering plants

Staminal sterility, also known in agronomic and biotechnological spheres as "male-sterility", consists in the lack of some stage of androsporogenesis and androgemetogenesis, which leads to the non-formation of a viable androphyte. A viable androphyte is considered to be a pollen grain morphologically typical and metabolically active that can emit a pollen tube (Dafni & Firmage 2000; Duarte-Silva et al. 2011). "Male sterility" would be a more appropriate term to designate only sterility events related to failures in androgametogenesis, without attributing sex to sporophytic phases (Cocucci & Mariath 1995). Since the term is used in the literature equally for any failure in the development of the anther and of the pollen grain, in the present study we will adopt the term 'staminal sterility' for failures in the initial stages of androsporogenesis (sporophytic sterility) and 'pollen sterility' for failures in stages after sporoderm formation (gametophytic sterility). The detection and investigation of staminal sterility in edible and medicinal plants are highly important, since they help improve the plant, because they are naturally free of self-pollination and therefore more easily manipulated in reproductive system experiments to produce strains with a given character of interest (Bhat et al. 2005). The study of androsporogenesis and androgametogenesis in cases of staminal sterility can determine the stage when spore development (in the sporophytic phase) or the pollen grain (in the gametophytic phase) cease. Besides, together with the tools of cytogenetics, immunocytochemistry, and transmission electron microscopy, it allows inferring the cause of this failure. Once the critical stage for the occurrence of staminal sterility has been identified, molecular biology studies can be performed to detect the genes involved in the expression of sterility. Embryological studies to investigate staminal sterility are common in widely sold edible plants, such as soy, wheat, rice, beans and maize, and little studied in medicinal plants used in the phytotherapeutic industry (Duarte-Silva et al. 2010).

Staminode formation is caused by different embryological events, motivated by equally diverse environmental and genetic factors. Different genes act on each stage of embryo development, and their failures may lead to the same result: stamen and pollen sterility.

Mutants *bam1* and *bam2,* of *Arabidopsis* do not develop the endothecium, middle layer and tapetum cells, and the mother cells of androspores, in turn, degenerate before meiosis (Hord et al., 2006).

Many cases of staminal sterility are related to tapetum problems. The function of the tapetum is related to the the synthesis of enzymes needed to separate the androspores from the tetrad and also to nourish the pollen grains (Goldberg et al., 1993). Tapetum degeneration occurs normally at the late stages of pollen grain development and it has been considered a process of programmed cell death or apoptosis (Papini et al., 1999; Li *et al.* 2006). However, apoptosis, early or late, leads to staminal sterility events, as in rice (*Oriza sativa* L.) where tapetum degradation occurs late, obliterating the anther locule and causing the androspores to collapse (Li et al., 2006). Already in mutant BR 97-17971, of *Glycine max,*

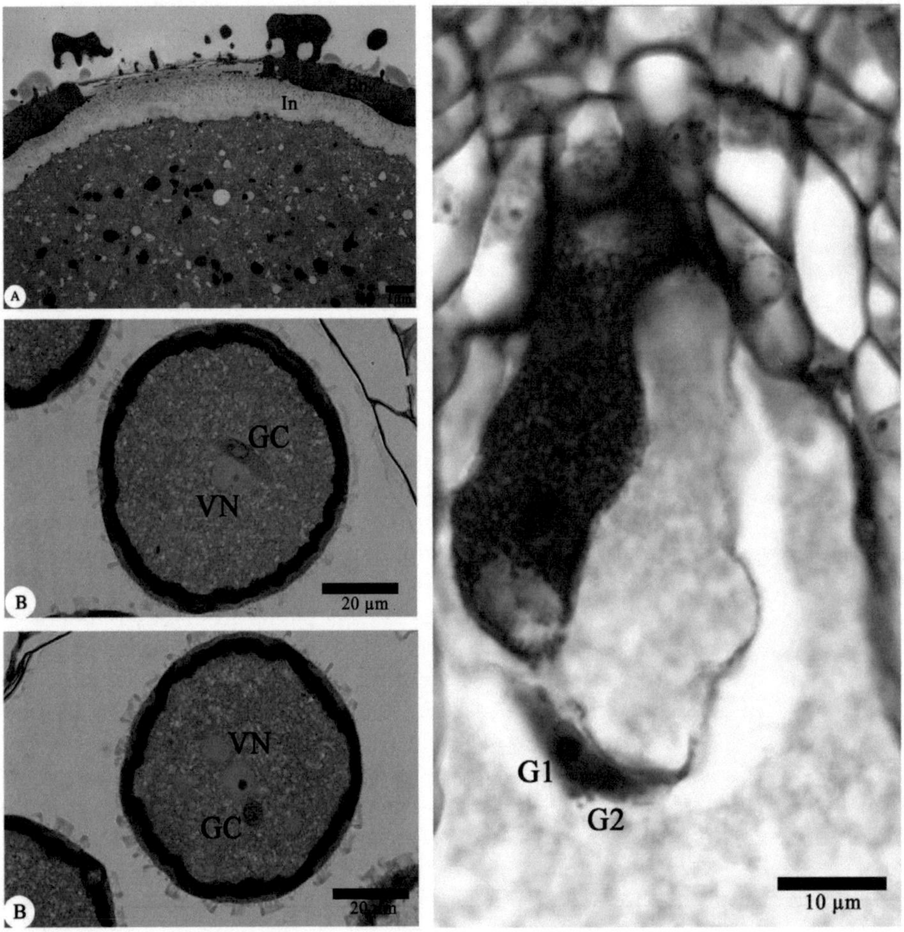


Fig. 4. Pollen grain of *Passiflora elegans.* (A) Eletron micrography of sporoderm (B) Slice of mature pollen grain with degenerative cell in a longitudinal section encompassed by the vegetative cell. (C) Slice of mature pollen cell at cross section. Generative cell enveloped by the vegetative cell. (D) Gametic cells (G1 and G2) after discharge of the pollen tube. (Ec) ectexine; (En) endexine; (In) Intine; (NV) nucleus of vegetative cell; (GC) generative cell, (G1 and G2) male gametes., (Si ) Synergid , (EC) Egg cell.

early degeneration of the tapetum occurs in telophase II of meiosis, with the absence or failure of cytokinesis of the androspore mother cells, forming a cenocyte, or, sometimes, a tetrad with some degenerated androspores (Bione et al., 2002). Another tapetum-related event is the abnormal vacuolation of tapetal cells in *Bidens cervicata* Sherff. (Asteraceae) which leads to the disintegration of the sporogenic tissue (Sun & Ganders 1987). In the case of maize (*Zea maiz* L., Poaceae), mutants for the *ms 23* and *ms 32* genes presented periclinal divisions in the tapetum layer followed by their non-differentiation, causing the cell death of the sporogenic tissue in prophase I of meiosis (Chaubal et al., 2000). In *Helianthus annus* L. (Asteraceae) disordered periclinal divisions occur, showing signs of disorganization in the organelles and in the cell wall. Thus, the androspore tetrads disintegrate (Horner, 1977).

Problems in the formation of the androspore tetrad also lead to sterility. In bean plants (*Phaseolus vulgaris* L., Leguminosae) abortions occur in the tetrad stage due to cytoplasmatic connections, which are maintained between the androspores, indicating incomplete or aberrant cytokinesis (Johns et al., 1998). A similar event occurs in pistillated flowers of *Valeriana scandens* (Caprifoliaceae). The androsporogenesis of pistillated flowers is the same as in perfect flowers until the androspore tetrad phase. In this stage the exine is deposited in the androspores, both in the primexine wall and in the aperture regions, forming connections between the androspores; as the callose degrades through the callase enzyme, the androspores are released in the locule in a tetrad shape; an exine continuum is formed among them; they undergo vacuolation and begin androgametogenesis, but become senescent, and only the exine of the sporoderm remains collapsed in the locule of the anther in anthesis (Figure 5A-B) (Duarte-Silva et al. 2010).

A mutant of strain 6492 of Arabidopsis (Brassicaceae), in the tetrad stage presents eight microspores enveloped by callose (Peirson et al., 1996). Two other mutants (strains 7219 and 7593) present tetrads with other sizes of microspores, with failures in callose production and in vacuole development, and also multinucleate cenocytes (Peirson et al., 1996). Disorders in the synthesis and degradation of callose, and in the timing at which these processes occur, lead to sterility. Mutant *ms32* of *Arabidopsis* presents early degradation of callose right after meiosis, because of the formation, in the same stage, as a large amount of rough

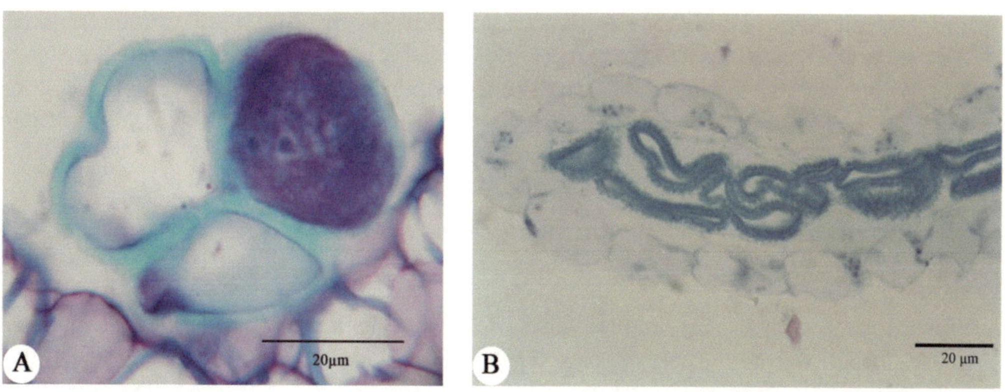


Fig. 5. (A) Malformed tetrad of *Valeriana scandens* (Caprifoliaceae). Observe the continuum of the exine between the tetrad androspores. (B) Sterile pollen in the anther in anthesis.

endoplasmic reticulum in the tapetum cells, probably responsible for callase synthesis and/or secretion in the anther locule (Fei & Sawhney 1999). On the other hand, in the mutant for gene *cals*5 of the same species, callose deposition practically does not occur in the mother cell of androspores and in the tetrad, causing androspore degeneration (Dong et al., 2005). Once the androspore tetrads have been formed, there are cases in which the androspores interrupt their development at this stage. In *Allium schoenoprasum*, two mutants for staminal sterility (*wi* e *st1*) do not present dissolution of the callose after microspore tetrad formation, causing the non-deposition of sporopollenin (Engelke et al. 2002).

Pollen grain abortion can also occur in the sporoderm development phase. The mutant *nef1* of *Arabidopsis thaliana* presents pollen grains with primexin and sporoderm without sporopollenin, synthetized and accumulated in the locule of the anther (Ariizumi et al. 2004). In mutants *cesa1* and *-6* of *Arabidopsis*, cellulose synthesis deficiency in the sporoderm leads to abortion of the pollen grain (Persson et al. 2007). Mutants *rip1* of *Oryza sativa* developed sterile pollen grains in consequence of no intine formation (Han et al. 2006). Also, in *Oryza sativa*, the presence of empty pollen grains is the result of allele interactions of loci *S-a*, *S-b* and *S-c* which lead to abnormalities in the migration of the androspore nucleus to the cell periphery, where asymmetric mitose occurs and the consequent formation of vegetative and generative cells (Zhang et al. 2006). In the same study, stained, but non viable pollen grains are listed among the failures of generative cell migration and of the vegetative nucleus to the center of pollen, as well as failures in sperm cell formation (Zhang et al. 2006). In *Arabidopsis*, the bicellular androphyte goes into programmed cell death after a deficiency in the division of the generative cells to form the gametic cells, due to the lack of the key enzyme 'SerinePalmitoyltransferase' (Teng et al. 2008).

The synthesis of reserve substances is a critical event in androphyte development. The synthesis and accumulation of starch were investigated in androphytes of *O. sativa* and six genes that act on the sucrose-starch metabolic pathway were identified (*Rsus, OSINV2,OsPGM, OsUGP,OsAGPL3* and *OsSSI*). Mutants for these genes are deficient in the production of amyloplasts and constitute a sterile class called HL type (Kong et al. 2008). *Arabidopsis* sporophytes recessive for the gene (*atatg6/atatg6*) develop morphologically typical androphytes that are incapable of emitting a pollen tube (Fujiki et al. 2007). On the other hand the transgenics of *Brassica campestris*, that do not have gene *BcMF2*, presented, in the sporoderm, the pectic proportion of the overdeveloped exintine and the underdeveloped endintine, causing in vitro development of balloon-shaped pollen tubes (Huang et al. 2009).

### 4.2 Cyperaceae and their uncommon microsporogenesis

#### 4.2.1 Ultrastructural and structural studies of pseudomonads in cyperaceae

Androsporogenesis in the Cyperaceae family follows a distinct pattern from that found in other Angiosperm groups. After meiosis, three of the four nuclei formed take up a defined region of the cell. They are isolated, degenerate and only one becomes the functional androspore. The four nuclei present a polarized distribution in an asymmetric cell known as pseudomonad (Figure 6A-B) (Selling 1947; Erdtman 1971; Strandhede 1973). In the development of the pseudomonad, all the cells come into contact with the tapetum inside the sporangium, in an arrangement known as peripheral (Kirpes et al. 1996). The pear-shaped pseudomonad has the broader region oriented toward the tapetum (abaxial region) and the narrower one oriented toward the center of the anther locule (adaxial region) (Figure 6b) (Strandhede, 1973). This spatial distribution, referring to the adaxial and abaxial aspects of a plant organ, may lead to mistaken interpretations, considering a entire sporangium, half of it oriented toward the adaxial aspect of the growth axis (rachila), while the other half is oriented toward its abaxial aspect. We suggest the orientation of these structures to the contiguous region, referring to the tapetum or locule.

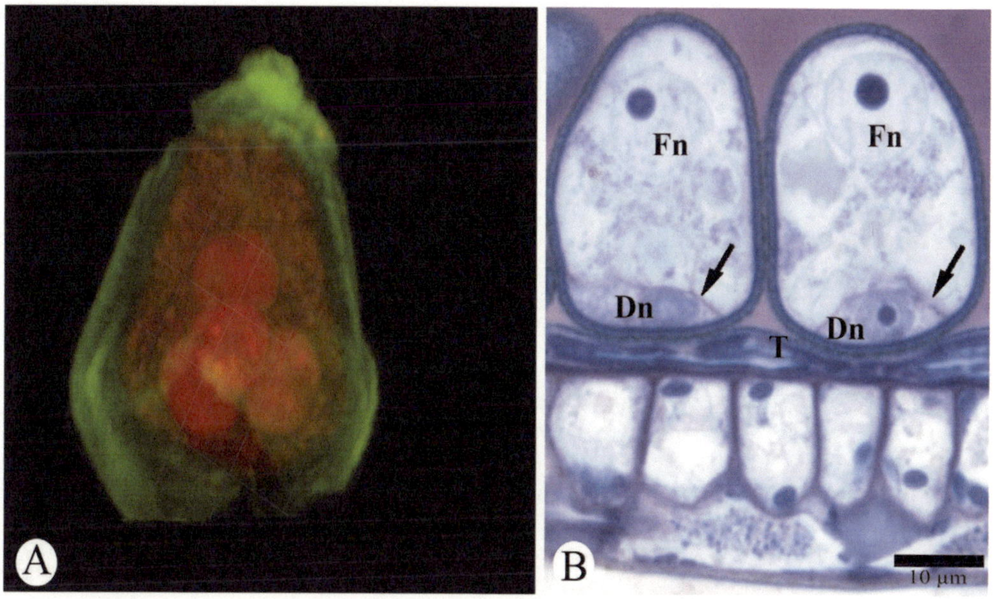


Fig. 6. (A) *Rhynchospora pubera* pseudomonad in confocal scanning microscopy showing the four nuclei in tetrahedral arrangement. The degenerative nuclei are located in a broad region of the cell, while the functional ones is placed in the central region. (B) Pseudomonad in contact with tapetum. The functional nucleus oriented toward the anther locule and the degenerative nucleus isolated by a thin inner cell wall (arrow). (Dn) degenerative nuclei; (Fn) functional nucleus; (T) tapetum.

In most genera of the Cyperaceae family, polarization follows a single pattern. The degenerative nuclei of the pseudomonad are oriented toward the locule, while the functional nucleus is oriented toward the tapetum region (Furness & Rudall 1999). This pattern of nuclear placement led to propose the "tapetum-pore" hypothesis. According to this hypothesis, the determining factor of the functional domain of the pseudomonad is due to the presence of the pollen pore close to the tapetum region (Strandhede 1973; Kirpes et al. 1996). This hypothesis can be applied to species of genus *Eleocharis* as shown in this chapter (see below). However, it cannot be applied to all Cyperaceae, since in *Rhynchospora* species the degenerative nuclei are found to be tapetum oriented and the functional nucleus is locule oriented (Figure 6B).

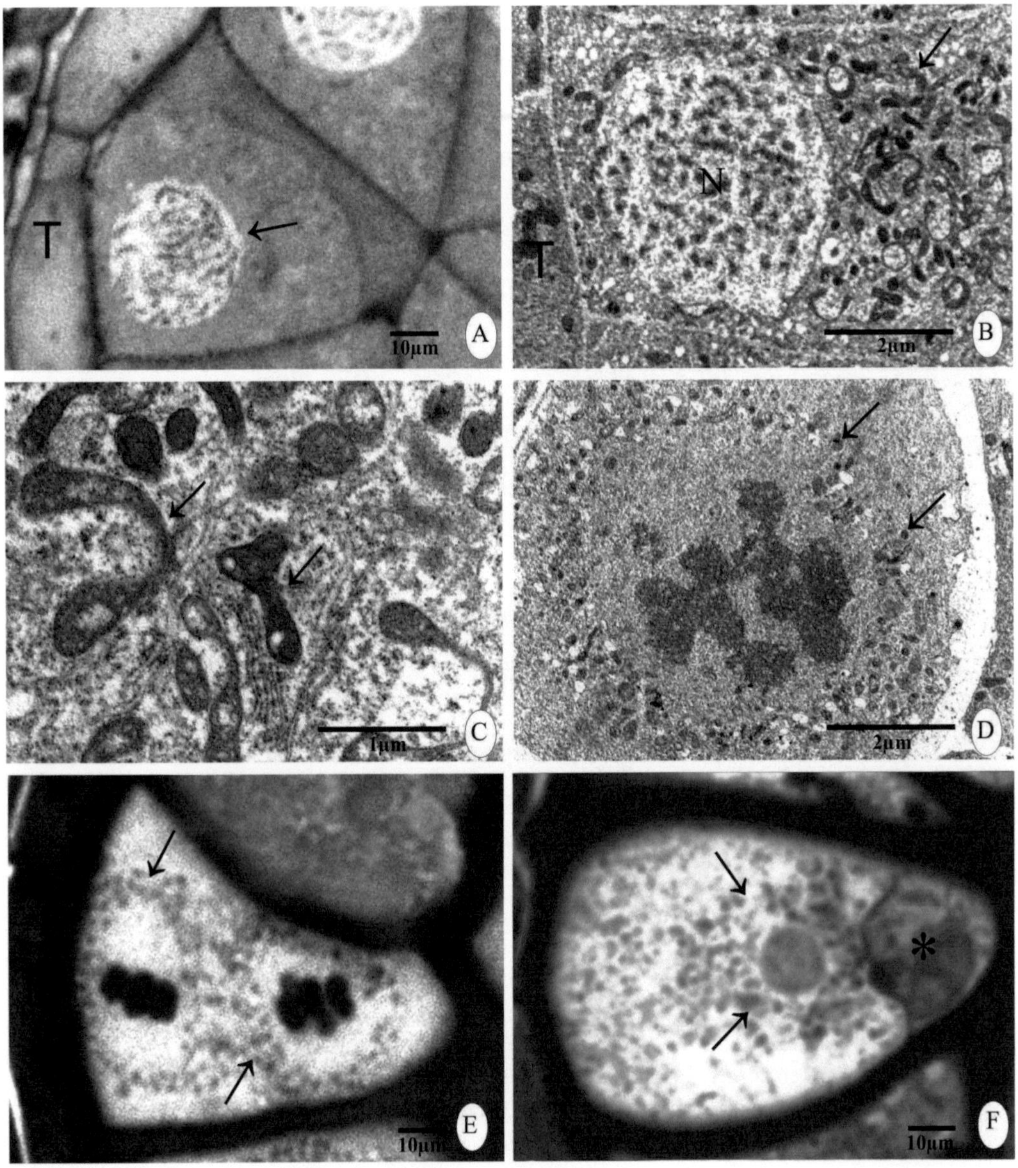


Fig. 7. Pseudomonads of *Eleocharis sellowiana*. (A) The nucleus is present in basal region of the androspore mother cell (arrow), during initial prophase. Toluidine blue 100X. (B) Electron micrograph of prophase I showing the organelles (arrow) located in the apical cytoplasm. (C) Detail of the figure 8B. Note organelles (arrow) in process of division, most of them are proplastids, mitochondria and rough endoplasmic reticulum. (D) Electron micrograph showing metaphase I. Arrows indicate organelles organized surrounding chromosomes. (E) Androspore mother cell during metaphase II exhibiting a cord of organelles (arrows) surrounding chromosomes. Toluidine blue. (F) Photomicrograph showing pseudomonad during final meiosis. The degenerative nuclei are at the cell apex (*). The arrows indicate remained organelles involving the functional nucleus. Toluidine blue. Tapetal cells (T). Nucleus (N).

In *Rhynchospora pubera* the androspores mother cell presents organelles with a polarized distribution, oriented towards the locule region, and the nucleus oriented towards the tapetal region (San Martin et al. 2009). These authors suggest that the pseudomonad undergoes a polarization process even before meiosis occurs. However, in *Carex blanda*, meiosis occurs with the nucleus of the androspore mother cell in the center of the cell and the three degenerative nuclei migrate to the pseudomonad region oriented toward the locule (Brown & Lemmon 2000). The reason why there is more than one type of polarization in the pseudomonads of Cyperaceae is still unknow. However, some cytoplasmic evidences indicate that this organization may be influenced by the behavior of organelles and cytoskeleton.

In *Eleocharis sellowiana*, as well as in other Cyperaceae, the androspores appears asymmetrically organized, culminating in pseudomonads polarized as found in *Carex*. However, in the early stages of meiosis the organelles develop an atypical arrangement around the chromosome complement. At prophase I, the nucleus occupy the basal region of the cell (Figure 7A-B) and the organelles increase in size and in number (Figure 7C). At metaphase I the organelles surround the chromosomes establishing a dense "Organelles Cord" (Figure 7D). This arrangement has not been documented for other Cyperaceae species, although it was reported in *Malva silvestris* (Kudlicka and Rodkiewicz 1990) and *Lavatera thuringiaca* (Tchórzewska *et al.* 2008). This "organelles cord" is held up sourrounding the chromosomes set until telophase I, when the phragmoplast is established. As meiosis progresses, the regions occupied by the phragmoplast are occupied by organelles cord, being one for each chromosome complement. These are held up until metaphase II / anaphase II (Figure 7E). There is evidence of organelles cord being maintained in one of the four nuclei after telophase II, and it is possibly important to select the functional nucleus. The functional one appears surrounded by an organelles cord in the pseudomonads in *E. sellowiana* (Figure 7F). The biological role of the organelles cord found in the *E. sellowiana* androspore mother cell remains uncertain, but the data suggest that it could influence in the delimitation of functional and degenerative nuclei at the transition from anaphase II to telophase II.

In *Rhynchospora pubera*, polarization occurs independent of the presence of organelles cord, and in the pseudomonads the functional nucleus appears directed to the anther locule. Toward the asymmetric and simultaneous cytokinesis, the degenerative nuclei are isolated after phragmoplast fusion and formation of an electron dense pectic wall (Figure 8A-B) (San Martin et al. 2011 in press). The degenerative nuclei are thus isolated with portions of cytoplasm containing organelles (Figure 8A-B). This shows the presence of two cell domains: one of them functional and the other degenerative. In this way, four androspores are formed, but three are eliminated (Figure 6A-B, 8A). This entire ensemble is contained in a single sporoderm with a maturating exine, constituted by tectum and columelle. (Figure 8A). In the cytoplasm of the functional domain, there are lipid droplets, which is not seen in the degenerative domain (Figure 8A). Vacuoles, mitochondria and other organelles are found both in the functional and in the degenerative domain (Figure 8A-B). Folded of rough endoplasmicc reticulum membranes are present in the functional cytoplasm, in some cases associated with lipid droplets (Figure 8C). The cytoplasm portions that envelop the degenerative androspores show signs of shrinkage, which does not occur in the cytoplasm of the functional androspore (Figure 8A-B). The degenerative androspore nuclei are small with more packed chromatin, seen both at light microscopy and at transmission electron microscopy. The chromatin in the functional nucleus is unpacked, indicating high metabolic activity (Figure 6B, 8A-B).

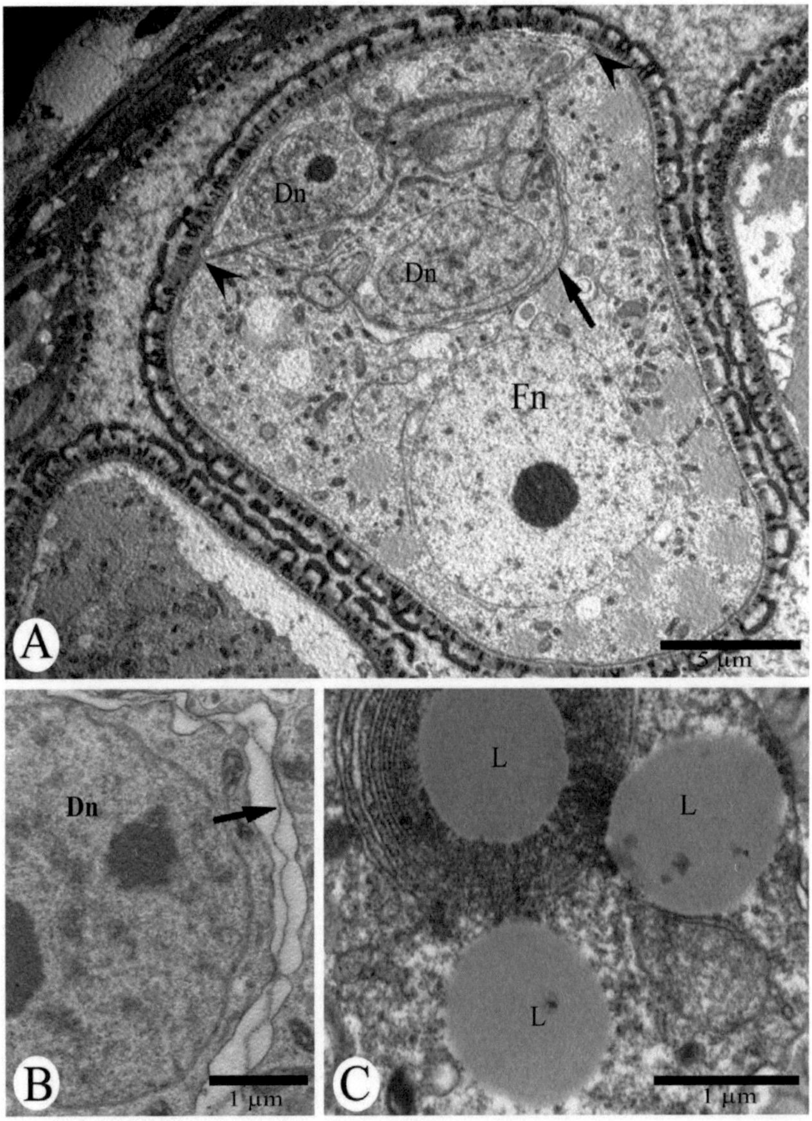


Fig. 8. Transmission electron micrographs of the pseudomonad of *Rhynchospora pubera*. (A) General view. Degenerative nuclei with chromatin packed and isolated by a wall (arrow), which establishes contact with intine (arrowhead). In the functional nucleus chromatin is unpacked. (B) Detail of inner cell wall isolating the degenerative androspores, arrows show the electrondense string in the inner of phragmoplast. (C) Free lipid droplets associated with folded membranes in the cytoplasm of functional androspore. (Dn) degenerative nucleus; (Fn) functional nucleus; (L) lipid droplet.

The degenerative androspores present ultrastructural characteristics of programmed cell death, highlighted by the packed chromatin, cytoplasmic shrinkage and vacuolation (Coimbra et al., 2004). On the other hand, the functional androspore shows characteristics of a cell during a phase of high molecule synthesis, evidenced by the unpacked chromatin, lipid droplets accumulation and presence of a well-developed rough endoplasmic reticulum. A crucial aspect in pseudomonad development in Cyperaceae is the occurrence of an asymmetrical cytokinesis after meiosis. This enables cell polarization and the isolation of the three degenerative androspores. In the same way, it allows the signalization to the programmed cell death, in degenerative domain, does not influences in the development of the functional domain.

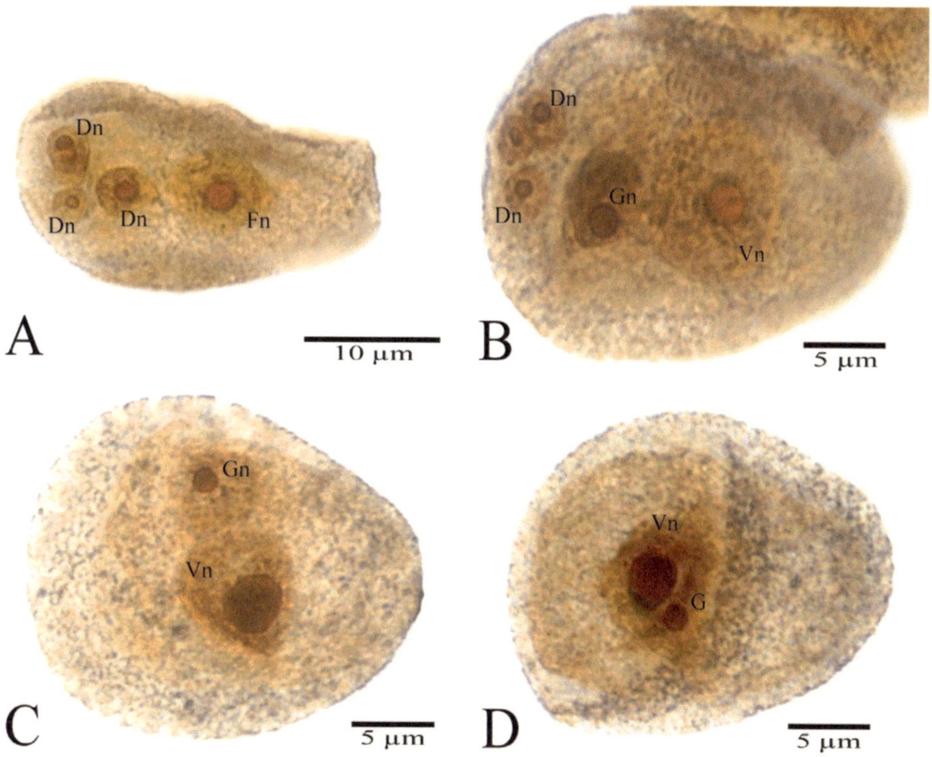


Fig. 9. Squash technique of the pseudomonad of *Rhynchospora pubera* stained with silver impregnation (AgNO3) to evidence ribonucleoproteins. (A) Four pseudomonad nuclei, three degenerative and one functional. (B) Gametophyte after first mitosis, showing the vegetative nucleus and the nucleus of the generative cell, in the presence of degenerative sporophytic nuclei. (C) After the complete PCD of the non-functional microspores, the generative cell and the vegetative nucleus are placed together in the central region of the pseudomonad. (D) Mature androphyte with vegetative cell and one gametic cell after generative cell mitosis. (Dn) Degenerative nucleus; (Fn) functional nucleus; (Gn) generative nucleus; (G) gametic cell; (Vn) vegetative nucleus.

Even in the presence of the degenerative androspores, the functional androspore undergoes mitosis giving rise to the vegetative and degenerative cell (Figure 9A-B), forming the young male gametophyte. After the complety elimination of the degenerative androspores , the generative cells gives rise to the gametic cells, through mitosis. Thus, the pollen grain (mature male gametophyte) is released from the anther in its tricellular form (Figure 9C-D).

The evolutionary history and adaptive advantage of developing a single functional androspore, instead of the four usual ones, remain unknown. A hypothesis would be that the increased volume of the cytoplasm would also increase the adaptive character of the cell (Ranganath & Nagashree 2000). This idea can be supported by the similarity of gynospore formation, where three of the four products of meiosis degenerate, resulting in an increased volume of the functional gynospore that will give rise to the female gametophyte.

Even so, some questions remain unanswered about androsporogenesis in the Cyperaceae family: 1) What is the biological reason for the degeneration of three of the four nuclei formed after meiosis? 2) Why does polarization occur differently in different genera? 3) Is the selection of functional and degenerative nuclei a chance phenomenon or not? 4) Does selection occur in favor of the functional nucleus or of the degenerative ones? 5) At what time during meiosis does the cellular signalling system act on the choice of nuclei?

### 4.2.2 Post-reductional meiosis in cyperaceae

Another poorly understood cytological feature about representatives of Cyperaceae, as well as, of holocentric chromosomes, is the post-reductional or inverted meiosis. This meiotic behavior was reported in *Carex* (Heilborn 1928) and it has been considered typical from members of Cyperaceae.

The inverted meiosis was also reported to *Luzula*, Juncaceae (Nordenskiöld 1951), and *Cuscuta*, Convolvulaceae (Guerra & Garcia 2004), as well as for some insect groups, but in the last case it was always associated with sex chromosomes and not with autosomes (Solari 1979; Pérez et al. 1997; Bongiorni et al. 2004). Besides holocentric chromosomes presented kinetic activity diffused along its major axis at mitosis (Nagaki et al. 2005), there is evidence of kinetic activity only in the terminal region of each chromatid, with spindle fibers attached directly to each one of the four chromatids (Vieira et al. 2009; Guerra et al. 2010). This arrangement could allow the formation of "box structures" of the bivalents (see Pazy & Plitmann 1987, Vanzela et al. 2000 and Guerra et al. 2010). However, there is no convincing image in the literature that shows a "box structure" directed to inverted meiosis, with the four chromatids completely individualized. Thus, we do not consider this enough to define the existence of inverted meiosis. In fact, it is very difficult to show if segregation of sister chromatids or homologous chromosomes has occurred using only conventional staining, unless there is a chromosome marker that allow to visualize each one of the chromatids. It is possible to univalents and sex chromosomes of insects (Hughes-Schrader & Schrader 1961; Vieira et al. 2009). The last author questioned the wide use of inverted meiosis for holocentric autosomes because reduction of part of the chromatid always occurs when there is chiasmate in bivalents, independent of orientation. This has been well documented in insects (Bongiorni et al. 2004; Nokkala et al. 2006), but not mentioned in plants (Nordenskiöld 1951, Strandhede 1965; Vanzela et al. 2000).

There are at least two excellent examples of inverted meiosis in plants. In the first case, Pazy (1997) showed the separation of sister chromatids in B-chromosomes in anaphase I of *Cuscuta babylonica*. In the second case, Da Silva et al. (2005) reported the separation of sister chromatids for all homologous of *Eleocharis subarticulata* (Cyperaceae). However, the two cases can be considered special situations due to the presence of a univalent B-chromosome and of a karyotype with multivalents rearranged by disploidy, respectively. But independent of these arguments, this atypical meiotic behavior has been referred only to organisms with holocentric chromosomes (Viera et al. 2009). Here we show evidence of reductional, or normal meiosis, in at least one chromosome pair of *Rhynchospora pubera*.

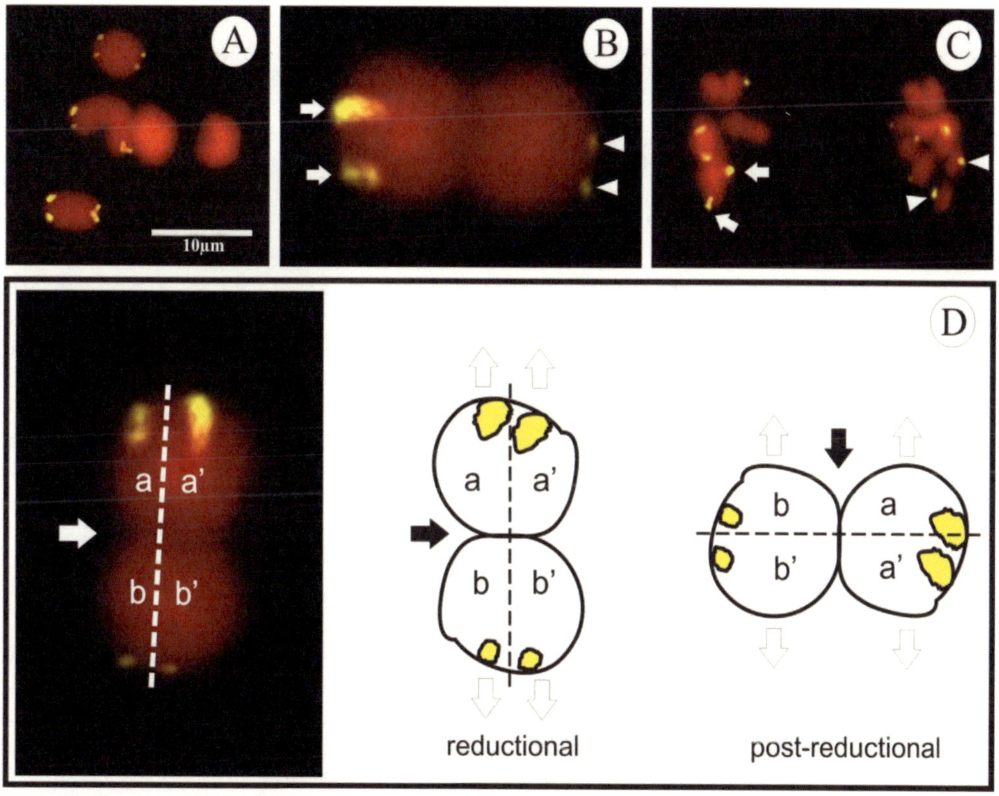


Fig. 10. Meiotic cells of *Rhynchospora pubera* hybridized with biotiniled 45S rDNA probe and detected with avidin-FITC. (A) Metaphase I showing pairs 1, 2 and 4 with terminal hybridizations signals. (B) Pair 2 isolated. Observe sister chromatids laterally joined while homologous are joined end-to-end. This bivalent shows a heteromorphism in the hybridization signals size (arrows and arrowshead). (C) Anaphase I and (D) Scheme with the second pair. Both images show segregation of homologous chromosomes and not sister chromatids. Arrows in (C) point out homologous of pair 2 with major signals and the arrowheads indicate the other homologous with minor hybridization signals. Thus, at least to pair 2 the meiosis was reductional and not inverted. The scheme in (D) was elaborated from pair 2 (on the left). The normal sense is the segregation of the homologues (center image), and not the segregation of sister chromatids in the first anaphase (on the right).

This event is enough to question the occurrence of inverted meiosis in all chromosomes and species of Cyperaceae. *R. pubera* exhibits six chromosomes with terminal 45S rDNA sites (Vanzela et al. 1998). Fortunately, we found one individual with a polymorphism in pair 2, which presents one of the homologous with a major hybridization signal after FISH with 45S rDNA probe. This event allowed accompanying the bivalent segregation in anaphase I and found the separation of homologous chromosomes, and not of sister chromatids (Figure 10).

This evidence raises doubts about some published images on bivalents in "box", which were interpreted as a conclusive diagnosis of post-reductional meiosis of all bivalents (Vanzela et al. 2000). At this time, there are no certainties as to whether all bivalents or part of them are oriented together or re-oriented independently, i. e., the post-reductional meiosis may occur but, is it necessary that all autosomes always behave the same way?

## 5. Acknowledgment

This work is part of doctoral thesis from Adriano Silvério and Érica Duarte-Silva, carried out at Programa de Pós-Graduação em Botânica da UFRGS. We thank CAPES, CNPq and FAPERGS for finnacial support, and the laboratories of Porto Alegre and Londrina for the use of the structure and tecnologies.

## 6. Conclusion

Firstly, based on Hofmeister's theory (1851), the life cycle of plants consists of two generations: sporophytic and gametophytic. In flowering plants, gametophytic generation is reduced to pollen (male gametophyte) and embryo sac (female gametophyte). In the sphere of studies on plant reproduction, is necessary limit the sexual terminology to the gametophytes, erradicating the sexual terminology applied to sporophytes, specially, the terms: male, female and hermophroditic flowers. In the second, the study of cellular and sub-cellular aspects of meiosis can improve the comprehension of plant meiosis process, particularly in cases of staminal or pollen sterility, as well as, in studies of uncommon types of meiosis, illustrated by pseudomonads in Cyperaceae.

## 7. References

Ainsworth, C. C. (1999) *Sex determination in plants*. BIOS Scientific Publishers Limited. ISBN:1859960421.USA.

APG III. (2009). Un update of the Angiosperm Phylogeny Group classification for the orders and families of flowering plants: APG III. *Botanical Journal of Linnean Society*. Vo. 161, No. 2, (October 2009), pp. 122-127, ISSN: 0024-4074.

Ariizumi, T.; Hatakeyama, K.; Hinata, K.; Inatsugi, R.; Nishida, I.; Sato, S.; Kato, T.; Tabata, S.; Toriyama, K. (2004). Disruption of the novel plant protein NEF1 affects lipid acumulation in the plastids of the tapetum and exine formation of pollen resulting in male sterility in Arabidopsis thaliana. *The Plant Journal*. Vo. 39, No. 2, (June 2004): pp. 170-181, ISSN: 0960-7412

Barrett, S. C. H. (2002). The evolution of plant sexual diversity. *Nature Genetics*. Vo. 3, (April 2001), pp. 274-284, ISSN: 1061-4036.

Bhat, V.; Dwivedi, K. K.; Khurana, J. P.; Sopory, S. K. (2005). Apomixis: An enigma with potencial applications. Special section: Embriology of flowering plants. *Current Science*. Vo. 89, No. 10, (December 2005), pp. 1879-1893, ISSN: 0011-3891.

Bione, N. C. P.; Pagliarini, M. S.; Almeida, L. A.; Seifert, A. L. (2002). An ms2 male sterile, female-fertile soybean sharing phenotypic expression with other ms mutant. *Plant Breeding*. Vo. 121, No. 4, (August 2002), pp. 307-313, ISSN: 0179-9541.

Blanvillain, R.; Boavida, L. C.; McCormick, S.; Ow., D. W. (2008). *EXPORTIN*1 genes are essential for development and function of the gametophytes in *Arabidopsis thaliana*. *Genetics*. Vo. 180, No. 3, (November 2008), pp. 1493-1500. ISSN: 0016-6731.

Boavida, L. C.; Vieria, A. M.; Becker, J. D.; Feijó, J. A. (2005). Gametophyte interaction and sexual reproduction: how plants make a zygote. *The International Journal of Developmental Biology*. Vo. 49, No. 5/6, pp. 615-632. ISSN: 0214-6282.

Bongiorni, S.; Fiorenzo, P.; Pippoletti, D.; Prantera, G. (2004). Inverted meiosis and meiotic drive in mealybugs. *Chromosoma*. Vo.112, No.7, (March 2004), pp331–341, ISSN: 0009-5915.

Brown, R. C.; Lemmon, B. E. (2000). The cytoskeleton and polarization during pollen development in *Carex blanda* (Cyperaceae). *American Journal of Botany*. Vo. 87, No. 1, pp. 1-11, ISSN: 0002-9122.

Camerarius, R. J. (1694). *De Sexu Plantarum Epistola*. Literis Erhardtianis.Tübingen, Germany.

Chaubal, R.; Zanella, C.; Trimnel, M.R.; Fox, T.W.; Albertsen, M.C.; Bedinger, P. (2000). Two male-sterile mutants of *Zea mays* (Poaceae) with an extra cell divison in the anther wall. *American Journal of Botany*. Vo. 87, No. 8, (August 2000), pp. 1193-1201. ISSN: 0002-9122.

Cocucci, A. E. (1969). El processo sexual en angiospermas. *Kurtziana*. Vo. 5, No. 5, (June 1969), pp. 407-423, ISSN: 1852-5962.

Cocucci, A. E. (1973). Some suggestions on the evolution of gametophytes of higher plants. *Phytomorphology*. Vo. 23, pp. 109-124, ISSN: 0031-9449.

Cocucci, A. E. (1980). Precisiones sobre la terminología sexológica aplicada a angiospermas. *Boletín de la Sociedad Argentina de Botánica*. Vo.11, No.1-2, (July 1980), pp. 75-81, ISSN: 0373-580X.

Cocucci, A. E.; Hunziker A. T. (1994). *Los ciclos biológicos en el reino vegetal* (2°ed.), Academia Nacional de Ciências, ISBN: 0325-3406, Argentina.

Cocucci, A. E.; Mariath, J. E. A. (1995) Sexualidade em plantas. *Ciência Hoje* Vo. 18, No. 106, pp. 51-61, ISSN: 0101-8515.

Cocucci, A. E. (2006). La embriologia e los sistemas reproductivos de Angiospermae. In: *Os Avanços da Botânica no início do século XXI*. Mariath, J. E. A.; Santos, R. P. p. 97-102. Sociedade Botânica do Brasil, ISBN: 8560428003. Brazil.

Coen, I. J. (2010). A case to which no parallel exists: the influence of Darwin's diferente forms of flowers. *American Journal of Botany*. Vo. 97, No. 5, (April 2010), pp.701-716, ISSN: 0002-9122.

Coimbra, S.; Torrao, L.; Abreu, I. (2004). Programmed cell death induces male sterility in *Actidia deliciosa* female flowers. *Plant physiologi and biochemistry*. Vo. 42, pp. 537-541. ISSN: 0981-9428

Cruden R. W.; Lloyd R. M. (1995). Embryophytes have equivalent sexual phenotypes and breeding systems: why not a common terminology to describe them? *American Journal of Botany*. Vo. 82. No. 6, (June 1995), pp. 816-825, ISSN: 0002-9122.

Da Silva, C. R. M.; González-Elizondo, M. S.; Vanzela, A. L. L. (2005). Reduction of chromosome number in *Eleocharis subarticulata* (Cyperaceae) by multiple translocation. *Botanical Journal of the Linnean Society*. Vo. 149, No. 4, (December 2005), pp.457–464, ISSN: 1095-8339.

Dafni A.; Firmage D. (2000). Pollen viability and longevity: practical, ecological and evolutionary implications. *Plant Systematics and Evolution*. Vo. 222, No. 1, (March 2000), pp. 113-132, ISSN: 0378-2697.

Duarte-Silva, E.; Vanzela, A. L. L.; Mariath, J. E. A. (2010). Developmental and cytogenetic analysis of pollen sterility in *Valeriana scandens* L. *Sexual Plant Reproduction*, Vo. 23, No. 2, (June 2010), pp. 105-113, ISSN 0934-0882.

Duarte-Silva, E.; Rodrigues, L. R.; Mariath, J. E. A. (2011). Contradictory results in pollen viability determination of Valeriana scandens L. *Gene Conserve, in press*. ISSN 1808-1878.

Darwin, C. R. (1877). *The different forms of flowers on plants of the same species*. Murray, England.

Dong, X.; Zonglie, H.; Sivaramakrishnan, M.; Mahfouz, M.; Verma, P. S. (2005). Callose synthase (CalS5) is required for exine formation during microgametogenesis and for pollen viability in *Arabidopsis*. *The Plant Journal*. Vo. 42, No. 3, (May 2005), pp. 315-328, ISSN: 0960-7412.

Engelke, T.; Hülsmann, S.; Tatlioglu T. (2002). A comparative study of microsporogenesis and anther wall development in different types of genic and citoplasmic male sterilities in chives. *Plant Breeding* Vo. 121, No. 3, (June 2002), pp. 254-258, ISSN: 0179-9541.

Fei H.; Sawhney V. K. (1999). MS32-regulated timing of callose degradation during microsporogenesis in Arabidopsis is associated with the accumulation of staked rough ER in tapetal cells. *Sexual Plant Reproduction.*Vo. 12, No. 3, (June 2002), pp. 188-193, ISSN: 0934-0882.

Fujiki, Y.; Yoshimoto, K.; Ohsumi, Y. (2007). An *Arabidopsis* homolog of yeast ATG6/VPS30 is essential for pollen germination. *Plant Physiology*. Vo. 143, No. 3, (March 2007), pp. 1132-1139, ISSN: 0032-0889.

Furness, C. A.; Rudall, P. J. (1999). Microsporogenesis in monocotyledons. *Annals of Botany* Vo. 84, pp. 475–499, ISSN: 1095-8290.

Guerra, M.; García, M. A. (2004). Heterochromatin and rDNA sites distribution in the holocentric chromosomes of *Cuscuta approximata* Bab. (Convolvulaceae). *Genome*. Vo. 47, No. 1, (February 2004), pp. 134–140, ISSN: 0831-2796.

Guerra, M.; Cabral, G.; Cuacos, M.; González-García, M.; González-Sánchez, M.; Vega, J.; Puertas, M. J. (2010). Neocentrics and Holokinetics (Holocentrics): Chromosomes out of the Centromeric Rules. Cytogenetic and Genome Research. Vo. 129, pp. 82–96, ISSN: 1662-3797.

Goldberg, R. B.; Beals, T. P.; Sanders, P. M. (1993). Anther development: basic principles and practical applications. *The Plant Cell*. Vo. 5, No. 10, (October 1993), pp. 1217-1229, ISSN: 1040-4651.

Greyson, R.I. (1994). *The development of flowers*. Oxford University Press, ISBN: 019506688X, England.

Han, M.; Jung, K.; Yi, G.; Lee, D.; An, G. (2006). *Rice immature pollen 1* (*RIP1*) is a regulator of late pollen development. *Plant and cell physiology*. Vo. 47, No. 11, (January 2007), pp. 1457-1472, ISSN: 0032-0781.

Heilborn, O. (1928). Chromosome studies in Cyperaceae. *Hereditas*. Vo. 11, pp. 182–192. ISSN: 0018-0661.

Hofmeister, W. (1862). On the germination, development and frutification of higher Cryptogamia ando n the frutification of Coniferae (English translation by F. Curry form the 1851 germany edition). London.

Hord, C.L.H.; Chen C.; DeYoung B.J.; Clark S.E.; Ma H. (2006). The *BAM1/BAM2* receptor-like kinases are importantt regulators of early *Arabidopsis* anther development. *Plant Cell*. Vo. 18, No. 7, (July 2006), pp.1667– 1680, ISSN: 1040-4651.

Horner, Jr., H. T. (1977). A Comparative Light- And Electron-Microscopic Study of Microsporogenesis in Male-Fertile and Cytoplasmic Male-Sterile Sunflower (Helianthus Annuus). *American Journal of Botany*. Vo. 64, No. 6, (July 1977), pp.745-759, ISSN: 0002-9122.

Huang, L.; Cao, J.; Zhang, A.; Ye, Y.; Liu, T. (2009). The Polygalacturonase gene BcMF2 from *Brassica campestris* is associated with intine development. *Journal of Experimental Botany*. Vo. 60, No. 1, (November 2008), pp. 301-313, ISSN: 0022-0957.

Johns, C.; Lu, M.; Lyznik, A.; Mackenzie, S. (1998). A mitochondrial DNA sequences isassociated with Abnormal Pollen Development in Cytoplasmic Male Sterile Bean Plants. *Genetics*. Vo. 150, No. 1, (September 1998), pp. 383-391, ISSN: 0016-6731.

Hughes-Schrader, S.; Schrader, F. (1961). The kinotochore of the Hemiptera. *Chromosoma.* Vo.12, pp.327 - 350. ISSN: 0009-5915.

Kaplan, D. R.; Cooke, T. J. (1996). The genius of Wilhelm Hofmeister: The origin of causal analytical research plant development. *American Journal of Botany.* Vo. 83, No. 12, (December 1996), pp. 1647-1660, ISSN: 0002-9122.

Karasawa, M.M.G. (2009). *Diversidade reprodutiva de plantas.* Sociedade Brasileira de Genética. ISBN:978-85-89265-12-6. Brazil.

Kaul, M.L.H. (1988). *Male sterility in higher plants. Monographs on the theoretical and applied genetics, 10.* Springer. ISBN: 0387179526. Germany.

Kirpes, C. C.; Clark, L. G.; Lersten, N. R. (1996). Systematic significance of pollenarrangement in microsporangia of Poaceae and Cyperaceae: review andobservations on representative taxa. *American Journal of Botany* Vo.83, pp1609–1622. ISSN: 0002-9122.

Li, N.; Da-Sheng, Z.; Hai-Sheng, L.; Xiao-xing, L.; Wan-qi, L.; Zheng, Y.; Huang-Wei, C.; Wang J.; Tie-Qiao, W.; Hai, H.; Luo, D.; Hong, M.; Da-Bing, Z. (2006). The rice tapetum degeneration retardation gene is required for tapetum degradation and anther development. *The Plant Cell.* Vo. 18, No. 2, (February 2006), pp. 2999-3014, ISSN: 1532-298X.

Linnaeus, C. (1810). *Système sexuel des végétaux: suivant les classes, les orders, les genres et les espèces, avec les caractères et les differences* (2° ed.). Arthus-Bertrand. France.

Nagaki, K.; Kashihara, K.; Murata, M. (2005). Visualization of diffuse centromeres with centromere-specific histone H3 in the holocentric plant *Luzula nivea. The Plant Cell.* Vo. 17, No. 7, (June 2005), pp. 1886–1893, ISSN: 1532-298X.

Nokkala, S.; Kuznetsova, V. G.; Maryanska-Nadachowska, A.; Nokkala, C. (2006). Holocentric chromosomes in meiosis. II. The modes of orientation and segregation of a trivalent. *Chromosome Research.* Vo. 14, No. 5, (March 2006), pp. 559-565, ISSN: 1573-6849.

Nordenskiöld, H. (1951). Cyto-taxonomical studies in the genus *Luzula* I. Somatic chromosomes and chromosomes numbers. *Hereditas.* Vo. 37, pp. 325-355, ISSN: 0018-0661.

Papini, A; Mosti, S.; Brighigna, L. (1999). Programmed-cell death events during tapetum development of angiosperms. *Protoplasma.* Vo. 207, No. 3-4, (September 1999), pp. 213-221, ISSN: 0033-183X.

Pazy, B. (1997). Supernumerary chromosomes and their behaviour in meiosis of the holocentric *Cuscuta babylonica* Choisy. *Botanical Journal of the Linnean Society* Vo.123, No. 2, (February 1997), pp. 173–17,. ISSN: 1095-8339.

Pérez, R.; Panzera, F.; Page, J.; Suja, J. A.; Rufas, J. S. (1997). Meiotic behaviour of holocentric chromosomes: orientation and segregation of autosomes in *Triatoma infestans* (Heteroptera). *Chromosome Research.* Vo. 5, No. 1, (February 1997), pp.47–56, ISSN: 1573-6849.

Peirson, B.N.; Owen H.A.; Feldmann K.A.; Makaroff, C.A. (1996). Characterization of three male sterile mutants of *Arabidopsis thaliana* exhibiting alterations in meiosis. *Sexual Plant Reproduction* Vo. 9, No. 1, pp. 1-16, ISSN: 0934-0882.

Ranganath, R. M.; Nagashee, N. R. (2000) Selective cell elimination during microsporogenesis in sedges. *Sexual Plant Reproduction.* Vo. 13, No. 1, (March 2000), pp. 53–60, ISSN: 0934-0882.

Quammen, D.; Shimitz, H. (2007). A passion for order. *National Geographic.* (June 2007). ISSN: 0027-9358.

San Martin, J. A. B.; Andrade, C. G. T. J.; Vanzela, A. L. L. (2009). Early meiosis in Rhynchospora pubera L. (Cyperaceae) is marked by uncommon ultrastructural features. *Cell Biology Interantional* Vo. 33, No. 10, (October 2009), pp. 1118-1122, ISSN: 106i5-6995.

San Martin, J. A. B.; Andrade, C. G. T. J; Mastroberti, A. A.; Mariath, J. E. A; Vanzela, A. L. L. (2011). Asymmetric tetrads and programmed cell death in the pseudomonads of Rhynchospora pubera (Cyperaceae). *Annals of Botany, in press.* ISSN: 1095-8290.

Selling, O. H. (1947). Studies in the Hawaiian pollen statistics. Part II. Thepollens of the Hawaiian phanerogams. *Bishop Museum Bulletin in Botany* Vo. 38, pp. 1–430, ISSN: 0893-3138.

Smith, M.B.; Palmer, R.G.; Horner, R.T. (2002). Microscopy of a citoplasmic male-sterile from an interspecific cross between Glycine max and G. soja (Leguminosae). *American Journal of Botany.* Vo. 89, No. 3, (March 2002), pp. 417-426, ISSN: 0002-9122.

Solari, A. J. (1979). Autosomal synaptonemal complex and sex chromosomes without axes in *Triatoma infestans* (Reduviidae, Hemiptera). *Chromosoma.* Vo. 72, pp. 225-240, ISSN: 0009-5915.

Strandhede, S. O. (1965). Chromosome studies in *Eleocharis*, subser. Palustres. *Opera Botanica.* Vo. 9, pp. 1–86. ISSN: 0078-5237.

Strandhede, S. O. (1973). Pollen development in the Eleocharis palustris group (Cyperaceae). II. Cytokinesisand microspore degeneration. *Botaniska Notiser.* Vo. 126, pp. 255–265. ISSN: 0006-8195

Sun, M.; Ganders, F.R. (1987). Microsporogenesis in male-sterile and hermaphroditic plants of nine gynodioecius taxa in Hawaiian *Bidens* (Asteraceae). *American Journal of Botany.* Vo. 74, No. 2, (February 1987), pp. 209-217, ISSN: 0002-9122.

Teng, C.; Dong, H.; Shi, L.; Deng, Y.; Mu, J.; Zhang, J.; Yang, X.; Zuo, J. (2008). Serine Palmitoyltransferase, a key enzyme for male gametophyte development in *Arabidopsis*. *Plant Physiology* Vo. 146, No. 3, (March 2008), pp. 1322- 1332, ISSN: 0032-0889.

Trelease, W. (1916). Two new terms cormophytaster and xeniophyte anxiomatically fundamental in botany. *Proccedings of the American Philosophical Society* Vo. 55, No. 3, pp. 237-242.ISSN: 0003-049X.

Vanzela, A. L. L.; Cuadrado, A.; Jouve, N.; Luceño, M.; Guerra, M. (1998) Multiple locations of the rDNA in species of *Rhynchospora* (Cyperaceae). *Chromosome Research* Vo.6, No.5, (March 1998), pp.345–349.

Vanzela A. L. L.; Luceño, M.; Guerra, M. (2000). Karyotype evolution and cytotaxonomy in Brazilian species of *Rhynchospora* Vahl (Cyperaceae). *Botanical Journal of the Linnean Society.* Vo.134, No.4 (June 2000), pp.557–566. ISSN: 1095-8339.

Viera, A.; Page, J.; Rufas, J. S. (2009). Inverted meiosis: the true bugs as a model to study. *Genome Dynamics.* Vo. 5, pp. 137–156, ISSN: 1662-3797.

Wagenitz, G. (1999). Botanical Terminology and Homology in Their Historical Context. *Plant Ecology and Evolution* Vo.68, No. 1/2 (March 1999), pp. 33-37, ISSN:1374-7886.

Zàrsky, V.; Tupy, J. (1995). A missed anniversary: 300 years after Rudolf Jacob Camerarius 'De sexu plantarum epistola'. *Sexual Plant Reproduction.* Vo. 8, No. 6, (November 1995), pp. 375-376, ISSN:0934-0882.

Zhang, Z.; Lu, Y.; Liu, X.; Feng, J.; Zhang, G. (2006). Cytological mechanism of pollen abortion resulting from allelic interaction of F1 pollen sterility locus in rice (*Oryza sativa* L.). *Genetica* Vo. 127, No. 1-3, (May 2006), pp. 295-302, ISSN: 0016-6707.

# 22

# Investigating Host Induced Meiosis in a Fungal Plant Pathogen

B. J. Saville, M. E. Donaldson and C. E. Doyle
*Trent University,*
*Canada*

## 1. Introduction

Fungal spores lend the smut and rust plant diseases their names. Smut fungi produce massive numbers of dark, dust like, thick walled teliospores and the name, smut, is derived from the older definition meaning dark smudge from soot, smoke or dirt. The rust fungi produce diseases characterised by the production of pustules erupting from the plant surface. They contain urediniospores which are often orange or rusty in colour. Spores are essential for fungal survival, providing a means of dispersal and often a structure to protect the fungus; they are also integral to fungal meiosis. Smut and rust fungi are biotrophs, meaning they derive their nutrients from living plant hosts. This interaction is very intimate, involving fungal penetration of the plant cell walls but not the plasma membranes (e.g. Snetselaar & Mims, 1992; Voegele & Mendgen, 2003). As such, most smut and rust fungi have only evolved to infect (and become meiotically competent within) one or a limited number of host species.

The economic impact of these pathogens is well illustrated by considering two crops significantly damaged by them: corn and wheat. According to Capitol Commodity Services (2011), corn remains the largest valued crop in the United States, totalling $67 billion in 2010. World-wide, corn crops were estimated at $163 billion in 2010 (U.S. Grains Council, 2010). The comparable numbers for wheat were $13 billion, and $140 billion, respectively (Capitol Commodity Services, 2011; U.S. Department of Agriculture, 2011). Although mitigated by varieties with partial resistance, the maize crop loss resulting from common smut of corn, caused by *Ustilago maydis*, is 2% annually, equivalent to ~$1 billion (Allen et al., 2011; Martinez-Espinoza et al., 2002). Wheat crop losses due to wheat leaf rust *Puccinia triticina* Eriks, which is the most common and widely distributed wheat rust, results in trace to 10% crop losses in many countries around the world. In the US, from 2000 to 2004, the loss was $350 million/year, and it can be $100 million/year in Canada. The production in China is more than twice that of the US and commonly suffers 10-30% crop loss per year (Huerta-Espino et al., 2011). There is also an extreme threat from emerging races of stripe rust of wheat (*Puccinia striiformis* f. sp. *tritici*) and wheat stem rust (*Puccinia graminis* f. sp. *tritici*). The emerging stem rust races are referred to collectively as UG99 after their location of origin (Uganda), and year of detection (1999). These races are virulent on the vast majority of wheat varieties cultivated around the world. It is predicted that if resistant varieties are not developed and utilized that the UG99 epidemic in Africa will become global (Singh et al., 2011).

The impact of smut and rust fungi is limited by deploying resistant crop varieties; however, the fungi overcome the resistance leading to cycles in which varieties with new resistances are released and fungi with new virulence genotypes arise. While new virulence alleles ultimately result from mutation, genotypic diversity is created through recombination. Some populations of leaf rust have a genetic structure consistent with an asexual dikaryotic population "within which stepwise mutation at avirulence or virulence loci regularly occurs" (Ordoñez & Kolmer, 2009). In contrast, greatly increased genetic diversity and epidemics of stem rust have been linked to sexual reproduction (Burdon & Reolfs, 1985; Jin, 2011) and eradicating the alternate host for stem rust, common barberry and other *Berberis* spp. on which sexual reproduction occurs, has provided substantial benefit in controlling wheat stem rust (Roelfs, 1982) and, inadvertently, stripe rust of wheat (Jin, 2011). Further, the corn smut pathogen *U. maydis* exists in predominantly out-crossing populations (Barnes et al., 2004). This suggests a key role for sexual reproduction in the emergence and maintenance of virulence genotypes.

The rust fungi are obligate biotrophs and cannot be cultured outside their hosts. The wheat rusts, as typified by stem rust, have five spore stages and require two completely unrelated hosts (Schumann & D'Arcy, 2009). The primary host is wheat and the alternative host is barberry. This complex and interesting life cycle will not be discussed in detail here except to note that, in the stem rust life cycle, meiosis likely initiates *in planta* followed by teliospore maturation (see paragraph below on rust teliospore microscopy). The diploid teliospores are produced late in the season on the primary host, wheat. They germinate and complete meiosis yielding basidiospores that infect the alternate host. In contrast to the rust fungi, the model fungal biotrophic pathogen *U. maydis* (Banuett, 1995; Brefort et al., 2009) is readily cultured in the laboratory on defined media and its sexual cycle can be completed within 28 days following injection of compatible haploid cells into seedlings of the host *Zea mays* (corn). *U. maydis* is amenable to genetic analysis and molecular manipulation, including homologous gene replacement, and several vectors are available for gene expression analysis. An annotated version of the genome sequence of *U. maydis* was released in 2007 (Kämper et al., 2006) and the annotation continues to be improved (e.g. Donaldson & Saville, 2008; Doyle et al., 2011; Ho et al., 2007; Kronstad, 2008; Morrison et al., in preparation). This allows molecular manipulation of *U. maydis* outside the host, followed by molecular analysis in the host.

The *U. maydis* life cycle (Figure 1) begins with teliospore germination and the completion of meiosis to create haploid basidiospores, which divide by budding. Compatible non-pathogenic haploids fuse to form the pathogenic filamentous dikaryon, which proliferates, branches, and penetrates the plant via the formation of specialised cells called appressoria. It grows within and between plant cells eliciting the formation of a tumour. Banuett and Herskowitz (1996) describe a series of developmental events that *U. maydis* undergoes in the tumour leading to teliospore formation. These events occur within the enlarged host cells and include: 1) the formation of hyphal branches at close intervals, 2) the production of a mucilaginous matrix in which the hyphae are embedded and the hyphal tips become lobed, 3) hyphae fragmentation, 4) rounding of fragmented hyphae and 5) the deposition of a pigmented thick cell wall. The pigmented teliospores enter a dormant state, the tumours disintegrate, and the teliospores are dispersed, continuing the cycle.

An overview of how meiosis proceeds in *U. maydis* was presented by Donaldson and Saville (2008). Since the early stages of meiosis occur *in planta* and meiosis is temporally linked to the formation of thick walled dormant teliospores, direct microscopic observation of meiotic events has not been possible. Therefore, it is informative to review how meiosis precedes in the related homobasidiomycete, *Coprinopsis cinerea*. This fungus can be induced to form mushrooms (fruiting bodies) in culture and, in these fruiting bodies, meiosis proceeds in a synchronous manner with over 60% of the approximately 10 million basidia in a given cap at the same stage (Pukkila et al., 1984). Kües, (2000) reviewed meiosis in *C. cinerea* and noted that chromatid duplication in premeiotic S phase is followed by karyogamy, and the cytological events of prophase I precede with the condensation and alignment of chromosomes (leptotene), synapsis (zygotene), and recombination nodule appearance (pachytene). This process, from post karyogamy to pachytene, is completed in six hours (Celerin et al., 2000). It is followed by desynapsis (diplotene) and the transition to metaphase (diakinesis). The second meiotic division occurs fairly rapidly following interphase, with prophase II through telophase II being completed in ~1 hour. The second division occurs in the same plane as the first, across the longitudinal axis of the basidium. Then, chromatid separation is followed by the four nuclei migrating toward the basidium tip where basidiospores form and the nuclei migrate into them then complete a round of mitosis. This overview of basidiomycete meiosis provides a framework for *U. maydis* investigations.

*U. maydis*, like other smut fungi, does not form a fruiting body. Instead, when teliospores germinate, basidia are formed in which meiosis is completed. So while a *C. cinerea* fruiting body has millions of basidia undergoing meiosis, in *U. maydis*, millions of teliospores are dispersed and each produces a basidium. What we know of the cytological events of meiosis in *U. maydis* is that when hyphae are enveloped in the mucilaginous matrix during teliospore formation, they contain a single nucleus, indicating karyogamy has occurred (Banuett & Herskowitz, 1996). If *U. maydis* meiosis follows the pathway of *C. cinerea*, then premeiotic S phase and the duplication of chromatids would have been completed before karyogamy occurred. The next meiotic event we are aware of in *U. maydis* is the germination of the teliospore when the nucleus is in late prophase I (O'Donnell & McLaughlin, 1984). Between karyogamy and germination the teliospore is dormant with extremely limited metabolic activity. This indicates that major meiotic events cannot be occurring; this leaves the possibility that, either there is a pause after karyogamy and meiosis continues with teliospore germination, or that prophase I and recombination events begin immediately after karyogamy and pause, perhaps at the pachytene checkpoint, when the teliospore becomes dormant. Following germination, the metaphase I spindles align with the longitudinal axis of the metabasidium, and a transverse septum forms, indicating the completion of telophase I and leading to the formation of two cells (O'Donnell & McLaughlin, 1984). This is rapidly followed by meiosis II, in which the nucleus in each cell migrates to a central location, divides and septa are formed, resulting in three haploid nuclei, each in a basidium cell. The fourth nucleus migrates to the base of the teliospore (Ramberg & McLaughlin, 1980). Basidospores form by budding, each basidium cell nucleus migrates into the respective basidiospore and divides, then one nucleus remains and the other migrates back into the basidium cell (Banuett, 1995). Basidiospores continue to divide by budding.

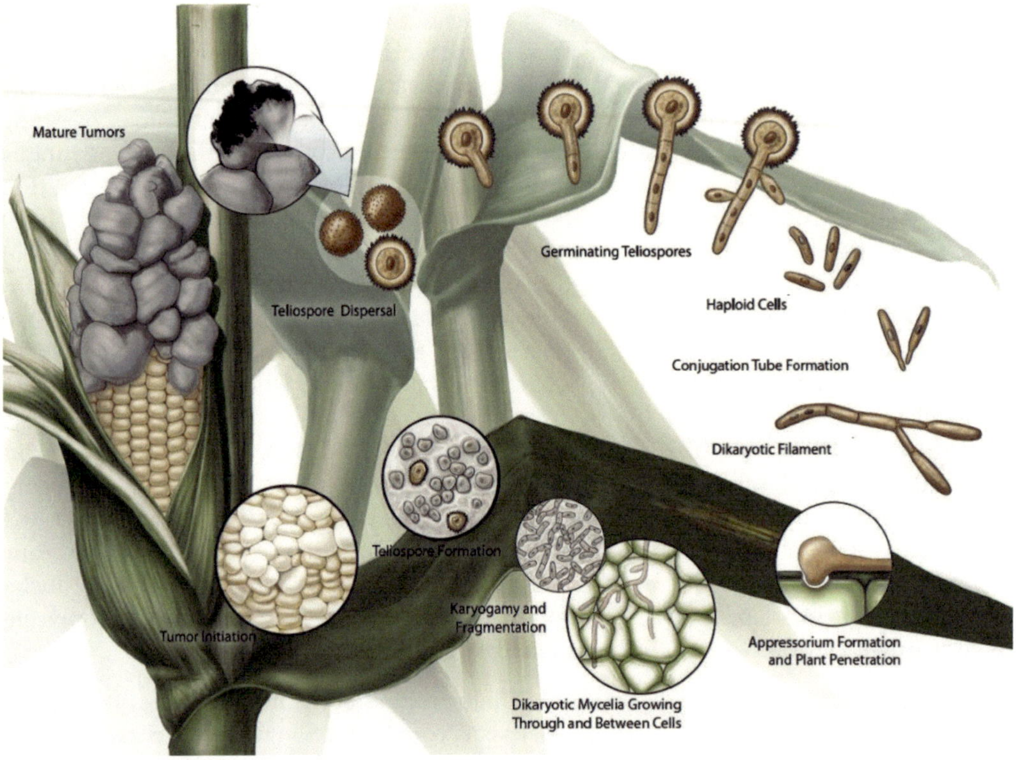


Fig. 1. The Life Cycle of *Ustilago maydis*. In this diagram, meiosis begins soon after karyogamy, pauses at pachytene during teliospore dispersal, and meiosis resumes during teliospore germination.

Support for the idea of meiosis proceeding immediately after karyogamy and pausing at pachytene comes from microscopic analysis of a number of rust fungi, notably *Coleosporium ipomoeae* (Mims & Richardson, 2005). This rust fungus, like other members of the *Coleosporium* genus, has thin cell walls which enable stained nuclei to be observed in developing, mature and germinating teliospores. Mims and Richardson (2005) observed synaptonemal complexes in a high percentage of the nuclei in unhydrated *C. ipomoeae* teliospores. This indicated that meiosis had begun soon after karyogamy and was interrupted or arrested at pachytene, where it remained until the teliospores were hydrated. Mims and Richardson (2005) also reported that synaptonemal complexes were observed in ungerminated teliospores of a number of other rust species including *Puccinia graminis* f.sp. *tritici* (Boehm et al., 1992). They report that: "arrested meiosis is common in teliospores of rust fungi and may, in fact, be the rule rather than the exception in these organisms."

The microscopically visible events of meiosis in *U. maydis,* and the model of meiosis beginning immediately after karyogamy and pausing at pachytene will be discussed further at different points throughout this review. However, the focus will switch to the discussions of environmental signals that trigger meiosis, transduction pathways that transmit these signals, control of gene expression, and an update of meiosis gene identification in *U. maydis,* with information on meiosis gene expression and evidence for post-transcriptional control mechanisms in *U. maydis*. In each section, relevant data from other fungal models, notably *Saccharomyces cerevisiae*, *Schizosaccharomyces pombe* and *C. cinerea*, will be reviewed for comparison and insight.

## 2. Signals triggering meiosis initiation in fungi: Genetic and environmental signals

The switch from mitotic division to meiosis involves a dramatic shift in cellular processes; in fact, this can be considered the most traumatic change a cell can undergo. Therefore, it is essential that entry into meiosis is tightly controlled, preventing the inappropriate execution of the meiotic program. The signals that trigger meiosis vary extensively between organisms, possibly due to a need for organisms to respond to the unique environmental niches in which they reside (Pawlowski et al., 2007). While the signals that trigger meiosis initiation are different, the timing is conserved from yeast to mice, occurring prior to the premeiotic S phase (Pawlowski et al., 2007). While this may seem obvious, the complex developmental processes that precede and accompany meiosis have obscured the timing until recently (Pawlowski et al., 2007). In this section, the nature and timing of signals leading to the initiation of meiosis in the model laboratory fungi *S. cerevisiae, S. pombe* and *C. cinerea* are reviewed and used as a reference in presenting hypotheses regarding meiotic initiation signals for the model plant pathogen *U. maydis*.

### 2.1 *Saccharomyces cerevisiae*

Meiosis in the ascomycete fungus *S. cerevisiae* has been extensively studied. For the purposes of this discussion, we will consider meiosis initiation as the first of three stages; the others being DNA replication, recombination, and the meiotic divisions leading to haploid products (Honigberg, 2003). This separation is interesting because it indicates an order of events different than that of *C. cinerea*.

In *S. cerevisiae*, meiosis initiation is triggered by environmental and genetic signals working in concert. To be receptive to the environmental signals, *S. cerevisiae* cells must be diploid and possess both MATa and MATα mating type alleles (reviewed in Piekarska et al., 2010). MATa and MATα encode components of the transcriptional repressor a1/α2, (Mitchell, 1994; Piekarska et al., 2010). The environmental signal involves three nutritional shifts: 1) the absence of an essential nutrient, 2) the presence of a non-fermentable carbon source, and 3) the absence of glucose (Honigberg, 2003). The essential nutrient typically eliminated in laboratory studies is nitrogen and, while there may also be a direct requirement for nitrogen sensing, limiting carbon, phosphates or sulphates can also provide the required signal to trigger meiosis initiation (Honigberg, 2003; Mitchell, 1994). The $CO_2$ produced through respiration, stimulated by the presence of a non-fermentable carbon source, results in the alkalization of the media, which may be a component of the 2$^{nd}$ shift (Honigberg, 2003). While respiration is a required signal throughout meiosis, the non-fermentable carbon source is only required prior to meiosis I (Honigberg, 2003; Piekarska et al., 2010). Finally, the presence of glucose can override the other signals and repress meiosis in *S. cerevisiae*, (Honigberg, 2003; Mitchell, 1994; Piekarska et al., 2010).

While the signal transduction pathways will be discussed later, other key aspects of meiosis initiation in *S. cerevisiae* are the timing of entry and the link between genetic and nutritional signals. A *S. cerevisiae* diploid cell commits to mitosis before DNA replication in the S phase.

It has been proposed that the commitment involves the separation of the spindle pole bodies (SPBs) during the cell cycle. In budding yeast cells where the SPBs are still together, the cells may arrest and enter the meiotic cycle, whereas after the SPBs have separated, the cell can no longer enter the meiotic cell cycle, and must complete mitosis (Simchen, 2009). Starvation for an essential nutrient results in the arrest of the cell in G1, when the SPBs are together (Honigberg, 2003; Piekarska et al., 2010), this specific arrest allows a switch to meiosis. The nutritional and genetic signals also converge to initiate meiosis through the transcriptional regulation of two main inducers of meiosis, *Ime1* (initiator of meiosis), which is a transcription factor that stimulates the expression of many early meiosis genes and *Ime2*, a serine/threonine protein kinase. The expression of *Ime1* is controlled by the a1/α2 repressor and by nutritional signals (Honigberg, 2003; Mitchell, 1994). Multiple nutritional signals converge on *Ime2* as well. The full expression of both of these genes is essential to the initiation and continuation of meiosis in *S. cerevisiae* (Honigberg, 2003; Mitchell, 1994).

### 2.2 *Schizosaccharomyces pombe*

Similar to *S. cerevisiae*, the initiation of meiosis in *S. pombe* requires diploid cells and nutrient starvation. However, *S. pombe* also requires pheromone signalling, whereas the *S. cerevisiae* pheromones are turned off after mating. In *S. pombe,* mating type is determined by the *mat1* locus. Each mating type allele codes two proteins, *mat1-P* codes *mat1-Pc* and *mat1-Pi,* while *mat1-M* codes *mat1-Mc* and *mat1-Mi. mat1-Mc* and *mat1-Pc* are essential for mating and meiosis, as they control pheromone and receptor production (Harigaya & Yamamoto, 2007; Yamamoto, 1996a). When compatible haploid cells are nitrogen starved, pheromone signalling is induced, which initiates cellular fusion and the formation of the diploids (Nielsen, 1993). These diploids grow mitotically, under rich nutrient conditions, but under nutrient starvation conditions they arrest in G1 and proceed to meiosis. As in *S. cerevisiae,* meiosis can only occur if the cells arrest in G1; beyond this point they are committed to mitosis (Harigaya & Yamamoto, 2007). However, meiosis in *S. pombe* will not proceed without the pheromone signal. Diploid cells lacking one pheromone receptor can still undergo meiosis but those lacking both cannot (Yamamoto, 1996a, 1996b).

The linkage to environmental signals in *S. pombe* comes through *Ste11*, a transcription factor expressed under nutrient starvation (Yamamoto, 1996a, 1996b). *Ste11* controls the expression of *mat1-Mc* and *mat1-Pc* along with other mating and meiosis genes. *Ste11* plays a similar role in *S. pombe* to *Ime1* in *S. cerevisiae,* as both transcription factors respond to environmental signals and lead to meiotic initiation. However, despite their functional similarities, these two proteins are not structurally similar (Burns et al., 2010a). *Mat1-Mc* and *Mat1-Pi* together stimulate the expression of *Mei3*, an inhibitor of *Pat1*, a serine/threonine protein kinase that itself inhibits meiotic initiation (Harigaya & Yamamoto, 2007; Willer et al., 1995). All of these signals converge on *Mei2,* an RNA binding protein which is essential for entry into, and continuation of, meiosis in fission yeast (Harigaya & Yamamoto, 2007).

### 2.3 *Coprinopsis cinerea*

*C. cinerea* is a filamentous, basidiomycete fungus that can be induced to form fruiting bodies (mushrooms) in the laboratory. As noted above, it is a model for the study of meiosis because the millions of basidia, the cells in which meiosis occurs, in a single cap develop synchronously. Initiation of meiosis in *C. cinerea* depends on light cues, not the nutritional cues used by *S. cerevisiae* and *S. pombe*. It has been hypothesized that linking fruiting body formation and meiosis to light/dark cycles provides a selective advantage because the fruiting bodies would be produced when animals are grazing, and *C. cinerea* depends upon animal ingestion for dispersal (Lu, 2000). This hypothesis is consistent with the concept of fungi responding to niche specific signals to initiate meiosis.

*C. cinerea* is well tuned to changes in lighting. Not only is light essential for karyogamy and the initiation of meiosis (Lu, 2000), but increasing the intensity of light speeds up the process, with less time being required to reach karyogamy under more intense light. It is proposed that the number of photons received is important in stimulating the progression of the cell into the premeiotic S phase and karyogamy (Lu, 2000). This timing is the same as the other fungi; therefore, although the signals are very different, the timing of commitment to meiosis is conserved, with the signal that initiates meiosis coming before the premeiotic S phase.

As may be expected, based on the different environmental triggers for initiation, *C. cinerea* has no orthologs to either *Ime1* or *Ste11*, the master meiotic regulators from *S. cerevisiae* and *S. pombe*, respectively. However, studies have shown that during meiosis, successive waves of transcription occur in *C. cinerea*, much like waves noted in both yeasts (Burns et al., 2010b). Hence, it may not be unreasonable to assume that there is a heretofore unidentified transcription factor that responds, directly or indirectly, to light signals and initiates this transcriptional program, making it similar in function, if not structure, to the regulators in budding and fission yeast.

### 2.4 *Ustilago maydis*

*U. maydis* is the model biotrophic basidiomycete plant pathogen (Banuett, 1995; Brefort et al., 2009). Like *S. cerevisiae* and *S. pombe*, there is a genetic and an environmental requirement for the initiation and completion of meiosis. *U. maydis* has two mating type loci, the multiallelic *b* locus and the diallelic *a* locus. The b locus codes a pair of homeodomain proteins that act as transcription factors when a heterodimeric protein consisting of polypeptides from different alleles is formed. The *a* locus codes for the pheromone and pheromone receptors. Alleles at each of these loci must be different in order for haploid cells to mate and for the maintenance of filamentous growth (reviewed in Banuett, 1995, 2002, 2010); however, only *b* locus heterozygosity is required for completion of meiosis (Banuett & Herskowitz, 1989). The environmental input required for meiosis is growth within the plant, and Banuett and Herskowitz (1996) suggested a peptide produced by the plant may stimulate karyogamy. In light of the earlier discussions here regarding a requirement for a signal to initiate premeiotic S phase and karyogamy, the suggestion by Banuett and Herskowitz (1996) could easily be extrapolated to suggest that the plant peptide stimulates premeiotic S phase and subsequent karyogamy in *U. maydis*. As reviewed by Banuett (2002), Kahmann and Kämper (2004), and Klosterman et al. (2007), the influence of the mating type loci is modulated by nutrition, pH, temperature, oxygen tension and plant signals, so it is possible that other factors influence meiosis in *U. maydis*.

To provide context for the possibility that nutritional conditions act as a signal influencing meiosis, Horst et al. (2010a) determined that, upon infection, *U. maydis* creates a strong nitrogen and carbon sink around the site of infection, and this stimulates the productivity of the remaining source leaves, allowing import of nutrients to the developing tumour tissue.

It is believed that the imported sucrose is used for building the tumour and for feeding *U. maydis*, and that the nitrogen may be fuelling both host defense protein synthesis and fungal growth (Horst et al., 2010b). This indicates that nutrition availability is an important aspect of the plant-pathogen interaction and that there is a competition for nutrients between the fungus and the plant. As an important part of its ecological niche, it is conceivable that changes in nutrient availability influence the progression of meiosis in *U. maydis*.

Genes that are involved in regulating the transition to meiosis have not yet been identified in *U. maydis*. Bioinformatic comparisons have determined that *U. maydis* does not possess an ortholog to *Ime1*, the master regulator of meiosis in *S. cerevisiae* (Donaldson & Saville, 2008). However, an ortholog to *Ste11*, the key transcription factor in *S. pombe*, is present in *U. maydis*. This putative ortholog is known as *Prf1* in *U. maydis* and its function has been previously characterized. Interestingly, it is a transcription factor that is involved in the sexual development of *U. maydis* in response to environmental signals, much like *Ste11*. *Prf1* is involved in regulating *a* and *b* mating type gene expression, resulting in high levels of pheromones and receptors during mating, and controlling *b* gene expression during pathogenesis (Hartmann et al., 1999). Four different environmental signals affect *Prf1*: the carbon source, pheromones, the *b* heterodimer and the cAMP pathway. These signals act to control *Prf1* transcriptionally and post-transcriptionally (Hartmann et al., 1999). This is similar to the function of *Ste11* in *S. pombe*, which controls pheromone gene expression in response to environmental signals, allowing for conjugation, the initiation of the sexual cycle and the commencement of meiosis. It is feasible that *Prf1* is also involved in initiating meiosis in *U. maydis*, possibly by stimulating the expression of a gene that controls further meiotic gene expression.

## 3. Signal transduction pathways and meiotic progression

The requirement for genetic and environmental signals to stimulate the entrance into meiosis implies there must be a way to transduce the environmental signals and integrate them with the genetic status of the cells. In this section we provide an overview of the signal transduction in *S. cerevisiae* and *S. pombe* and then, with this background, we link what is known about pathogenic signal transduction in *U. maydis* to its potential role in meiosis. Since research on these organisms has historically emphasized different levels of the signal transduction pathways, the focus in each section varies. In *S. cerevisiae*, major regulators are known and the focus has been on transcriptional control, and as such the overview will focus on signalling as it influences transcription. In *S. Pombe*, the major regulator is also known, but the emphasis has not been as strongly focused on transcription so this section is somewhat more pathway oriented. In *U. maydis*, the master regulators are not known so the knowledge of signal transduction in pathogenesis is reviewed and a model is presented for how this may stimulate the initiation of meiosis.

### 3.1 *Saccharomyces cerevisiae*

The initiation and continuation of meiosis are linked to environmental cues through multiple signal transduction pathways in *Saccharomyces cerevisiae*. The master controller of meiosis is the gene *Ime1*. The influences on this gene primarily result in changes in its transcription, which is controlled by the genetic and environmental signals. *Ime1* has an unusually large promoter region of 2,100bp, which is divided into 4 different Upstream Controlling Sequences, UCS1-4. These UCSs respond to different signals. Nutritional signals affect UCS1 and 2, with UCS2 promoting the transcription of *Ime1* and UCS1 inhibiting it. Cell-type signals affect UCS3 and 4, repressing the expression of *Ime1* in MAT-insufficient cells (Sagee et al., 1998). This section will focus on how these different signals are relayed to influence the transcription of this master controller.

### 3.1.1 Genetic control

The cell-type signals that control *Ime1* are transmitted through a repressor, *Rme1,* and an activator, *Ime4*. In haploid *S. cerevisiae,* the RME1 protein inhibits meiosis by repressing the expression of *Ime1*. It does so by binding to the *Rme1* Repressor Element (RRE), within UCS4 of the *Ime1* promoter (Covitz & Mitchell, 1993; Sagee et al., 1998). In diploid MATa/MATα cells, the proteins a1, a MATa product, and α2, a MATα product, form the a1/α2 heterodimer. This heterodimer binds upstream of *Rme1* and directly represses its transcription (Covitz et al., 1991). Repression of *Rme1* results in the de-repression of *Ime1,* as RME1 is no longer available to bind to the RRE, and in this way *Rme1* transmits the cell-type signal directly to *Ime1*. IME4 expression is necessary for the full expression of *Ime1* (Shah & Clancy, 1992). The a1/α2 heterodimer regulates *Ime1* expression by repressing the transcription of *Ime4* antisense and allowing the transcription of *Ime4* sense transcript (discussed further in section 6.4). The MATa/MATα cell-type signal also regulates *Ime1* expression through the UCS3 repressor region, however the protein involved has not been identified (Sagee et al., 1998). The status of the diploid cell is determined by the mating type loci, and the outlined transcriptional control pathways ensure that *Ime1* is only expressed, and meiosis can only proceed, in diploid MATa/MATα cells.

### 3.1.2 Nutritional control

The nutritional signals that control meiotic initiation in *S. cerevisiae* are transmitted through a signalling network composed of the RAS, cAMP and TOR pathways, all of which regulate the expression of transcription factor *Ime1* and kinase *Ime2* (reviewed in Piekarska et al., 2010).

While nitrogen limitation is often described as a requirement for meiosis in *S. cerevisiae,* starvation of any essential nutrient can stimulate meiosis. In each case, nutrient starvation may not have a direct effect; rather, it may act indirectly since nutrient limitation results in G1 arrest, and G1 arrest is required for meiosis initiation (Honigberg & Purnapatre, 2003). The response to nitrogen starvation is mediated, in part, by the TOR pathway. This pathway controls the expression of metabolism genes and, as such, its role in meiosis is also proposed to be indirect, because *Tor2* causes changes in metabolism that result in G1 arrest (Honigberg & Purnapatre, 2003). G1 arrest is essential to meiosis initiation, as we have discussed. CLN3 is a G1 cyclin that is part of the mitotic G1 to S phase transition. In nitrogen deprived cells, CLN3 is strongly down-regulated (Gallego et al., 1997). G1 cyclins, like CLN1, 2 and 3 down-regulate *Ime1* in cells grown in nutrient rich medium. This, in turn, represses the initiation of meiosis until cells are starved (Colomina et al., 1999). Starvation triggers a reduction in G1 cyclin levels resulting in the cells arresting at G1 (Colomina et al., 1999; Gallego et al., 1997). Lowered cyclin levels allow IME1 to be transferred to the nucleus, where it initiates meiosis by stimulating transcription of early meiotic genes (Zaman et al.,

2008). Apart from the indirect effects of nitrogen limitation, *Ime1* transcription may be directly influenced by nitrogen limitation, since deletion of the UCS1 upstream controlling sequence allows meiosis in the presence of nitrogen (Kassir et al., 2003). This nitrogen signal is transmitted through *Cdc25*, a positive regulator of the cAMP/PKA and MAPK pathways. The pathway involved in the transduction of *Cdc25*'s effect on *Ime1* is currently unknown (Kassir et al., 2003).

Carbon source is another essential element in the regulation of *Ime1* activity, both in repressing its function under non-favourable conditions and in activating its function under favourable conditions. Carbon source signals act on UCS2, the only controlling region that possess upstream activating sequences (UAS). In the presence of glucose, *Ime1* transcription is repressed at UCS2, preventing *Ime1* expression. UCS1 is also a target for repressing *Ime1* when glucose is present (Kassir et al., 2003). However, UCS2's promoter activity is stimulated in the presence of a non-fermentable carbon source (Sagee et al., 1998; Kassir et al., 2003). So when glucose is absent, *Ime1* expression is stimulated, but it is opposed by the constitutive repressor elements of USC2 and UCS1, unless nitrogen is also limited, which results in a high level of *Ime1* expression, inducing meiosis (Govin & Berger, 2009; Kassir et al., 2003).

The cAMP/PKA pathway is known to transmit the glucose signal to *Ime1* in many ways. Glucose is sensed by the G coupled receptor, GPR1, which activates GPA2, a component of a transmembrane heterotrimeric G protein that activates PKA through adenylyl cyclase (reviewed in Honigberg & Purnapatre, 2003). Adenylyl cyclase activity increases the level of cAMP in the cell, and increased cAMP leads to repression of *Ime1* (Kassir et al., 2003). Repression is mediated through transcription factor MSN2 which stimulates *Ime1* transcription, but with increased cAMP levels it is not transmitted to the nucleus, preventing *Ime1* activation (Kassir et al., 2003). SOK2 is another DNA binding protein that mediates the response of *Ime1* to glucose through the cAMP/PKA pathway. SOK2 functions as a repressor by associating with MSN2. When glucose is not present, SOK2 is converted to an activator (Shenhar & Kassir, 2001). As a further control, *Sok2* expression is dependent on glucose, when cells are growing in a non-fermentable carbon source, SOK2 levels drop dramatically, alleviating its repression of *Ime1* (Shenhar & Kassir, 2001). RIM15 is a serine/threonine protein kinase that is inactivated by PKA phosphorylation when cells are growing in glucose rich media and is increased in acetate media. RIM15 promotes the disassembly of the *Ume6* repressor complex, contributing to the activation of *Ime1* (Zaman et al., 2008). Intracellular acidification of yeast cells also plays into the cAMP pathway. Lowered pH inside the cell stimulates *Ras2*, which stimulates cAMP synthesis (Thevelein & De Winde, 1999). Outside of the cAMP/PKA pathway, glucose sensing also affects *Ime1* through the *Snf1* signal transduction pathway. Glucose inhibits the SNF1 protein kinase, which is necessary for full expression of *Ime1*. However, this is not the only use for SNF1; it also plays a role in *Ime2* regulation and spore formation (Honigberg & Lee, 1998).

It is clear that the regulation of *Ime1* integrates multiple factors to control meiotic initiation in response to environmental cues. However, *Ime1* is not the only target of nutritional regulation; *Ime2* is a meiosis specific protein kinase that is the second major regulator of meiosis in *S. cerevisiae*. It affects multiple stages of meiotic progression, and its transcription and activity are controlled by nitrogen and carbon source signals. *Ime2* activity is inhibited by glucose through GPA2, the α subunit of the heterotrimeric G-protein (a component of the cAMP/PKA pathway). When active GPA2 interacts with the C terminus of IME2, this interaction represses the activity of IME2, which in turn inhibits entry into meiosis (Donzeau & Bandlow, 1999). Glucose also modifies the protein stability of IME2 through the glucose sensors SNF3 and RGT2 (Rubin-Bejerano et al., 1996). UME6 binds to the *Ime2* promoter, repressing transcription in the presence of glucose and nitrogen. During vegetative growth, *Ime2* expression is repressed, like many early meiosis genes, by the UME6-SIN3-RPD3 complex. Under meiotic conditions, UME6 disassociates from SIN3 and RPD3, forming a complex with IME1, which activates the transcription of *Ime2* (Honigberg & Purnapatre, 2003; Purnapatre et al., 2005). The stabilization of this UME6-IME1 complex requires starvation for both nitrogen and glucose. The stabilization is mediated through phosphorylation by RIM11, a glycogen synthase kinase (Chung et al., 2001; Purnapatre et al., 2005) and RIM15, a protein kinase. The expression of RIM15 is repressed when glucose is present in the media and the activity of RIM15 and RIM11 are repressed through the cAMP/PKA pathway, which destabilizes the UME6-IME1 complex (Honigberg & Purnapatre, 2003; Piekarska et al., 2010; Xiao & Mitchell, 2000). Finally, media alkalization effects the expression of *Ime2* through the activation of the UME3-UME5 complex, which has been shown to be required for the full expression of *Ime2* (Cooper & Strich, 2002; Honigberg & Purnapatre, 2003). Thus it is clear that carbon and nitrogen nutritional signals converge on both *Ime1* and *Ime2* in order to control the initiation of meiosis.

### 3.2 *Schizosaccharomyces pombe*

In *S. pombe,* the master controller of meiosis is *Ste11*, a transcription factor that stimulates both mating and meiosis. It triggers the expression of both mating type loci and *Mei2*, another key meiosis control gene (Sugimoto et al., 1991). Regulation of both *Ste11* and *Mei2* integrates cell type and environmental signals that lead to initiation of meiosis in *S. pombe*. This section will focus on how these signals are conveyed to the regulators of meiosis through signal transduction pathways, and how these pathways are required for the initiation of meiosis.

#### 3.2.1 Genetic control

A requirement for meiosis in *S. pombe* is that cells are diploid and contain mating type loci *mat1-P* which codes *mat1-Pc* and *mat1-Pi*, as well as *mat1-M*, which codes *mat1-Mc* and *mat1-Mi*. The genes *mat1-Mc* and *mat1-Pc* stimulate pheromone signalling and are essential for both mating and meiosis (Willer et al., 1995). The expression of these two genes requires STE11 (Yamamoto, 1996a) and *Ste11* is only expressed under nutrient starvation conditions (see next prargraph). The pheromones produced bind to their respective receptors (Yamamoto, 1996b). A G protein α subunit, GPA1, is coupled to the pheromone receptors, transmitting the signal downstream (Obara et al., 1991). This activates a MAP kinase cascade including: MAPKKK BYR2, MAPKK BYR1 and MAPK SPK1 (reviewed in Yamamoto, 1996b). Signals received at SPK1 are transmitted to stimulate expression of *mat1-Pi* and *mat1-Mi*. These gene products then allow for the initiation of meiosis by stimulating the expression of *Mei3* (Willer et al., 1995; Yamamoto, 1996b). Another GTP binding protein, RAS1, helps to regulate the MAPK cascade through activating BYR2. RAS1 binds to BYR2 and controls its translocation to the plasma membrane (Bauman et al., 1998). Interestingly, a Ras homolog in *S. cerevisiae*, *Ras1,* is also involved in meiotic initiation, but by repressing it through the cAMP/PKA pathway (Honigberg & Purnapatre, 2003). This is another example of how similar signals are utilized in different ways by divergent organisms. The requirement for starvation to stimulate *Ste11,* which stimulates expression at the mating type loci, provides a link between environmental signals and genetic status of the cells.

### 3.2.2 Nutritional control

Sexual development in *S. pombe* requires nutrient starvation; with nitrogen starvation, in particular, playing an essential role. Starvation initiates mating, which is typically immediately followed by meiosis. The nutritional signals are linked to meiosis through the cAMP/PKA pathway. In *S. pombe,* similar to *S. cerevisiae,* increased levels of intracellular cAMP inhibit meiosis progress, while lower levels lead to its initiation (reviewed in Yamamoto, 1996a). When cells are growing in nutrient rich media, cAMP levels are high, but when they are transferred to nitrogen-free media, the cAMP levels decrease by approximately 50% before meiosis occurs. The cAMP then increases to a level greater than or equal to those in nutrient rich media during sporulation (the last stage of meiosis). When the cAMP level is artificially elevated in the cells, it results in sterility (Mochizuki & Yamamoto, 1992). Carbon starvation also results in a decrease in intracellular cAMP levels and can contribute to the initiation of meiosis (Isshiki et al., 1992). The cAMP levels in *S. pombe* are controlled by GPA2, the ortholog of GPA2 in *Saccharomyces cerevisiae,* a heterotrimeric G protein which controls the activity of adenylate cyclase. *Gpa2* null mutants had low levels of intracellular cAMP and were able to mate and sporulate, even in rich media (Honigberg & Purnapatre, 2003; Isshiki et al., 1992). GPA2 is necessary for the cell to be able to increase cAMP levels upon glucose stimulation, indicating that it is directly involved in sensing carbon starvation. The ability of the GPA2 mutant to sporulate, even on nitrogen rich media, may also indicate its involvement in nitrogen sensing (Isshiki et al., 1992). Changes in cAMP levels alter the activity of Protein Kinase A (PKA). PKA controls the expression of the major meiosis control gene *Ste11* through its impact on RST2 (Kunitomo et al., 2000). RST2 binds to an upstream *cis*-element, inducing *Ste11* expression. Phosphorylation of RST2 by PKA suppresses its ability to induce transcription of *Ste11.* PKA activity also controls the nuclear localization of RST2, where high levels of PKA result in RST2 being mostly located in the cytoplasm, while low levels result in it being found in the nucleus (Higuchi et al., 2002). When nutritional starvation results in the decrease in cAMP, and thus PKA activity, this results in the activation of RST2, which in turn stimulates *Ste11* expression, leading to meiotic gene expression. In addition to control over *Ste11,* the cAMP signalling pathway also acts to control *Mei2,* another crucial regulator of meiosis initiation. As with *Ste11,* increased cAMP levels inhibit the expression of *Mei2* (Y. Watanabe et al., 1988). MEI3 inactivates PAT1, which inhibits both MEI2 and STE11 through phosphorylation. When MEI3 is expressed, its inactivation of PAT1 results in the accumulation of unphosphorylated and active *Mei2.* The active MEI2 stimulates the continuation of meiosis. In fact, the expression of *Mei3* can bypass both nutritional and genetic requirements and result in ectopic meiosis (Peng et al., 2003). MEI3, is a substrate of PKA; however, decreased phosphorylation does not affect MEI3's ability in inactivate PAT1 (Peng et al., 2003). Regardless of this remaining uncertainty, this information clearly indicates that the cAMP pathway transmits the nutritional starvation signal and influences the initiation of meiosis on multiple levels in *S. pombe.*

The cAMP/PKA pathway is not the only signal transduction pathway for nutritional sensing. The TOR pathway transmits signals involved in nitrogen source availability. Genes induced by TOR2, a component of the TORC1 complex, include those induced by nitrogen starvation. *Tor2* is a negative regulator of meiosis, with *Tor2* inhibition increasing meiosis (Matsuo et al., 2007). TOR2 forms a complex with, and inhibits the function of both *Ste11* and *Mei2,* leading to the repression of meiosis (Álvarez & Moreno, 2006). The TOR pathway interacts with the PKA pathway; both are used as a means to drive cell growth and inhibit sporulation. They also work together to regulate *Ste11* expression and localization within the cell. STE11 is located throughout the cell, but under meiosis conditions, it builds up in the nucleus. PKA appears to have a controlling role in nuclear localization, when PKA is absent, STE11 localizes to the nucleus, even in the presence of TOR2; the absence of TOR2 also results in nuclear localization of STE11 (Valbuena & Moreno, 2010). Cells with constitutively active *Tor2* are impaired in mating, but they regain functional mating when PKA is deactivated, suggesting that PKA is a more potent regulator. When PKA is at a high level in the cell, RST2 represses *Ste11* transcription, and mating and meiosis are inhibited (Valbuena & Moreno, 2010). This indicates that the cAMP/PKA pathway interacts with the TOR pathway to control expression and localization of STE11. This, in turn, controls the initiation of meiosis.

There is one additional pathway that transmits nutrient starvation signals to *Ste11,* the stress response pathway (SRP). Stress includes starvation, the typical trigger for meiosis initiation in *S. pombe.* The SRP includes the MAPKK WIS1 and MAPK STY1 that play a role in meiosis initiation and stress response in the cell (Kato et al., 1996; Shiozaki & Russell, 1996; Wilkinson et al., 1996). STY1 phosphorylates and modifies the activity of the transcription factor, ATF1 (Shiozaki & Russell, 1996; Wilkinson et al., 1996). ATF1 is necessary for the expression of *Ste11* during nutrient starvation (Takeda et al., 1995). Therefore, nutrient starvation signals are also transmitted through the stress response pathway to control *Ste11* expression and meiosis in *S. pombe.* This is notably different from what occurs in *S. cerevisiae,* where the closest homolog to STY1 is HOG1, which in budding yeast responds only to osmotic stress, not stress in general (Wilkinson et al., 1996).

### 3.3 *Ustilago maydis*

In *U. maydis* research, the focus has been on signals leading to pathogenesis. A look at the life cycle of this fungus (Figure 1) illustrates how closely pathogenesis is tied to the events of sexual reproduction. There are differences given *U. maydis* is a basidiomycete, for example, when compatible haploid cells fuse they form a filamentous dikaryon and not a diploid. This dikaryon is the pathogenic form and persists for some time before karyogamy is stimulated and meiosis ensues. Recall this is also the situation in the model basidiomycete mushroom, *C. cinerea.* However, like the yeasts, the proteins coded at the *U. maydis* mating type loci interact with the output of signal transduction pathways to influence continued development toward meiosis. In order to integrate signals from the mating type loci with environmental signals it is reasonable to expect that, in *U. maydis,* these signals converge on a given gene or gene(s). These genes have not yet been identified. In the following discussion, the signal transduction pathways, as they are currently understood, will be outlined. There are interesting similarities to signalling pathways in the yeasts and this enables hypotheses to be generated regarding the signalling leading to meiosis in *U. maydis*.

### 3.3.1 Host/environmental control

Mating, morphogenesis and pathogenicity depend on the cAMP/PKA and MAPK pathways in *U. maydis*. While each pathway transmits signals independently, there is crosstalk between them. The cAMP pathway, as it has been elucidated thus far, begins with a heterotrimeric G protein for which the α subunit and the β subunit have been identified. The α submit is GPA3, the only one of four α subunits coded by *U. maydis* that influences the cAMP pathway. GPA3 mutants are sterile and unable to respond to pheromone signalling, thus unable to mate (Regenfelder et al., 1997). GPA3 associates with the β subunit BPP1 and together they convey the signal to adenylate cyclase, UAC1, the next component of the pathway (Muller et al., 2004). Adenylate cyclase produces cAMP, which activates protein kinase A (PKA) by causing its regulatory subunit, UBC1, to dissociate from the catalytic subunit, ADR1 (Feldbrugge et al., 2004; Gold et al., 1997). cAMP signalling in *U. maydis* has several roles. Its influences: 1) alter the expression of *a* and *b* mating type genes in response to pheromone signalling (Kaffarnik et al., 2003), 2) direct the switch from budding to filamentous growth (Lee et al., 2003), and 3) control pathogenic development (Gold et al., 1997). The influence on filamentous growth is linked to cAMP levels and thus PKA activity. Lower levels of cAMP or altered PKA activity, such as is the case with a defective ADR1 subunit, results in constitutive filamentous growth, while high cAMP/PKA levels result in a budding phenotype (Lee et al., 2003). The influence of the cAMP pathway on pathogenic development was determined through mutation of *Ubc1* (the PKA regulatory subunit), which resulted in high PKA activity. *U. maydis* strains with these mutations were able to colonize the plant, but were unable to form tumours or teliospores. *Uac1* mutants, with low PKA activity, are non-pathogenic (Gold et al., 1997). This suggests that tight control of PKA is required for proper progression of pathogenesis, with low PKA being required for filamentous growth, followed by increased PKA activity needed for infection of the plant, and then lowered PKA once again for tumour and teliospore formation (Gold et al., 1997). Consistent with the requirement for tight control, *U. maydis* strains carrying a constitutively active *Gpa3* can infect corn, leading to tumour formation but not teliospore development (Krüger et al., 2000). It was suggested that the difference between the *Uac1* and the *Gpa3* mutant phenotype is due to different levels of PKA activity in the two mutants, with the *Gpa3* mutant likely representing a less active version with a less defective pathogenic cycle (Krüger et al., 2000). Thus, carefully regulated levels of cAMP appear to be required throughout sexual development, and pathogenesis.

In addition to cAMP signalling, mating and pathogenesis are also regulated by a MAPK signalling cascade. The pathway consists of MAPKKK *Ubc4/Kpp4*, MAPKK *Ubc5/Fuz7* and MAPK *Ubc3/Kpp2* and it may respond to signals transmitted through *Ras2*, a *U. maydis* homolog of the *S. pombe Ras1* (Muller et al., 2003). Evidence supports the pheromone signal being transmitted through a single MAPK pathway, which is also similar to *S. pombe* (Muller et al., 2003). In a parallel pathway to pheromone response, the MAPK cascade is necessary for appressorium formation and function, as well as filamentous growth in the plant. While *Kpp2* is required for appressorium formation, a second MAPK, *Kpp6*, is involved in plant penetration (Muller et al., 2003). Unlike *S. pombe*, no known G-protein α subunit plays a role in the *U. maydis* MAPK cascade; however, a plant signal likely influences this pathway through some means, since the maintenance of *U. maydis* filamentous growth requires the host plant. One possibility is through the link with another pathway. This is suggested because disruption of the MAPK pathway resulted in repression of the constitutive filamentous growth phenotype that is caused by *Adr1* mutation (Muller et al., 2003), recall ADR1 is the catalytic subunit of PKA which is activated by cAMP.

Exploration of the links between the cAMP/PKA and MAPK pathways revealed crosstalk through proteins that are putative orthologs to two major meiotic regulators discussed above. The first is CRK1, which is an IME2 related protein kinase. *Ime2* is a key meiotic regulator and target of environmental signals in *S. cerevisiae*. The second is *Prf1*, a putative ortholog of *Ste11*, a key regulator of meiosis in *S. pombe*. *Crk1* is a target of environmental stimuli in *U. maydis*: *Crk1* mutants are impaired in their response to environmental signals, and *Crk1* is highly expressed when cells are grown in nutrition stress conditions (Garrido & Pérez-Martín, 2003). *Crk1* also plays a role in mating and pathogenesis since *Crk1* mutants are unable to mate on plates and have attenuated pathogenesis producing few tumours and no observed black teliospores (Garrido et al., 2004). *Crk1* is also involved in cell morphogenesis. When *Crk1* is overexpressed, it causes filamentous growth. When *Crk1* is inactivated, it suppresses the constitutive filamentous growth that results from *Adr1* and *Gpa3* mutants. This indicates that it acts downstream of these cAMP pathway genes, however high levels of *Crk1* cannot repress the budding phenotype of a *Ubc1* mutant, indicating it cannot override all cAMP mediated responses (Garrido & Pérez-Martín, 2003). The expression of *Crk1* is regulated by both the cAMP and MAPK pathways, which have antagonistic effects on its transcription. *Crk1* is transcriptionally repressed by the cAMP pathway, with high PKA levels resulting in a low level of *Crk1* expression and vice versa (Garrido & Pérez-Martín, 2003). The MAPK pathway, conversely, positively regulates *Crk1* expression, with *Kpp2* (a MAPK) mutants resulting in much lower levels of *Crk1* in the cell (Garrido & Pérez-Martín, 2003). KPP2 also interacts physically with CRK1, and is required for the role of CRK1 in cell morphogenesis (Garrido et al., 2004). In addition, *Fuz7* (a MAPKK) is required for activation of *Crk1*. FUZ7 phosphorylates CRK1, activating it (Garrido et al., 2004). Thus *Crk1* is clearly involved in the integration of the cAMP and MAPK signalling pathways. However, many of the phenotypes of *Crk1* mutants appear to result from an effect on *Prf1*, since *Crk1* controls the transcription of *Prf1*.

PRF1 is an HMG protein that controls the expression of mating type genes, which regulate mating, pathogenesis and cell morphology. PRF1 binds to the pheromone response element, or PRE, upstream in the *a* and *b* loci, stimulating their expression (Hartmann et al., 1996). Therefore, a *Prf1* mutant strain is unable to mate because it is unable to produce or respond to pheromones. The receptor and pheromone are coded by the *a* mating type locus. Through its control of the *b* mating-type locus *Prf1* influences filamentous growth and pathogenesis. A solopathogenic *Prf1* mutant is unable to cause tumours when it infects the plant (Hartmann et al., 1996). It is possible that *Prf1* acts as a mediator for response to plant signals during pathogenic growth. PRF1 is controlled through the cAMP/PKA and MAPK pathways, facilitating control by pheromones and environmental signals. PRF1 has phosphorylation sites for both MAPK and PKA, and mutations in either of these sites impede mating. This indicates that both MAPK and PKA phosphorylation are required for proper function of PRF1 in sexual development (Kaffarnik et al., 2003). Interestingly, these phosphorylation sites also determine which genes are activated by PRF1, with MAPK phosphorylation being necessary for *b* gene expression, but not for *a*, while PKA phosphorylation is required for both (Kaffarnik et al., 2003). The MAPK pathway may also have a role in inducing the transcription of *Prf1*, as a constitutively active *Fuz7* can increase *Prf1* levels (Kaffarnik et al., 2003). Beyond these post-translational controls, *Prf1* has a cis-regulatory element in its promoter that is termed the UAS, an upstream activator sequence. The *Prf1* UAS appears to regulate transcription of *Prf1* in response to cAMP and carbon source signals. Glucose or sucrose stimulates *Prf1* transcription via the UAS (Hartmann et al., 1999). High cAMP levels repress *Prf1* transcription though the UAS. It is important to note that this is a separate mechanism from the post-transcriptional activation of *Prf1* by PKA, and this seemingly contradictory activity of the cAMP pathway results in increase in *a* gene expression at moderate cAMP levels, but repression through transcriptional control at higher levels (Hartmann et al., 1999). This emphasizes the fine scale control imparted by cAMP levels. The cAMP pathway could also mediate the carbon source signal, or it could be mediated by a separate pathway; this is not yet elucidated (Hartmann et al., 1999).

The link between PRF1 and CRK1 is that CRK1 is required for transcriptional activation of *Prf1* through the UAS (Garrido et al., 2004). This provides another avenue for *Prf1* control by MAPK and cAMP. Kaffarnik et al. (2003) theorized that the cAMP and MAPK paths may be required to control mating because mating typically occurs on the plant, and if sensing the plant results in increased cAMP levels, this would be sufficient to increase *a* gene expression, increasing pheromone expression and making mate detection easier, then pheromone signalling would feed back into the cAMP and MAPK pathways. The MAPK pathway would then initiate conjugation tube formation and mating (Muller et al., 2003), and the cAMP and MAPK pathways would increase the transcription and the activity of *Prf1*, triggering *b* gene expression, and pathogenesis. Thus it is clear that the integration between the two signalling pathways provides a mechanism whereby a plant signal received before penetration could lead to the subsequent events of pathogenesis; however, what triggers meiosis?

The discovery that a decrease in cAMP level is required for the completion of teliospore development suggests that the fungus must lower cAMP levels during pathogenesis to allow teliospores to form. This could be in response to a signal received from the plant. Interestingly, as we discussed above, a decrease in cAMP/PKA levels is necessary to stimulate meiosis in both *S. cerevisiae* and *S. pombe*. Since, in *U. maydis*, meiosis initiation begins around the time of teliospore formation, it is compelling to link the arrest of teliospore development, resulting from elevated cAMP levels, to meiosis. This mutation-stimulated arrest occurs sometime between when the hyphae form lobed tips, and when they fragment and begin rounding and swelling (Krüger et al., 2000). Interestingly, this is very shortly after the time that karyogamy occurs during normal pathogenic development, recall karyogamy occurs before hyphal fragmentation, but after the cells are imbedded in the mucilaginous matrix (Banuett & Herskowitz, 1996). These findings can be integrated in a model where the *U. maydis* dikaryon infects the plant and grows within and between cells, stimulating the initiation of tumour formation, and then it receives a signal from the plant which leads to the fungal cells entering premeiotic S phase and karyogamy, concomitant with the reduction of cAMP, allowing teliospore formation to proceed. The signals for karyogamy and teliospore formation must at least be interrelated, as these two processes need to proceed simultaneously to avoid crucial disruptions in both developmental pathways. As meiosis proceeds, the teliospore develops such that when it enters a dormant state, meiosis arrests at pachytene. This could be the result of reaching the end of a developmental cascade initiated by the plant signals, or a response to another plant signal.

## 4. Control of meiotic gene expression

The signals received from the environment are transduced through the pathways noted above and result in cascades of transcription that guide meiosis. These waves of transcription have been well studied in *S. cerevisiae* and *S. pombe*. In this section, knowledge of these transcriptional cascades is reviewed and compared. The existing data regarding transcription during meiosis in *U. maydis* is then presented and compared to that of the yeasts.

### 4.1 *Saccharomyces cerevisiae*

In *S. cerevisiae*, the stages of meiosis have been defined by the waves of genes expressed in a transcriptional cascade. Typically these genes are classified as early, middle and late, depending upon their time of expression during meiosis. Some researchers have found it necessary to further subdivide expression, and, as such, genes may be referred to as belonging to an intermediate expression time; for example, mid-late genes are expressed before late genes, but after the typical middle gene expression (Chu et al., 1998; Mitchell, 1994). In this section we provide an overview of the transcriptional waves, with information on the control of transcription and the relationship of expression to meiotic progression.

#### 4.1.1 Initiation of meiosis

The master regulator of meiosis in *S. cerevisiae* is IME1, a transcription factor that initiates the transcriptional cascade. It is the point of integration of environmental signals and directly controls the expression of early meiosis genes. Under meiotic conditions, IME1 interacts with UME6. UME6 was first identified as a repressor of meiotic genes under vegetative growth conditions. It binds at the upstream repression sequence 1 (URS1) found in target genes (Mitchell, 1994). However, during meiotic growth, UME6 forms a complex with IME1, and this complex activates early meiotic genes, often through the URS1 (Chu et al., 1998; Mitchell, 1994; Rubin-Bejerano et al., 1996). URS1 is a weak upstream activator sequence, and as such, the signal to initiate transcription is often augmented by binding of activator ABF1 at a distinct recognition sequence (Vershon & Pierce, 2000). Based on their expression patterns, early genes have been subdivided into three groups: early (I) induction, early (II) induction and early-middle induction (Chu et al., 1998). These early genes are involved in controlling DNA replication and the events of prophase I: chromosome pairing, homologous recombination and spindle pole body movements (Chu et al., 1998; reviewed in Piekarska et al., 2010). Interestingly, though the early-middle phase genes grouped with other early genes, most lack the URS1, indicating that they are unlikely to be controlled by IME1/UME6. Instead, about half of these genes possess the MSE (middle sporulation element) indicating expression is controlled by NDT80 (Chu et al., 1998). *Ime2* is a key early gene whose transcription is initiated by IME1. IME2 acts through a second pathway that does not directly involve IME1. So there is an IME1 dependant pathway that does not involve IME2 and an IME2 dependant pathway (Mitchell et al., 1990; Mitchell, 1994). IME2 is a cdk-like protein kinase, which plays a key role in transitions in meiosis. It acts to amplify transcription of meiosis genes including itself, activates NDT80 to trigger middle meiosis gene expression and stabilizes Clb cyclins through its inhibition of the APC/C (anaphase promoting complex/cyclosome), which in turn controls chromosome segregation (Marston & Amon, 2004; reviewed in Piekarska et al., 2010). IME2 also targets SIC1, resulting in its degradation, triggering the initiation of the S phase and premeiotic DNA replication (Piekarska et al., 2010). Additionally, IME2 phosphorylates IME1, which then signals it for destruction by the proteasome (Guttmann-Raviv et al., 2002). In this way, IME1 initiates meiosis and IME2 reinforces this and enables it to proceed to the next stage of meiosis, middle gene expression.

### 4.1.2 Commitment and continuation

Fully active NDT80 is necessary for the full expression of middle meiosis genes and thus for the continuation of meiosis in *S. cerevisiae*. These middle meiosis genes are required for meiotic divisions, and include genes such as B-type cyclins and those involved in spore morphogenesis (Chu & Herskowitz, 1998). NDT80 binds to the conserved MSE element, found upstream of 70% of middle meiosis genes (Chu et al., 1998; Chu & Herskowitz, 1998). NDT80 competes for some of the MSEs with another transcription factor, SUM1, which acts as a repressor of middle meiosis genes during vegetative growth and early meiosis. NDT80 and SUM1 bind to overlapping, yet different, sequences within the MSE, resulting in MSEs that function as *Sum1* repressors, *Ndt80* activators, or both simultaneously (Pierce et al., 2003). A combination of upstream elements also controls the expression of *Ndt80*. While *Ndt80* is a middle meiosis gene, it is expressed slightly before the rest of the middle meiosis genes. This expression pattern, termed pre-middle, results from two URS1s and two MSEs, located upstream of *Ndt80* (Pak & Segall, 2002a). During vegetative growth, expression of *Ndt80* is repressed by both UME6 and SUM1 acting on URS1 and MSE respectively. After the initiation of meiosis, the UME6 repressor complex is replaced with UME6-IME1, but expression is still repressed by the MSE (Pak and Segall, 2002a). IME2 and CDK1 phosphorylate SUM1, leading to its release from the MSE and relieving its repression of *Ndt80* (Ahmed et al., 2009; Pak & Segall, 2002a; Shin et al., 2010). This allows for low level *Ndt80* expression, stimulated by IME1 at URS1. The expressed NDT80 then binds to the MSE in its own promoter region, stimulating expression, leading to full middle gene expression and progression into the first meiotic divisions. However, both *Sum1* and *Ndt80* expression are also controlled by the pachytene checkpoint, which can prevent the expression of middle meiotic genes. Middle gene expression is essential for the cell to exit from the pachytene checkpoint and enter into meiotic divisions. The pachytene checkpoint, or meiotic recombination checkpoint, is part of a surveillance system in eukaryotic cells that arrests the cell cycle in response to defects. To ensure the integrity of the events of meiosis, this checkpoint prevents the cell from exiting the pachytene stage of prophase I and entering into meiotic divisions before the completion of recombination (Roeder & Bailis, 2000). Cells arrested at pachytene are not yet committed to meiosis, meaning they can revert to mitotic growth if conditions are adjusted. This is the last point at which the cell can return to mitotic growth, as after the transition to the first meiotic divisions, the cell is committed to meiosis

(Shuster & Byers, 1989). This makes the pachytene checkpoint the "point of no return" for the cell, allowing one last chance for the cell to arrest and abort meiotic progression, and revert to mitotic growth. In *Dmc1* mutants, DSB repair is impaired, in *Zip1* mutants SC formation is impaired and in *Hop2* mutants, synapsis is defective. Each of these mutants trigger pachytene arrest (Roeder & Bailis, 2000). Checkpoint arrest is mediated through proteins that monitor synapsis and recombination and exert their effects on downstream targets of checkpoint regulation. The checkpoint targets and stabilizes SWE1, a kinase that inactivates CDC28, preventing exit from the pachytene, and SUM1, which represses the expression of *Ndt80* (Pak & Segall, 2002b; Roeder & Bailis, 2000). The checkpoint machinery also directly inhibits the activity of NDT80 by inhibiting its phosphorylation (Hepworth et al., 1998; Pak & Segall, 2002b; Tung et al., 2000). The CDC28/Clb complex allows cell cycle progression past the pachytene checkpoint and into meiotic divisions (Tung et al., 2000). Fully active NDT80 then allows for the expression of middle meiosis genes, leading to meiotic divisions and spore formation and full commitment to meiosis.

The final waves of meiotic gene expression are mid-late and late genes. These genes are involved in spore wall formation and spore maturation, but the transcription factors that initiate their expression are not currently known (Chu et al., 1998; Vershon & Pierce, 2000). In the mid-late genes, 36% have at least one MSE located upstream, indicating that these may be regulated by NDT80, SUM1 or both. Their delay in expression is theorized to be due to other negative regulatory elements (NREs) present in the promoter region that delay expression until the mid-late phase. The factor that acts on these regulatory elements is not known; however, there is evidence that it requires a co-repressor complex of SSN6 and TUP1 (Chu et al., 1998; Vershon & Pierce, 2000). The late genes do not contain either of the previously identified regulatory elements and the control of their expression is not yet understood (Vershon & Pierce, 2000). What is known, however, is that it requires two separate pathways, one involving SPS1 and SMK1, part of a MAPK cascade, and one involving SWM1, a middle meiosis gene that is part of the anaphase promoting complex (Piekarska et al., 2010; Vershon & Pierce, 2000). *Smk1* transcription is regulated through the APC, which links the completion of meiosis to spore formation and maturation, as controlled by the late genes, and through the RAS/cAMP pathway; indicating that nutritional control is still having an effect on spore formation, even after the full commitment to meiosis is made (reviewed in Piekarska et al., 2010). There is still much to learn about the control of meiotic gene expression in *Saccharomyces cerevisiae*, but is it clear that tightly controlled waves of transcription, coupled with a key meiotic checkpoint, ensure that each stage of this transcriptional cascade proceeds only when the cell is prepared to proceed.

### 4.2 *Schizosaccharomyces pombe*

In *Schizosaccharomyces pombe*, meiosis is controlled by the key transcription factor *Ste11* and the RNA binding protein, MEI2. As in *S. cerevisiae*, many genes are differentially expressed once meiosis is initiated. Mata et al. (2002), proposed four temporal classes; starvation/pheromone induced genes, early genes, middle genes, and late genes. While this progression is similar to *S. cerevisiae*, the control of meiosis in *S. cerevisiae* and *S. pombe* are highly divergent. There are few conserved genes among these species and the regulatory machinery differs. A transcription analysis of *S. pombe* with comparison to the core meiotic transcriptome from two strains of *S. cerevisiae* identified 75 shared genes (Mata et al., 2002). This compares to hundreds of genes with meiosis specific expression in each species (Mata et al., 2002). As such, one would expect differences in the transcriptional control of meiosis between *S. cerevisiae* and *S. pombe*. Here we provide an overview of how transcription triggered by *Ste11* initiates meiosis, how *Mei2* then controls meiotic progression, and how the transcription factors control different waves of transcription during meiosis in *S. pombe*.

### 4.2.1 Initiation of meiosis

The first genes induced during *S. pombe* meiosis are those that act in response to starvation, including nitrogen transporters, metabolism and mating type regulators. This is followed by the expression of genes involved in pheromone signalling and entry into meiosis, including *Ste11* and *Mei2*. STE11 is a transcription factor that is essential to the initiation of meiosis. It controls the transcription of several key genes, including *Mei2* and the mating type genes *mat1-Pc* and *mat1-Mc*, required for the initiation and continuation of meiosis (Mata et al., 2002). STE11 is an HMG-box protein, responsible for the expression of nitrogen responsive genes during starvation conditions. Ectopic expression of *Ste11* in vegetative growth conditions triggers mating and meiosis, while *Ste11* disruptions result in sterility (Sugimoto et al., 1991). This indicates an essential role for *Ste11* in *S. pombe* meiosis. STE11 binds DNA at TR (T-rich) boxes, present in varying copy numbers upstream of target genes including *matP*, *matM* , *Mei2* and *Ste11* itself (Sugimoto et al., 1991). The mating type genes are required for pheromone signalling which stimulates *Ste11* activity (Harigaya & Yamamoto, 2007). STE11 also binds to the TR box upstream of its gene, stimulating its own expression. This positive feedback loop reinforces the cell's commitment to meiosis (Kunitomo et al., 2000). *Ste11* activity is inhibited by CDK phosphorylation and since STE11 is highly unstable, the protein rapidly disappears if it is not able to stimulate its own expression (Kjærulff et al., 2007). This provides a means to tightly control expression of *Ste11*. CDK activity is low in the beginning of G1, and then increases through S and into G2. When CDK activity increases, STE11 is phosphorylated and degraded, this restricts STE11 function to G1 (Kjærulff et al., 2007). This is similar to the regulation in *S. cerevisiae* of IME1 by G1 cyclins in response to nutrient signals, which trigger arrest at the G1 phase (Colomina et al., 1999). This may indicate that CDK phosphorylation of a transcription factor plays a role in restricting meiosis initiation to the G1 phase in many organisms.

The stimulation of *Mei2*, *mat1-Pc* and *mat1-Mc* expression by STE11 leads to another level of meiotic control. Mating-type loci gene expression leads to pheromone production which stimulates *Mei3* expression. MEI3 inactivates *Pat1*, which functions to prevent the expression of both *Ste11* and *Mei2* during vegetative growth and in haploid cells (Yamamoto, 1996a). In this way, STE11 is responsible for the expression of both itself and *Mei2* in two different ways; directly through stimulation at the TR box, and indirectly through the pheromone response pathway which leads to the expression of *Mei3*. MEI2, expression leads to the induction of meiosis (Yamamoto, 1996a). Early genes are expressed after the initiation of meiosis, they are involved in S phase, chromosome pairing and recombination. Many of the genes expressed at this time contain an upstream element, the MluI box, which suggests they are controlled by the CDC10, RES2, REP1 transcription complex (Mata et al., 2002).

### 4.2.2 Commitment and continuation

*Mei2* is critical for the mitotic-meiotic switch in fission yeast and for the commitment of the cell to meiosis (Y. Watanabe et al., 1988). Like *S. cerevisiae, S. pombe* makes the critical decision to enter meiosis before the premeiotic S phase (Marston & Amon, 2004). However, unlike budding yeast, once *Mei2* is active, *S. pombe* is fully committed to meiosis, and the cell cannot be induced to revert to mitosis (Y. Watanabe et al., 1988). It should be noted that *Mei2* is also required for meiosis I (reviewed in Yamamoto, 1996b). MEI2 contains three RNA recognition motifs and this RNA binding capability is essential for its function in stimulating meiotic initiation and continuation through meiosis I. The RNA that interacts with MEI2 to promote premeiotic DNA synthesis is currently unknown; however, it has been found that MEI2 must interact with meiRNA, the non-functional RNA product of *Sme2,* to successfully promote entry into meiosis I (Watanabe & Yamamoto, 1994, cited in Yamamoto, 1996b). meiRNA is required for the import of *Mei2* into the nucleus before meiosis I (Yamashita et al., 1998). *Mei2* is located in the cytoplasm of the cell during vegetative growth, but it condenses into a single spot within the nucleus during meiotic prophase. These dots can be identified in the nucleus even before premeiotic DNA synthesis and then they fade away after the first meiotic division (Yamashita et al., 1998). The formation of this dot requires MEI2 and meiRNA association, un-associated MEI2 and meiRNA remain in the cytoplasm. Once in the nucleus, MEI2 forms the dot and promotes meiosis I. meiRNA is then no longer required for the function of MEI2 in promoting meiosis I; however, MEI2 binding to other RNAs is crucial (Yamashita et al., 1998). Once in the nucleus, MEI2 promotes meiosis I by modifying the availability of meiosis specific mRNA transcripts. In vegetatively growing cells, meiosis specific mRNAs are selectively eliminated by the MMI1 RNA binding protein, which interacts with an RNA element termed the DSR (determinant of selective removal) (Harigaya et al., 2006). During meiosis, MMI1 changes its localization within the nucleus, from several spots to a single dot, which overlaps the MEI2 dot. It is believed that MEI2 sequesters MMI1, preventing it from eliminating meiosis specific genes, resulting in their stable expression (Harigaya et al., 2006). One of these stabilized genes is *Mei4,* a transcription factor involved in controlling middle meiosis genes and necessary for meiosis I (Harigaya et al., 2006; Yamamoto, 2010).

*Mei4* is a meiosis specific transcription factor that binds to an element upstream of its target genes termed FLEX-D, which activates their transcription. It is part of the cascade that controls meiosis in *S. pombe* and *Mei4* mutants arrest in prophase I (Horie et al., 1998). *Mei4* is key to the expression of genes during middle meiosis in *S. pombe,* the genes involved in meiotic divisions, as well as its own expression. *Mei4 is* autoregulated, and it possesses two FLEX-like sequences in its 5′ upstream region, so low levels of *Mei4* expression result in greater transcription (Abe & Shimoda, 2000). Middle genes include cell cycle regulators like *Cdc25,* kinases, components of the SPB and other genes required for progression through the cell cycle. Also represented were genes involved in cell morphogenesis, membrane trafficking, and possibly spore formation (Mata et al., 2002). Interestingly, two of the genes controlled by *Mei4, Mde3* and *Pit1,* are homologs to *S. cerevisiae Ime2.* These genes are involved in sporulation and asci formation, but they do not seem to delay meiotic progression (Abe & Shimoda, 2000). This makes sense, based on their different timing of expression, as *Ime2*'s role in early and middle meiosis requires it to be expressed in early meiosis, not middle meiosis like *Mde3* and *Pit1.* The upstream regions of more than half of these genes have elements similar to the *Mei4* binding motif and 90% of known *Mei4* target genes are found to be up-regulated in the middle phase of meiosis, (Mata et al., 2002). In this way, *Mei4* demonstrates some functional similarities to the *S. cerevisiae Ndt80*, which is also expressed during middle meiosis, where it regulates its own expression, promotes the expression of other middle meiosis genes and is essential for progression to the first meiotic divisions. Therefore, although they are not related proteins, NDT80 and MEI4 seem to fulfil functionally equivalent roles, indicating that this post-initiation/premeiotic division stage is a conserved component of meiotic completion.

Late meiosis genes in *S. pombe* are involved in spore formation and they are expressed after the meiotic divisions. These include stress response, cell cycle regulation and cell wall formation genes (Mata et al., 2002). Many late genes have a binding site for Atf transcription factors and over half of late genes are regulated by ATF21 and ATF31. These transcription factors are expressed during the middle phase of meiosis, and induce late gene expression (Mata et al., 2002). The conservation of transcriptional waves in *S. pombe* and *S. cerevisiae* as well as *C. cinerea* (Burns et al., 2010b) suggests this may be a wide spread mechanism to ensure that the orderly progression of meiosis.

### 4.3 *Ustilago maydis*

The *Ustilago maydis* meiotic transcriptional program has not been elucidated; however, initial data in this area is available in the form of transcript profiling during periods of sexual development and bioinformatic analysis comparing *U. maydis* genes to known meiotic genes in other organisms. Here we will review and update the results of these past analyses, reflect on what they suggest regarding transcriptional control of meiosis in *U. maydis* and propose future experiments.

Zahiri et al. (2005) used cDNA microarray hybridization experiments to investigate changes in gene expression during teliospore germination. They selected two time points for investigation: 4 hrs and 11 hrs post induction of germination. Transcript levels at these time points were compared to those in the dormant teliospore. To provide context, recall that *U. maydis* teliospores germinate at late prophase I (O'Donnell & McLaughlin, 1984). Therefore, by the time teliospores germinate, the early stages of meiosis are completed and the stage is set for completion of meiosis I. Early biochemical experiments showed that, during teliospore germination, total RNA increased steadily; however, protein synthesis did not proceed at a measurable level until approximately 6 hrs after inducing germination. From 6hrs onward, protein synthesis increased linearly with time (Tripathi & Gottlieb, 1974). Zahiri et al. (2005) identified genes whose transcript levels decreased upon germination and proposed that these transcripts were stored in the dormant spore and degraded as germination proceeded, possibly following translation. These transcripts were proposed to code proteins required early in the germination process, or for reinitiating meiosis before visible signs of germination were evident. Genes involved in early meiosis would be expected to be captured in this study, and Zahiri et al. (2005) identified those involved in recombination, DNA repair, transcription, translation, protein turnover and assembly, stress response, and metabolism. The interpretation of Zahiri et al. (2005) was that the array of genes found was consistent with change from a state of dormancy to one of physiological activity, and with the events of early meiosis, notably DNA recombination and repair. Upon re-examination, two of the genes in this category, *Rad51* and *Brh2*, in addition to their role in meiosis, are required for teliospore germination. Null mutants of *Rad51* and *Brh2* are unable to produce basidia (Kojic et al 2002). Transcript presence for these genes in the dormant teliospore, therefore, may or may not support the occurrence of the early stages of meiosis in the early stages of teliospore germination. Interestingly, *Rad51* transcript level decreases as germination proceeds, while the *Brh2* transcript level increases. *Brh2* expression is consistent with it having an ongoing role in the events of germination and/or meiosis. This data also showed evidence of waves of transcription. Zahiri et al. (2005) noted that genes upregulated at the later stage of germination and meiosis included: DNA repair, protein turnover, cell wall synthesis and metabolism. Cell wall synthesis genes are involved in basidium formation, which would fit with genes typically expected to be expressed during late meiosis. The increased expression of genes involved in protein turnover is believed to indicate the physiological transition and we now see that *Brh2*, a gene thought to be only involved in DNA repair, may have other roles during teliospore germination. Zahiri et al. (2005) proposed that the dormant teliospore is in a premeiotic state and that it begins meiosis immediately upon induction of germination. However, Donaldson and Saville (2008) proposed that DNA replication occurred before karyogamy, while the cell is still *in planta*. This means that the initial steps of meiosis up to prophase I would occur before the teliospore enters dormancy, with the cell arresting at the pachytene checkpoint (Donaldson & Saville, 2008). This would be consistent with the observation that as the basidium forms, the cell is already in late prophase I, clearing the pachytene checkpoint and beginning meiotic divisions only a short time after induction of germination, and before any new protein synthesis has been detected in the teliospore (Donaldson & Saville, 2008). The reinterpretation of the Zahiri et al. (2005) data, with the knowledge of alternate roles for some genes otherwise considered to be meiosis genes (Banuett, 2010), indicates that the Donaldson and Saville (2008) interpretation is more likely correct.

Donaldson and Saville (2008) performed comparative genomic analysis between *U. maydis,* and *S. cerevisiae, S. pombe,* and *N. crassa*. They identified 164 potential *U. maydis* orthologs to meiosis genes found in other fungi, of which 66 genes overlapped with the core meiotic genes conserved between *S. cerevisiae* and *S. pombe* (Mata et al., 2002). Potential orthologs were identified to several key meiotic genes, including: *Ime2, Ndt80, Ume6,* and *Ste11.* Notably absent, however, were *U. maydis* orthologs to *Mei4, Ime1, Atf21* and *Atf31* (Donaldson & Saville, 2008). Of the orthologs that were identified, the *Ime2* and *Ste11* orthologs, *Crk1* and *Prf1,* respectively, have been well characterized in *U. maydis.* Although both *Crk1* and *Prf1* are involved in mating and pathogenic development of *U. maydis* (discussed earlier in this chapter), a direct link to meiotic initiation has not been shown for either gene. This could indicate that these two proteins perform a different role in *U. maydis;* influencing mating, but not directly influencing meiosis; or that the role in meiosis could simply be obscured by the fact that *Crk1* and *Prf1* mutants prevent pathogenesis, arresting development before meiosis occurs. Distinguishing between these possibilities will require further investigation.

*Ndt80* in *U. maydis* (hereinafter referred to as *UmNdt80*) is highly divergent from its *S. cerevisiae* ortholog. It was identified based on similarity with a *N. crassa* gene that had a low level of similarity to *S. cerevisiae Ndt80* (Donaldson & Saville, 2008; Borkovich et al., 2004). *U. maydis* strains in which *UmNdt80* is deleted are capable of mating, pathogenesis, tumour formation and teliospore production. However, *UmNdt80* mutant teliospores are tan coloured, in contrast to the dark brown teliospores formed by a wild-type *U. maydis* infection. These *UmNdt80* mutant teliospores are meiotically deficient, with up to 95% germinating as diploids, suggesting that they failed to complete meiosis (Doyle & Saville, unpublished). These initial analyses of *UmNdt80*, a potential meiotic control gene, suggest that it plays an essential role in teliospore formation and meiotic completion. *UmNdt80* appears to play a role after mating and initiation of pathogenesis is complete, affecting the later events of meiosis and spore formation. This is similar to the role of NDT80 in *S. cerevisiae*, which is interesting when one considers that NDT80 and UmNDT80 are highly divergent proteins, with only the NDT80-PhoG active site showing similarity. From this, we infer that *UmNdt80* functions as a transcription factor involved in meiotic progression and teliospore formation, but its expression is not regulated like *S. cerevisiae Ndt80*. *U. maydis* is a fungal pathogen that achieves meiotic competence and forms teliospores only *in planta*, it is clear that the environmental signals leading to meiosis and teliospore formation are different than those involved with meiosis in *S. cerevisiae*. Consistent with this, *U. maydis* lacks the main transcription factor (*Ime1*) that stimulates the expression of *Ndt80* in *S. cerevisiae* and the *U. maydis Ime2* ortholog, *Crk1* (Donaldson & Saville, 2008) does not have the direct link to meiosis exhibited by the *S. cerevisiae, Ime2*.

While the bioinformatic and functional analyses of transcription factors in *U. maydis* have revealed some interesting possibilities concerning meiotic control, further wet lab experiments are required. The focus of these experiments will be to understand the progression of gene expression during *U. maydis* meiosis and the role of UmNDT80 in this process. We will investigate the functions of *U. maydis* orthologs for *S. cerevisiae* genes involved in meiosis, including *Spo11*, and *Rim11*. We are also investigating the upstream control of *UmNdt80*, with a goal of working back to find transcription factors involved in the initiation of meiosis and teliospore formation. These, and other studies underway, will provide the tools to identify the environmental (plant) signals required for meiotic initiation.

## 5. Meiosis gene presence and function in fungi

In this section we provide an overview on how meiosis genes can be identified in organisms with a sequenced genome. We then provide a comparative analysis of the presence and absence of "core meiosis genes" in select pathogenic and non-pathogenic fungi and close with a transcriptional analysis of predicted *U. maydis* meiosis genes. The transcriptional analysis section contains a brief discussion of the possible post transcriptional events that control meiosis gene expression in *U. maydis*.

### 5.1 Identification of meiosis genes in fungi

The use of DNA microarrays facilitated the identification of a large number of genes involved in meiosis and sporulation in *S. cerevisiae* and *S. pombe*. Chu et al. (1998) identified over 1000 *S. cerevisiae* genes with differential expression (induced or repressed) during meiosis, representing nearly 16% of the budding yeast transcriptome. Genes were grouped based on their temporal expression into 7 distinct clusters; fine-tuning the previously identified early, middle, mid-late, and late meiotic- and sporulation-specific gene clusters (Mitchell, 1994). Primig et al. (2000) identified strain-dependent meiosis-specific genes by comparing the meiotic transcriptome of two yeast strains (SK1 and W303), which differ in their rates of sporulation. A core set of 900 genes with strain-independent meiotic expression was observed and the inventory of meiosis- and sporulation-specific genes in budding yeast was expanded with the identification of 650 previously unreported meiosis-specific genes. In both studies, the functions of uncharacterized genes were inferred as meiotic- or sporulation-specific, based on their temporal expression (Chu et al., 1998; Primig et al., 2000). Schlecht and Primig (2003) further defined a set of 75 core meiotic- and sporulation-specific genes for *S. cerevisiae*. Mata et al. (2002) identified approximately 1000 *S. pombe* genes with a fourfold increase in expression during meiotic growth conditions compared to vegetative growth conditions. Mata et al. (2002) compared the meiosis-specific fission yeast genes to the core strain-independent meiosis-specific genes (Primig et al., 2000) and identified 75 genes upregulated during meiosis in both budding and fission yeast. This core group of shared genes between the two diverged yeast species contained genes related to the process of meiosis and sporulation (*Rec8*, *Dmc1*, and *Hop2* for example) but lacked genes related to the timing of their expression; indicating the control of meiosis evolved after budding and fission yeast diverged from a common ancestor (Mata et al., 2002). Mata and Bahler (2003) expanded their analysis of *S. pombe* and observed that organism-specific genes (orphans) were over-represented during meiosis and sporulation, particularly in meiotic prophase. Mata and Bahler (2003) noted that meiotic structural proteins are poorly conserved, contrasting the identification of core recombination proteins among eukaryotes (Villeneuve & Hillers, 2001).

Information gained from the DNA microarray studies in budding yeast and fission yeast was used to identify meiotic orthologs in the filamentous ascomycete *Neurospora crassa* and the basidiomycete pathogen *U. maydis* (Borkovich et al., 2004; Donaldson & Saville, 2008). Putative orthologs for the majority (~77%) of core meiotic genes shared between *S. cerevisiae* and *S. pombe* were identified in *U. maydis*. The inability to detect all of the core meiotic genes indicates that either meiosis genes have diverged beyond sequence recognition using blastp-analysis in *U. maydis* relative to the yeasts, or there are basidiomycete- or *U. maydis*-specific meiosis genes that replace the functions of identified yeast genes (Donaldson & Saville, 2008).

### 5.2 The core eukaryotic meiosis-specific machinery

Much attention has been given to the identification of a conserved set of core meiotic proteins across eukaryotes. Villeneuve and Hillers (2001) identified meiotic recombination proteins shared between animals, plants and fungi; presumably stemming from a common ancestor. Key components of the conserved meiotic recombination machinery include: SPO11, RAD50/MRE11, DMC1, RAD51, MSH4/MSH5, and MLH1. While analyzing the *Giardia lamblia* genome, Ramesh et al. (2005) augmented the list of core meiotic proteins identified by Villeneuve and Hillers (2001) to include HOP1, HOP2, MND1, RAD52, MSH2, MSH6, MLH2, MLH3, and PMS1. While identifying meiotic homologs in *Trichomonas vaginalis*, Malik et al. (2007) added RAD1, MER3, SMC1-5, RAD18, RAD21, REC8, PDS5, and SCC3 to the list of core meiotic proteins conserved across a wide range of plants, animals and fungi. Of the 29 proteins conserved across eukaryotes, only SPO11, HOP1, HOP2, MND1, DMC1, MSH4, MSH5, MER3, and REC8 are reported to be functional solely during meiosis (Malik et al., 2007). Interestingly, when looking at the phylogenetic distribution of the 29 core meiotic proteins across the fungi studied by Malik et al. (2007), one can observe that the loss of key meiosis proteins is restricted to the 9 proteins only functional during meiosis (with the exception of MLH2 and MLH3 in some fungi).

Table 1 shows the presence and absence of these 9 proteins across the model yeasts *S. cerevisiae* and *S. pombe,* the model basidiomycete mushroom, *C. cinereus,* and fungal plant pathogens, including: *Gibberella zeae* (wheat head blight fungus), *Magnaporthe grisea* (rice blast fungus), *Sporisorium reilianum* (maize head smut), and *U. maydis* (common smut of corn). We will focus our discussion on the loss of HOP2, MND1, DMC1 and HOP1.

The absence of an ortholog to DMC1 is coincident with a loss of MND1, and HOP2 (reviewed in Neale & Keeney, 2006). *G. zeae, M. grisea, S. reilianum,* and *U. maydis* lack clear orthologs to DMC1, MND1, and HOP2 (Table 1). Loss of DMC1, MND1, and HOP2 is not unique to the fungal plant pathogens as it has been reported in *Drosophila melanogaster, Caenorhabditis elegans,* and *N. crassa* (Malik et al., 2007). Recently in a comparison of eight *Candida* genomes, these genes were absent in *C. guilliermondii* and *C. lusitaniae* (Butler et al., 2009). In an excellent review of the homologous recombination system in *U. maydis,* Holloman et al. (2008) concluded BRH2, RAD51, and REC2, a paralog to RAD51, efficiently mediate homologous pairing during meiosis in a RAD51-dependent manner (in the absence of DMC1, MND1, and HOP2). Additionally, given its capacity to promote DMC1-like DNA strand exchange, it was speculated that REC2 evolved as a substitute for DMC1 in *U. maydis* (Holloman et al., 2008). While the *U. maydis* REC2 is a weak ortholog to *S. cerevisiae* REC57 (e-value = 4-e4; reported in Holloman et al., 2008), there is a clear ortholog in *S. reilianum* (e-value = 0.0). Therefore, it would not be surprising for REC2 to compensate for the loss of DMC1 in *S. reilianum* as well.

A recognizable ortholog to HOP1 is absent in *G. zeae, M. grisea, S. reilianum,* and *U. maydis* (Table 1). This loss is not unique to the fungal plant pathogens, as *D. melanogaster, N. crassa, C. guilliermondii* and *C. lusitaniae* lack clear HOP1 orthologs (Butler et al., 2009; Malik et al., 2007). HOP1 is a structural component of the synaptonemal complex (SC), a tripartite structure which holds homologous chromosomes together during meiosis (reviewed in Loidl, 2006). The absence of clear orthologs to other synaptonemal complex proteins: ZIP1, ZIP2, ZIP3, and RED1, coupled with the inability to observe SCs microscopically (Fletcher, 1981), has brought into question whether SC formation occurs in *U. maydis* (Donaldson & Saville, 2008; Holloman et al., 2008). It should be noted that, with the exception of HOP1, SC proteins show great sequence divergence between organisms (Loidl, 2006). Additionally, SC formation may occur in *U. maydis* during teliospore development (*in planta*), or prior to teliospore germination when the thick cell wall interferes with SC visualization (Fletcher, 1981). Therefore, SC formation in *U. maydis* may occur. Conversely, SC formation may not occur in *U. maydis,* as is the case in *Aspergillus nidulans,* and *S. pombe* (Loidl, 2006). In *S. pombe,* linear elements (LinEs) are formed in the absence of SCs. It has been suggested that the low chromosome number in *S. pombe* enables an abridged version of the SC machinery to efficiently pair and recombine chromosomes during meiosis (Loidl, 2006). In this mechanism, an ortholog to *S. cerevisiae* RED1 (*S. pombe* REC10) is essential for the formation of LinEs, while HOP1, and MEK1 are active in their formation, but not required (Loidl, 2006). *U. maydis* contains an ortholog only to MEK1 (Donaldson & Saville, 2008), suggesting that it is unable to form LinEs.

| Protein | *S. cerevisiae*[1] | *S. pombe*[1] | *C. cinereus*[2] | *G. zeae*[1] | *M. grisea*[1] | *S. reilianum*[3] | *U. maydis*[4] | *S. cerevisiae* function[5] |
|---|---|---|---|---|---|---|---|---|
| **SPO11** | + | + | + | + | + | + | + | Meiosis-specific protein that initiates meiotic recombination by catalyzing the formation of double-strand breaks in DNA via a transesterification reaction; required for homologous chromosome pairing and synaptonemal complex formation |
| **HOP1** | + | + | + | - | - | - | - | Meiosis-specific DNA binding protein that displays Red1p dependent localization to the unsynapsed axial-lateral elements of the synaptonemal complex; required for homologous chromosome synapsis and chiasma formation |
| **HOP2** | + | + | + | - | - | - | - | Meiosis-specific protein that localizes to chromosomes, preventing synapsis between nonhomologous chromosomes and ensuring synapsis between homologs; complexes with Mnd1p to promote homolog pairing and meiotic double-strand break repair |
| **MND1** | + | + | + | - | - | - | - | Protein required for recombination and meiotic nuclear division; forms a complex with Hop2p, which is involved in chromosome pairing and repair of meiotic double-strand breaks |
| **DMC1** | + | + | + | - | - | - | - | Meiosis-specific protein required for repair of double-strand breaks and pairing between homologous chromosomes; homolog of Rad51p and the bacterial RecA protein |
| **MSH4** | + | - | + | + | + | + | + | Protein involved in meiotic recombination, required for normal levels of crossing over, colocalizes with Zip2p to discrete foci on meiotic chromosomes, has homology to bacterial MutS protein |
| **MSH5** | + | - | + | + | + | + | + | Protein of the MutS family, forms a dimer with Msh4p that facilitates crossovers between homologs during meiosis; msh5-Y823H mutation confers tolerance to DNA alkylating agents; homologs present in C. elegans and humans |
| **MER3** | + | - | + | - | + | + | + | Meiosis specific DNA helicase involved in the conversion of double-stranded breaks to later recombination intermediates and in crossover control; catalyzes the unwinding of Holliday junctions; has ssDNA and dsDNA stimulated ATPase activity |
| **REC8** | + | + | + | + | + | + | + | Meiosis-specific component of sister chromatid cohesion complex; maintains cohesion between sister chromatids during meiosis I; maintains cohesion between centromeres of sister chromatids until meiosis II; homolog of S. pombe Rec8p |

[1]Data retrieved from Malik et al. (2007). [2]Data retrieved from Burns et al. (2010a). [3]Data retrieved from the Munich Information center for Protein Sequences *Sporisorium reilianum* Database (Schirawski et al., 2010). [4]Data retrieved from Donaldson and Saville (2008). [5]Protein function retrieved from the *Saccharomyces* Genome Database (2011).

Table 1. Core meiosis-specific genes conserved among model fungi and select fungal plant pathogens. Putative loss of protein is highlighted in grey.

### 5.3 Core meiosis-specific gene expression in *U. maydis*

In order to gain insight into the timing of meiosis *in planta,* we investigated the expression of four core meiosis-specific genes in *U. maydis* (Table 1). We included a fifth gene, *Mre11,* a key component in the MRE11-RAD50-XRS2 (MRX) complex, which processes double strand break ends prior to homologous recombination (Holloman et al., 2008). Schlecht and Primig (2003) identified *Mre11* as being meiosis and sporulation specific in *S. cerevisiae.* Using a combination of statistical analysis and PCR, Ho et al. (2007) identified a conserved hypothetical gene (*Um01426*) to be highly expressed in the dormant teliospore, compared to haploid cells grown in rich media. This gene was included in our analysis to estimate the timing of teliospore maturation in the *in planta* time course expression analysis. Glyceraldehyde 3-phosphate dehydrogenase (*UmGapd*) is constitutively expressed in *U. maydis* and its expression was used to detect the presence of *U. maydis* cells *in planta.*

Golden Bantam seedlings were infected with compatible *U. maydis* haploids (FB1, FB2) and leaf samples were taken 2, 4, 6, 8, 10, and 14 days post infection (dpi). RNA was isolated from these six leaf time-points, as well as dikaryotic and forced diploid mycelia grown filamentously, teliospores isolated from mature tumours on infected ears of corn, and individual compatible haploids. Equal amounts of RNA were used as template for reverse transcriptase reactions primed with oligo-d$(T)_{16}$. The resulting cDNA was diluted and equal amounts were used as template for PCR. When possible, primers were designed to flank introns (*UmSpo11, Um01426,* and *UmGapd*), to clarify the difference in sizes of the amplified products between PCRs with cDNA as template and genomic DNA as template (Figure 2a). The results presented as "leaf" represent a combination of plant and fungal RNA isolated from infected leaves while the *U. maydis* cell type results are RT-PCR results from pure fungal RNA. Therefore, the results are displayed as two separate panels (leaf samples, or *U. maydis* cell-types; Figure 2a). Given that the amount of RNA going into first strand synthesis was equivalent in each panel, the resulting RT-PCR product viewed on the ethidium-bromide stained agarose gel may be interpreted as representing the relative expression for each transcript. Comparison between panels is not valid. We estimated the relative expression of the meiosis-specific transcripts for each gene individually, for the leaf and *U. maydis* cell-types (Figure 2b).

Banuett and Herskowitz (1996) provide an excellent framework for a comparison between the initiation of meiosis and homologous recombination in relation to hyphal development and teliospore formation *in planta.* It should be cautioned that differences in the timing of *U. maydis* development may arise due to the type of maize variety infected, and plant growth conditions (Banuett & Herskowitz, 1996). The total RNA isolated from leaf samples is expected to contain RNA from *U. maydis* cells at different stages of development since *U. maydis* development is asynchronous *in planta.* Additionally, changes in transcript levels does not necessarily imply changes in the respective protein levels, especially since meiosis genes are known to be post-transcriptionally regulated (Burns et al., 2010b). We will attempt to determine the timing of meiosis initiation and homologous recombination relative to the *in planta* development of *U. maydis.* Given that we used a different maize variety and infected corn seedlings 2 days later than Banuett and Herskowitz (1996), we might expect inconsistencies between the molecular and morphological studies. Nonetheless, it is interesting that the expression of *Um01426,* a gene highly expressed in mature teliospores (Ho et al., 2007) is upregulated 6-8 dpi, in line with the time that teliospore formation is initiated, and its expression peaks 14 dpi when mature teliospores are visible (Figure 2a,b; Banuett & Herskowitz, 1996).

a)

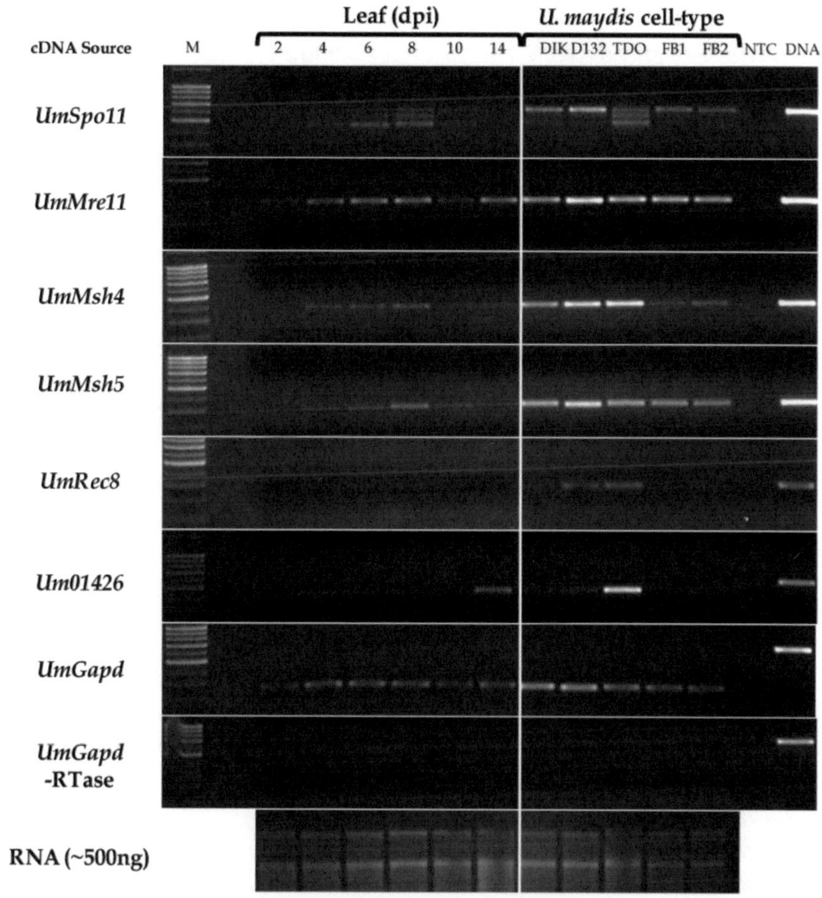


b)

| | Relative level of expression[1]: Leaf (days post infection) | | | | | | Relative level of expression[2]: *U. maydis* cell-type | | | | |
|---|---|---|---|---|---|---|---|---|---|---|---|
| Gene | 2 | 4 | 6 | 8 | 10 | 14 | DIK | D132 | TDO | FB1 | FB2 |
| *UmSpo11* | - | + | ++ | +++ | + | - | + | + | +++ | + | + |
| *UmMre11* | + | ++ | +++ | +++ | + | +++ | + | +++ | ++ | ++ | ++ |
| *UmMsh4* | - | ++ | ++ | ++ | + | + | ++ | +++ | +++ | + | + |
| *UmMsh5* | - | + | ++ | +++ | ++ | - | ++ | +++ | ++ | + | + |
| *UmRec8* | - | + | + | + | - | - | + | ++ | +++ | + | + |
| *Um01426* | - | + | ++ | ++ | + | +++ | ++ | ++ | +++ | + | + |

Fig. 2. Semi-quantitative RT-PCR analysis of core meiotic gene expression in *U. maydis*. a) The cellular origins of the cDNA templates were: Leaf samples taken at 2, 4, 6, 8, 10, and 14 days post infection (dpi); DIK, dikaryotic filamentous mycelia; D132, diploid filamentous mycelia; TDO, dormant teliospore; FB1, haploid cell (*a1 b1*); FB2 haploid cell (*a2 b2*); NTC, no template control; DNA, genomic DNA; M, FullRanger 100 bp DNA Ladder (Norgen Biotek). RNA quality was accessed by glyoxal agarose gel electrophoresis. b) Relative levels of gene expression were estimated on a gene-by-gene basis independently for the [1]leaf and [2]cell-type specific RT-PCR groupings; -, no expression; +, low expression; ++, mid expression; +++, high expression.

*Spo11* expression has been used to signal the transition between non-meiotic and meiotic cells in *S. cerevisiae* and *S. pombe* (Burns et al., 2010b). We detected unspliced *UmSpo11* at 2 dpi where filaments have been observed on the leaf epidermal surface (Banuett & Herskowitz, 1996). A discussion on the implications of alternatively spliced *UmSpo11* will follow; however, if the spliced variant detected at 4 dpi (Figure 2a) yields a protein that is responsible for double strand break formation at a time where dikaryotic filaments penetrate through the stomata and branch within the plant cells, then the dikaryotic filament may be prepped to initiate the transition from mitotic to meiotic cells directly after karyogamy occurs (9-10 dpi; Banuett & Herskowitz, 1996). Premeiotic DNA replication in C. cinerea occurs prior to karyogamy (reviewed in Burns et al., 2010b). In U. maydis, the timing of premeiotic DNA replication, relative to karyogamy is unknown. The expression of many genes involved in homologous recombination (*UmMre11, UmMsh4, UmMsh5,* and *UmRec8*) prior to the time-points suggested for hyphal fragmentation and karyogamy is intriguing. We may have detected so-called "leaky" transcription, but due to the deleterious effects of leaky transcription, it is more likely that the transcript is present and the protein is not functional at the time we detected. In a comparison of the meiotic expression profiles of shared orthologs between *S. pombe, S. cerevisiae,* and *C. cinerea,* Burns et al. (2010b) note that the expression of *Spo11* and *Rec8* peak late in meiosis, prior to the first meiotic division, past the time-point when the protein is functional. We observed that, while the expression of core genes involved in homologous recombination in *U. maydis* are detectable 4 dpi, they peak in-between 6-10 dpi, coincident with teliospore formation, hyphal fragmentation and karyogamy (Figure 2a,b; Banuett & Herskowitz, 1996). Given this expression of the core meiotic genes responsible for homologous recombination, and using expression of *Um01426* (discussed above) as a reference, we propose cells are prepped for meiosis prior to teliospore maturation.

### 5.4 Post-transcriptional control of Spo11 and controlled meiotic splicing in *S. cerevisiae* and *S. pombe*

Under specific conditions in budding yeast, regulated splicing can affect translation by introducing frame shift mutations or nonsense codons, producing non-functional proteins (Juneau et al., 2007). Using high-density tiling arrays, Juneau et al. (2007) discovered 13 intronic meiosis-specific genes that undergo regulated splicing in *S. cerevisiae*. Using RT-PCR, it was observed that the transcripts *Ama1, Hfm1, Hop2, Mnd1, Rec107, Rec114, Rec102, Pch2, Spo22, Dmc1, Mei4, Sae3,* and *Spo1* spliced more efficiently (>84%) during sporulation compared to vegetative growth (Juneau et al., 2007). Therefore, regulated splicing of select meiotic-specific transcripts could help the cell overcome the deleterious effects of leaky meiotic gene expression during mitosis.

Similarly, meiosis-specific splicing has been noted in *S. pombe*. In a random sampling of 96 intronic meiosis-specific genes, Averbeck et al. (2005) used RT-PCR to identify 12 transcripts (including *Crs1, Meu13, Rec8, Spo4, Spo6,* and *Mfr1*) that underwent meiosis-specific splicing and correlated with the temporal waves of meiotic-gene expression (early, middle, late) observed during meiotic progression (Mata et al., 2002). Overexpression of *Crs1* (cyclin-like protein regulated via splicing), was toxic to vegetative cells, highlighting the requirement of mitotically growing cells to have tight regulation of meiosis-specific genes. Moldon et al. (2008) showed *Rem1* encodes two proteins with different functions, depending on the regulated splice form. During vegetative growth, full-length *Rem1* affects recombination in the premeiotic S phase, while spliced *Rem1* acts as a cyclin during meiosis I (whose expression is toxic in mitotic cells). Control of *Rem1* splicing is guided by two forkhead transcription factors, *Fkh2* and *Mei4*. During vegetative growth, FKH2 binds the *Rem1* promoter and *Rem1* is not spliced. During meiosis, MEI4 binds the *Rem1* promoter, and recruits the spliceosome, leading to a spliced variant of *Rem1* (Moldon et al., 2008). The prevalence of meiosis-specific splicing in *S. pombe* adds additional levels of meiotic posttranscriptional gene regulation.

Interestingly, in our analysis of the expression of *UmSpo11*, we detected three different PCR products of varying sizes ranging from ~400bp to ~600bp (Figure 2a). The ~600bp product co-migrated with the amplification using genomic DNA as template. We ruled out genomic DNA as a source of contamination due to the absence of amplification in PCR using RNA as template (minus reverse transcriptase) and the presence, in RT-PCR reactions of other intron containing genes (*Um01426*, and *UmGapd*), of only PCR products of a size consistent with the mature (spliced) transcripts. The primers designed for the *UmSpo11* PCR flanked an intron, and the expected amplicon size for processed transcripts, based on the current genome annotation, was ~350bp. No expressed sequence tag data is available for the *UmSpo11* region in question so it is possible that the current online annotation in the *Ustilago maydis* database for *UmSpo11* does not correctly predict the intron size (Mewes et al., 2008). Experiments are underway to determine whether or not the transcripts represented by the ~400bp or ~500bp amplicons contain an uninterrupted ORF. It is tempting to speculate that *UmSpo11* has transcripts of different sizes that code for proteins with distinct functions, and/or that the *UmSpo11* transcript undergoes meiosis-specific splicing. In mice and humans, two SPO11 isoforms are produced by alternative splicing (Romanienko & Camerini-Otero, 1999). The two isoforms in mice, SPO11β and SPO11α, are translated from a transcript containing all 13 exons and a transcript which skips the second exon, respectively (Bellani et al., 2010). Bellani et al. (2010) studied SPO11 isoform expression levels in mouse meiocytes and determined SPO11β initiates double strand breaks in early spermatocytes and SPO11α is present in pachytene/diplotene spermatocytes where it might act as a topoisomerase.

One final possibility is that one, or more of the *UmSpo11* amplicons represents a natural antisense transcript (NAT) and not an alternatively spliced transcript. NATs are polyadenylated in *U. maydis* (Ho et al., 2007) and therefore could be represented as a cDNA product in the presented reverse transcriptase reactions. If present, the NAT cDNA from the *UmSpo11* locus could then serve as template in the PCR. This is not without precedent as an antisense transcript overlaps the 3' end of the *Arabidopsis thaliana AtSpo11-2* locus (Hartung & Puchta, 2000). Three different isoforms of *AtSpo11-2* were observed, varying in their 3'UTR length and in the presence of an intron in the 3'UTR. While it is possible that the antisense transcript to *AtSpo11-2* elicits the RNA silencing pathway, it may be possible that the antisense transcript regulates the splicing of *AtSpo11-2* by masking the splice sites in the 3'UTR. Given the absence of a functional RNAi pathway in *U. maydis*, if one of the alternative splice forms seen for *UmSpo11* is an antisense transcript, it may act to regulate the splicing of *UmSpo11*. Experiments are underway to characterize all UmSpo11 transcripts.

It is noteworthy that Heimel et al. (2010) recently showed that *UmCib1*, a transcription factor required for pathogenic development, is predominantly unspliced during saprophytic growth, but undergoes splicing during biotrophic growth. Therefore, it is highly likely that other biological roles for alternate splicing in *U. maydis* remain to be discovered.

## 6. A regulatory role for fungal noncoding RNAs in meiosis

This section will begin with a broad overview of noncoding RNA (ncRNA) function in eukaryotes. There is very limited information on ncRNAs in other smuts and rusts; therefore, we will highlight the prevalence of meiosis-specific ncRNAs in *S. cerevisiae* and *S. pombe*, including putative functional roles for their expression. We will review specific examples of how ncRNAs function in controlling gene expression and conclude with knowledge that our laboratory is accumulating on ncRNAs and long natural antisense transcripts (NATs) in *U. maydis*.

### 6.1 Introduction to noncoding RNAs in eukaryotes

Recent estimates are that >90% of eukaryotic genomes are transcribed, but protein-coding transcripts only account for ~2-3% of eukaryotic genome transcription (reviewed in Costa, 2010). The difference is comprised of noncoding RNAs, some of which have a role in controlling gene expression. Thus, at least a portion of these so-called ncRNAs actually have a function that adds to the complexity of gene expression. Noncoding RNAs are divided into classes depending on their size and origin. For example, short ncRNAs (~20-31nt) include microRNAs (miRNAs), piwi-interacting RNAs (piRNAs), and small interfering RNAs (siRNAs). Long ncRNAs (>200nt) include, but are not limited to, long intergenic transcripts, and natural antisense transcripts (NATs). NATs are RNA molecules transcribed from the DNA strand complementary to that which codes the mRNA (reviewed in Costa, 2010; Faghihi & Wahlestedt 2009; Tisseur et al., 2011). Noncoding RNAs exert their function at the transcriptional or post-transcriptional level using a wide range of regulatory mechanisms including: RNA interference (RNAi), transcriptional interference, RNA masking (affecting mRNA-splicing, -transport, -polyadenylation, -translation, or -stability), RNA editing, X chromosome inactivation, imprinting, and chromatin remodelling (Costa, 2005; reviewed in Lavorgna et al., 2004; Munroe & Zhu, 2005). Notably, while most plants, animal and fungi contain functional RNA silencing machinery, phylogenetic analyses have revealed select ascomycetes (*S. cerevisiae* and *Candida lusitaniae*) and *U. maydis* lack the canonical RNAi machinery. The expression of ncRNAs, especially NATs in fungi that do not contain the canonical RNAi machinery sets the stage for discovering new mechanisms of controlling meiotic gene expression.

### 6.2 Global expression of meiosis-specific ncRNAs in *S. cerevisiae* and *S. pombe*

Yassour et al. (2011) created a strand-specific cDNA library using RNA isolated from *S. cerevisiae* cells during mid-log growth in rich media. Next-generation (Illumina) sequencing revealed transcript units that had an antisense orientation to 1,103 annotated transcripts. It was concluded that these antisense transcripts may be functional, given there was little evidence they arose from unterminated transcription, bi-directional transcription initiated from divergent promoters, or potential nucleosome-free regions (Yassour et al., 2010). A subset of sense-antisense transcript pairs was examined using strand-specific quantitative real-time PCR (qRT-PCR) and their expression patterns were inversely related, supporting a model where antisense transcripts interfere with sense transcript expression (Yassour et al., 2010). Additionally, the expression levels of six sense-antisense transcript pairs were studied across five yeast species using qRT-PCR. In some instances, both antisense transcript presence and differential expression were conserved, further supporting a functional role for antisense transcripts in *S. cerevisiae* (Yassour et al., 2010). 85 genes expressed at 8 hours post induction of sporulation were associated with antisense transcripts during *S. cerevisiae* mid-log phase growth. For example, the meiosis genes encoding *Ime4, Ndt80, Rec102, Gas2, Sps19, Slz1, Rim9,* and *Smk1* were all associated with long antisense transcripts. Overall, antisense units were prevalent in processes repressed during mid-log phase growth, leading Yassour et al. (2010) to hypothesize that NAT expression in *S. cerevisiae* may be involved in a global repression of stress, stationary phase, and meiosis genes when cells are grown in rich conditions. As a whole, in *S. cerevisiae,* and other yeast species, differentially expressed sense-antisense transcript pairs provide a means of controlling gene expression in response to environmental conditions and in some cases, enable the transition from mid-log phase- to meiotic-growth conditions.

Meiosis-specific genes were identified by T. Watanabe et al. (2001) using a subtractive cDNA library enriched for meiotic gene expression in heterozygous *S. pombe* diploid cells grown in nitrogen starvation conditions. This approach identified 31 *Meu* (meiotic expression upregulated) transcripts, 5 of which were ncRNAs. Notably, *Meu16* encodes an antisense ncRNA overlapping *Mde6* (a *Mei4*-dependent protein). The function of this antisense is not known. Additionally, individual RACE experiments uncovered ncRNAs at the *Rec7* (required for early steps of meiotic recombination) and *Spo6* (required for progression of meiosis II and sporulation) loci (Molnar et al., 2001; Nakamura et al., 2000). Specifically, three antisense transcripts (*Tos1, Tos2* and *Tos3*), of varying lengths, were discovered at the *Rec7* locus. It has been suggested that the *Tos* RNAs may indicate the location of dsDNA break formation (DSB; see below) at the *Rec7* locus (Wahls et al., 2008). *Spo6-L,* encodes a constitutively expressed bidirectional transcript in reverse orientation to the meiosis-specific *Spo6* gene. The function of *Spo6-L* remains unknown (Nakamura et al., 2000).

Subsequently, Wilhelm et al. (2008) studied the transcriptome of *S. pombe* from cells grown in rich media and from five stages of meiotic development under nitrogen limiting conditions.

Their investigation yielded 426 previously unannotated ncRNAs, including 58 ncRNAs (34 of which overlapped known genes in antisense orientation) upregulated under meiotic growth conditions. Many of the ncRNAs appear to be expressed in waves similar to meiosis-specific gene expression in *S. pombe* (Mata et al., 2002, 2007). Ni et al. (2010) created a strand-specific cDNA library using RNA isolated from *S. pombe* cells grown in rich media with or without heat shock. Next generation (Illumina) sequencing revealed ncRNA transcript units that did not overlap with previously defined protein-coding genes. Some loci in *S. pombe,* absent of protein-coding genes, had a comparable number of ncRNA transcripts on both strands, indicating that unlike *S. cerevisiae,* ncRNAs in *S. pombe* may function via the formation of double-stranded RNA, possibly eliciting chromatin remodelling, or posttranscriptional gene silencing. Additional differences that Ni et al. (2010) found between budding and fission yeast include: that antisense transcription is commonly driven through bidirectional promoters in *S. pombe* but not in *S. cerevisiae* and, while the majority of antisense transcripts in *S. pombe* are independently regulated, sense-antisense transcript levels are coordinated in *S. cerevisiae*. This may imply that antisense-mediated gene regulation in *S. pombe* occurs at the posttranscriptional level, or in *trans*, without affecting the relative levels of the sense transcript (Ni et al., 2010). It was observed that differentially expressed genes had a higher abundance of antisense transcripts than constitutively expressed genes, indicating that antisense RNAs may be involved in a targeted control of gene expression (Ni et al., 2010). In total, 2,409 *S. pombe* genes had overlapping antisense transcripts under normal or heat shock conditions. Gene ontology analysis revealed, like *S. cerevisiae*, *S. pombe* is enriched for antisense transcription at 68 loci involved in meiosis, meiotic chromosome segregation, meiotic recombination and ascospore formation. It was hypothesized that antisense transcripts may repress "leaky" meiotic genes under vegetative conditions at the transcriptional or posttranscriptional level (Ni et al., 2010). Using RNA-Seq, the transcriptomes of the fission yeasts *S. pombe*, *S. octosporus*, *S. cryophilus*, and *S. japonicus* were compared under growth conditions including log-phase, glucose starvation, early stationary phase, and heat shock (Rhind et al., 2011). This comparison identified conserved antisense transcripts among some of the fission yeasts. Additionally, for meiotic genes with antisense transcripts, the level of the antisense transcript was higher than the sense transcript (Rhind et al., 2011). For example, meiosis-upregulated genes (*Mug5*, *Mug7*, *Mug27*, *Mug28*, *Mug97*), MEI4 dependent genes (*Mde2*, *Mde3*, *Mde4*, *Mde7*), genes involved in meiotic recombination (*Rec7*, *Rec15*, *Rec24*, *Rec27*) and sporulation-specific genes (*Spo4*, *Spo6*) had higher levels of antisense transcript than sense transcript (Rhind et al., 2011, Supporting online material S21). Notably, antisense transcripts detected towards the core eukaryotic meiosis genes *Hop1* and *Dmc1*, were higher than sense transcript levels, while an antisense transcript level lower than that of the sense transcript was observed for *Rec8*. Strand-specific northern blotting was used to detect relative levels of *S. pombe Spo4*, *Spo6*, *Mde2*, *Mde7*, and *Mug8* sense-antisense transcript pairs. This revealed that antisense transcription of meiotic genes did not share an inverse relationship to sense transcription during log-phase growth, reinforcing the findings of Ni et al. (2010). Taken together, these findings suggest that antisense transcription during log-phase growth does not directly inhibit the transcription of sense transcripts as in *S. cerevisiae*, but elicits the formation of double-stranded RNA to recruit RNAi machinery to destroy "leaky" meiotic transcripts during mitotic growth (Rhind et al., 2011).

### 6.3 Rrp6 controls global expression of meiosis-specific ncRNAs in *S. cerevisiae*

Additional mechanisms of regulating the timing of ncRNA expression during meiosis in *S. cerevisiae* have been discovered. Degradation of ncRNAs in *S. cerevisiae* was linked to RRP6, a key component of the nuclear exosome complex responsible for RNA processing and degradation (Wyers et al., 2005). Deep transcriptome analyses identified cryptic unstable transcripts (CUTs) that accumulate in ΔRrp6 vegetative cells (Neil et al., 2009; Xu et al., 2009). Separately, high-resolution oligonucleotide tiling arrays identified meiotic unannotated transcripts (MUTs), ncRNAs that accumulate in meiotic but not fermenting or respiring cells, and rsSUTs, ncRNAs exhibiting peak expression during respiring or sporulating *MAT* **a**/α diploids (Lardenois et al., 2011). MUTs and rsSUTs were observed to overlap sense mRNAs in an antisense orientation, known promoter regions, or autonomously replicating sequences (ARSs). Lardenois et al. (2011) found that a subset of MUTs and rsSUTs, previously characterized as CUTs (Neil et al., 2009; Xu et al., 2009), are targeted by the nuclear exosome for degradation during vegetative growth conditions. Moreover, Rrp6 expression was observed across all cell-types; but RRP6 levels dropped dramatically as cells switched from mitotic to meiotic growth. During this transition, the decrease in RRP6 levels paralleled the increase in MUTs. Additionally, Δ*Rrp6* cells were unable to proceed with premeiotic DNA replication or to undergo meiosis and spore formation. The progression through meiosis may be facilitated by the accumulation of MUTs transcribed at mitotically active loci (such as *Chs2*, *Cln3*, and *Hug1*); MUT expression would interfere with the transcription of some mitotic genes during meiosis (Lardenois et al., 2011). Yassour et al. (2011) observed an increased level of antisense transcription in Δ*Rrp6* mutants, associated with a small decrease in complementary sense mRNA levels. Additionally, the transcription of the MUT, itself, may interfere with promoter regions required for proper transcription of select mRNAs or ARS elements required for DNA replication during specific cell-stages. For example, MUT expression was detected towards the *Cln2* promoter region. CLN2 is a repressor of IME1; therefore, *Cln2* levels decrease during meiosis, possibly facilitated through a promoter-interference mechanism where MUT transcription hinders promoter activity (Lardenois et al., 2011).

### 6.4 *S. cerevisiae IME4* and *ZIP1* ncRNA functions

*S. cerevisiae MAT* **a**/α diploids require full activation of *IME1* which is mediated by IME4 expression. Therefore, *Ime4* expression during nutrient starvation is pivotal in determining whether or not the cell initiates meiosis. Hongay et al. (2006) observed cell-type specific sense and antisense transcription at the *Ime4* locus. Haploids expressed an antisense transcript to *Ime4*, called *Rme2* (regulator of meiosis 2; Gelfand et al., 2011), and *MAT* **a**/α diploids expressed *Ime4* sense RNA. In *MAT* **a**/α diploids, the **a**1-α2 protein heterodimer silences expression of *Rme2*, enabling the expression of *Ime4*, full expression of *Ime1*, and entry into meiosis. Their findings were consistent with a transcriptional interference mechanism, since transcription of *Rme2* in haploid cells only interfered with *Ime4* sense expression in *cis* (Hongay et al., 2006). Similarly, *Zip2*, a meiosis-specific protein involved in synaptonemal complex formation, shows cell-type specific sense and antisense expression (Gelfand et al., 2011). Haploids express an antisense transcript to *Zip2*, called *Rme3* (regulator of meiosis 3) and *MAT* **a**/α diploids express *Zip2* sense RNA. The **a**1-α2 protein heterodimer silences expression of *Rme3* in *MAT* **a**/α diploids, enabling expression of *Zip2*. Gelfand et al. (2011) expanded on previous research to show that *Rme2* extension through the *Ime4* promoter region was not required for *Ime4* repression and *Rme3* does not extend through the entire *Zip2* ORF, indicating that both *Rme2* and *Rme3* do not interfere with TATA-binding proteins or polymerase binding in the promoter regions. Additionally, a 450 bp region within *Ime4* was essential for *Rme2*-mediated repression. This suggested that the 450 bp region may only be transcribed in a single direction at one time, or that extension of the transcript is terminated by specific protein complexes which bind this region, or chromatin remodelling occurs at this site. Overall, transcriptional interference may be prevalent in controlling yeast gene expression (Gelfand et al., 2011). Such mechanisms may be useful in fine-tuning condition-specific gene expression, especially when "leaky" expression of certain genes may be harmful to the cell.

### 6.5 *S. pombe* meiRNA function: The mei2-meiRNA complex

*S. pombe* MEI2 is an RNA-binding protein required for premeiotic DNA replication and the initiation of meiosis I (Y. Watanabe & Yamamoto, 1994; reviewed in Yamamoto et al., 2010). This protein has been discussed in detail in "4.2.2 Commitment and Continuation". In the context of this section, the role of a 0.5kb ncRNA transcribed at the *Sme2* locus (dubbed meiRNA) will be discussed. meiRNA binds to MEI2 and this ncRNA-protein complex is transported to the nucleus (Y. Watanabe & Yamamoto, 1994). Two scenarios have been described whereby meiRNA determines the nuclear localization of MEI2; meiRNA either interferes with MEI2 export from the nucleus, or facilitates MEI2 import into the nucleus (Sato et al., 2001). This nuclear MEI2-meiRNA complex binds MMI1, a protein that targets meiotic transcripts containing DSR motifs for degradation, during mitosis. This interaction interferes with MMI1, stabilizing transcripts required for the progression of S. pombe cells through meiosis I (Yamamoto et al., 2010). From this overview one can see that ncRNAs control the mitosis-meiosis switch in the divergent S. pombe and S. cerevisiae; however, they do so by very different mechanisms.

### 6.6 *S. pombe* meiotic hotspots

In *S. pombe*, the dsDNA breaks (DSBs) that initiate recombination, cluster to 194 prominent and 159 weak DSB peaks that favour intergenic regions (IGRs, Cromie et al., 2007). T. Watanabe et al. (2002) identified 68 polyadenylated ncRNAs from a random sampling of cDNAs originating from *S. pombe* cells in mitotic or meiotic growth phase. By cross referencing the aforementioned studies, it was determined that 24 polyadenylated ncRNAs were located entirely within a DSB peak (Wahls et al., 2008). Overall, Wahls et al. (2008) concluded that meiotic DSB hotspots preferentially form at loci that express long polyadenylated ncRNAs, many of which are expressed solely during meiosis. There are two mechanisms by which ncRNAs may guide meiotic recombination proteins to DSB hotspots: 1) the ncRNAs make DNA accessible to DSB formation through meiotically induced chromatin remodelling, and 2) ncRNA-DNA hybrids (R-loops) guide the meiotic recombination machinery to the DSB sites (Wahls et al., 2008).

### 6.7 *U. maydis* ncRNA/antisense transcription

RNA-seq has not been performed on *U. maydis* cell-types, but limited strand-specific expression data is available from the creation of EST libraries from various cell-types and nutritional conditions. To help facilitate *U. maydis* genome annotation, cDNA libraries were constructed from cell-types, including: germinating and dormant teliospores (Sacadura & Saville, 2003; Ho et al., 2007), filamentous diploids (Nugent et al., 2004) and dikaryons (Morrison et al., in preparation). Recall that teliospore formation and germination are temporally linked to meiosis in *U. maydis* (reviewed in Donaldson & Saville, 2008). Of the 319 uniESTs that did not match an annotated gene model in the *U. maydis* genome, 108 uniquely represented RNAs expressed in the dormant or germinating teliospores. This corresponds to 34% of the identified ncRNAs, while these two cDNA libraries account for only 17% of the total ESTs from all cell-types (Saville, unpublished). In total, ~250 NATs have been identified in *U. maydis*, including NATs expressed in the dormant and germinating teliospores (55 and 12, respectively). The function of the NATs and ncRNAs in *U. maydis* is under investigation. Ten teliospore-specific NATs, annotated during analysis of the dormant teliospore cDNA library, have been verified as teliospore-specific, using strand-specific RT-PCR (Ho et al., 2010). Unlike *S. cerevisiae* and *S. pombe*, the *U. maydis* NATs expressed in the dormant and germinating teliospore are not enriched for mitosis-specific genes and the NATs expressed during vegetative growth are not enriched for meiosis-specific genes. Additionally, inverse expression patterns have not been observed for sense-antisense transcript pairs; precluding transcriptional interference as the principal mechanism of action for NATs in *U. maydis*. Therefore, their function in the dormant and germinating teliospores appears to be unique to *U. maydis*.

## 7. Conclusion

This chapter provides an overview of meiotic events in the model fungal species *Saccharomyces cerevisiae*, *Schizosaccharomyces pombe* and *Coprinopsis cinerea* as a means of providing context for an exploration of meiosis in the model plant pathogen *Ustilago maydis*. Like the yeast fungi, *U. maydis* has set genetic requirements for entry into meiosis; it must be diploid and contain complementary alleles at the b mating type locus. With this genetic background, the fungus is able to accept an environmental signal that triggers entry into meiosis. This signal comes from the plant host and an exploration of the stages of pathogenic development led us to hypothesize that the stage before hyphal fragmentation, and after the cells become embedded in a mucilaginous matrix, is the time it must receive a signal from the plant to trigger entry into premeiotic S phase and undergo karyogamy. We uncover similarities between the role of the MAPK and cAMP/PKA pathways in mating and meiosis initiation in yeasts and the mating and pathogenesis signal transduction pathways in *U. maydis*. This is very relevant because of the requirement for growth within the host for *U. maydis* to become meiotically competent. These comparisons emphasized that the *U. maydis* genes *Crk1* and *Prf1*, which are orthologs of the major meiosis control genes *Ime2* in *S. cerevisiae* and *Ste11* in *S. pombe* respectively, provide a means whereby mating type and environmental signals could be transduced to influence meiosis. This led to a model of how meiosis is triggered in *U. maydis* and its linkage with teliospore development. We present an overview of waves in transcription in the yeasts and present evidence for potential waves of transcription in *U. maydis*. The identification of *U. maydis* meiosis genes by bioinformatic analyses is updated with an identification of the conserved absence of core meiosis genes in plant pathogenic fungi. We also present data that identifies *UmNdt80* as the first gene known to be required for meiosis completion in *U. maydis*. The timing of expression of six core meiosis genes in *U. maydis* is followed during *in planta* development. This uncovered support for the model that *U. maydis* enters meiosis very soon after karyogamy and then arrests during pachytene, when the teliospore matures and enters a dormant state. This information also identified transcriptional and posttranscriptional control of *Spo11* as potential key transitions in *U. maydis* meiotic progression. The final portion of the chapter highlights new data on the bioinformatic discovery of ncRNAs and NATs in *U. maydis* and their overrepresentation among ESTs in the teliospore and germinating teliospore libraries. In the context of the emerging role for these RNAs in controlling aspects of meiosis in *S. cerevisiae* and *S. pombe,* the discovery and confirmation of these RNAs in *U. maydis* is compelling. This chapter identifies several areas where further research will provide tremendous insight regarding meiosis initiation and progression in *U. maydis*.

During proofing, gametogenesis initiation (van Werven & Amon, 2011) and RNAi-independent roles for antisense transcripts in controlling meiotic genes (Chen & Neiman, 2011) in budding and fission yeasts were reviewed.

## 8. Acknowledgement

We would like to acknowledge Natalie Pearson for her excellent artwork in Figure 1, thank Laura Peers for fact finding and organizational support, and thank Christine Russell for assistance in proofing this manuscript. We also acknowledge funding from NSERC of Canada, and the Ontario Ministry of Research and Innovation's Ontario Research Fund-Research Excellence program.

## 9. References

Abe, H. & Shimoda, C. (2000). Autoregulated expression of Schizosaccharomyces pombe meiosis-specific transcription factor Mei4 and a genome-wide search for its target genes. *Genetics,* Vol.154, No.4, (April 2000), pp. 1497-1508, ISSN 0016-6731

Ahmed, N.T., Bungard, D., Shin, M.E., Moore, M. & Winter, E. (2009). The Ime2 protein kinase enhances the disassociation of the Sum1 repressor from middle meiotic promoters. *Molecular and cellular biology,* Vol.29, No.16, (August 2009), pp. 4352-4362, ISSN 1098-5549

Allen, A., Islamovic, E., Kaur, J., Gold, S., Shah, D. & Smith, T.J. (2011). Transgenic maize plants expressing the Totivirus antifungal protein, KP4, are highly resistant to corn smut. *Plant biotechnology journal,* (February 2011), ISSN 1467-7652

Alvarez, B. & Moreno, S. (2006). Fission yeast Tor2 promotes cell growth and represses cell differentiation. *Journal of cell science,* Vol.119, No.Pt 21, (November 2006), pp. 4475-4485, ISSN 0021-9533

Averbeck, N., Sunder, S., Sample, N., Wise, J.A. & Leatherwood, J. (2005). Negative control contributes to an extensive program of meiotic splicing in fission yeast. *Molecular cell,* Vol.18, No.4, (May 2005), pp. 491-498, ISSN 1097-2765

Banuett, F. (2010). *Ustilago maydis* and Maize: a Delightful Interaction, In: Cellular and Molecular Biology of Filamentous Fungi, K.A. Borkovich & D.J. Ebbole, (Ed.), 622-644, ASM Press, ISSN 978-1-55581-473-1, Washington, USA

Banuett, F. (2002). Pathogenic development in *Ustilago maydis*: A progression of morphological transitions that results in tumor formation and teliospore production, In: Molecular biology of fungal development, H.D. Osiewacz, (Ed.), 349-398, Marcel Dekker, ISSN 0824707443, New York, USA

Banuett, F. & Herskowitz, I. (1996). Discrete developmental stages during teliospore formation in the corn smut fungus, Ustilago maydis. *Development,* Vol.122, No.10, (October 1996), pp. 2965-2976, ISSN 0950-1991

Banuett, F. (1995).Genetics of *Ustilago maydis*, a fungal pathogen that induces tumors in maize.*Annual Review of Genetics,* Vol.29, (n.d.), pp. 179-208, ISSN 0066-4197

Banuett, F. & Herskowitz, I. (1989). Different a alleles of Ustilago maydis are necessary for maintenance of filamentous growth but not for meiosis. *Proceedings of the National Academy of Sciences of the United States of America,* Vol.86, No.15, (August 1989), pp. 5878-5882, ISSN 0027-8424

Barnes, C.W., Szabo, L.J., May, G. & Groth, J.V. (2004). Inbreeding levels of two Ustilago maydis populations. *Mycologia,* Vol.96, No.6, (November 2004), pp. 1236-1244, ISSN 0027-5514

Bauman, P., Cheng, Q.C. & Albright, C.F. (1998). The Byr2 kinase translocates to the plasma membrane in a Ras1-dependent manner. *Biochemical and biophysical research communications,* Vol.244, No.2, (March 1998), pp. 468-474, ISSN 0006-291X

Bellani, M.A., Boateng, K.A., McLeod, D. & Camerini-Otero, R.D. (2010). The expression profile of the major mouse SPO11 isoforms indicates that SPO11beta introduces double strand breaks and suggests that SPO11alpha has an additional role in prophase in both spermatocytes and oocytes. *Molecular and cellular biology,* Vol.30, No.18, (September 2010), pp. 4391-4403, ISSN 1098-5549

Boehm, E.W.A., Wenstrom, J.C., McLaughlin, D.J., Szabo, L.J., Roelfs, A.P. & Bushnell, W.R. (1992). An ultrastructural pachytene karyotype for Puccinia graminis f. sp. tritici. *Canadian Journal of Botany,* Vol.70, (n.d.), pp. 401-4113, ISSN 0008-4026

Borkovich, K.A., Alex, L.A., Yarden, O., Freitag, M., Turner, G.E., Read, N.D., Seiler, S., Bell-Pedersen, D., Paietta, J., Plesofsky, N., Plamann, M., Goodrich-Tanrikulu, M., Schulte, U., Mannhaupt, G., Nargang, F.E., Radford, A., Selitrennikoff, C., Galagan, J.E., Dunlap, J.C., Loros, J.J., Catcheside, D., Inoue, H., Aramayo, R., Polymenis, M., Selker, E.U., Sachs, M.S., Marzluf, G.A., Paulsen, I., Davis, R., Ebbole, D.J., Zelter, A., Kalkman, E.R., O'Rourke, R., Bowring, F., Yeadon, J., Ishii, C., Suzuki, K., Sakai, W. & Pratt, R. (2004). Lessons from the genome sequence of Neurospora crassa: tracing the path from genomic blueprint to multicellular organism. *Microbiology and molecular biology reviews,* Vol.68, No.1, (March 2004), pp. 1-108, ISSN 1092-2172

Brefort, T., Doehlemann, G., Mendoza-Mendoza, A., Reissmann, S., Djamei, A. & Kahmann, R. (2009). Ustilago maydis as a Pathogen. *Annual Review of Phytopathology,* Vol.47, (n.d.), pp. 423-445, ISSN 0066-4286

Burdon, J.J. & Roelfs, A.P. (1985). The effect of sexual and asexual reproduction on the isozyme structure of populations of Puccinia graminis. *Phytopathology,* Vol.75, (n.d.), pp. 1068-1073, ISSN 0031-949X

Burns, C., Pukkila, P.J. & Miriam, Z.E. (2010a). Meiosis, In: Cellular and Molecular Biology of Filamentous Fungi, K.A. Borkovich & D.J. Ebbole, (Ed.), 81-95, ASM Press, ISSN 978-1-55581-473-1, Washington, USA

Burns, C., Stajich, J.E., Rechtsteiner, A., Casselton, L., Hanlon, S.E., Wilke, S.K., Savytskyy, O.P., Gathman, A.C., Lilly, W.W., Lieb, J.D., Zolan, M.E. & Pukkila, P.J. (2010b). Analysis of the Basidiomycete Coprinopsis cinerea reveals conservation of the core meiotic expression program over half a billion years of evolution. *PLoS genetics,* Vol.6, No.9, (September 2010), pp. e1001135, ISSN 1553-7404

Butler, G., Rasmussen, M.D., Lin, M.F., Santos, M.A., Sakthikumar, S., Munro, C.A., Rheinbay, E., Grabherr, M., Forche, A., Reedy, J.L., Agrafioti, I., Arnaud, M.B., Bates, S., Brown, A.J., Brunke, S., Costanzo, M.C., Fitzpatrick, D.A., de Groot, P.W., Harris, D., Hoyer, L.L., Hube, B., Klis, F.M., Kodira, C., Lennard, N., Logue, M.E., Martin, R., Neiman, A.M., Nikolaou, E., Quail, M.A., Quinn, J., Santos, M.C., Schmitzberger, F.F., Sherlock, G., Shah, P., Silverstein, K.A., Skrzypek, M.S., Soll, D., Staggs, R., Stansfield, I., Stumpf, M.P., Sudbery, P.E., Srikantha, T., Zeng, Q., Berman, J., Berriman, M., Heitman, J., Gow, N.A., Lorenz, M.C., Birren, B.W., Kellis,

M. & Cuomo, C.A. (2009). Evolution of pathogenicity and sexual reproduction in eight Candida genomes. *Nature,* Vol.459, No.7247, (June 2009), pp. 657-662, ISSN 1476-4687

Capitol Commodity Services. (February, 2011). U.S. crop values jumped 22% in 2010, 04.09.2011, Available from <http://www.ccstrade.com/futures-news/grains/story/u-s-crop-values-jumped-22-in-2010-800410457/>

Celerin, M., Merino, S.T., Stone, J.E., Menzie, A.M. & Zolan, M.E. (2000). Multiple roles of Spo11 in meiotic chromosome behavior. *The EMBO journal,* Vol.19, No.11, (June 2000), pp. 2739-2750, ISSN 0261-4189

Chen, H.M. & Neiman, A.M. (2011). A conserved regulatory role for antisense RNA in meiotic gene expression in yeast. *Current opinion in microbiology,* Vol.14, No.6, (December 2011), pp. 655-659, ISSN 1879-0364

Chu, S., DeRisi, J., Eisen, M., Mulholland, J., Botstein, D., Brown, P.O. & Herskowitz, I. (1998). The transcriptional program of sporulation in budding yeast. *Science,* Vol.282, No.5389, (October 1998), pp. 699-705, ISSN 0036-8075

Chu, S. & Herskowitz, I. (1998). Gametogenesis in yeast is regulated by a transcriptional cascade dependent on Ndt80. *Molecular cell,* Vol.1, No.5, (April 1998), pp. 685-696, ISSN 1097-2765

Chung, K.S., Won, M., Lee, S.B., Jang, Y.J., Hoe, K.L., Kim, D.U., Lee, J.W., Kim, K.W. & Yoo, H.S. (2001). Isolation of a novel gene from Schizosaccharomyces pombe: stm1+ encoding a seven-transmembrane loop protein that may couple with the heterotrimeric Galpha 2 protein, Gpa2. *The Journal of biological chemistry,* Vol.276, No.43, (October 2001), pp. 40190-40201, ISSN 0021-9258

Colomina, N., Gari, E., Gallego, C., Herrero, E. & Aldea, M. (1999). G1 cyclins block the Ime1 pathway to make mitosis and meiosis incompatible in budding yeast. *The EMBO journal,* Vol.18, No.2, (January 1999), pp. 320-329, ISSN 0261-4189

Cooper, K.F. & Strich, R. (2002). Saccharomyces cerevisiae C-type cyclin Ume3p/Srb11p is required for efficient induction and execution of meiotic development. *Eukaryotic cell,* Vol.1, No.1, (February 2002), pp. 66-74, ISSN 1535-9778

Costa, F.F. (2010). Non-coding RNAs: Meet thy masters. *BioEssays: news and reviews in molecular, cellular and developmental biology,* Vol.32, No.7, (July 2010), pp. 599-608, ISSN 1521-1878

Costa, F.F. (2005). Non-coding RNAs: new players in eukaryotic biology. *Gene,* Vol.357, No.2, (September 2005), pp. 83-94, ISSN 0378-1119

Covitz, P.A. & Mitchell, A.P. (1993). Repression by the yeast meiotic inhibitor RME1. *Genes & development,* Vol.7, No.8, (August 1993), pp. 1598-1608, ISSN 0890-9369

Covitz, P.A., Herskowitz, I. & Mitchell, A.P. (1991). The yeast RME1 gene encodes a putative zinc finger protein that is directly repressed by a1-alpha 2. *Genes & development,* Vol.5, No.11, (November 1991), pp. 1982-1989, ISSN 0890-9369

Cromie, G.A., Hyppa, R.W., Cam, H.P., Farah, J.A., Grewal, S.I. & Smith, G.R. (2007). A discrete class of intergenic DNA dictates meiotic DNA break hotspots in fission yeast. *PLoS genetics,* Vol.3, No.8, (August 2007), pp. e141, ISSN 1553-7404

Donaldson, M.E. & Saville, B.J. (2008). Bioinformatic identification of Ustilago maydis meiosis genes. *Fungal genetics and biology,* Vol.45, Suppl 1, (August 2008), pp. S47-53, ISSN 1096-0937

Donzeau, M. & Bandlow, W. (1999). The yeast trimeric guanine nucleotide-binding protein alpha subunit, Gpa2p, controls the meiosis-specific kinase Ime2p activity in response to nutrients. *Molecular and cellular biology,* Vol.19, No.9, (September 1999), pp. 6110-6119, ISSN 0270-7306

Doyle, C.E., Donaldson, M.E., Morrison, E.N. & Saville, B.J. (2011). Ustilago maydis transcript features identified through full-length cDNA analysis. *Molecular genetics and genomics,* Vol.286, No.2, (August 2011), pp. 143-159, ISSN 1617-4623

Faghihi, M.A. & Wahlestedt, C. (2009). Regulatory roles of natural antisense transcripts. *Nature reviews molecular cell biology,* Vol.10, No.9, (September 2009), pp. 637-643, ISSN 1471-0080

Feldbrugge, M., Kamper, J., Steinberg, G. & Kahmann, R. (2004). Regulation of mating and pathogenic development in Ustilago maydis.*Current opinion in microbiology,* Vol.7, No.6, (December 2004), pp. 666-672, ISSN 1369-5274

Fletcher, H.L. (1981). A search for synaptonemal complexes in Ustilago maydis. *Journal of cell science,* Vol.50, (August 1981), pp. 171-180, ISSN 0021-9533

Gallego, C., Gari, E., Colomina, N., Herrero, E. & Aldea, M. (1997). The Cln3 cyclin is down-regulated by translational repression and degradation during the G1 arrest caused by nitrogen deprivation in budding yeast. *The EMBO journal,* Vol.16, No.23, (December 1997), pp. 7196-7206, ISSN 0261-4189

Garrido, E., Voss, U., Muller, P., Castillo-Lluva, S., Kahmann, R. & Perez-Martin, J. (2004). The induction of sexual development and virulence in the smut fungus Ustilago maydis depends on Crk1, a novel MAPK protein. *Genes & development,* Vol.18, No.24, (December 2004), pp. 3117-3130, ISSN 0890-9369

Garrido, E. & Perez-Martin, J. (2003). The crk1 gene encodes an Ime2-related protein that is required for morphogenesis in the plant pathogen Ustilago maydis. *Molecular microbiology,* Vol.47, No.3, (February 2003), pp. 729-743, ISSN 0950-382X

Gelfand, B., Mead, J., Bruning, A., Apostolopoulos, N., Tadigotla, V., Nagaraj, V., Sengupta, A.M. & Vershon, A.K. (2011). Regulated antisense transcription controls expression of cell-type-specific genes in yeast. *Molecular and cellular biology,* Vol.31, No.8, (April 2011), pp. 1701-1709, ISSN 1098-5549

Gold, S.E., Brogdon, S.M., Mayorga, M.E. & Kronstad, J.W. (1997). The Ustilago maydis regulatory subunit of a cAMP-dependent protein kinase is required for gall formation in maize. *The Plant cell,* Vol.9, No.9, (September 1997), pp. 1585-1594, ISSN 1040-4651

Govin, J. & Berger, S.L. (2009). Genome reprogramming during sporulation. *The International journal of developmental biology,* Vol.53, No.2-3, (n.d.), pp. 425-432, ISSN 1696-3547

Guttmann-Raviv, N., Martin, S. & Kassir, Y. (2002). Ime2, a meiosis-specific kinase in yeast, is required for destabilization of its transcriptional activator, Ime1. *Molecular and cellular biology,* Vol.22, No.7, (April 2002), pp. 2047-2056, ISSN 0270-7306

Harigaya, Y. & Yamamoto, M. (2007). Molecular mechanisms underlying the mitosis-meiosis decision. *Chromosome research: an international journal on the molecular, supramolecular and evolutionary aspects of chromosome biology,* Vol.15, No.5, (n.d.), pp. 523-537, ISSN 0967-3849

Harigaya, Y., Tanaka, H., Yamanaka, S., Tanaka, K., Watanabe, Y., Tsutsumi, C., Chikashige, Y., Hiraoka, Y., Yamashita, A. & Yamamoto, M. (2006). Selective elimination of messenger RNA prevents an incidence of untimely meiosis. *Nature,* Vol.442, No.7098, (July 2006), pp. 45-50, ISSN 1476-4687

Hartmann, H.A., Kruger, J., Lottspeich, F. & Kahmann, R. (1999). Environmental signals controlling sexual development of the corn Smut fungus Ustilago maydis through the transcriptional regulator Prf1. *The Plant cell,* Vol.11, No.7, (July 1999), pp. 1293-1306, ISSN 1040-4651

Hartmann, H.A., Kahmann, R. & Bolker, M. (1996). The pheromone response factor coordinates filamentous growth and pathogenicity in Ustilago maydis. *The EMBO journal,* Vol.15, No.7, (April 1996), pp. 1632-1641, ISSN 0261-4189

Hartung, F. & Puchta, H. (2000). Molecular characterisation of two paralogous SPO11 homologues in Arabidopsis thaliana. *Nucleic acids research,* Vol.28, No.7, (April 2000), pp. 1548-1554, ISSN 1362-4962

Heimel, K., Scherer, M., Schuler, D. & Kamper, J. (2010). The Ustilago maydis Clp1 protein orchestrates pheromone and b-dependent signaling pathways to coordinate the cell cycle and pathogenic development. *The Plant cell,* Vol.22, No.8, (August 2010), pp. 2908-2922, ISSN 1532-298X

Hepworth, S.R., Friesen, H. & Segall, J. (1998). NDT80 and the meiotic recombination checkpoint regulate expression of middle sporulation-specific genes in Saccharomyces cerevisiae. *Molecular and cellular biology,* Vol.18, No.10, (October 1998), pp. 5750-5761, ISSN 0270-7306

Higuchi, T., Watanabe, Y. & Yamamoto, M. (2002). Protein kinase A regulates sexual development and gluconeogenesis through phosphorylation of the Zn finger transcriptional activator Rst2p in fission yeast. *Molecular and cellular biology,* Vol.22, No.1, (January 2002), pp. 1-11, ISSN 0270-7306

Ho, E.C., Donaldson, M.E. & Saville, B.J. (2010). Detection of antisense RNA transcripts by strand-specific RT-PCR, In: RT-PCR Protocols,2nd Edition, N. King, (Ed.), 125-138, Humana Press, ISSN 1940-6029, New York, USA

Ho, E.C., Cahill, M.J. & Saville, B.J. (2007). Gene discovery and transcript analyses in the corn smut pathogen Ustilago maydis: expressed sequence tag and genome sequence comparison. *BMC genomics,* Vol.8, No.1, (September 2007), pp. 334, ISSN 1471-2164

Holloman, W.K., Schirawski, J. & Holliday, R. (2008). The homologous recombination system of Ustilago maydis. *Fungal genetics and biology,* Vol.45, Suppl 1, (August 2008), pp. S31-9, ISSN 1096-0937

Hongay, C.F., Grisafi, P.L., Galitski, T. & Fink, G.R. (2006). Antisense transcription controls cell fate in Saccharomyces cerevisiae. *Cell,* Vol.127, No.4, (November 2006), pp. 735-745, ISSN 0092-8674

Honigberg, S.M. & Purnapatre, K. (2003). Signal pathway integration in the switch from the mitotic cell cycle to meiosis in yeast. *Journal of cell science,* Vol.116, No.Pt 11, (June 2003), pp. 2137-2147, ISSN 0021-9533

Honigberg, S.M. & Lee, R.H. (1998). Snf1 kinase connects nutritional pathways controlling meiosis in Saccharomyces cerevisiae. *Molecular and cellular biology,* Vol.18, No.8, (August 1998), pp. 4548-4555, ISSN 0270-7306

Horie, S., Watanabe, Y., Tanaka, K., Nishiwaki, S., Fujioka, H., Abe, H., Yamamoto, M. & Shimoda, C. (1998). The Schizosaccharomyces pombe mei4+ gene encodes a meiosis-specific transcription factor containing a forkhead DNA-binding domain. *Molecular and cellular biology,* Vol.18, No.4, (April 1998), pp. 2118-2129, ISSN 0270-7306

Horst, R.J., Doehlemann, G., Wahl, R., Hofmann, J., Schmiedl, A., Kahmann, R., Kamper, J., Sonnewald, U. & Voll, L.M. (2010a). Ustilago maydis infection strongly alters organic nitrogen allocation in maize and stimulates productivity of systemic source leaves. *Plant physiology,* Vol.152, No.1, (January 2010), pp. 293-308, ISSN 1532-2548

Horst, R.J., Doehlemann, G., Wahl, R., Hofmann, J., Schmiedl, A., Kahmann, R., Kamper, J. & Voll, L.M. (2010b). A model of Ustilago maydis leaf tumor metabolism. *Plant signaling & behavior,* Vol.5, No.11, (November 2010), pp. 1446-1449, ISSN 1559-2324

Huerta-Espino, J., Singh, R.P., German, S., McCallum, B.D., Park, R.F., Chen, W.Q., Bhardway, S.C. & Goyeau, H. (2011). Global status of wheat leaf rust caused by Puccinia triticina. *Euphytica,* Vol.179, (n.d.), pp. 143-160, ISSN 0014-2336

Isshiki, T., Mochizuki, N., Maeda, T. & Yamamoto, M. (1992). Characterization of a fission yeast gene, gpa2, that encodes a G alpha subunit involved in the monitoring of nutrition. *Genes & development,* Vol.6, No.12B, (December 1992), pp. 2455-2462, ISSN 0890-9369

Jin, Y. (2011). Role of Berberis spp. as alternate hosts in generating new races of Puccinia graminis and P. striiformis. *Euphytica,* Vol.179, (n.d.), pp. 105-108, ISSN 0014-2336

Juneau, K., Palm, C., Miranda, M. & Davis, R.W. (2007). High-density yeast-tiling array reveals previously undiscovered introns and extensive regulation of meiotic splicing. *Proceedings of the National Academy of Sciences of the United States of America,* Vol.104, No.5, (January 2007), pp. 1522-1527, ISSN 0027-8424

Kaffarnik, F., Muller, P., Leibundgut, M., Kahmann, R. & Feldbrugge, M. (2003). PKA and MAPK phosphorylation of Prf1 allows promoter discrimination in Ustilago maydis. *The EMBO journal,* Vol.22, No.21, (November 2003), pp. 5817-5826, ISSN 0261-4189

Kahmann, R. & Kamper, J. (2004). *Ustilago maydis*: how its biology relates to pathogenic development. *New Phytologist,* Vol.164, (n.d.), pp. 31-42, ISSN 1469-8137

Kamper, J., Kahmann, R., Bolker, M., Ma, L.J., Brefort, T., Saville, B.J., Banuett, F., Kronstad, J.W., Gold, S.E., Muller, O., Perlin, M.H., Wosten, H.A., de Vries, R., Ruiz-Herrera, J., Reynaga-Pena, C.G., Snetselaar, K., McCann, M., Perez-Martin, J., Feldbrugge, M., Basse, C.W., Steinberg, G., Ibeas, J.I., Holloman, W., Guzman, P., Farman, M., Stajich, J.E., Sentandreu, R., Gonzalez-Prieto, J.M., Kennell, J.C., Molina, L., Schirawski, J., Mendoza-Mendoza, A., Greilinger, D., Munch, K., Rossel, N., Scherer, M., Vranes, M., Ladendorf, O., Vincon, V., Fuchs, U., Sandrock, B., Meng, S., Ho, E.C., Cahill, M.J., Boyce, K.J., Klose, J., Klosterman, S.J., Deelstra, H.J., Ortiz-Castellanos, L., Li, W., Sanchez-Alonso, P., Schreier, P.H., Hauser-Hahn, I., Vaupel, M., Koopmann, E., Friedrich, G., Voss, H., Schluter, T., Margolis, J., Platt, D., Swimmer, C., Gnirke, A., Chen, F., Vysotskaia, V., Mannhaupt, G., Guldener, U., Munsterkotter, M., Haase, D., Oesterheld, M., Mewes, H.W., Mauceli, E.W., DeCaprio, D., Wade, C.M., Butler, J., Young, S., Jaffe, D.B., Calvo, S., Nusbaum, C., Galagan, J. & Birren, B.W. (2006). Insights from the genome of the biotrophic fungal plant pathogen Ustilago maydis. *Nature,* Vol.444, No.7115, (November 2006), pp. 97-101, ISSN 1476-4687

Kassir, Y., Adir, N., Boger-Nadjar, E., Raviv, N.G., Rubin-Bejerano, I., Sagee, S. & Shenhar, G. (2003).Transcriptional regulation of meiosis in budding yeast. *International review of cytology,* Vol.224, (n.d.), pp. 111-171, ISSN 0074-7696

Kato, T.,Jr, Okazaki, K., Murakami, H., Stettler, S., Fantes, P.A. & Okayama, H. (1996). Stress signal, mediated by a Hog1-like MAP kinase, controls sexual development in fission yeast. *FEBS letters,* Vol.378, No.3, (January 1996), pp. 207-212, ISSN 0014-5793

Kjaerulff, S., Andersen, N.R., Borup, M.T. & Nielsen, O. (2007). Cdk phosphorylation of the Ste11 transcription factor constrains differentiation-specific transcription to G1. *Genes & development,* Vol.21, No.3, (February 2007), pp. 347-359, ISSN 0890-9369

Klosterman, S.J., Perlin, M.H., Garcia-Pedrajas, M., Covert, S.F. & Gold, S.E. (2007). Genetics of morphogenesis and pathogenic development of Ustilago maydis. *Advances in Genetics,* Vol.57, (n.d.), pp. 1-47, ISSN 0065-2660

Kojic, M., Kostrub, C.F., Buchman, A.R. & Holloman, W.K. (2002). BRCA2 homolog required for proficiency in DNA repair, recombination, and genome stability in Ustilago maydis. *Molecular cell,* Vol.10, No.3, (September 2002), pp. 683-691, ISSN 1097-2765

Kronstad, J.W. (2008). Mining the genome of the biotrophic fungal pathogen Ustilago maydis. *Fungal genetics and biology,* Vol.45 Suppl 1, (August 2008), pp. S1-2, ISSN 1096-0937

Kruger, J., Loubradou, G., Wanner, G., Regenfelder, E., Feldbrugge, M. & Kahmann, R. (2000). Activation of the cAMP pathway in Ustilago maydis reduces fungal proliferation and teliospore formation in plant tumors. *Molecular plant-microbe interactions,* Vol.13, No.10, (October 2000), pp. 1034-1040, ISSN 0894-0282

Kues, U. (2000). Life history and developmental processes in the basidiomycete Coprinus cinereus. *Microbiology and molecular biology reviews,* Vol.64, No.2, (June 2000), pp. 316-353, ISSN 1092-2172

Kunitomo, H., Higuchi, T., Iino, Y. & Yamamoto, M. (2000). A zinc-finger protein, Rst2p, regulates transcription of the fission yeast ste11(+) gene, which encodes a pivotal transcription factor for sexual development. *Molecular biology of the cell,* Vol.11, No.9, (September 2000), pp. 3205-3217, ISSN 1059-1524

Lardenois, A., Liu, Y., Walther, T., Chalmel, F., Evrard, B., Granovskaia, M., Chu, A., Davis, R.W., Steinmetz, L.M. & Primig, M. (2011). Execution of the meiotic noncoding RNA expression program and the onset of gametogenesis in yeast require the conserved exosome subunit Rrp6. *Proceedings of the National Academy of Sciences of the United States of America,* Vol.108, No.3, (January 2011), pp. 1058-1063, ISSN 1091-6490

Lavorgna, G., Dahary, D., Lehner, B., Sorek, R., Sanderson, C.M. & Casari, G. (2004). In search of antisense. *Trends in biochemical sciences,* Vol.29, No.2, (February 2004), pp. 88-94, ISSN 0968-0004

Lee, N., D'Souza, C.A. & Kronstad, J.W. (2003). Of smuts, blasts, mildews, and blights: cAMP signaling in phytopathogenic fungi. *Annual Review of Phytopathology,* Vol.41, (n.d.), pp. 399-427, ISSN 0066-4286

Loidl, J. (2006). S. pombe linear elements: the modest cousins of synaptonemal complexes. *Chromosoma,* Vol.115, No.3, (June 2006), pp. 260-271, ISSN 0009-5915

Lu, B.C. (2000). The control of meiosis progression in the fungus Coprinus cinereus by light/dark cycles. *Fungal genetics and biology,* Vol.31, No.1, (October 2000), pp. 33-41, ISSN 1087-1845

Malik, S.B., Pightling, A.W., Stefaniak, L.M., Schurko, A.M. & Logsdon, J.M.,Jr. (2007). An expanded inventory of conserved meiotic genes provides evidence for sex in Trichomonas vaginalis. *PloS one,* Vol.3, No.8, (August 2007), pp. e2879, ISSN 1932-6203

Marston, A.L. & Amon, A. (2004). Meiosis: cell-cycle controls shuffle and deal. *Nature reviews. Molecular cell biology,* Vol.5, No.12, (December 2004), pp. 983-997, ISSN 1471-0072

Martinez-Espinoza, A.D., Garcia-Pedrajas, M.D. & Gold, S.E. (2002). The Ustilaginales as plant pests and model systems. *Fungal genetics and biology,* Vol.35, No.1, (February 2002), pp. 1-20, ISSN 1087-1845

Mata, J., Wilbrey, A. & Bahler, J. (2007).Transcriptional regulatory network for sexual differentiation in fission yeast. *Genome biology,* Vol.8, No.10, (October 2007), pp. R217, ISSN 1465-6914

Mata, J. & Bahler, J. (2003). Correlations between gene expression and gene conservation in fission yeast. *Genome research,* Vol.13, No.12, (December 2003), pp. 2686-2690, ISSN 1088-9051

Mata, J., Lyne, R., Burns, G. & Bahler, J. (2002). The transcriptional program of meiosis and sporulation in fission yeast. *Nature genetics,* Vol.32, No.1, (September 2002), pp. 143-147, ISSN 1061-4036

Matsuo, T., Otsubo, Y., Urano, J., Tamanoi, F. & Yamamoto, M. (2007). Loss of the TOR kinase Tor2 mimics nitrogen starvation and activates the sexual development pathway in fission yeast. *Molecular and cellular biology,* Vol.27, No.8, (April 2007), pp. 3154-3164, ISSN 0270-7306

Mewes, H.W., Dietmann, S., Frishman, D., Gregory, R., Mannhaupt, G., Mayer, K.F., Munsterkotter, M., Ruepp, A., Spannagl, M., Stumpflen, V. & Rattei, T. (2008). MIPS: analysis and annotation of genome information in 2007. *Nucleic acids research,* Vol.36, No.Database issue, (January 2008), pp. D196-201, ISSN 1362-4962

Mims, C.W. & Richardson, E.A. (2005). Light and electron microscopy of teliospores and teliospore germination in the rust fungus Coleosporium ipomoeae. *Canadian Journal of Botany,* Vol.83, No.5, (May 2005), pp. 451-458, ISSN 0008-4026

Mitchell, A.P. (1994). Control of meiotic gene expression in Saccharomyces cerevisiae. *Microbiological reviews,* Vol.58, No.1, (March 1994), pp. 56-70, ISSN 0146-0749

Mitchell, A.P., Driscoll, S.E. & Smith, H.E. (1990). Positive control of sporulation-specific genes by the IME1 and IME2 products in Saccharomyces cerevisiae. *Molecular and cellular biology,* Vol.10, No.5, (May 1990), pp. 2104-2110, ISSN 0270-7306

Mochizuki, N. & Yamamoto, M. (1992). Reduction in the intracellular cAMP level triggers initiation of sexual development in fission yeast. *Molecular & general genetics,* Vol.233, No.1-2, (May 1992), pp. 17-24, ISSN 0026-8925

Moldon, A., Malapeira, J., Gabrielli, N., Gogol, M., Gomez-Escoda, B., Ivanova, T., Seidel, C. & Ayte, J. (2008). Promoter-driven splicing regulation in fission yeast. *Nature,* Vol.455, No.7215, (October 2008), pp. 997-1000, ISSN 1476-4687

Molnar, M., Parisi, S., Kakihara, Y., Nojima, H., Yamamoto, A., Hiraoka, Y., Bozsik, A., Sipiczki, M. & Kohli, J. (2001). Characterization of rec7, an early meiotic recombination gene in Schizosaccharomyces pombe. *Genetics,* Vol.157, No.2, (February 2001), pp. 519-532, ISSN 0016-6731

Muller, P., Leibbrandt, A., Teunissen, H., Cubasch, S., Aichinger, C. & Kahmann, R. (2004). The Gbeta-subunit-encoding gene bpp1 controls cyclic-AMP signaling in Ustilago maydis. *Eukaryotic cell,* Vol.3, No.3, (June 2004), pp. 806-814, ISSN 1535-9778

Muller, P., Weinzierl, G., Brachmann, A., Feldbrugge, M. & Kahmann, R. (2003). Mating and pathogenic development of the Smut fungus Ustilago maydis are regulated by one mitogen-activated protein kinase cascade. *Eukaryotic cell,* Vol.2, No.6, (December 2003), pp. 1187-1199, ISSN 1535-9778

Munroe, S.H. & Zhu, J. (2006). Overlapping transcripts, double-stranded RNA and antisense regulation: a genomic perspective. *Cellular and molecular life sciences,* Vol.63, No.18, (September 2006), pp. 2102-2118, ISSN 1420-682X

Nakamura, T., Kishida, M. & Shimoda, C. (2000). The Schizosaccharomyces pombe spo6+ gene encoding a nuclear protein with sequence similarity to budding yeast Dbf4 is required for meiotic second division and sporulation. *Genes to cells: devoted to molecular & cellular mechanisms,* Vol.5, No.6, (June 2000), pp. 463-479, ISSN 1356-9597

Neale, M.J. & Keeney, S. (2006). Clarifying the mechanics of DNA strand exchange in meiotic recombination. *Nature,* Vol.442, No.7099, (July 2006), pp. 153-158, ISSN 1476-4687

Neil, H., Malabat, C., d'Aubenton-Carafa, Y., Xu, Z., Steinmetz, L.M. & Jacquier, A. (2009). Widespread bidirectional promoters are the major source of cryptic transcripts in yeast. *Nature,* Vol.457, No.7232, (February 2009), pp. 1038-1042, ISSN 1476-4687

Ni, T., Tu, K., Wang, Z., Song, S., Wu, H., Xie, B., Scott, K.C., Grewal, S.I., Gao, Y. & Zhu, J. (2010). The prevalence and regulation of antisense transcripts in Schizosaccharomyces pombe. *PloS one,* Vol.5, No.12, (December 2010), pp. e15271, ISSN 1932-6203

Nielsen, O. (1993). Signal transduction during mating and meiosis in S. pombe. *Trends in cell biology,* Vol.3, No.2, (February 1993), pp. 60-65, ISSN 0962-8924

Nugent, K.G., Choffe, K. & Saville, B.J. (2004). Gene expression during Ustilago maydis diploid filamentous growth: EST library creation and analyses. *Fungal genetics and biology,* Vol.41, No.3, (March 2004), pp. 349-360, ISSN 1087-1845

Obara, T., Nakafuku, M., Yamamoto, M. & Kaziro, Y. (1991). Isolation and characterization of a gene encoding a G-protein alpha subunit from Schizosaccharomyces pombe: involvement in mating and sporulation pathways. *Proceedings of the National Academy of Sciences of the United States of America,* Vol.88, No.13, (July 1991), pp. 5877-5881, ISSN 0027-8424

O'Donnell, K.L. & McLaughlin, D.J. (1984). Ultrastructure of Meiosis in *Ustilago maydis. Mycologia,* Vol.76, No.3, (May 1984), pp. 468-485, ISSN 0027-5514

Ordonez, M.E. & Kolmer, J.A. (2009). Differentiation of molecular genotypes and virulence phenotypes of Puccinia triticina from common wheat in North America. *Phytopathology,* Vol.99, No.6, (June 2009), pp. 750-758, ISSN 0031-949X

Pak, J. & Segall, J. (2002a). Regulation of the premiddle and middle phases of expression of the NDT80 gene during sporulation of Saccharomyces cerevisiae. *Molecular and cellular biology,* Vol.22, No.18, (September 2002), pp. 6417-6429, ISSN 0270-7306

Pak, J. & Segall, J. (2002b). Role of Ndt80, Sum1, and Swe1 as targets of the meiotic recombination checkpoint that control exit from pachytene and spore formation in Saccharomyces cerevisiae. *Molecular and cellular biology,* Vol.22, No.18, (September 2002), pp. 6430-6440, ISSN 0270-7306

Pawlowski, W.P., Sheehan, M.J. & Ronceret, A. (2007). In the beginning: the initiation of meiosis. *BioEssays: news and reviews in molecular, cellular and developmental biology,* Vol.29, No.6, (June 2007), pp. 511-514, ISSN 0265-9247

Peng, Z., Wang, W., Schettino, A., Leung, B. & McLeod, M. (2003). Inactivation of Ran1/Pat1 kinase bypasses the requirement for high-level expression of mei2 during fission yeast meiosis. *Current genetics,* Vol.43, No.3, (June 2003), pp. 178-185, ISSN 0172-8083

Piekarska, I., Rytka, J. & Rempola, B. (2010). Regulation of sporulation in the yeast Saccharomyces cerevisiae. *Acta Biochimica Polonica,* Vol.57, No.3, (n.d.), pp. 241-250, ISSN 1734-154X

Pierce, M., Benjamin, K.R., Montano, S.P., Georgiadis, M.M., Winter, E. & Vershon, A.K. (2003). Sum1 and Ndt80 proteins compete for binding to middle sporulation element sequences that control meiotic gene expression. *Molecular and cellular biology,* Vol.23, No.14, (July 2003), pp. 4814-4825, ISSN 0270-7306

Primig, M., Williams, R.M., Winzeler, E.A., Tevzadze, G.G., Conway, A.R., Hwang, S.Y., Davis, R.W. & Esposito, R.E. (2000). The core meiotic transcriptome in budding yeasts. *Nature genetics,* Vol.26, No.4, (December 2000), pp. 415-423, ISSN 1061-4036

Pukkila, P.J., Yashar, B.M. & Binninger, D.M. (1984). Analysis of meiotic development in Coprinus cinereus. *Symposia of the Society for Experimental Biology,* Vol.38, (n.d.), pp. 177-194, ISSN 0081-1386

Purnapatre, K., Gray, M., Piccirillo, S. & Honigberg, S.M. (2005). Glucose inhibits meiotic DNA replication through SCFGrr1p-dependent destruction of Ime2p kinase. *Molecular and cellular biology,* Vol.25, No.1, (January 2005), pp. 440-450, ISSN 0270-7306

Ramberg, J.E. & McLaughlin, D.J. (1980). Ultrastructural study of promycelial development and basidiospore initiation in Ustilago maydis. *Canadian Journal of Botany,* Vol.58, No.14, (n.d.), pp. 1548-1561, ISSN 0008-4026

Ramesh, M.A., Malik, S.B. & Logsdon, J.M.,Jr. (2005). A phylogenomic inventory of meiotic genes; evidence for sex in Giardia and an early eukaryotic origin of meiosis. *Current biology,* Vol.15, No.2, (January 2005), pp. 185-191, ISSN 0960-9822

Regenfelder, E., Spellig, T., Hartmann, A., Lauenstein, S., Bolker, M. & Kahmann, R. (1997). G proteins in Ustilago maydis: transmission of multiple signals? *The EMBO journal,* Vol.16, No.8, (April 1997), pp. 1934-1942, ISSN 0261-4189

Rhind, N., Chen, Z., Yassour, M., Thompson, D.A., Haas, B.J., Habib, N., Wapinski, I., Roy, S., Lin, M.F., Heiman, D.I., Young, S.K., Furuya, K., Guo, Y., Pidoux, A., Chen, H.M., Robbertse, B., Goldberg, J.M., Aoki, K., Bayne, E.H., Berlin, A.M., Desjardins, C.A., Dobbs, E., Dukaj, L., Fan, L., FitzGerald, M.G., French, C., Gujja, S., Hansen, K., Keifenheim, D., Levin, J.Z., Mosher, R.A., Muller, C.A., Pfiffner, J., Priest, M., Russ, C., Smialowska, A., Swoboda, P., Sykes, S.M., Vaughn, M., Vengrova, S., Yoder, R., Zeng, Q., Allshire, R., Baulcombe, D., Birren, B.W., Brown, W., Ekwall, K., Kellis, M., Leatherwood, J., Levin, H., Margalit, H., Martienssen, R., Nieduszynski, C.A., Spatafora, J.W., Friedman, N., Dalgaard, J.Z., Baumann, P., Niki, H., Regev, A. & Nusbaum, C. (2011). Comparative functional genomics of the fission yeasts. *Science,* Vol.332, No.6032, (May 2011), pp. 930-936, ISSN 1095-9203

Roeder, G.S. & Bailis, J.M. (2000). The pachytene checkpoint. *Trends in genetics,* Vol.16, No.9, (September 2000), pp. 395-403, ISSN 0168-9525

Roelfs, A.P. (1982). Effects of barberry eradication on stem rust in the United States. *Plant Disease,* Vol.66, No.2, (n.d.), pp. 177-181, ISSN 0191-2917

Romanienko, P.J. & Camerini-Otero, R.D. (1999). Cloning, characterization, and localization of mouse and human SPO11. *Genomics,* Vol.61, No.2, (October 1999), pp. 156-169, ISSN 0888-7543

Rubin-Bejerano, I., Mandel, S., Robzyk, K. & Kassir, Y. (1996). Induction of meiosis in Saccharomyces cerevisiae depends on conversion of the transcriptional represssor Ume6 to a positive regulator by its regulated association with the transcriptional activator Ime1. *Molecular and cellular biology,* Vol.16, No.5, (May 1996), pp. 2518-2526, ISSN 0270-7306

Sacadura, N.T. & Saville, B.J. (2003). Gene expression and EST analyses of Ustilago maydis germinating teliospores. *Fungal genetics and biology,* Vol.40, No.1, (October 2003), pp. 47-64, ISSN 1087-1845

Saccharomyces Genome Database. (August, 2011). Saccharomyces Genome Database, 17.08.2011, Available from <http://www.yeastgenome.org/>

Sagee, S., Sherman, A., Shenhar, G., Robzyk, K., Ben-Doy, N., Simchen, G. & Kassir, Y. (1998). Multiple and distinct activation and repression sequences mediate the regulated transcription of IME1, a transcriptional activator of meiosis-specific genes in Saccharomyces cerevisiae. *Molecular and cellular biology,* Vol.18, No.4, (April 1998), pp. 1985-1995, ISSN 0270-7306

Sato, M., Shinozaki-Yabana, S., Yamashita, A., Watanabe, Y. & Yamamoto, M. (2001). The fission yeast meiotic regulator Mei2p undergoes nucleocytoplasmic shuttling. *FEBS letters,* Vol.499, No.3, (June 2001), pp. 251-255, ISSN 0014-5793

Schirawski, J., Mannhaupt, G., Munch, K., Brefort, T., Schipper, K., Doehlemann, G., Di Stasio, M., Rossel, N., Mendoza-Mendoza, A., Pester, D., Muller, O., Winterberg, B., Meyer, E., Ghareeb, H., Wollenberg, T., Munsterkotter, M., Wong, P., Walter, M., Stukenbrock, E., Guldener, U. & Kahmann, R. (2010). Pathogenicity determinants in smut fungi revealed by genome comparison. *Science,* Vol.330, No.6010, (December 2010), pp. 1546-1548, ISSN 1095-9203

Schlecht, U. & Primig, M. (2003). Mining meiosis and gametogenesis with DNA microarrays. *Reproduction,* Vol.125, No.4, (April 2003), pp. 447-456, ISSN 1470-1626

Schumann, G.L. & D'Arcy, J.D. (2009). What Are the Causes of Plant Diseases?, In: *Essential Plant Pathology, Second Edition,* pp. 21-39, American Phytopathological Society Press, ISSN 978-0-89054-381-8, Minnesota, USA

Shah, J.C. & Clancy, M.J. (1992). IME4, a gene that mediates MAT and nutritional control of meiosis in Saccharomyces cerevisiae. *Molecular and cellular biology,* Vol.12, No.3, (March 1992), pp. 1078-1086, ISSN 0270-7306

Shenhar, G. & Kassir, Y. (2001). A positive regulator of mitosis, Sok2, functions as a negative regulator of meiosis in Saccharomyces cerevisiae. *Molecular and cellular biology,* Vol.21, No.5, (March 2001), pp. 1603-1612, ISSN 0270-7306

Shin, M.E., Skokotas, A. & Winter, E. (2010). The Cdk1 and Ime2 protein kinases trigger exit from meiotic prophase in Saccharomyces cerevisiae by inhibiting the Sum1 transcriptional repressor. *Molecular and cellular biology,* Vol.30, No.12, (June 2010), pp. 2996-3003, ISSN 1098-5549

Shiozaki, K. & Russell, P. (1996). Conjugation, meiosis, and the osmotic stress response are regulated by Spc1 kinase through Atf1 transcription factor in fission yeast. *Genes & development,* Vol.10, No.18, (September 1996), pp. 2276-2288, ISSN 0890-9369

Shuster, E.O. & Byers, B. (1989). Pachytene arrest and other meiotic effects of the start mutations in Saccharomyces cerevisiae. *Genetics,* Vol.123, No.1, (September 1989), pp. 29-43, ISSN 0016-6731

Simchen, G. (2009). Commitment to meiosis: what determines the mode of division in budding yeast? *BioEssays: news and reviews in molecular, cellular and developmental biology,* Vol.31, No.2, (February 2009), pp. 169-177, ISSN 1521-1878

Singh, R.P., Hodson, D.P., Huerta-Espino, J., Jin, Y., Bhavani, S., Njau, P., Herrera-Foessel, S., Singh, P.K., Singh, S. & Govindan, V. (2011). The Emergence of Ug99 Races of the Stem Rust Fungus is a Threat to World Wheat Production. *Annual Review of Phytopathology,* Vol.49, (September 2011), pp. 465-481, ISSN 0066-4286

Snetselaar, K.M. & Mims, C.W. (1992). Sporidial fusion and infection of maize seedlings by the smut fungus *Ustilago maydis*. *Mycologia,* Vol.84, (n.d.), pp. 193-203, ISSN 0027-5514

Sugimoto, A., Iino, Y., Maeda, T., Watanabe, Y. & Yamamoto, M. (1991). Schizosaccharomyces pombe ste11+ encodes a transcription factor with an HMG motif that is a critical regulator of sexual development. *Genes & development,* Vol.5, No.11, (November 1991), pp. 1990-1999, ISSN 0890-9369

Takeda, T., Toda, T., Kominami, K., Kohnosu, A., Yanagida, M. & Jones, N. (1995). Schizosaccharomyces pombe atf1+ encodes a transcription factor required for sexual development and entry into stationary phase. *The EMBO journal,* Vol.14, No.24, (December 1995), pp. 6193-6208, ISSN 0261-4189

Thevelein, J.M. & de Winde, J.H. (1999). Novel sensing mechanisms and targets for the cAMP-protein kinase A pathway in the yeast Saccharomyces cerevisiae. *Molecular microbiology,* Vol.33, No.5, (September 1999), pp. 904-918, ISSN 0950-382X

Tisseur, M., Kwapisz, M. & Morillon, A. (2011). Pervasive transcription - Lessons from yeast. *Biochimie,* Vol.93, No.11, (November 2011), pp. 1889-1896, ISSN 1638-6183

Tripathi, R.K. & Gottlieb, D. (1974). Sequential biosynthesis of ribonucleic acids during germination of teliospores of Ustilago maydis. *Mycologia,* Vol.66, No.3, (May-Jun 1974), pp. 413-421, ISSN 0027-5514

Tung, K.S., Hong, E.J. & Roeder, G.S. (2000). The pachytene checkpoint prevents accumulation and phosphorylation of the meiosis-specific transcription factor Ndt80. *Proceedings of the National Academy of Sciences of the United States of America,* Vol.97, No.22, (October 2000), pp. 12187-12192, ISSN 0027-8424

U.S. Department of Agriculture. (August, 2011). Wheat Data: Yearbook Tables, World and U.S. wheat production, exports, and ending stocks, 06.09.2011, Available from <http://www.ers.usda.gov/data/wheat/YBtable04.asp>

U.S. Grains Council.(November, 2010). Corn, 06.09.2011, Available from <http://www.grains.org/corn>

Valbuena, N. & Moreno, S. (2010). TOR and PKA pathways synergize at the level of the Ste11 transcription factor to prevent mating and meiosis in fission yeast. *PloS one,* Vol.5, No.7, (July 2010), pp. e11514, ISSN 1932-6203

van Werven, F.J. & Amon, A. (2011). Regulation of entry into gametogenesis. *Philosophical Transactions of the Royal Society B: Biological Sciences,* Vol.366, No.1584, (December 2011), pp. 3521-3531, ISSN 0962-8436

Vershon, A.K. & Pierce, M. (2000). Transcriptional regulation of meiosis in yeast. *Current opinion in cell biology,* Vol.12, No.3, (June 2000), pp. 334-339, ISSN 0955-0674

Villeneuve, A.M. & Hillers, K.J. (2001). Whence meiosis? *Cell,* Vol.106, No.6, (September 2001), pp. 647-650, ISSN 0092-8674

Voegele, R.T. & Mendgen, K. (2003). Rust haustoria: nutrient uptake and beyond. *New Phytologist,* Vol.159, (n.d.), pp. 93-100, ISSN 1469-8137

Wahls, W.P., Siegel, E.R. & Davidson, M.K. (2008). Meiotic recombination hotspots of fission yeast are directed to loci that express non-coding RNA. *PloS one,* Vol.3, No.8, (August 2008), pp. e2887, ISSN 1932-6203

Watanabe, T., Miyashita, K., Saito, T.T., Nabeshima, K. & Nojima, H. (2002). Abundant poly(A)-bearing RNAs that lack open reading frames in Schizosaccharomyces pombe. *DNA research: an international journal for rapid publication of reports on genes and genomes,* Vol.9, No.6, (December 2002), pp. 209-215, ISSN 1340-2838

Watanabe, T., Miyashita, K., Saito, T.T., Yoneki, T., Kakihara, Y., Nabeshima, K., Kishi, Y.A., Shimoda, C. & Nojima, H. (2001). Comprehensive isolation of meiosis-specific genes identifies novel proteins and unusual non-coding transcripts in Schizosaccharomyces pombe. *Nucleic acids research,* Vol.29, No.11, (June 2001), pp. 2327-2337, ISSN 1362-4962

Wilhelm, B.T., Marguerat, S., Watt, S., Schubert, F., Wood, V., Goodhead, I., Penkett, C.J., Rogers, J. & Bahler, J. (2008). Dynamic repertoire of a eukaryotic transcriptome surveyed at single-nucleotide resolution. *Nature,* Vol.453, No.7199, (June 2008), pp. 1239-1243, ISSN 1476-4687

Watanabe, Y. & Yamamoto, M. (1994). S. pombe mei2+ encodes an RNA-binding protein essential for premeiotic DNA synthesis and meiosis I, which cooperates with a novel RNA species meiRNA. *Cell,* Vol.78, No.3, (August 1994), pp. 487-498, ISSN 0092-8674

Watanabe, Y., Lino, Y., Furuhata, K., Shimoda, C. & Yamamoto, M. (1988). The S. pombe mei2 gene encoding a crucial molecule for commitment to meiosis is under the regulation of cAMP. *The EMBO journal,* Vol.7, No.3, (March 1988), pp. 761-767, ISSN 0261-4189

Wilkinson, M.G., Samuels, M., Takeda, T., Toone, W.M., Shieh, J.C., Toda, T., Millar, J.B. & Jones, N. (1996). The Atf1 transcription factor is a target for the Sty1 stress-activated MAP kinase pathway in fission yeast. *Genes & development,* Vol.10, No.18, (September 1996), pp. 2289-2301, ISSN 0890-9369

Willer, M., Hoffmann, L., Styrkarsdottir, U., Egel, R., Davey, J. & Nielsen, O. (1995). Two-step activation of meiosis by the mat1 locus in Schizosaccharomyces pombe. *Molecular and cellular biology,* Vol.15, No.9, (September 1995), pp. 4964-4970, ISSN 0270-7306

Wyers, F., Rougemaille, M., Badis, G., Rousselle, J.C., Dufour, M.E., Boulay, J., Regnault, B., Devaux, F., Namane, A., Seraphin, B., Libri, D. & Jacquier, A. (2005). Cryptic pol II transcripts are degraded by a nuclear quality control pathway involving a new poly(A) polymerase. *Cell,* Vol.121, No.5, (June 2005), pp. 725-737, ISSN 0092-8674

Xiao, Y. & Mitchell, A.P. (2000). Shared roles of yeast glycogen synthase kinase 3 family members in nitrogen-responsive phosphorylation of meiotic regulator Ume6p. *Molecular and cellular biology,* Vol.20, No.15, (August 2000), pp. 5447-5453, ISSN 0270-7306

Xu, Z., Wei, W., Gagneur, J., Perocchi, F., Clauder-Munster, S., Camblong, J., Guffanti, E., Stutz, F., Huber, W. & Steinmetz, L.M. (2009). Bidirectional promoters generate pervasive transcription in yeast. *Nature,* Vol.457, No.7232, (February 2009), pp. 1033-1037, ISSN 1476-4687

Yamamoto, M. (2010). The selective elimination of messenger RNA underlies the mitosis-meiosis switch in fission yeast. *Proceedings of the Japan Academy:Series B, Physical and biological sciences,* Vol.86, No.8, (n.d.), pp. 788-797, ISSN 1349-2896

Yamamoto, M. (1996a). The molecular control mechanisms of meiosis in fission yeast. *Trends in biochemical sciences,* Vol.21, No.1, (January 1996), pp. 18-22, ISSN 0968-0004

Yamamoto, M. (1996b). Regulation of meiosis in fission yeast. *Cell structure and function,* Vol.21, No.5, (October 1996), pp. 431-436, ISSN 0386-7196

Yamashita, A., Watanabe, Y., Nukina, N. & Yamamoto, M. (1998). RNA-assisted nuclear transport of the meiotic regulator Mei2p in fission yeast. *Cell,* Vol.95, No.1, (October 1998), pp. 115-123, ISSN 0092-8674

Yassour, M., Pfiffner, J., Levin, J.Z., Adiconis, X., Gnirke, A., Nusbaum, C., Thompson, D.A., Friedman, N. & Regev, A. (2010). Strand-specific RNA sequencing reveals extensive regulated long antisense transcripts that are conserved across yeast species. *Genome biology,* Vol.11, No.8, (n.d.), pp. R87, ISSN 1465-6914

Zahiri, A.R., Babu, M.R. & Saville, B.J. (2005). Differential gene expression during teliospore germination in Ustilago maydis. *Molecular genetics and genomics,* Vol.273, No.5, (June 2005), pp. 394-403, ISSN 1617-4615

Zaman, S., Lippman, S.I., Zhao, X. & Broach, J.R. (2008). How Saccharomyces responds to nutrients. *Annual Review of Genetics,* Vol.42, (n.d.), pp. 27-81, ISSN 0066-4197